PAIN MEDICINE AND MANAGEMENT

Just the Facts

MW00837378

Notice

Medicine is an ever-changing science. As new research and clinical experience broaden our knowledge, changes in treatment and drug therapy are required. The authors and the publisher of this work have checked with sources believed to be reliable in their efforts to provide information that is complete and generally in accord with the standards accepted at the time of publication. However, in view of the possibility of human error or changes in medical sciences, neither the authors nor the publisher nor any other party who has been involved in the preparation or publication of this work warrants that the information contained herein is in every respect accurate or complete, and they disclaim all responsibility for any errors or omissions or for the results obtained from use of the information contained in this work. Readers are encouraged to confirm the information contained herein with other sources. For example and in particular, readers are advised to check the product information sheet included in the package of each drug they plan to administer to be certain that the information contained in this work is accurate and that changes have not been made in the recommended dose or in the contraindications for administration. This recommendation is of particular importance in connection with new or infrequently used drugs.

PAIN MEDICINE AND MANAGEMENT
Just the Facts

Second Edition

Editors

Peter S. Staats, MD, MBA

Department of Anesthesiology and Critical Care Medicine
Johns Hopkins University
Baltimore, Maryland

Mark S. Wallace, MD

Professor of Clinical Anesthesiology
Chair, Division of Pain Medicine
Department of Anesthesiology
University of California, San Diego

New York Chicago San Francisco Athens London Madrid
Mexico City Milan New Delhi Singapore Sydney Toronto

Pain Medicine and Management: Just the Facts, Second Edition

Copyright © 2015 by the McGraw-Hill Education. All rights reserved. Printed in the United States of America. Except as permitted under the United States Copyright Act of 1976, no part of this publication may be reproduced or distributed in any form or by any means, or stored in a database or retrieval system, without the prior written permission of the publisher.

Previous edition copyright © 2005 by the McGraw-Hill Companies, Inc.

1 2 3 4 5 6 7 8 9 0   QVS/QVS   20 19 18 17 16 15

ISBN 978-0-07-181745-5
MHID 0-07-181745-X

This book was set in Minion Pro Regular by MPS Limited.
The editors were Brian Belval and Peter J. Boyle.
The production supervisor was Richard Ruzycka.
Project management was provided by Asheesh Ratra, MPS Limited.
The art manager was Armen Ovsepyan.
The designer was Alan Barnett.
Quad Graphics Versailles was printer and binder.

This book was printed on acid-free paper.

Cataloging-in-publication data for this book is on file at the Library of Congress

McGraw-Hill books are available at special quantity discounts to use as premiums and sales promotions, or for use in corporate training programs. To contact a representative please e-mail us at bulksales@mcgraw-hill.com.

We would like to dedicate this book to the millions of patients suffering from pain worldwide, and the physicians and health care providers who care for them. We would also like to make a special thank you to the authors of this text. In drafting our wish list for authors, we searched for experts around the globe to help us gather the most relevant information on the management of pain. Many of you helped us with the first edition of this book, and your dedication has made the process seamless. We intend for this book to be a broad resource on the management of pain, as well as a tool for those studying for their board examination or seeking to further their knowledge base in pain management.

There are so many influential leaders who have contributed to the advancement of caring for patients with pain. While we cannot list everyone who has helped or influenced us, we would like to make a special thank you to our leaders and mentors in the field of pain for their sage counsel and advice over the years. Two great men, Dr. Sam Hassenbusch and Dr. John Oakley, deserve special mention. They were great friends and leaders, true heroes of pain management, and both gave tirelessly to the field of pain management. Tragically, we lost them both much too early. Sam and John, while you are no longer physically with us, your influence is still felt across the globe. We thank you and miss you.

To our parents: You gave us the foundation and compass to begin this journey, along with continued love and support along the way. We understand, now that we are parents, all the sacrifices and care you provided, and are truly appreciative.

To our spouses, Nancy and Anne: You will never know how deeply we need your support and counsel. We appreciate all that you do for us to try to do something that matters to improve the care of patients across the globe.

To our children, Alyssa, Dylan, Rachel, Zachary, and Dominick, the next generation: You are entering such an exciting time in the evolution of medicine and the history of mankind. The advances that will come during your lifetime will seem almost like magic to a previous generation. We encourage you to embrace your dreams and hopes, and use your energy to improve the lives of others and the world in some way.

Peter S. Staats, MD, MBA

Mark S. Wallace, MD

CONTENTS

CONTRIBUTORS

Stephen E. Abram, MD, Professor of Anesthesiology, Medical College of Wisconsin, Milwaukee, Wisconsin, *Chapter 1*

Raimy R. Amasha, MD, Johns Hopkins University School of Medicine, Baltimore, Maryland, *Chapters 41, 60*

Charles E. Argoff, MD, Albany Medical Center, Albany, New York, *Chapter 58*

Gerald M. Aronoff, MD, Medical Director, Carolina Pain Associates, PA, and North American Pain and Disability Group, Charlotte, North Carolina, *Chapter 79*

Miroslav "Misha" Bačkonja, MD, Medical Director Neuroscience, CRI Lifetree Research, Department of Neurology, University of Wisconsin, Madison, Wisconsin, *Chapters 11, 19*

Zahid Bajwa, MD, Director, Boston Headache Institute, Director, Clinical Research at Boston Pain Care Center, Waltham, Massachusetts, *Chapter 9*

Allan J. Belzberg, MD, FRCSC, Clinical Director, Neurosurgery Pain Research Institute, Associate Professor of Neurological Surgery, Johns Hopkins University School of Medicine, Baltimore, Maryland, *Chapter 32*

Ramsin Benyamin, MD, President, Millennium Pain Center, Bloomington, Illinois; Clinical Assistant Professor of Surgery, College of Medicine, University of Illinois, Urbana-Champaign; Adjunct Professor, Department of Biological Sciences, Illinois State University, Normal, Illinois, *Chapter 77*

Ira M. Bernstein, MD, Department of Obstetrics and Gynecology, University of Vermont College of Medicine, Burlington, Vermont, *Chapter 49*

T. Joel Berry, MD, Pain Fellow, Department of Pain, MD Anderson Cancer Center, Houston Texas, *Chapter 39*

Niteesh Bharara, MD, Interventional Pain Management Specialist, Virginia Spine Institute, Reston, Virginia, *Chapter 34*

Brian M. Block, MD, PhD, President, Baltimore Spine Center, Lutherville, Maryland, *Chapter 14*

Richard G. Bowman, MD, Center for Pain Relief, Inc, Charleston, West Virginia, *Chapter 68*

Allen W. Burton, MD, Houston Pain Centers, Houston Texas, *Chapter 39*

Michael G. Byas-Smith, MD, Associate Professor, Department of Anesthesiology, Emory University School of Medicine, Emory University Hospital, Atlanta, Georgia, *Chapter 40*

Martin D. Cheatle, PhD, Director, Pain and Chemical Dependency Program, Center for Studies of Addiction, Perelman School of Medicine, University of Pennsylvania, Philadelphia, Pennsylvania, *Chapter 53*

Faride Chejne-Gomez, MD, Professor of Pain Medicine and Palliative Care, Universidad Nacional Autónoma de México (UNAM), Instituto Nacional de Cancerología, American British Cowdray Medical Center, México DF, México, *Chapter 36*

Paul J. Christo, MD, MBA, Johns Hopkins University School of Medicine, Baltimore, Maryland, *Chapter 41*

Michael R. Clark, MD, MPH, MBA, Associate Professor and Vice Chair, Department of Psychiatry and Behavioral Sciences, Director, Pain Treatment Program, Johns Hopkins University School of Medicine, Baltimore, Maryland, *Chapter 18*

Steven P. Cohen, MD, Professor, Director of Medical Education and Quality Improvement for Pain Management, Division of Pain Medicine, Department of Anesthesiology and Critical Care Medicine, Johns Hopkins School of Medicine, Baltimore, Maryland; Walter Reed National Military Medical Center, Bethesda, Maryland; Uniformed Services University of the Health Sciences, Bethesda, Maryland, *Chapter 64*

Arnaldo Neves Da Silva, MD, Neurologist, Michigan Headache and Neurological Institute, Ann Arbor, Michigan, *Chapter 31*

Elizabeth J. Dansie, PhD, Department of Anesthesiology and Pain Medicine, University of Washington, Seattle, Washington, *Chapter 8*

Miles R. Day, MD, Associate Professor of Anesthesiology and Pain Management, Texas Tech University Health Sciences Center, Lubbock, Texas, *Chapter 78*

Timothy R. Deer, MD, President and CEO, Center for Pain Relief, Inc, Charleston, West Virginia, *Chapter 68*

Richard Derby, MD, Medical Director, Spinal Diagnostics and Treatment Center, Daly City, California, *Chapter 76*

Anjuli Desai, MD, Capitol Pain Institute, Austin, Texas, *Chapter 34*

Sudhir Diwan, MD, DABIPP, Chairman, New York Society Interventional Pain Physicians, New York, New York, *Chapter 33*

Michael J. Dorsi, MD, Neurosurgeon, Community Memorial Hospital and St. John's Regional Medical Center, Ventura, California, *Chapter 32*

Michel Y. Dubois, MD, Joyce H. Lowinson Professor in Pain Medicine and Palliative Care, Professor of Anesthesiology, New York University School of Medicine and Langone Medical Centers, New York, New York, *Chapter 7*

Maxim S. Eckmann, MD, Associate Professor, Anesthesiology and Pain Management, Director, Pain Medicine, University of Texas Health Science Center at San Antonio, San Antonio, Texas, *Chapter 65*

Robert R. Edwards, PhD, Associate Professor, Department of Anesthesia, Harvard Medical School, Clinical Psychologist, Pain Management Center, Brigham and Women's Hospital, Boston, Massachusetts, *Chapter 13*

Juan Egas, MD, Pain Medicine Fellow, Pain Medicine Division, Department of Anesthesiology, Perioperative and Pain Medicine, Stanford University Pain Management Center, Redwood City, California, *Chapter 27*

Bradley A. Eli, DMD, MS, Director, San Diego Headache and Facial Pain Center, Director, Sleep Treatment and Research Institute, Assistant Professor, Anesthesiology, University of California, San Diego, La Jolla, California, *Chapter 35*

Mazin Ellias, MD, FRCA, Medical Director, Advanced Pain Management, Wausau, Wisconsin, *Chapter 74*

Michael A. Erdek, MD, Johns Hopkins University School of Medicine, Baltimore, Maryland, *Chapter 60*

Frank Falco, MD, Adjunct Associate Professor, Temple University Medical School; Director, Temple University Hospital's Pain Management Fellowship Program, Philadelphia, Pennsylvania, *Chapter 34*

Roger B. Fillingim, PhD, Professor, University of Florida College of Dentistry, Director, Pain Research and Intervention Center of Excellence, Gainesville, Florida, *Chapter 4*

Kenneth A. Follett, MD, PhD, Professor and Chief, Division of Neurosurgery, University of Nebraska Medical Center, Omaha, Nebraska, *Chapter 66*

Kristin D. Forner, MD, Assistant Clinical Professor, Department of Medicine, University of California, San Diego, California, *Chapter 70*

Timothy Furnish, MD, Assistant Clinical Professor, Director, Pain Fellowship, Division of Pain Medicine, Department of Anesthesiology, University of California, San Diego, California, *Chapter 24*

Bradley S. Galer, MD, President, Pain Group, Nuvo Research Inc, West Chester, Pennsylvania, *Chapter 16*

Rollin M. Gallagher, MD, MPH, Deputy National Program Director for Pain Management, VA Central Office, Director for Pain Policy Research and Primary Care, Penn Pain Medicine, Philadelphia VA Medical Center, Philadelphia, Pennsylvania, *Chapter 53*

Arnold R. Gammaitoni, PharmD, VP, Scientific Affairs, Nuvo Research Inc, West Chester, Pennsylvania, *Chapter 16*

Rodolfo Gebhardt, MD, Associate Professor, Department of Pain, MD Anderson Cancer Center, Houston Texas, *Chapter 39*

Harold J. Gelfand, MD, Assistant Professor of Anesthesiology, Johns Hopkins University School of Medicine, Baltimore, Maryland, *Chapter 48*

Robert D. Gerwin, MD, Johns Hopkins University School of Medicine, Baltimore, Maryland, *Chapter 43*

F. Michael Gloth III, MD, FACP, AGSF, Chief Medical Officer, Moorings Park Healthy Living, Naples, Florida; Associate Professor of Medicine, Division of Geriatric Medicine and Gerontology, Johns Hopkins University School of Medicine; Adjunct Associate Professor, Department of Epidemiology and Public Health, University of Maryland School Medicine, Baltimore, Maryland, *Chapter 42*

Theodore S. Grabow, MD, Adjunct Assistant Professor, Department of Anesthesiology and Critical Care Medicine, Johns Hopkins University School of Medicine, Baltimore, Maryland, *Chapter 14*

Robert S. Greenberg, MD, Departments of Anesthesiology and Critical Care Medicine, Johns Hopkins Medical Institutions, Baltimore, Maryland, *Chapter 44*

Eric Grigsby, MD, MBA, Neurovations Research, Napa, California, *Chapter 69*

Jorge Guajardo-Rosas, MD, Assistant Professor of Anesthesiology and Pain Medicine, Universidad Nacional Autónoma de México (UNAM); Coordinator of Department, Pain Clinic, Instituto Nacional de Cancerología, American British Cowdray Medical Center, México DF, México, *Chapter 36*

Anita Gupta, DO, PharmD, Associate Professor, Medical Director, University Pain Institute, Division of Pain Medicine and Regional Anesthesiology, Department of Anesthesiology and Perioperative Medicine, Drexel University College of Medicine, Philadelphia, Pennsylvania, *Chapter 64*

Steven R. Hanling, MD, Naval Medical Center San Diego, San Diego, California, *Chapter 46*

Oliver van Hecke, MBChB, Medical Research Institute, University of Dundee, Dundee, Scotland, United Kingdom, *Chapter 3*

Andrew Albert Indresano, MD, Resident, University of California, San Diego, California, *Chapter 30*

Gordon Irving, MD, Medical Director, Swedish Pain Center, Swedish Medical Center, Seattle, Washington; Associate Professor, Anesthesiology Department, University of Washington School of Medicine, Seattle, Washington, *Chapter 75*

Mohammed A. Issa, MD, Instructor, Department of Anesthesia, Harvard Medical School, Pain Management Center, Brigham and Women's Hospital, Boston, Massachusetts, *Chapter 13*

Leonard Kamen, DO, Physiatrist, MossRehab, Elkins Park, Pennsylvania; Clinical Associate Professor, Department of Physical Medicine and Rehabilitation, Temple University Hospital, Philadelphia, Pennsylvania, *Chapter 51*

Arthur Kavanaugh, MD, Division of Rheumatology, Allergy, Immunology, University of California, San Diego, La Jolla, California, *Chapter 38*

Nicole Khetani, MD, Resident in Anesthesiology, Thomas Jefferson University Hospital, Philadelphia, Pennsylvania, *Chapter 26*

Kenneth L. Kirsh, PhD, Millennium Research Institute Laboratories, San Diego, California, *Chapter 52*

Elliot S. Krames, MD, Private practice, San Francisco, California, *Chapter 28*

Michael Kurisu, DO, Clinical Director, Center for Integrative Medicine, University of California, San Diego, La Jolla, California, *Chapter 61*

Erin Lawson, MD, Department of Anesthesiology, Center for Pain Medicine, University of California, San Diego, La Jolla, California; Lexington Interventional Pain Management, Lexington Medical Center, West Columbia, South Carolina, *Chapter 19*

Sang-Heon Lee, MD, PhD, Associate Professor, Department of Physical Medicine and Rehabilitation, Korea University College of Medicine, Seoul, South Korea, *Chapter 76*

Imanuel R. Lerman, MD, Assistant Clinical Professor, Department of Anesthesiology, University of California, San Diego, La Jolla, California, *Chapter 56*

Albert Y. Leung, MD, Clinical Professor of Anesthesiology, Center for Pain Medicine, Department of Anesthesiology, University of California, San Diego, La Jolla, California, *Chapter 57*

Sean Li, MD, Premier Pain Centers, LLC, Shrewsbury, New Jersey, *Chapter 59*

Felix Linetsky, MD, Prolotherapy Florida, Clearwater, Florida, *Chapter 71*

Michael W. Loes, MD, Southwest Pain Management Associates, Phoenix, Arizona, *Chapter 17*

John D. Loeser, MD, Professor Emeritus, Department of Neurological Surgery and Anesthesia and Pain Medicine, University of Washington, Seattle, Washington, *Chapter 6*

Sean Mackey, MD, PhD, Redlich Professor, Chief, Pain Medicine Division, Department of Anesthesiology, Perioperative and Pain Medicine, Stanford University Pain Management Center, Redwood City, California, *Chapter 27*

Laura MacNeil, University of Guelph, Guelph, Ontario, Canada, *Chapter 12*

Irina Melnik, MD, Staff Physician, Spinal Diagnostics and Treatment Center, Daly City, California, *Chapter 76*

Matthew Meunier, MD, Professor, Orthopedic Surgery, University of California, San Diego, California, *Chapter 29*

Robert Scott Meyer, MD, Professor, Orthopedic Surgery, University of California, San Diego, California, *Chapter 30*

Mikiko Murakami, DO, Department of Physical Medicine and Rehabilitation, Icahn School of Medicine, Mount Sinai Hospital, New York, New York, *Chapter 33*

Kieran J. Murphy, MD, Professor, Department of Medical Imaging, University of Toronto, Toronto, Ontario, Canada, *Chapter 12*

Richard B. North, MD, Neurological Surgeon, private practice, Baltimore, Maryland, *Chapter 63*

Einar Ottestad, MD, Clinical Assistant Professor, Director, Acute Pain Service, Pain Medicine Division, Department of Anesthesiology, Perioperative and Pain Medicine, Stanford University Pain Management Center, Redwood City, California, *Chapter 27*

Sunil J. Panchal, MD, President, National Institute of Pain, Lutz, Florida, *Chapter 67*

Marco Pappagallo, MD, Director, Comprehensive Pain Treatment Center, Associate Professor of Neurology, New York University School of Medicine, Hospital for Joint Diseases, New York, New York, *Chapter 21*

Steven D. Passik, PhD, Millennium Research Institute Laboratories, San Diego, California, *Chapter 52*

Amol Patwardhan, MD, Assistant Professor, Anesthesiology and Pharmacology, Co-Director, Comprehensive Pain Management, Arizona Health Sciences Center, University of Arizona, Tucson, Arizona, *Chapter 49*

Richard Payne, MD, Esther Colliflower Professor of Medicine and Divinity, Duke University, Durham, North Carolina; John B. Francis Chair in Bioethics, Center for Practical Bioethics, Kansas City, Missouri, *Chapter 50*

Annie Philip, MBBS, Associate Professor of Anesthesiology and Physical Medicine and Rehabilitation, University of Rochester School of Medicine and Dentistry, Rochester, New York, *Chapter 47*

Ricardo Plancarte, MD, PhD, Professor of Anesthesiology and Pain Medicine, Universidad Nacional Autónoma de México (UNAM), Coordinator of Department, Pain Clinic, Instituto Nacional de Cancerología, American British Cowdray Medical Center, México DF, México, *Chapter 36*

Gregory R. Polston, MD, Associate Professor of Clinical Anesthesiology, Center for Pain Medicine, University of California, San Diego, La Jolla, California, *Chapter 5*

Jason E. Pope, MD, Center for Pain Relief, Inc, Charleston, West Virginia, *Chapter 68*

Carmen M. Quinones, MD, Premier Pain Centers, Shrewsbury, New Jersey, *Chapter 72*

Gabor Racz, MD, Chair Emeritus, Department of Anesthesiology, School of Medicine, Texas Tech University Health Sciences Center, Lubbock, Texas, *Chapter 78*

P. Prithvi Raj, MD, Founder and Past President, World Institute of Pain, Winston-Salem, North Carolina, *Chapter 37*

Srinivasa N. Raja, MD, Johns Hopkins University School of Medicine, Baltimore, Maryland, *Chapter 41*

Somayaji Ramamurthy, MD, Professor, Anesthesiology and Pain Management, University of Texas Health Science Center at San Antonio, San Antonio, Texas, *Chapter 65*

James P. Rathmell, MD, Department of Anesthesiology Harvard Medical School, Boston, Massachusetts, *Chapter 49*

Richard L. Rauck, MD, Center for Clinical Research, LLC, Winston-Salem, North Carolina, *Chapter 54*

Ignacio Reyes-Torres, MD, Fellow, Interventional Pain Management, Universidad Nacional Autónoma de México (UNAM), Instituto Nacional de Cancerología, México, *Chapter 36*

Juan Carlos Robles, MD, Clinical Instructor, Department of Physical Medicine and Rehabilitation, New York University School of Medicine, New York, New York, *Chapter 72*

Eric Roeland, MD, Assistant Clinical Professor, Department of Medicine, University of California, San Diego, California, *Chapter 70*

Nathan J. Rudin, MD, MA, Associate Professor (CHS), Department of Orthopedics and Rehabilitation, University of Wisconsin School of Medicine and Public Health, Madison, Wisconsin, *Chapter 10*

Matthew A. Ruehle, BA, Millennium Research Institute Laboratories, San Diego, California, *Chapter 52*

Lloyd Saberski, MD, Advanced Diagnostic Pain Treatment Center, New Haven, Connecticut, *Chapters 62, 71*

Joel R. Saper, MD, Director, Michigan Headache and Neurological Institute, Ann Arbor, Michigan, *Chapter 31*

Michael Saulino, MD, PhD, Physiatrist, Moss Rehab, Elkins Park, Pennsylvania; Assistant Professor, Department of Rehabilitation Medicine, Thomas Jefferson University Hospital, Philadelphia, Pennsylvania, *Chapter 51*

Anne M. Savarese, MD, Division Head, Pediatric Anesthesiology, Assistant Professor of Anesthesiology and Pediatrics, University of Maryland School of Medicine, Baltimore, Maryland, *Chapter 25*

Devon Schmidt, BA, Neurovations Research, Napa, California, *Chapter 69*

Jennifer Schneider, PhD, MD, Private practice, Tucson, Arizona, *Chapter 17*

David M. Schultz, MD, Anesthesiologist, Medical Advanced Pain Specialists (MAPS), Minneapolis, Minnesota, *Chapter 55*

Daniel A. Schwarz, MD, Pain Recovery Specialists, Southfield, Michigan, *Chapter 15*

Blair H. Smith, MD, Medical Research Institute, University of Dundee, Dundee, Scotland, United Kingdom, *Chapter 3*

Michael T. Smith, PhD, Professor, Psychiatry and Behavioral Sciences, Johns Hopkins University School of Medicine, Baltimore, Maryland, *Chapter 13*

Linda S. Sorkin, PhD, Department of Anesthesiology, University of California, San Diego, La Jolla, California, *Chapter 2*

Dmitri Souzdalnitski, MD, PhD, Center for Pain Medicine, Western Reserve Hospital, Cuyahoga Falls, Ohio, *Chapter 56*

Kevin Sperber, MD, Clinical Instructor, Pain Medicine Specialist, New York University School of Medicine, Director of Inpatient Services, Comprehensive Pain Treatment Center, Hospital for Joint Diseases, New York, New York, *Chapter 21*

Peter S. Staats, MD, MBA, Department of Anesthesiology and Critical Care Medicine, Johns Hopkins University, Baltimore, Maryland, *Chapter 73*

Michael Stanton-Hicks, MB, BS, Department of Pain Management, Center for Neurological Restoration, Cleveland Clinic, Cleveland, Ohio, *Chapter 71*

Michelle Stern, MD, Assistant Clinical Professor of Physical Medicine and Rehabilitation, Columbia University College of Physician and Surgeons, New York Presbyterian Hospital, New York, New York, *Chapter 21*

Richard L. Stieg, MD, MHS, Private practice, Denver, Colorado, *Chapter 80*

Anand C. Thakur, MD, Clinical Assistant Professor, Department of Anesthesiology, Wayne State University School of Medicine; Medical Director, ANA Pain Management, Detroit, Michigan, *Chapter 23, 45*

Rajbala Thakur, MBBS, Associate Professor of Anesthesiology and Physical Medicine and Rehabilitation, University of Rochester School of Medicine and Dentistry, Rochester, New York, *Chapter 47*

Andrea M. Trescot, MD, Pain and Headache Center, Eagle River, Alaska, *Chapter 15*

Dennis C. Turk, PhD, Professor, Department of Anesthesiology and Pain Medicine, John and Emma Bonica Chair, Anesthesiology and Pain Research, Professor, University of Washington School of Medicine, Seattle, Washington, *Chapter 8*

Ralph E. Tuttle, DO, Naval Medical Center San Diego, San Diego, California, *Chapter 46*

Zuhre Tutuncu, MD, Division of Rheumatology, Allergy, Immunology, University of California, San Diego, La Jolla, California, *Chapter 38*

Christopher M. Viscomi, MD, Department of Anesthesiology, Harvard Medical School, Boston, Massachusetts, *Chapter 49*

Eugene R. Viscusi, MD, Professor of Anesthesiology, Director, Acute Pain Management, Thomas Jefferson University, Philadelphia, Pennsylvania, *Chapter 26*

Mark S. Wallace, MD, Professor of Clinical Anesthesiology, Chair, Division of Pain Medicine, Department of Anesthesiology, University of California, San Diego, *Chapters 11, 20, 24, 73*

Ajay D. Wasan, MD, MSc, Vice Chair for Pain Medicine, Department of Anesthesiology, University of Pittsburgh Medical Center; Visiting Professor of Anesthesiology and Psychiatry, University of Pittsburgh School of Medicine, Pittsburgh, Pennsylvania, *Chapter 13*

Brian G. Wilhelmi, MD, JD, Johns Hopkins University School of Medicine, Baltimore, Maryland, *Chapter 41*

Christopher L. Wu, MD, Professor of Anesthesiology, Johns Hopkins University School of Medicine, Baltimore, Maryland, *Chapter 48*

Tony L. Yaksh, PhD, Department of Anesthesiology, University of California, San Diego, La Jolla, California, *Chapters 2, 22*

Hong Yang, MD, PhD, Division of Rheumatology, Allergy, Immunology, University of California, San Diego, La Jolla, California, *Chapter 38*

Jon Y. Zhou, MD, Resident in Anesthesiology, Thomas Jefferson University Hospital, Philadelphia, Pennsylvania, *Chapter 26*

PREFACE

We edited the first *Pain Medicine and Management: Just the Facts* over ten years ago, and it has served as a valuable tool for physicians who need a brief review on a topic, and those studying for the examination process. Over the past ten years a tremendous amount has changed in the health care arena, while some things have remained largely unchanged. Pain remains one of the greatest health care crises affecting American citizens and citizens of the world. Uncontrolled pain remains a major cause of disability, lost productivity, increased health care costs, and decreased quality of life. In 2011, the Institute of Medicine (IOM) published their landmark report "Relieving Pain in America: A Blueprint for Transforming Prevention, Care, Education, and Research." The fact that the IOM took on this effort speaks to the growing public opinion on the impact chronic pain has on everyday life. The report led to the National Pain Strategy (NPS) charged with providing the Secretary of Health recommendations on the future of pain care in America. One likely focus of the report will be on the importance of using a biopsychosocial approach to pain management. Like our first edition, the second edition of *Pain Medicine and Management: Just the Facts* has a chapter devoted to this topic.

Over these past ten years we have also learned that opioids, while they may control some pains, can be fraught with problems including overutilization, abuse, diversion, and addiction. In 1995, the American Pain Society voiced that pain should be considered *the fifth vital sign*. In 1999, noting the tremendous problem with pain, the JCAHO endorsed the fifth vital sign as a mandatory component of a patient's evaluation. As an outgrowth, physicians were told that they must treat pain, and hospitals depend on patient satisfaction scores to determine reimbursement rates. While this may seem like a progressive and appropriate approach at first glance, unfortunately, no clear evidence-based algorithm was provided to physicians or hospitals. Uncontrolled pain soon became equated with "give more opiates." Opioid treatment guidelines were initially intended for acute pain management, but guidelines emerged for their use in chronic pain and rapidly became the standard for (chronic and cancer) outpatient settings as well. Without adequate training, physicians relied on increased use of opioids, believing that opioids were uniformly effective. This approach has recently been challenged, and a more thoughtful risk-benefit analysis has been advocated as it relates to opioid management with more emerging evidence favoring harm than benefit. In order to help address these concerns, a specific chapter on the clinical role of opiates in chronic pain was added to this edition, along with updates on substance abuse and the roles of urine toxicology and appropriate monitoring. Many alternatives to opiates are also provided throughout the text and are in line with the long favored biopsychosocial approach to chronic pain.

In addition, the Affordable Care Act has improved access to care for many, which of course every physician wants; however, there may be unintended consequences as well. If physicians are not provided adequate resources and tools to provide that care, we may see problems with over-utilization of pharmaceutical drugs or inappropriate referrals for more invasive procedures. Insurance companies have been given unparalleled power to deny appropriate care, which frequently involves interventional care. Ironically, in some settings this drives physicians to more expensive or possibly riskier pharmacologic strategies. This text is intended to be one of many tools that physicians can use to help diagnose and manage their patients with chronic pain.

This second edition of *Pain Medicine and Management: Just the Facts* includes 14 new chapters and 66 updated chapters that reflect the evolving practice of pain medicine. We omitted six chapters that were out-of-date. Each chapter is not intended to be an exhaustive, reference-based source, rather a quick resource to help health care providers and their patients with appropriate strategies. Although each chapter presents individual topics, it should not distract from the integration of multidisciplinary assessment and treatment using a biopsychosocial model. Whether brief or extensive, we believe that all chronic pain patients need to be evaluated in this context before initiating treatment.

1 TEST PREPARATION
AND PLANNING

Stephen E. Abram, MD

SUBSPECIALTY CERTIFICATION EXAMINATION IN PAIN MEDICINE

- There are several examinations from several organizations
  - The American Board of Anesthesiology (ABA)
    - A written examination in pain medicine designed to test the presence of knowledge that is essential for a physician to function as a pain medicine practitioner.
    - The only board examination that is recognized by the American Board of Medical Specialties.
    - The only board that requires completion of an American Counsel on Graduate Medical Education Accredited Pain Fellowship.
    - Serves as the Pain Medicine subspecialty examination for the American Board of Physical Medicine and Rehabilitation (ABPMR) and for the American Board of Psychiatry and Neurology (ABPN).
    - Certification awarded by these Boards on successful completion of the examination is time limited and expires in 10 years, and a pain medicine recertification examination is offered to provide maintenance of certification as well.
    - As of the year 2012, nearly 5000 ABA, over 1500 ABPMR, and nearly 300 ABPN diplomates have received initial certification, and over 2500 physicians have completed the recertification process.
    - In 2010, the program of Maintenance of Certification in Anesthesiology for Subspecialties (MOCA-SUBS) was initiated.
      - Beginning in 2017, all ongoing certification will be carried out through the MOCA-SUBS process for all of the specialties involved in the certification process.
      - As of the writing of this chapter in 2013, the process for the three specialties has not been completely defined, but it is likely that a recertification examination will continue to be part of the process.
  - American Board of Pain Medicine
    - Offers a Pain Medicine board examination through the American Academy of Pain Medicine
  - American Board of Interventional Pain Physicians (ABIPP)
    - Offers an examination process for interventional pain physicians through the American Society of Interventional Pain Physicians (ASIPP).
  - The World Institute of Pain (WIP) offers an examination for international physicians who are not eligible for the United States ABME-approved fellowship training.
- The examination required for the Certificate of Added Qualifications in Pain Management was initially offered in 1993 by the ABA, 1 year after the Accreditation Council for Graduate Medical Education approved the first accredited pain fellowship programs. Entrance into the examination up until 1998 was dependent on either completion of a 1-year fellowship in pain management or the equivalent of at least 2 years of full-time pain management practice. Subsequent to the 1998 exam, ABA diplomates were required to complete an ACGME-approved pain fellowship. The name of the certification process has recently been changed to Subspecialty Certification in Pain Medicine.
- Beginning with the year 2000 examination, the ABA Pain Medicine Examination was made available to diplomates of the ABPN and the ABPMR. For a

period of 5 years, physicians from these specialties were admitted to the examination system on the basis of temporary criteria similar to the process in place for ABA diplomates during the first 5 years of the examination system. Since 2005, successful completion of an ACGME-approved fellowship in pain medicine has been required. Candidates from the ABPN and the ABPMR are awarded subspecialty certification by their respective boards, not by the ABA, on successful completion of the examination. The ABPMR offers subspecialty certification to any physician who is a diplomate of an American Board of Medical Specialties (ABMS)-approved board, and who has completed an ACGME-approved pain fellowship training program. This process has provided the opportunity for physicians in any discipline, including primary care physicians, to obtain certification in pain medicine, provided they are able to obtain fellowship training. With the expansion of the examination system to diplomates of the other boards, there was a broadening of the scope of the examination. Question writers and editors from Neurology, Psychiatry, and PM&R were added to the examination preparation process. Although previous examinations included material from all aspects of pain management practice, the infusion of new expertise produced a more diverse question bank. The examination should, and does, contain information from all the disciplines involved in the multidisciplinary treatment of pain. The areas of knowledge that are tested can be found in the ABA Pain Medicine Certification Examination Content Outline. This document is revised periodically and can be found on the ABA website, http://www.abanes.org.

- The ABA Pain Medicine Certification Examination is a comprehensive 200-question exam, administered by computer. The examination now uses only the A-type question format. The A-type question is a "choose the best answer" format with four or five possible answers.
- The ABA, ABPMR, and ABPN certificates in pain medicine are limited to a period of 10 years, after which diplomates are required to pass a recertification examination. The recertification process uses the 200-question certification exam. The success rates for ABA diplomates from 2005 through 2012 are as follows:

	2005	2006	2007	2008	2009	2010	2011	2012
Certification	83%	86%	78%	89%	89%	89%	80%	86%
Recertification	93%	88%	89%	92%	86%	91%	100%	77%

The pass rate for ABPMR diplomates for 2012 was 86% for initial certification and 85% for recertification. For ABPN diplomates, it was 91% for initial certification and 85% for recertification.

- The ABA began offering a Pain Medicine In-Training Examination in 2013. This is a 3-hour, 150-question examination that offers Pain Medicine Fellows the opportunity to experience this type of computer-based examination in their subspecialty and gives them information regarding their areas of knowledge strengths and weaknesses. It also provides fellowship training programs some feedback on how well they are preparing their trainees for exam preparation.

PREPARING FOR THE EXAM

- A reasonable first step in the study process is to identify areas of weakness.
- The ABA Content Outline (available through the ABA website or through each of the other two primary boards).
  - Provides a detailed and comprehensive list of topics that pain fellows need to study in order to understand the scientific basis of pain management, to provide good patient care, and to do well on the certification exam.
  - The order of topics is not designed to be a curriculum to be followed for the year of fellowship training. Rather the Content Outline is useful in assuring that all of the areas of knowledge are adequately covered during the fellowship and as a study guide for exam preparation.
  - This text covers a large portion of the required knowledge base for successful completion of the examination.
- Selection of study materials is always a dilemma.
  - A useful source is the *Core Curriculum for Professional Education in Pain*, published by the International Association for the Study of Pain (IASP).
    - Available for purchase through the IASP website (www.iasp-pain.org) and is also available as PDF downloads at that site.
    - It is organized somewhat differently than the ABA Core Curriculum, and has a less extensive list of topics.
    - Emphasizes the important aspects of each area of study, and provides concise information about each target area as well as extensive bibliographies for each section.
    - The latest version is the third edition, published in 2005.
    - While some of the references will be out of date and supplanted by more recent publications, there are many classic references that are still quite relevant.
  - There are a growing number of textbooks on pain medicine, each with its own strengths and weaknesses.

- It is reasonable to use comprehensive textbooks as a study source, keeping in mind that, by definition, information is somewhat outdated by the time a large textbook is printed and that there are strong and weak chapters in any given textbook.
- While the examination tends not to use extremely new findings, there is an effort to keep information current, particularly if there are strong data from multiple sources.
- It may be helpful to supplement the use of textbooks with recent review articles, particularly for topics in fields that are changing rapidly, such as the basic sciences related to pain.
  - Available through medical literature search instruments, such as Medline, which can be limited to English language, review articles, and, where appropriate, discussions of human subjects or patients.
  - Some students retain information best from written material, others from spoken lectures.
    - A combination of both sources results in the most effective retention.
    - Participation in pain medicine review courses provides both visual and auditory inputs.
      - Offered by:
        - American Pain Society
        - IASP
        - American Society of Regional Anesthesia and Pain Medicine
        - American Academy of Pain Medicine. Many of the specialty societies offer topics in acute, chronic, and cancer pain management at their annual meetings as well.
        - ASIPP annual meeting
      - High-quality courses are also offered by both academic and private practice groups.
      - Many review courses offer audio tapes of lectures. A major advantage of this medium is the ability to use commuting time to review pertinent topics. Hearing material that has previously been read tends to solidify one's learning.
- Perhaps the best learning method is to review the available information regarding a patient one is currently managing.
  - For many practitioners, application of this knowledge in the clinical setting is the best way to learn new information and to retain knowledge.
  - Review the available literature on a given condition in anticipation of a particular patient coming into the clinic or hospital with that condition or shortly after seeing a patient with the condition.
- Problem-based learning sessions, which are becoming more prevalent in clinical meetings and symposia, are also effective in focusing on a clinical condition and linking that clinical situation to a knowledge base.

- Question-and-answer textbooks may be helpful in identifying gaps in knowledge and, if self-testing is done periodically, may be a measure of study progress. Practice examinations increase one's confidence in the test-taking process and increase familiarity with the format.

GENERAL STUDY TECHNIQUE

PLANNING MATERIAL TO COVER

- The material to be studied will depend to a great extent on the range and depth of material covered in residency and fellowship training, and the time period from which training has been completed.
- Study of material covered in depth during training need only be reviewed briefly, while material covered only superficially needs to be studied in depth. Much of this decision is dictated by the candidate's specialty.
  - An anesthesiologist probably needs to spend considerable time on headache management or rehabilitation of the spinal cord-injured patient, while a neurologist needs to study indications of and techniques for nerve blocks.
  - As noted above, a grid, such as the ABA Core Curriculum, can be used to select topics for review versus in-depth study.

PLANNING STUDY TIME

- Once you begin the study process, it is helpful to evaluate the amount of time available for study and to schedule your available time.
  - Very short study sessions tend to be ineffective, whereas 1- to 2-hour sessions are probably optimal.
  - Daily sessions of an hour or two are more productive than weekly sessions of 5 or 6 hours.
  - According to Sherman and Wildman, the best schedule is an hour or two daily for many days, ending in a concentrated review session shortly before the examination.
  - Early in the study process, considerable time should be devoted to surveying the material to be learned, whereas later in the process, reading and reviewing material should be used more frequently.
  - It is helpful to develop a routine for each study session. An example follows:
    - Briefly review previously studied material.
    - Survey new material to study.
    - Review study questions on the topic, or create study questions.
    - Study the material.
    - Review the material studied.

STUDY SKILLS

- Look for the main ideas in what you read.
- When reading about the management of a specific syndrome, what is the principal treatment modality?
- For a chronic condition, the primary goal may be regaining strength and flexibility, while many of the specific treatments merely provide the means to achieve this primary goal.
- Understanding the pathophysiology of a specific condition helps you remember the clinical features and management principles of the disorder. Assess your confidence in your knowledge and understanding of a topic. If you feel good about that material, go on to a different topic. If not, continue to read and review.
- Write out a brief summary of the material you have studied. Include the main ideas and the most important details.
- If possible, discuss the material with other trainees or with colleagues. Ask others about their understanding of a topic. If their ideas conflict with yours, reread the material. Read additional material on important topics. This will reinforce learning and may uncover areas where controversy and differences of opinion exist. A variety of techniques have been devised to help us remember important information.
  - One helpful technique is to organize information being learned. The Content Outline can be helpful in organizing information by topic.
  - There are a number of specific techniques for aiding memory and recall.
    - Overlearning refers to the repetitive study of a topic that is already familiar.
    - As stated previously, listening to an audio tape of a lecture subsequent to reading about the topic can reinforce learning.
    - Analogies can be helpful. You can compare a topic being learned to a topic with which one is familiar. For instance, you might think of certain types of neuropathic pain caused by an ectopic focus of nociceptor activity as analogous to a seizure. Such an analogy may be particularly useful, as both conditions may benefit from the same type of drugs.
    - Imagery can be a powerful memory technique. Creation of a visual image that describes a condition, a theory, or a treatment can be a very effective aid to learning and recall.
    - Some students find the use of acronyms helpful. I occasionally find myself using mnemonics and acronyms I learned many years ago in medical school. The ones that are a bit risqué seem to be the easiest to remember.

- Recitation of material aloud multiple times is an effective way of improving retention. If the recited material rhymes or is connected to a vivid mental picture, it will be still easier to remember.
- If you are in an academic setting, teaching the material you have just learned to other trainees can be an extremely powerful technique, as it requires organization as well as understanding of the material.
- Restating information, such as rewriting certain key aspects of a learned topic, can be a powerful tool. Restating a concept in your own words is most effective.
- Quiz yourself on the material. This is particularly important for auditory learners.
- Note taking is particularly important for visual learners. Notes should be brief, clear, and succinct. This is much more effective than underlining, and notes can be reviewed shortly after the reading session, and may be used for self-testing.
- Review should be done immediately after completion of a learning session. Practice should then be repeated periodically.
- Intent to learn is important.
  - Reading and listening to new information with the active intent to learn is key to the memory process.
  - Some of the techniques stated above should be coupled with this active intent to remember.
- Attention and interest are critical.
  - As the pain medicine examination covers material that is vitally important to future practice, interest should be given.
  - There may, however, be material outside your proposed area of expertise or practice that stirs little interest.
  - Consider situations in which such material might become important to your practice.
- There are a number of reasons why we forget learned material.
  - We may not have learned the material well. During the learning process, the material must be given interest and attention.
  - Subsequently, questioning oneself about the material and periodically reviewing are critical.
    - Disuse leads to loss of memory.
      - We forget the most in the first 24 hours after learning, and it is during this period that review is most helpful.
      - Interference is another source of forgetting.
        - Interference may be related to anxiety, distraction, emotional disturbance, and intellectual interference.

- ◆ Intellectual interference, or mental over-crowding, is related to loss of memory during subsequent intellectual activity.
  - ◆ This can be minimized by reflecting on what has just been learned, and by synthesizing and organizing the material before moving on to other topics.
  - ○ Another strategy is to follow a learning session with sleep or nonintellectual activities, such as exercise, and recreation.
  - ○ A lack of attention or effort during the learning process is very detrimental. There must be concentration without distraction during the learning process, and a conscious effort to learn and remember.

STRESS AND ANXIETY

- Stress that occurs during preparation for an exam is related primarily to anxiety over the possibility of failing the exam and the consequences of that failure. The best way to deal with this is through adequate preparation and the use of practice tests to demonstrate preparedness.
- There are a number of techniques for dealing with the remaining anxiety and stress.
  - ○ If anxiety interferes with the study process, meditation, relaxation exercises, and massage can be helpful.
  - ○ Many individuals find that aerobic exercise works best.
  - ○ If you begin to panic during test preparation or the test itself, it is helpful to focus your attention away from the anxiety-provoking topic.
  - ○ Breathing exercises, with concentration on breathing alone, can be beneficial.
- Another technique is to concentrate on a muscle group, first contracting then relaxing those muscles. Make a tight fist, hold it for a few seconds, then open and relax your hand, watching the blood return to the palm. Negative thoughts about the exam or about poor performance ("catastrophizing") can increase anxiety and fear, increase catecholamine levels, and interfere with performance.
  - ○ Mental practice or mental rehearsal, a technique often used by athletes, can replace negative thoughts, and can be adapted to the examination process.
  - ○ Visualize yourself sitting in the exam setting calmly and confidently, focusing all your attention on the examination. You will thus create a vivid mental image of positive outcomes, such as successfully answering a question. The technique needs to be repeated on multiple occasions. It is most successful when it is preceded by relaxation exercises.

TAKING THE EXAM

- Reviewing of important information the day before the exam can be beneficial, but keep the sessions to an hour or two and do not let them compete with needed recreation, relaxation, and sleep.
- Eat regular, moderate-sized meals.
- Use stress-reducing techniques.
- If you do aerobic exercise regularly, continue it the day before the exam.
- On the day of the exam, avoid last-minute cramming. It is probably best not to study at all in the last hours before the exam.
- You may want to avoid caffeine, even if you use it regularly, as the combination of examination anxiety and caffeine may produce over-stimulation.
- Arrive at the examination site early enough that you are not rushed or stressed.
- Assess the number of questions on the exam and calculate the amount of time you can spend per question. Read the directions carefully.
- Computer-based exams usually provide a brief practice exam that can be used prior to the start of the actual exam. Be sure to participate in this exercise.
- Read each question or stem carefully. Note questions asking for "all are correct except" answers.
- Think of your own answer or answers to the questions before reading the examination answers and choose responses that are closest to yours.
- Eliminate choices that you know are incorrect.
- Read all the possible responses before selecting an answer. Some questions ask for the *best* answer among responses that may have more than one correct answer.
- For examinees who are prone to test anxiety, it may be helpful to read through but not answer difficult questions initially, answering the easier questions first. This technique provides momentum and confidence to complete the exam initially. Later items may provide cues for answering skipped items.
- Answer all the questions unless there is a penalty for wrong responses (this should be made clear from the test instructions).
- Use all of the allotted time.
- Rework difficult questions and look for errors on easy questions, such as selection of the wrong letter or misreading of the stem.

BIBLIOGRAPHY

Charlton JE, ed. *Core Curriculum for Professional Education in Pain*. 3rd ed. Seattle, Wash: IASP Press; 2005.

Davies D. *Maximizing Examination Performance. A Psychological Approach*. London: Kogan Page; 1986.

Longman DC, Atkinson RH. *College Learning and Study Skills.* 3rd ed. Minneapolis, Minn: West; 1993.

Sherman TM, Wildman TM. *Proven Strategies for Successful Test Taking.* Columbus, Oh: Charles E. Merrill; 1982.

Suinn RM. *Psychology in Sports.* Minneapolis, Minn: Burgess; 1980.

ONLINE RESOURCES

Dartmouth Academic Skills Center http://www.dartmouth.edu/admin/acskills/

Study Skills Assessment Instrument http://www.hhpublishing.com/_assessments/LASSI/index.html

University of Minnesota Learning and Academic Skills Center http://www.ucs.umn.edu/lasc/OnlineLearn.htmlx

University of New Mexico Center for Academic Program Support http://www.unm.edu/~caps/strategies.html

University of South Australia Learning Connection http://www.unisanet.unisa.edu.au/learningconnection/students.htm http://www.unisanet.unisa.edu.au/examsuccess/

2   A BRIEF REVIEW OF THE BASIC PHYSIOLOGY OF PAIN PROCESSING

Linda S. Sorkin, PhD
Tony L. Yaksh, PhD

PAIN—MULTIPLE FACETS

- "Pain" as defined by the International Association for the Study of Pain: "An unpleasant sensory and emotional experience associated with actual or potential tissue damage, or described in terms of such damage."
- The psychophysical experience of pain may be divided into sensory-discriminative ("I hurt here on a scale of 1–10") and motivational-affective ("I really don't like this experience and will try to avoid it in the future") components.
- The so-called prefrontal lobotomies carried out in the last century had no effect upon sensations associated with chronic pain (eg, head and neck cancer), but altered the affective component of the pain state. This is taken as support of this orthogonal dichotomy.

NOCICEPTIVE PAIN

BEHAVIORAL CHARACTERISTICS

- "Nociceptive pain" is secondary to real or threatened damage to non-neural tissue and subsequent nociceptor activation.
- The nociceptive message is initiated by high intensity, potentially tissue-injuring stimuli (thermal, mechanical, and/or chemical products, including both endogenous locally derived agents, eg, kinins, prostaglandins (PGs), and exogenous chemical products)

applied to or released near non-neural tissues (skin, muscle, viscera, etc.).
- A nociceptive stimulus typically evokes a constellation of responses with increasingly complex levels of organization:
  - local flexion (withdrawal) of the stimulated limb, which may be spinally mediated (local reflexes);
  - autonomic responses (increased pituitary-sympathetic outflow, respiratory rate/blood pressure/heart rate) mediated by outflow organized at the brainstem level;
  - organized escape behavior; and
  - emotive/affective expressions organized at the cortical level.

NOCICEPTIVE PAIN PATHWAYS

- As spinal cord lesions restricted to one side produce deficits in contralateral pain (the Brown Sequard syndrome and identified by William Gower to be important for pain in humans), pain is said to be a "crossed pathway." (This is the basis for the classic ventrolateral cordotomy for pain.)
- The simplest anatomic pathway underlying the encoding of the nociceptive stimulus involves three neurons:
  - Primary afferent neuron that goes from skin to spinal cord with the cell body in the dorsal root ganglia (DRG),
  - Spinal cord projection neuron with the cell body in the dorsal horn that projects to the contralateral lateral thalamus via the ventrolateral quadrant (eg, the spinothalamic), and
  - Thalamocortical neuron that projects to the ipsilateral primary somatosensory cortex.
- This three-neuron system displays a high degree of somatotopic organization: for example, stimulation of the left big toe activates specific neuronal populations

in the ipsilateral spinal cord and contralateral thalamic and cortical levels. This system is thought to underlie the sensory discriminative component of the nociceptive experience.

- Spinal neurons also project via the brainstem, medial thalamus, and/or midbrain areas to anterior cingulate gyrus. This system is thought to underlie the affective-motivational component of the nociceptive experience. This system is phylogenetically older, involves more neurons, and is slower than the sensory discriminative pathway.

- There is also a multisynaptic system projecting though the brainstem reticular formation (spinoreticulotract) that is believed to serve in complex pathways contributing to the autonomic response and to spinal–brainstem–spinal loops (see below) for modulation and/or integration of the nociceptive message.

TISSUE INJURY PAIN—UNDERLYING MECHANISMS

- Nociceptive pain is initiated by tissue injury; it can be secondary to incision (acute trauma), inflammation, or disease.

- As will be reviewed in more detail below, there are several populations of primary afferent fibers, characterized by morphology, conduction velocity, and importantly the nature of the stimulus that can produce activity (action potentials).

- Potentially tissue-damaging stimuli—mechanical, thermal, or chemical—can activate specific populations of primary afferents as determined by their receptors; collectively they are called "nociceptors." While some nociceptive afferent fibers are specific to one modality (eg, cold or a particular chemical such as histamine or bradykinin), a majority of axon terminals are studded with multiple types of receptors and thus, are "polymodal" and respond to multiple inputs, which "match" their receptors.

- Tissue injury initiates a cascade of local events.
  - Plasma extravasation (capillary leak).
  - Infiltration of inflammatory cells (macrophages, neutrophils, and mast cells).
  - Release of a wide variety of "active factors" from plasma (bradykinin) and from local injured (eg, K^+ and H^+) and inflammatory (eg, histamine, cytokines, and prostanoids) cells.
  - Release of peptides from collaterals of activated nociceptive nerve terminals (eg, substance P [sP], calcitonin gene–related peptide [CGRP], and glutamate). These neuropeptides induce vasodilation, increased vascular permeability, and further escape of plasma proteins into the tissue. This

vascular leak causes edema at the injury site and the surrounding flare (indicating precapillary dilation).

- The local chemical; milieu initiates two events:
  - Activation of receptors on peripheral terminals of "pain fibers" (nociceptors), which initiates action potentials, whose frequency is related to local concentrations of inflammatory products.
  - In addition to exciting nociceptors, these products act via second messenger cascades involving several kinases to sensitize nociceptors by lowering the threshold of, or increasing, the open time of individual ion channel containing receptors. If the thermal threshold is reduced such that body temperature or other normal physiological processes initiates neural activity, this would appear to be spontaneous pain. Reduction of thresholds of nociceptors to temperature and pressure within the innocuous range is manifested as allodynia and is also called primary hyperalgesia (eg, a lowering of threshold to produce afferent discharge).

PRIMARY AFFERENT FIBERS

- Primary afferent fibers are divided into classes based on morphology: myelinated versus unmyelinated and axonal diameter ($A\beta > A\delta > C$) and their corresponding conduction velocities ($A\beta > A\delta > C$).

- Most fibers that transmit acute nociceptive pain are $A\delta$ (small myelinated) or C (unmyelinated) fibers. Not all $A\delta$ and C fibers transmit pain information; many code for innocuous temperature, itch, and touch.

- Some afferent fibers, "silent or sleeping nociceptors," signal only after there has been an overt tissue damage. Chemicals released by injury/inflammation can sensitize these receptors. Accordingly, many of these are thought to play a prominent role in arthritis pain and other diseases associated with tissue damage or chronic inflammation. Viscera contain a particularly large proportion of silent nociceptors.

- Parallel experiments comparing electrophysiological data in single C nociceptive fibers to human psychophysical data show a high correlation between activity in primary afferent fibers and a pain sensation. This suggests that afferent fiber activity mediates pain and that inhibition of this activity diminishes pain.

- In many cases, transduction mechanisms for stimuli activating afferent terminals have been identified. Within the cutaneous C nociceptive fiber population, fibers containing TRPV1 receptors are typically activated by high temperatures (>48°C). Importantly, these channels are also activated by the chemical capsaicin and decreases in pH (acidity). These axons contain a variety of neuropeptides.

- Other C nociceptors are positive for the surface lectin IB4 and are capsaicin-insensitive. The IB4+ fibers tend to have sensitivity to mechanical stimuli.
- Both classes of C fibers have monosynaptic terminations in laminae I and II of the spinal dorsal horn, with the peptidergic ones being more superficial (see below).
- Aδ nociceptors primarily terminate in laminae I and V of the dorsal horn (see below).
- C fibers have polysynaptic connections with neurons in lamina V as well as with neurons in deeper dorsal horn. Many nociceptive afferents from viscera have monosynaptic input to lamina X around the central canal as well as bilaterally throughout the spinal dorsal horn.

SPINAL CORD SENSORY ORGANIZATION

- Primary afferent fibers terminate either directly or indirectly through interneurons onto spinal cord transmission cells that convey their information to supraspinal sites. Some neurons project to various midbrain and thalamic nuclei that serve as way stations for the discriminative and affective components of pain. These ascending pathway nuclei are predominantly crossed and ascend in the anterolateral quadrant of the spinal cord contralateral to the cell body and the innervated body part.
- Other neurons project to brainstem autonomic centers in the reticular formation that regulate increases in cardiovascular function and respiration in tandem with affective components of nociceptive transmission; these pathways tend to be bilateral. In addition to ascending pathways, intrinsic pathways in the spinal cord connect to motor neurons that participate in reflex motor activity.
- Given that nociceptive afferent fibers terminate in laminae I and II, it is understandable that the neurons in lamina I are largely activated by high-threshold stimuli and are termed "nociceptive specific." Conversely, many cells that are found in deeper dorsal horn laminae send dendrites toward the superficial layers and receive high-threshold afferent input on their distal dendrites, but they also receive low-threshold input on their cell bodies and ascending dendrites. These cells thus respond to low-threshold stimuli and to high-threshold input. These cells are said to receive convergent input, in which they fire more action potentials; as the intensity of the stimulation increases, they are called "wide dynamic range (WDR)" neurons.
- In the case of both nociceptive-specific and WDR neurons, action potential firing frequency is dependent upon the intensity of the afferent stimulus, with nociceptive-specific neurons showing an increased discharge starting at noxious stimulus intensities, whereas WDR neurons begin to discharge at low non-noxious stimulus intensities and progressively increase firing rates as intensity rises.
- Interestingly, in the face of high-frequency C-fiber input, many WDRs show a marked increase in their response to a given stimulus intensity. This results in repeated mild stimuli producing a disproportionately high level of discharge, a phenomena called "wind up."
- Many WDR neurons are multimodal and respond to both mechanical and thermal inputs. Others respond exclusively to noxious heat or cold. There are also cells that respond only to chemical stimulation, including histamine release in the skin (and thus likely mediate itch). A small population of nociception-specific cells is located in deep dorsal horn.
- Convergence of input from the outer body surface (skin) and from viscera onto individual spinal neurons also occurs. Thus, when activity is initiated in viscera, pain is referred to the portion of the body surface that "shares" those neurons. This is one explanation for "referred pain."

SPINAL CORD PHARMACOLOGY

- Afferent nociceptive fibers release glutamate and peptides from their central terminals in the spinal cord. Some peptides are released along with the glutamate only when the afferent fibers fire action potentials at high frequencies (equivalent to severe injury). The postsynaptic effects may usefully be thought of as having: (i) acute, (ii) early onset/short duration, (iii) delayed onset/intermediate duration, and (iv) slow onset, long duration.
- *Acute onset postsynaptic events.* Glutamate produces a fast response (depolarization) in the spinal neurons via receptors linked to ion channels. These are called non-N-methyl-D-aspartate (NMDA)–type glutamate receptors and consist of amino-3-hydroxy-5-methly-4-isoxazole-proprionic acid (AMPA) and kainate receptors, which increase membrane permeability to Na+, yielding a prominent but transient depolarization. This linkage accounts for the majority of the acute response produced by brief activation of low- and high-threshold afferents.
- As noted, in the face of on-going high-threshold/high-frequency input, the input–output function of dorsal horn neurons is altered. This change in gain may be broadly considered in terms of events that occur acutely, lasting milliseconds to seconds, events that are longer lasting (seconds to minutes), and events that are very long lasting (hours to days).

- *Early onset/short-duration postsynaptic events.* Brief events such as wind-up, discussed previously, occur secondary to high-frequency bursts of C-fiber input resulting from the release of peptides, such as sP, which serve to prolong the initial depolarization. This leads to changes in transmembrane voltage that remove a voltage-dependent "Mg^{2+} block" from a subtype of glutamate receptor, the NMDA receptor, which is then capable of being activated. NMDA receptors are ligand-gated calcium channels, which allow influx of Ca^{2+} in addition to Na^+. Increased intracellular calcium leads to a magnification of the incoming response via second messenger cascades involving various kinases, such that each incoming signal results in successively more output.

- *Delayed onset/intermediate-duration postsynaptic events.* If high-frequency C-fiber activity persists, other more enduring intracellular biochemical cascades occur that also magnify and enhance the afferent response to yield a long-lasting spinal sensitization. One such cascade includes Ca^{2+} activation of the enzyme phospholipase A_2 (PLA_2); this frees arachadonic acid from plasma membranes, thus making it available as a substrate for the enzyme cyclooxygenase (COX) and results in the production of PGs. These lipids act on specific PG receptors to increase the amount of neurotransmitter released per action potential invading the terminal. PGs also act via specific PG receptors on glia to activate them and cause them to release additional neuroactive substances including proinflammatory cytokines.

- Other enzymes, including nitric oxide synthetase (NOS), are activated by Ca^{2+} in a similar manner, also resulting in a magnification of the transmitted response.

- *Slow-onset, long-duration postsynaptic events.* Increases in intracellular Ca^{2+} lead to the activation of a variety of transcription factors that activate protein synthesis. Proteins made are often key elements in proinflammatory cascades such as COX-2 and NOS. This leads to long-term changes in sensitization of the dorsal horn as the result of a burst of high-frequency small-afferent input.

- The above scenario along with the findings that general anesthetics do not block primary afferent transmitter release provides a rationale behind the premise of "preemptive analgesia." One class of agents that reduce the likelihood of such sensitization are the opiates.

- Spinal opiates inhibit C fiber-mediated nociceptive activity. They bind to μ opiate receptors on the central terminal of nociceptive primary afferent fibers (presynaptic) and, by reducing Ca^{2+} entry when the action potential invades the terminal, reduce the amount of neurotransmitter released per action potential. Opiates also bind postsynaptically (on the dorsal horn neurons). Here, opiates increase permeability to K^+, which hyperpolarizes the neurons and results in an inhibition of acute nociceptive transmission. Aβ fibers do not have presynaptic opiate receptors. Thus, if Aβ (touch) fibers mediate pain (allodynia), spinal opiates have only a postsynaptic action and exert less analgesic effect than they would on C fiber-mediated pain. This is one theory of why Aβ-mediated pain is relatively opiate resistant.

- Serotonin and norepinephrine also inhibit nociceptive transmission both pre- and postsynaptically. These monoamines are released primarily from axons whose cell bodies are located in the brainstem. Analgesic actions are potentiated by monoamine re-uptake (tricyclic antidepressants) inhibitors and are synergistic with morphine.

- Low-threshold afferent input to many nociceptive dorsal horn neurons is under tonic GABAergic and glycinergic inhibition, which selectively reduces postsynaptic responses to light touch. Note that WDR neurons respond to Aβ input, but such input is not considered noxious. Removal of the glycinergic/GABAergic receptor activation removes the *inhibition* otherwise activated by Aβ input. This leads to a strongly enhanced response of the WDR neurons. Removal of this inhibition results in high-frequency responses to innocuous stimuli that are thus interpreted as pain.

SPINOFUGAL PROJECTIONS

- There is a strong projection from both superficial and deep dorsal horn to the contralateral lateral thalamus (spinothalamic tract). This "classical" pathway projects to somatosensory (S1) cortex and is postulated to be integral to sensory discrimination of pain, that is, where exactly is it?, is it sharp?, is it hot?, and so on.

- Superficial (lamina I) dorsal horn has a unique projection to posterior thalamus (VMpo) within the posterior complex; this nucleus, in turn, projects to posterior insula cortex. This area has recently been proposed to be a unique cortical pain center as well as to be involved in homeostatic control of the internal environment, including tissue integrity.

- The ventrocaudal portion of the medial dorsal thalamus (MDvc) also receives an exclusive input from lamina I. This area projects to the anterior cingulate cortex. This medial pathway is likely to mediate the motivational-affective component of pain.

- Other pathways contribute to changes in autonomic function concomitant with pain, including the spinoreticular and spinomesencephalic tracts.

- The postsynaptic dorsal column pathway projects to posterolateral thalamus via a dorsal column nucleus relay and is thought to be specific for visceral pain. Lesioning the axons of these spinal cord neurons has been used clinically for pelvic pain secondary to cancer.

NEUROPATHIC PAIN

BEHAVIORAL CHARACTERISTICS

- After a variety of injuries to the peripheral and central components of the somatosensory projection system, animals and humans can develop a stereotypical pattern of pain symptomatology broadly called "neuropathic pain."
- Frequent components of this evolving syndrome are:
  - ongoing sharp shooting sensations referred to the peripheral distribution of the injured peripheral nerve, and
  - abnormal painful sensations in response to light touch applied to the relevant body surface. The latter phenomenon is called tactile or mechano-allodynia.
- This constellation of sensory events was first formally recognized by Silas Weir Mitchell in the 1860s .
- The psychophysics of the allodynia and the differential effects of limb ischemia and local anesthetics emphasize that the pain is evoked by the activation of low-threshold mechanoreceptors (Aβ afferents), although C-tactile afferents also play a role in allodynia development.
- The ability of *low-threshold* afferent fibers to evoke this anomalous pain state is de facto evidence that the peripheral nerve injury has led to a reorganization of central processing; that is, it is not a simple case of peripheral sensitization of otherwise high-threshold afferent fibers.
- In addition to these behavioral changes, the neuropathic pain condition may display other contrasting anomalies, including, on occasion, an ameliorating effect of sympathectomy of the affected limb and an attenuated responsiveness to analgesics such as opiates.

NERVE INJURY EVOKED CHANGES IN STRUCTURE AND FUNCTION

- Following peripheral nerve injury, several events occur that signal long-term changes in peripheral and central processing.
- In the periphery, there is an acute dying back (retrograde chromatolysis) that proceeds for some interval at which time the axon begins to develop growth cones and sprout.
- Growth cones frequently fail to make contact with their old targets, the sprouts form tangled structures known as neuromas.
- Ectopic activity is generated from neuromas and the cell bodies (DRG) of injured axons. Importantly, this includes not only mechanically injured axons, but also axons exposed to proinflammatory injury products.
- Dorsal horn neurons exhibit spontaneous activity and an exaggerated response to normally innocuous afferent input as well as increased receptive fields.

MECHANISMS UNDERLYING NEUROPATHIC PAIN PHENOTYPE

SPONTANEOUS PAIN

- Under normal conditions, primary afferents exhibit little spontaneous activity.
- Following an acute injury to the nerve, afferent axons display an initial burst of firing secondary to the injury followed by a variable interval of electrical silence.
- Over time, both myelinated- and unmyelinated-injured axons develop measurable levels of spontaneous afferent traffic.
- This afferent discharge is believed to contribute to ongoing pain sensations.
- An important organizing principle is that the spontaneous activity appears to arise first in the neuroma followed by ongoing activity arising from the DRG of axons either directly injured or affected by the local inflammatory milieu.
- After nerve injury, there are "massive" changes in the expression of various proteins within the DRG. We will focus only on a few classes of protein that represent the importance of such changes.
  - Ion channel expression
    - *Sodium channels (Na_v).* Voltage-sensitive sodium channels mediate action potential propagation in myelinated and unmyelinated axons.
    - There are seven populations of Na_v in peripheral nerve, differing in their current activation properties and structure. One major difference is sensitivity to tetrodotoxin (TTX), the two TTX-sensitive subtypes are associated with nociceptors.
    - Several lines of evidence support the importance of Na_v channels in neuropathic pain:
      - Increased expression of Na_v in neuroma and DRG after nerve injury with a consequent increased neuronal excitability.
      - Ability of systemic lidocaine to reduce allodynic states in human and animals.
      - Mutations that cause gain of function in individual Na_v subtypes, particularly the Na_v 1.7 subtype, are associated with congenital

syndromes reported in humans to result in a variety of severe pain states (eg, erthromyalgia) while loss-of-function mutations can lead to a profound congenital insensitivity to pain.

- *Voltage-sensitive potassium channel.* Potassium channels (K_v) have many subtypes after nerve injury, many K_vs show a downregulation, leading to increased excitability.
- *Voltage-sensitive calcium channels (Ca_v).* There are a wide variety of voltage-sensitive Ca_vs. Neurotransmitter release from the primary afferent is largely mediated by the "N-type calcium channel." Increased expression of this channel has been identified after nerve injury. Of particular interest, these channels possess an extracellular auxiliary protein—the $\alpha 2\delta$ subunit. This is also increased in the DRG after nerve injury. Importantly, this is the proposed binding site for the gabapentin type drugs, known to have efficacy in nerve injury pain states.

○ Receptor expression
- Regenerating nerve terminals and neuromas have growth cones that possess transduction properties not found in the naïve axon. Additionally, the DRG neurons express new chemical receptors and changes in sensory thresholds.
- Thus, injured afferent fibers may develop sensitivity to a number of humoral factors, such as prostanoids, catecholamines, and proinflammatory cytokines such as tumor necrosis factor.

○ Change in DRG cell profiles
- DRG neurons begin to express a variety of transcription factors believed to contribute to the pronounced changes in protein expression briefly noted above.
- Satellite cells (the glia of the DRG) become activated and macrophages infiltrate the DRG. Satellite cells and macrophages release active factors, which can result in sensitization and in the DRG becoming an "ectopic" action potential generator.

○ Sympathetic-dependent generation of afferent activity
- After peripheral nerve injury, the peripheral neuroma becomes innervated by postganglionic sympathetic terminals.
- There is a prominent growth of postganglionic sympathetic terminals into the DRG of the injured axons, which form baskets around the cell bodies of the nerve fibers.
- Several properties of this innervation are interesting: (i) invests all sizes of ganglion cells, but particularly type A (large) ganglion cells; and (ii) innervation occurs in both ipsilateral and contralateral DRG.

- Stimulation of preganglionic efferents, directly activates both the neuroma and the DRG in a manner blocked by intravenous phentolamine (an α-preferring antagonist) emphasizing an adrenergic effect.

EVOKE ALLODYNIC PAIN

- The observation that low-threshold tactile stimulation yields pain states has been the subject of considerable interest.
- Several underlying mechanisms have been proposed to account for this seemingly anomalous linkage.
  ○ DRG cell cross-talk
  - Following nerve injury, there is evidence suggesting that "cross-talk" develops between populations of afferent fibers in the DRG and in the neuroma.
  - Depolarizing currents in one axon may generate a depolarizing voltage and action potentials in an adjacent quiescent axon.
  - This depolarization would result in activity in one axon driving activity in a second.
  - In this manner, it is hypothesized that activity in a large low-threshold afferent could drive activity in an adjacent high-threshold afferent.
  - Alternatively, it is appreciated that DRG cells in vitro can release a variety of transmitters and express excitatory receptors.
  ○ Afferent sprouting in spinal cord
  - Under normal circumstances, large myelinated ($A\beta$) afferents project into lamina IV of the dorsal horn.
  - Small afferents ($A\delta$ and C fibers) tend to project more superficially, into spinal laminae I and II, a region with many nocisponsive neurons.
  - Following peripheral nerve injury, it has been argued that central terminals of the large myelinated afferents ($A\beta$ fibers) sprout into lamina II of the spinal cord.
  - The degree to which this sprouting occurs remains controversial, and although it may occur, it is far less prominent than originally reported.
  ○ Spinal glutamate release
  - There is little doubt that spinal glutamate release plays a major role in the post-nerve injury pain state.
  - Studies have emphasized that after nerve injury there is a significant enhancement of resting spinal glutamate release.
  - Spinal glutamate has multiple sources:
    □ increased spontaneous release from the primary afferent,

- a loss of intrinsic inhibition that may serve to modulate resting glutamate secretion from both central terminals of afferent fibers and dorsal horn neurons, and
- impairment of glutamate removal due to down-regulation of astrocytic glutamate transporters (see below).

- Physiological significance of glutamate release is emphasized by two convergent observations:
  - intrathecally delivered glutamate evokes prominent tactile allodynia and thermal hyperalgesia though activation of spinal NMDA and non-NMDA receptors, and
  - spinal delivery of NMDA antagonists attenuate hyperalgesia generated in animal models of nerve injury without altering acute nociception.
- NMDA receptor activation mediates facilitation of neuronal excitability.
- In addition, the NMDA receptor is a calcium ionophore that, when activated, leads to prominent increases in intracellular calcium.
- Increased intracellular calcium initiates a cascade of events that includes the activation of a variety of enzymes (kinases), some of which phosphorylate membrane proteins (eg, calcium channels and NMDA receptors), and others, such as the mitogen-activated protein kinases (MAPK), which mediate the intracellular signaling leading to altered expression of a variety of proteins and peptides (eg, COX and dynorphin).

○ Non-neuronal cells and nerve injury
- Following nerve injury (section or compression), there is a significant increase in activation of spinal microglia and astrocytes in spinal segments receiving input from the injured nerves. Specific blockade of glial activation reduces pain behavior.
- Astrocytes are activated by a variety of neurotransmitters and growth factors including fractalkine, cytokines, and complement components.
- Astrocytes are enriched with glutamate transporter molecules that remove glutamate from the synapse, these play a critical role in glutamate homeostasis and the development of neuropathic pain.
- Importantly, Aβ-fiber activity is necessary for microglial activation following nerve injury.
- Glial activation leads to increased spinal expression of COX/NOS/glutamate transporters/proteinases, substances that play an important role in the facilitated state.

○ Loss of intrinsic GABAergic/glycinergic inhibitory control
- The most prevalent cell population in spinal cord are interneurons. Inhibitory interneurons contain and release GABA and/or glycine.

- GABA/glycine–containing terminals are frequently presynaptic to central terminals of Aβ and Aδ afferent fibers and form distinctive complexes containing reciprocal synapses, while GABAergic axosomatic connections on spinothalamic cells have also been identified.
- Accordingly, these amino acids normally exert important tonic and evoked inhibitory control over the activity of Aβ primary afferent terminals and second-order neurons in the spinal dorsal horn.
- Relevance of this intrinsic inhibition is clear because intrathecal delivery of GABA-A or glycine receptor antagonists leads to a powerful behaviorally defined tactile allodynia in the absence of injury. This hyperexcitability/allodynia is not affected by spinal opiates.
- Similarly, animals genetically lacking glycine binding sites often display a high level of spinal hyperexcitability.
- These observations led to the consideration that following nerve injury, there may be a loss of GABAergic neurons. But, this loss is now known to be minimal.
- More recent observations now suggest a second, more viable alternative. After nerve injury, spinal neurons may regress to a neonatal phenotype in which GABA-A activation becomes excitatory. This excitatory effect is secondary to reduced activity of plasma membrane Cl$^-$ transporters, which changes the reversal current for Cl$^-$ conductance. Following these changes, release of GABA and glycine, membrane Cl$^-$ conductance increases as before, but now action results in membrane depolarization and excitation.

BIBLIOGRAPHY

Bennett GJ, Xie YK. A peripheral mononeuropathy in rat that produces disorders of pain sensation like those seen in man [see comments]. *Pain*. 1988;33:87–107.

Burchiel KJ, Ochoa JL. Pathophysiology of injured axons. *Neurosurg Clin N Am*. 1991;2:105–116.

Carlton SM, Hayes ES. Light microscopic and ultrastructural analysis of GABA-immunoreactive profiles in the monkey spinal cord. *J Comp Neurol*. 1990;300:162–182.

Chen L, Huang LY. Protein kinase C reduces Mg^{2+} block of NMDA-receptor channels as a mechanism of modulation. *Nature*. 1992;356:521–523.

Craig AD. Interoception: the sense of the physiological condition of the body. *Curr Opin Neurobiol*. 2003;13:500–505.

Craig AD. Distribution of trigeminothalamic and spinothalamic lamina I terminations in the macaque monkey. *J Comp Neurol*. 2004;477:119–148.

Dabby R. Pain disorders and erythromelalgia caused by voltage-gated sodium channel mutations. *Curr Neurol Neurosci Rep.* 2012;12:76–83.

Decosterd I, Woolf CJ. Spared nerve injury: an animal model of persistent peripheral neuropathic pain. *Pain.* 2000;87:149–158.

Devor M, Wall PD. Cross-excitation in dorsal root ganglia of nerve-injured and intact rats. *J Neurophysiol.* 1990;64:1733–1746.

Furlan AD, Lui PW, Mailis A. Chemical sympathectomy for neuropathic pain: does it work? Case report and systematic literature review. *Clin J Pain.* 2001;17:327–336.

Gao YJ, Ji RR. Chemokines, neuronal–glial interactions, and central processing of neuropathic pain. *Pharmacol Ther.* 2010;126:56–68.

Gold MS, Weinreich D, Kim CS, Wang R, Treanor J, Porreca F, Lai J. Redistribution of Na(V)1.8 in uninjured axons enables neuropathic pain. *J Neurosci.* 2003;23:158–166.

Gundlach AL. Disorder of the inhibitory glycine receptor: inherited myoclonus in Poll Hereford calves. *FASEB J.* 1990;4:2761–2766.

Hirshberg RM, Al-Chaer ED, Lawand NB, Westlund KN, Willis WD. Is there a pathway in the posterior funiculus that signals visceral pain? *Pain.* 1996;67:291–305.

Hu P, McLachlan EM. Macrophage and lymphocyte invasion of dorsal root ganglia after peripheral nerve lesions in the rat. *Neuroscience.* 2002;112:23–38.

Hughes DI, Scott DT, Todd AJ, Riddell JS. Lack of evidence for sprouting of Abeta afferents into the superficial laminas of the spinal cord dorsal horn after nerve section. *J Neurosci.* 2003;23:9491–9499.

Jensen TS, Gottrup H, Sindrup SH, Bach FW. The clinical picture of neuropathic pain. *Eur J Pharmacol.* 2001;429:1–11.

Kajander K, Waikaka S, Bennett G. Spontaneous discharge originates in the dorsal root ganglion at the onset of a painful peripheral neuropathy in the rat. *Neurosci Lett.* 1992;138:225–228.

Kim SH, Chung JM. An experimental model for peripheral neuropathy produced by segmental spinal nerve ligation in the rat. *Pain.* 1992;50:355–363.

Liljencrantz J, Bjornsdotter M, Morrison I, et al. Altered C-tactile processing in human dynamic tactile allodynia. *Pain.* 2013;154:227–234.

Liu B, Li H, Brull SJ, Zhang JM. Increased sensitivity of sensory neurons to tumor necrosis factor alpha in rats with chronic compression of the lumbar ganglia. *J Neurophysiol.* 2002;88:1393–1399.

McLachlan EM, Janig W, Devor M, Michaelis M. Peripheral nerve injury triggers noradrenergic sprouting within dorsal root ganglia. *Nature.* 1993;363:543–546.

Michaelis M, Habler HJ, Jaenig W. Silent afferents: a separate class of primary afferents? *Clin Exp Pharmacol Physiol.* 1996;23:99–105.

Parsons CG. NMDA receptors as targets for drug action in neuropathic pain. *Eur J Pharmacol.* 2001;429:71–78.

Polgar E, Todd AJ. Tactile allodynia can occur in the spared nerve injury model in the rat without selective loss of GABA or GABA(A) receptors from synapses in laminae I-II of the ipsilateral spinal dorsal horn. *Neuroscience.* 2008;156:193–202.

Price TJ, Cervero F, de Koninck Y. Role of cation-chloride-cotransporters (CCC) in pain and hyperalgesia. *Curr Top Med Chem.* 2005;5:547–555.

Raja SN, Dickstein RE, Johnson CA. Comparison of postoperative analgesic effects of intraarticular bupivacaine and morphine following arthroscopic knee surgery. *Anesthesiology.* 1992;77:1143–1147.

Rasband MN, Park EW, Vanderah TW, Lai J, Porreca F, Trimmer JS. Distinct potassium channels on pain-sensing neurons. *Proc Natl Acad Sci U S A.* 2001;98:13373–13378.

Rudomin P. Selectivity of the central control of sensory information in the mammalian spinal cord. *Adv Exp Med Biol.* 2002;508:157–170.

Russell N, Schaible H-G, Schmidt R. Opiates inhibit the discharges of fine afferent units from inflamed knee joint of the cat. *Neurosci Lett.* 1987;76:107–112.

Schafers M, Lee DH, Brors D, Yaksh TL, Sorkin LS. Increased sensitivity of injured and adjacent uninjured rat primary sensory neurons to exogenous tumor necrosis factor-alpha after spinal nerve ligation. *J Neurosci.* 2003;23:3028–3038.

Shehab SA, Spike RC, Todd AJ. Evidence against cholera toxin B subunit as a reliable tracer for sprouting of primary afferents following peripheral nerve injury. *Brain Res.* 2003;964:218–227.

Shinder V, Govrin-Lippmann R, Cohen S, et al. Structural basis of sympathetic-sensory coupling in rat and human dorsal root ganglia following peripheral nerve injury. *J Neurocytol.* 1999;28:743–761.

Shir Y, Seltzer Z. A-fibers mediate mechanical hyperesthesia and allodynia and C-fibers mediate thermal hyperalgesia in a new model of causalgiform pain disorders in rats. *Neurosci Lett.* 1990;115:62–67.

Sorkin LS, Puig S. Neuronal model of tactile allodynia produced by spinal strychnine: effects of excitatory amino acid receptor antagonists and a mu-opiate receptor agonist. *Pain.* 1996;68:283–292.

Stephenson FA. Subunit characterization of NMDA receptors. *Curr Drug Targets.* 2001;2:233–239.

Stoll G, Jander S, Myers RR. Degeneration and regeneration of the peripheral nervous system: from Augustus Waller's observations to neuroinflammation. *J Peripher Nerv Syst.* 2002;7:13–27.

Sung B, Lim G, Mao J. Altered expression and uptake activity of spinal glutamate transporters after nerve injury contribute to the pathogenesis of neuropathic pain in rats. *J Neurosci.* 2003;23:2899–2910.

Suter MR, Berta T, Gao YJ, Decosterd I, Ji RR. Large A-fiber activity is required for microglial proliferation and p38 MAPK activation in the spinal cord: different effects of resiniferatoxin and bupivacaine on spinal microglial changes after spared nerve injury. *Molecular Pain.* 2009;5:53.

Todd AJ, Anatomy of primary afferents and projection neurones in the rat spinal dorsal horn with particular emphasis on substance P and the neurokinin 1 receptor. *Exp Physiol.* 2002;87:245–249.

Tong YG, Wang HF, Ju G, Grant G, Hokfelt T, Zhang X. Increased uptake and transport of cholera toxin B-subunit in dorsal root ganglion neurons after peripheral axotomy: possible implications for sensory sprouting. *J Comp Neurol.* 1999;404:143–158.

Watkins LR, Maier SF. Beyond neurons: evidence that immune and glial cells contribute to pathological pain states. *Physiol Rev.* 2002;82:981–1011.

Wiesenfeld-Hallin Z, Aldskogius H, Grant G, Hao JX, Hokfelt T, Xu XJ. Central inhibitory dysfunctions: mechanisms and clinical implications. *Behav Brain Sci.* 1997;20:420–425; discussion 435–513.

Willis WD, Jr., Westlund KN. The role of the dorsal column pathway in visceral nociception. *Curr Pain Headache Rep.* 2001;5:20–26.

Woolf CJ, Shortland P, Coggeshall RE. Peripheral nerve injury triggers central sprouting of myelinated afferents. *Nature.* 1992;355:75–78.

Wu G, Ringkamp M, Hartke TV, et al. Early onset of spontaneous activity in uninjured C-fiber nociceptors after injury to neighboring nerve fibers. *J Neurosci.* 2001;21:RC140.

Yaksh TL. Behavioral and autonomic correlates of the tactile evoked allodynia produced by spinal glycine inhibition: effects of modulatory receptor systems and excitatory amini acid antagonists. *Pain.* 1989;37:111–123.

Yarnitsky D, Simone DA, Dotson RM, Cline MA, Ochoa JL. Single C nociceptor responses and psychophysical parameters of evoked pain: effect of rate of rise of heat stimuli in humans. *J Physiol.* 1992;450:581–592.

3 THE EPIDEMIOLOGY OF CHRONIC PAIN

Oliver van Hecke, MBChB
Blair H. Smith, MD

PAIN: ACUTE AND CHRONIC

- Pain is a subjective and individual experience with enormous societal impact. It is both, a signpost that helps as a diagnostic tool in many different diseases and, at the same time, a symptom in its own right.
- In the acute phase, its function is to warn us of actual or impending tissue damage. Acute pain thus can be useful and adaptive.
- Persistent (ie, chronic) pain is generally pathological or maladaptive, and represents an ongoing pathology, a dysfunctional healing process, or an inappropriate response. This persistence of pain includes physical, behavioral, and cognitive dimensions that tend to dominate the experience of pain.
- Chronic, noncancer pain and its epidemiology form the main subject of this chapter.

CHRONIC PAIN: CONCEPT AND DEFINITION

- Chronic pain is more than just a comorbidity of other identifiable diseases or injury. Chronic pain is acknowledged as a condition with its own agreed set of definitions and taxonomy.
- The International Association for the Study of Pain (IASP) has characterized chronic pain as *"pain which has persisted beyond normal tissue healing time,"* which, *"in the absence of other criteria,"* is taken to be 3 months. However, some signs of chronic pain are evidenced well before 3 months.
- The IASP definition of chronic pain includes pain of any severity and is not specific to a particular diagnosis or body site.
- The difference between acute and chronic pain is more than just duration. A more specific definition of chronic pain should also include a measure of the significance or impact of pain on daily activities.

EPIDEMIOLOGY: DEFINITION

- Epidemiology is the "study of the distribution and determinants of health-related states or events in specified populations and the applications of this study to control health problems."
- This is the study of groups or communities (rather than individuals) with chronic pain that gives insight into its occurrence, incidence, and prevalence, and aims to identify risk factors, that is, factors that lead to or favor chronicity.

WHY IS EPIDEMIOLOGY OF CHRONIC PAIN IMPORTANT?

The important aims of chronic pain epidemiology are listed in Table 3-1.

TABLE 3-1 The Benefits of Epidemiological Study of Chronic Pain

Good epidemiological data on chronic pain will provide information on:
- Its distribution in the community, those in greatest need of treatment or the greatest likelihood of improvement
- Factors associated with chronic pain that lead to chronicity
- Preventive measures
- Improving prognosis to limit pain severity and minimize disability
- Impact of quality of life
- Evaluation of treatment strategies
- Allocation of health care service and educational resources

Source: Adapted, with permission, from Smith BH, Torrance N. Epidemiology of chronic pain. In: McQuay HJ, Kalso E, Moore RA, eds. *Systematic Reviews in Pain Research: Methodology Refined.* Seattle, Wash: IASP Press; 2008. pp. 247-273.

ESTIMATES OF PREVALENCE OF CHRONIC PAIN

- The range of population prevalence estimates of chronic pain (ie, the proportion of the population affected) is wide (7%–64%), in part, because of differences in the precise definition of chronic pain used, methods of data collection (eg, lower prevalence rates for phone surveys than those that used postal questionnaires), and differences in sampled population groups.
- The largest study ($n = 46,000$) found a chronic pain prevalence of 20% in Europe. Overall, the collated evidence suggests a mean prevalence of chronic pain of 20%–25%. Prevalence estimates of severe disabling chronic pain lie between 5% and 15%.
- It is beyond the scope of this chapter to report the prevalence of every individual chronic pain condition or syndrome. Some are listed in Table 3-2.

INCIDENCE OF CHRONIC PAIN

- The incidence of chronic pain (ie, the proportion of the population developing new chronic pain) is difficult to measure. From the available but limited evidence, the incidence of chronic pain (overall) is probably between 5% and 10% per year.

FACTORS ASSOCIATED WITH CHRONIC PAIN

- Although chronic pain in an individual may have a single primary cause (eg, trauma or herpes zoster), there are other factors that influence the duration, intensity,

TABLE 3-2   Estimated Prevalence of Common Chronic Pain Conditions in the General Population

Chronic lower back pain	23%
Symptomatic osteoarthritis knee[a]	UK: 12%–16% US: 10%–35%
Pain with neuropathic characteristics	7%–8%
Postherpetic neuralgia	2.6%–7.2% of those with herpes zoster
Postsurgical pain	10%–30% of those having surgery
Chronic headache	3%–4%
Complex regional pain syndrome	0.2%
Chronic chest pain	6%
Central poststroke pain	1%–12% of those having a stroke
Fibromyalgia	0.7%–3.3%
Chronic functional abdominal pain syndrome	2%

[a]Increasing prevalence in older age groups.

TABLE 3-3   Factors Associated with Chronic Pain

A. Modifiable	Pain
	Mental health (particularly anxiety and depression)
	Other comorbidities
	Smoking
	Obesity
	Sleep
	Employment status and occupational factors
B. Nonmodifiable	Age
	Sex
	Cultural background
	Socioeconomic background
	History of trauma or injury (including surgery)
	History of interpersonal violence or abuse
	Heritable factors (including genetic)

Source: Data from Van Hecke O, Torrance N, Smith BH. Chronic pain epidemiology and its clinical relevance. *Br J Anaesth.* 2013 July;111:13-18.

and spectrum (physical, psychological, social, and emotional) of these effects.
- An understanding of the risk factors associated with the presence and development of chronic pain is important to guide clinical management, reducing pain severity and minimizing disability.
- At a population level, factors known to be associated with chronic pain include physical, psychological, and social variables and are summarized in Table 3-3.
- Some risk factors are amenable to medical intervention, others not (eg, age and sex).

MODIFIABLE FACTORS ASSOCIATED WITH CHRONIC PAIN

Pain

- The most important clinical risk factor for chronic pain is pain itself—either acute pain or chronic pain at another site.
- The more severe the acute pain, and the greater the number of pain sites, the more likely it is that severe chronic pain will develop.
- Anatomical changes within the brain are likely to occur in the early stages of pain (before pain could be labeled as chronic). This suggests that early intervention will be important in preventing chronicity.

Mental Health

- Anxiety, depression, and catastrophizing beliefs about pain are associated with a poorer prognosis in people with various chronic pain conditions.
- It is likely that this relationship is *bi-directional*—pain causing depression and vice versa. This reinforces how

factors, such as depression and anxiety associated with chronic pain, become part of the overall condition itself and augment the pain experience.

- Pain outcomes are more favorable when depressive symptoms are addressed together with appropriate pain management.

Multimorbidity in Chronic Pain

- The prevalence of chronic pain is higher in those with other chronic diseases than those without. For example, up to a third of people with coronary heart disease also have chronic pain, and a similar percentage of people with chronic obstructive pulmonary disease have chronic pain.
- Individuals with severe chronic pain were up to three times more likely to die from ischemic heart disease compared to those with no chronic pain.
- The comorbidity, co-prescribing, and co-occurrence of disability lead to greater challenges in managing each condition and reducing impact. Chronic pain cannot be managed in isolation.

Smoking

- Heavy smokers tend to report more pain locations and also increased pain intensity compared to those who have never smoked. However, the evidence for a direct causal relationship between smoking and pain is lacking.
- It remains unanswered whether smoking cessation improves pain. Nonetheless, smoking remains a major risk factor for cardiovascular disease, which is a common comorbidity and cause of mortality among people with chronic pain.

Obesity

- The relationship between chronic pain and obesity is more complex than simply one of mechanical overload. Community-based twin studies have demonstrated that familial (ie, genetic and environmental) factors were significant contributors to the association.
- The impact of pain on functional status and health-related quality of life is greater in obese individuals than in those with a normal body mass index, although the direct effect of weight on these measurements remains unclear.
- Reducing or preventing chronic pain by weight loss has yet to be demonstrated beyond that of osteoarthritis and other mechanical etiology.
- Secondary prevention may be more important in reducing cardiovascular risk and overall impact than simply reducing pain severity per se.

Sleep Problems

- A Norwegian prospective study involving only women over a 17-year period found that disrupted sleep was a risk factor for the onset of chronic pain and predictive for pain persistence (but not worsening of pain).
- Addressing sleep problems in chronic pain patients may lessen the risk of developing depressive illness, which is associated with a poorer pain prognosis.

Employment Status and Occupational Factors

- Evidence shows that individuals who were not able to work due to illness or disability were more likely to report chronic pain than those who were employed.
- The influence of poor job control, expectations for return to work, and fear of re-injury all contribute to occupational risk factors for the onset or persistence of pain.

NONMODIFIABLE FACTORS ASSOCIATED WITH CHRONIC PAIN

Older Age

- The occurrence of *disabling* chronic pain continues to rise with age. Although the onset of pain per se does not have a clear relationship with age, there is generally a higher prevalence of chronic pain in older age.

Female Sex

- Chronic pain syndromes generally have a higher prevalence in women with more women than men seeking treatment for it.
- Consistent themes emerge: women are found to have lower pain thresholds, experience greater unpleasantness (or intensity) with pain, and have different analgesic sensitivity.

Ethnicity and Cultural Background

- The prevalence of chronic pain is similar between developed and developing countries according to the WHO World Mental Health Surveys.
- There is also some evidence that ethnocultural differences in (experimental) pain perception correlate with clinical pain indices in a range of pain conditions, often with undertreatment in ethnic minority groups.

Socioeconomic Background

- Chronic pain prevalence is inversely related to socioeconomic status.

- People living in poorer socioeconomic circumstances not only experience more pain, but also experience more *severe* pain.
- The onset of pain interfering with daily activities has been shown to be associated with neighborhood deprivation, low levels of education, and (perceived) income inequalities.

Trauma, Injury, and Surgery

- Chronic postsurgical pain is a potential but substantial risk of certain surgical procedures.
- Between 10% and 30% of patients undergoing common surgical procedures report persistent or intermittent pain of varying severity at 1-year postoperatively with higher rates (>40%) after major thoracic surgery and breast cancer surgery.
- There is little evidence to support the theory that the more severe the surgical insult or tissue damage, the greater the risk of persistent pain.
- There is evidence that severe acute postoperative pain and surgery lasting more than 3 hours predicts increased pain and poor functional outcome at 6 months post surgery.

History of Abuse or Interpersonal Violence

- Pain is more common among people of any age who report a previous history of abuse or violence, in either a domestic or a public setting.

Genetic Risk Factors and Heritability

- Birth cohort studies have shown that chronic pain conditions "run in families," and children of parents with chronic pain conditions are more likely to develop pain conditions themselves.
- The reporting of pain itself is likely a heritable phenotype, that is, partly determined by genes, the shared environment and their interaction.
- No unique "pain" gene is likely to be discovered, but rather a complex combination of genetic factors interacts with psychosocial and lifestyle factors to produce chronic pain.
- Animal studies have discovered hundreds of genes relevant to pain pathway, but only a smaller number have been demonstrated in humans.
- The most studied gene in relation to pain is catechol-*O*-methyltransferase (*COMT*), an enzyme that degrades neurotransmitters including dopamine. However, the nature and the extent of association remain to be clarified.
- Other genes, such as *CYP4502D6*, are important in determining response to analgesics.
- Genetic studies are likely to underestimate the contribution of the "shared environment" in chronic

TABLE 3-4   Impact of Chronic Pain on Populations

Poor general and mental health
Increased mortality
Activity limitations (leisure, social, work, and sexual)
Impaired health-related quality of life
Increased healthcare use (consultations, investigations, drug adverse events, addiction, etc.)
Financial difficulties
Economic (productivity loss and disability benefit)
Social (poverty, deprivation, and isolation)

pain. Addressing these nongenetic aspects (eg, pain behavior) as part of a pain management program is thus important.

IMPACT OF CHRONIC PAIN

- The vast majority of people with chronic pain never attend a specialist pain clinic but are seen in primary care.
- Every measured dimension of health is adversely affected by chronic pain (Table 3-4).
- The financial cost to society is huge; estimates include €300 billion per annum in Europe, and up to $635 billion per annum in the United States in 2008.

FUTURE RESEARCH

- Sociodemographic, clinical, and genetic factors associated with chronic pain are important in identifying, designing, and targeting relevant interventions in chronic pain.
- Chronic pain management focusing exclusively on pharmacological interventions will fail to address the role of activity, psychological, and social factors in maintaining daily function.
- Better recognition of chronic pain is required, followed by dedicated coding within routinely collected data sources and disease registries.
- Research that ignores population-level factors and intervenes exclusively in high-risk individuals (eg, specialist pain clinics) restricts the options for reducing the overall community burden of chronic pain.
- The existence of both individual- and population-level risk factors for chronic pain suggests that multiple opportunities for intervention exist.

BIBLIOGRAPHY

Barnett K, Mercer SW, Norbury M, Watt G, Wyke S, Guthrie B. Epidemiology of multimorbidity and implications for health care, research, and medical education: a cross-sectional study. *Lancet.* 2012;380:37–43.

Breivik H, Collett B, Ventafridda V, Cohen R, Gallacher D. Survey of chronic pain in Europe: Prevalence, impact on daily life, and treatment. *Eur J Pain.* 2006;10:287–333.

Diatchenko L, Nackley A, Tchivileva I, Shabalina S, Maixner W. Genetic architecture of human pain perception. *TRENDS in Genetics.* 2007;23:605–613.

Elliott A, Smith B, Hannaford P, Smith W, Chambers W. The course of chronic pain in the community: results of a 4-year follow-up study. *Pain.* 2002;99:299–307.

Elliott A, Smith B, Penny K, Smith W, Chambers W. The epidemiology of chronic pain in the community. *Lancet.* 1999;354:1248–1252.

Ellsberg M, Jansen H, Heise L, et al. Intimate partner violence and women's physical and mental health in the WHO multi-country study on women's health and domestic violence: an observational study. *Lancet.* 2008;371:1165–1172.

Greenspan J, Craft R, LeResche L. Studying sex and gender differences in pain and analgesia. A consensus report. *Pain.* 2007;132:S26–S45.

Hocking LJ, Generation S, Morris AD, Dominiczak AF, Porteous DJ, Smith BH. Heritability of chronic pain in 2195 extended families. *Eur J Pain.* 2012;16:1053–1063.

IASP. *Classification of Chronic Pain. Descriptions of Chronic Pain Syndromes and Definitions of Pain Terms.* Lyon, France: IASP Press; 1986.

Institute of Medicine of the National Academies. *Relieving Pain in America: A Blueprint for Transforming Prevention, Care, Education, and Research.* Washington, DC: Institute of Medicine of the National Academies; 2011.

John U, Hanke M, Meyer C, Volzke H, Baumeister SE, Alte D. Tobacco smoking in relation to pain in a national general population survey. *Prev Med.* 2006;43:477–481.

Jones G, Silman A, Power C, Macfarlane G. Do common symptoms in childhood increase the risk of chronic widespread pain in adults? Data from the 1958 British Birth Cohort Study. *Am J Epidemiol.* 2006;163:S14.

Kehlet H, Jensen TS, Woolf CJ. Persistent postsurgical pain: risk factors and prevention. *Lancet.* 2006;367:1618–1625.

Kroenke K, Bair M, Damush T, et al. Optimized antidepressant therapy and pain self-management in primary care patients with depression and musculoskeletal pain: a randomized controlled trial. *JAMA.* 2009;301:2099–2110.

Last R. *A Dictionary of Epidemiology.* 4th ed. Oxford, United Kingdom: International Epidemiological Association; 2001.

Nittera AK, Pripp AH, Forsetha KØ. Are sleep problems and non-specific health complaints risk factors for chronic pain? A prospective population-based study with 17 year follow-up. *Scand J Pain.* 2012;3:210–217.

Poleshuck E, Green C. Socioeconomic disadvantage and pain. *Pain.* 2008;136:235–238.

Shaw W, Linton S, Pransky G. Reducing sickness absence from work due to low back pain: how well do intervention strategies match modifiable risk factors?. *J Occup Rehabil.* 2006;16:591–605.

Smith BH, Torrance N. Epidemiology of chronic pain. In: McQuay HJ, Kalso E, Moore RA, eds. *Systematic Reviews in Pain Research: Methodology Refined.* Seattle, Wash: IASP Press; 2008:247–273.

Torrance N, Elliott A, Lee A, Smith B. Severe chronic pain is associated with increased 10 year mortality. A cohort record linkage study. *Eur J Pain.* 2010;14:380–386.

van Hecke O, Torrance N, Smith BH. Chronic pain epidemiology and its clinical relevance. *Br J Anaesth.* 2013 Jul;111:13–18.

van Hecke O, Torrance N, Smith BH. Chronic pain epidemiology—where do lifestyle factors fit in?. *Br J Pain.* In press.

4 SEX, GENDER, AND PAIN

Roger B. Fillingim, PhD

HISTORICAL AND CONCEPTUAL ISSUES

- Research regarding sex, gender, and pain has grown dramatically in the last three decades. While publications regarding "pain" increased by 500% from 1980 to 2008, publications regarding sex, gender, and pain increased by more than 3000% over the same time period.
- The terms sex and gender have different connotations. Sex refers to one's biological sex based on chromosomal complement and genital anatomy, while gender includes not only sex, but also sociocultural influences, such as stereotypic gender roles.
- McCarthy recently noted three types of sex differences:
  - Sexual dimorphism in which the endpoint exists in different forms in males and females.
  - Sex differences (ie, quantitative differences) in which the endpoint exists on a continuum and males and females, on average, differ in their responses.
  - Sex convergence and divergence (ie, qualitative sex differences) in which males and females show the same response on the endpoint, but the neural mechanisms underlying the responses differ across sex.

SEX DIFFERENCES IN CLINICAL PAIN

- Epidemiologic studies investigating the prevalence of chronic pain (eg, pain on most days lasting longer than 6 months) consistently demonstrate higher prevalence among women, though the magnitude of the sex difference varies across studies (Table 4-1).
- Numerous studies have also examined sex differences in the prevalence of specific pain conditions. In general, females show greater prevalence for most of the more common chronic pain conditions.
- Research addressing whether women and men differ in their reported clinical pain severity provides inconsistent results.

TABLE 4-1 Summary of Findings Regarding Sex Differences in Clinical and Experimental Pain Conditions

PAIN TYPE	PATTERN OF FINDINGS	COMMENTS
Prevalence of Chronic Pain	Higher prevalence in females for most pain conditions	Effects are quite consistent across most common chronic pain conditions. Female:male ratio is greater in the clinical setting than in the general population.
Severity of Chronic Clinical Pain	Mixed findings, no clear pattern	Most findings derive from clinical samples, which are biased toward individuals with more severe pain.
Severity of Acute Clinical Pain	Mixed results, trend toward slightly but significantly greater pain among women	Most findings are based on postoperative and procedural pain, which can be confounded by responses to analgesics.
Experimental Pain	Greater pain sensitivity in females across all stimulus modalities.	Direction of findings is strikingly significant across all pain measures and stimulus modalities. Magnitude of the difference varies across studies and pain measures.

○ *Acute pain.* Studies of acute postoperative and procedural pain show mixed results. Some investigators report greater pain among women, others report greater pain among men, and some others report no sex differences. Of course, pain intensity in such studies is influenced by analgesic interventions, which may also vary by sex (see below), complicating interpretation of these findings.

■ A recent study explored electronic medical record data to examine sex differences in pain intensity in more than 11,000 patients with numerous diagnoses. The findings indicated consistently higher clinical pain ratings among women compared to men.

○ *Transition from acute to chronic pain.* Several prospective studies have indicated increased risk for transition to chronic pain among women compared to men, for conditions such as temporomandibular disorders, whiplash, postherpetic neuralgia, and chronic postoperative pain.

○ *Chronic pain.* Research in clinical samples of patients experiencing chronic pain also reveals inconsistent findings regarding sex differences in pain severity. Several studies report no sex differences in pain severity, while other find that women report greater clinical pain compared to men.

■ It is important to recognize that selection biases influence the severity of chronic pain in the clinical setting, because patients with less severe pain are less likely to seek treatment. Indeed, for most pain conditions that show female predominance, the female:male ratio is substantially greater in clinical samples than in the general population, suggesting that a greater proportion of women than men with the condition seek health care.

SEX DIFFERENCES IN LABORATORY PAIN SENSITIVITY

• Sex differences in clinical pain could be, in part, driven by sex differences in processing of nociceptive information. Thus, laboratory pain assessment has been used to characterize sex differences in responses to carefully controlled painful stimuli. A wide variety of stimulus modalities and pain measures has been investigated (Table 4-2).

TABLE 4-2 Common Experimental Pain Modalities and Pain Measures that Have Been Used to Study Sex Differences

PAIN MODALITIES	CHARACTERISTICS
Electrical Pain	Brief, cutaneous, or muscle, typically stimulates all afferent classes
Heat Pain	Brief or tonic, cutaneous or immersion, can activate afferent classes selectively
Cold Pain	Brief or tonic, cutaneous or immersion, activates a-delta and C fibers
Mechanical Pain	Generally brief, cutaneous, muscle, or viscera, can be blunt or punctate, can activate a-delta or C fibers
Ischemic Pain	Tonic, muscle pain, predominantly C fiber-mediated, clinically relevant
Chemical Pain	Tonic, cutaneous, subcutaneous, or muscle, typically C fiber-mediated, examples include capsaicin, glutamate, and hypertonic saline
Pain Measures	**Description**
Pain Threshold	The lowest level of stimulation required to produce pain
Pain Tolerance	The greatest level of stimulation the participant is willing or able to withstand
Pain Ratings	Magnitude estimates of the intensity or unpleasantness of suprathreshold stimuli
Temporal Summation of Pain	Increases in perceived pain as a function of repetitive administration of a suprathreshold stimulus
CPM	A measure of pain inhibitory function typically operationalized as the reduction in the painfulness of one stimulus that occurs when administered concurrently in the presence of a second stimulus at a remote body site

- Across multiple stimulus modalities, women consistently exhibit lower pain threshold and pain tolerance than men. In addition, ratings of suprathreshold painful stimuli are consistently higher for women than men (see Table 4-1). While the pattern of these sex differences is quite consistent, it is important to note that the magnitude of the sex difference varies across studies.
- Temporal summation refers to an increase in pain with repeated stimulation at the same stimulus intensity, which represents the perceptual manifestation of windup, a form of transient central sensitization. Multiple studies have demonstrated increased temporal summation of pain in women than men in response to both thermal and mechanical stimuli.
- In addition to assessing basal pain responses, laboratory methods can characterize pain inhibitory function. The most commonly used method for this purpose is conditioned pain modulation (CPM; also known as diffuse noxious inhibitory controls (DNIC)). With CPM, the experimenter determines the extent to which one painful stimulus (the conditioning stimulus) influences the intensity of another painful stimulus applied to a remote body site (the test stimulus). Greater inhibitory function is inferred from the extent to which the conditioning stimulus reduces the painfulness of the test stimulus. A recent meta-analysis of studies examining sex differences in CPM reported consistently higher CPM among men than women.
- Overall, laboratory pain research clearly demonstrates greater pain sensitivity, increased pain facilitation, and reduced pain inhibition among women compared to men. While increasing evidence supports the clinical relevance of laboratory pain assessment, the degree to which sex differences in experimental pain sensitivity contribute to sex differences in clinical pain remains unknown.

SEX DIFFERENCES IN TREATMENT RESPONSES

- Sex differences in responses to opioid analgesics have been investigated primarily in acute clinical and experimental pain models. A recent meta-analysis of these findings produced the following conclusions (Table 4-3).
  - For clinical studies (primarily postoperative pain), no sex differences in μ-opioid analgesia emerged overall. However, when restricting analyses to patient-controlled analgesia (PCA), women consumed lower amounts of μ-opioid medication, with the largest effect emerging for PCA morphine studies

TABLE 4-3 Summary of Findings Regarding Sex Differences in Analgesic Responses to Opioids

MEDICATION CLASS	CLINICAL STUDIES	EXPERIMENTAL STUDIES
All μ-Opioid Agonists	No sex difference	Women show great analgesia than men (small to medium effect)
μ-Opioid Agonists PCA Only	Opioid consumption lower in women than men (small effect)	N/A
Morphine Studies	No sex difference	Women show great analgesia than men (small to medium effect)
Morphine PCA Only	Opioid consumption lower in women than men (medium effect)	N/A
Mixed-Action Agonist-Antagonists	Women show great analgesia than men (large effect)	No sex difference

Source: Reproduced, with permission, from Niesters M, Dahan A, Kest B, et al. Do sex differences exist in opioid analgesia? A systematic review and meta-analysis of human experimental and clinical studies. *Pain.* 2010;151:61-68.

(a moderate effect size). It is important to note that these studies actually assessed opioid consumption rather than pain relief, which may be influenced by factors other than analgesia (eg, side effects).
  - Studies investigating μ-opioid analgesics tested against experimentally induced pain demonstrated greater morphine analgesia for women. This effect size was also moderate in magnitude.
  - For mixed-action opioid agonist-antagonist medications (eg, butorphanol, nalbuphine, and pentazocine), women exhibit significantly greater analgesia than men in clinical studies, with a large effect size.
  - In contrast, no sex-dependent effects were found for analgesic responses to mixed action opioids in studies of experimentally induced pain.
  - Both clinical and experimental studies also report that women experience significantly more adverse side effects of μ-opioids and mixed-action opioids compared to men.
- Research examining sex differences in analgesic responses to nonopioid medications has been more limited.
  - Studies of sex differences in responses to NSDAIDs have produced mixed results, with no clear evidence of a sex difference emerging.
  - One study of pressure pain thresholds showed that lidocaine produced greater cutaneous anesthesia in men than women.
  - Several studies suggest that males show a more robust placebo response than females, particularly

when using an intentional placebo manipulation that induces analgesic expectancies.

- Whether men and women respond differently to non-pharmacologic pain treatments has been investigated in a few studies, but no clear pattern of sex differences has emerged.
- In addition to whether treatments are differentially effective in women versus men, several studies have investigated whether the predictors of treatment outcome vary as a function of sex.
  - In chronic pain patients undergoing multiple pain treatments, higher pretreatment anxiety was associated with greater treatment-associated pain reductions for men but not women.
  - Another study found that higher pretreatment pain tolerance more strongly predicted reductions in pain severity and pain-related interference following interdisciplinary pain treatment among women than men.
  - Regarding predictors of response to physical therapy treatments, baseline levels and duration of pain symptoms predicted outcomes in women, whereas type of treatment and fear-avoidance beliefs predicted treatment response among men.
  - Thus, additional research to identify sex-specific predictors of outcomes from various pain treatments is warranted.
- Gender bias in pain treatment has been investigated in a large number of studies, and clinical wisdom often suggests that women are at greater risk for undertreatment of pain. However, a recent review of this literature concluded that while women and men are often treated differently, this disparity sometimes favors women and sometimes favors men.

MECHANISMS UNDERLYING SEX DIFFERENCES

- Factors contributing to sex differences are often separated into "biological" versus "psychosocial" mechanisms; however, this distinction is artificial as psychosocial processes exert their influences via biological mechanisms and biological factors produce psychosocial effects. The following "biological" factors contribute to sex difference in pain.

"BIOLOGICAL" FACTORS

- *Hormonal influences.* Gonadal hormonal influences on pain include both organizational and activational effects, which refer to long-term developmental influences versus transient effects in adulthood, respectively. Also, hormonal influences on pain are

complex and can depend on: (1) the dose and timing of hormonal exposure; (2) the type of pain; (3) the entire hormonal complement (ie, the presence of multiple hormonal factors); and (4) the site of action of the hormones (eg, peripheral vs. spinal vs. supraspinal).

- Clinical and experimental pain responses have been shown to vary across the menstrual cycle, with greater clinical pain and pain sensitivity observed during the premenstrual and menstrual phases. Although, on average, these effects are modest in magnitude.
- Exogenous hormone use, especially estrogen replacement among postmenopausal women, has been associated with increased risk for clinical pain and increased experimental pain sensitivity.
- *Genetic influences.* Several findings suggest sex-dependent genetic influences on pain. These are examples of qualitative sex differences, and they suggest that certain aspects of the pain or analgesic circuitry are fundamentally different for women and men.
  - The A118G single-nucleotide polymorphism (SNP) of the μ-opioid receptor gene (OPRM1) was found to be associated with pressure pain sensitivity in men but not women. Also, the rare allele was associated with increased heat pain sensitivity among women but decreased heat pain sensitivity in men. Parallel findings were recently observed in a clinical population; women with the rare allele showed poorer recovery from lumbar disc herniation, whereas the rare allele predicted enhanced recovery among men.
  - The melanocortin-1 receptor (MC1R) gene (ie, the "redhead" gene) was associated with "kappa" opioid analgesia in a sex-dependent manner. Specifically, women with two variant alleles of the gene showed greater analgesic responses to pentazocine than compared to women without two variant alleles; however, MC1R genotype was not associated with pain among men.
- *Endogenous opioids.* Sex differences in endogenous opioid function have been reported. At rest, women showed higher μ-opioid receptor binding than men in several brain regions, while men exhibited greater brain μ-opioid receptor binding in response to experimentally induced muscle pain. Also, sex hormones influenced brain μ-opioid receptor binding in women.

PSYCHOSOCIAL FACTORS

- Multiple "psychosocial" factors contribute to sex differences in pain.
  - Gender roles, which are sculpted by both biology and social learning, have been associated with pain responses. In general, higher levels of masculinity and femininity are associated with lower and higher

pain sensitivity, respectively. Also, both males and females consider women more sensitive to pain, less able to endure pain, and more willing to report pain compared to men. Also, some evidence suggests that pain responses are influenced by experimenter gender, with individuals typically reporting less pain to an opposite sex versus a same sex experimenter. While gender role measures are correlated with experimental pain sensitivity, they rarely completely explain observed sex differences in pain responses.

- Sex differences in pain coping have been documented, with women reporting more frequent coping attempts and employing a wider array of coping strategies compared to men. Of particular importance, women report higher levels of pain catastrophizing, a maladaptive cognitive response to pain, characterized by hopelessness, rumination, and magnification, which is associated with poorer pain outcomes. Pain catastrophizing has mediated sex differences in clinical and experimental pain in some studies.

- In general, women report higher levels of affective distress than men, including anxiety and depression, and both anxiety and depression are associated with increased risk of pain. Interestingly, several studies suggest that anxiety may be more strongly associated with pain among men than women. In contrast, among individuals with depression, women are more likely to reported pain than men.

CLINICAL IMPLICATIONS

- The direct clinical implications of sex differences in pain are somewhat limited, and the currently available evidence does not support sex-specific pain evaluation or treatment. However, several general recommendations can be made.
  - First, given the abundant evidence of sex differences in both the prevalence and the neurobiology of pain, any vestigial biases against women who present with pain in the clinical setting should be immediately expunged.
  - Given the increased risk for pain among women, pain prevention programs for many clinical conditions should consider tailoring toward women.
  - There is evidence of sex differences in responses to opioids, both in terms of analgesia and side effects. While sex-specific medication selection or doing is not recommended, providers should recognize the potential for these differences and be prepared to adjust treatment accordingly. As always, treatment should be individualized based on the patient's characteristics, including but not limited to their sex.

CONCLUSIONS

- Sex differences in clinical pain are well documented, with women at increased risk for many chronic pain conditions compared to men.
- Sex differences in responses to opioids have also been reported, such that women appear to show greater analgesia in response to morphine and mixed action opioids, but women report greater side effects as well.
- Multiple biopsychosocial mechanisms contribute to sex differences in pain and analgesia.

BIBLIOGRAPHY

Bernardes SF, Keogh E, Lima ML. Bridging the gap between pain and gender research: a selective literature review. *Eur J Pain.* 2008;12:427–440.

Cepeda MS, Farrar JT, Baumgarten M, et al. Side effects of opioids during short-term administration: effect of age, gender, and race. *Clin Pharmacol Ther.* 2003;74:102–112.

Edwards RR, Augustson E, Fillingim RB. Differential relationships retween anxiety and treatment-associated pain reduction among male and female chronic pain patients. *Clin J Pain.* 2003a;19:208–216.

Edwards RR, Doleys DM, Lowery D, Fillingim RB. Pain tolerance as a predictor of outcome following multidisciplinary treatment for chronic pain: differential effects as a function of sex. *Pain.* 2003b;106:419–426.

Edwards RR., Sarlani E, Wesselmann U, Fillingim RB. Quantitative assessment of experimental pain perception: multiple domains of clinical relevance. *Pain.* 2005;114:315–319.

Fillingim RB, Kaplan L, Staud R, et al. The A118G single nucleotide polymorphism of the mu-opioid receptor gene (OPRM1) is associated with pressure pain sensitivity in humans. *J Pain.* 2005;6:159–167.

Fillingim RB, King CD, Ribeiro-Dasilva MC, et al. Sex, gender, and pain: a review of recent clinical and experimental findings. *J Pain.* 2009;10:447–485.

Garofalo JP, Gatchel RJ, Wesley AL, Ellis E. Predicting chronicity in acute temporomandibular joint disorders using the research diagnostic criteria. *J Am Dent Assoc.* 1998;129:438–447.

George SZ, Fritz JM, Childs JD, Brennan GP. Sex differences in predictors of outcome in selected physical therapy interventions for acute low back pain. *J Orthop Sports Phys Ther.* 2006;36:354–363.

Gialloreti LE, Merito M, Pezzotti P, et al. Epidemiology and economic burden of herpes zoster and post-herpetic neuralgia in Italy: a retrospective, population-based study. *BMC Infect Dis.* 2010;10:230.

Kehlet H, Jensen TS, Woolf CJ. Persistent postsurgical pain: risk factors and prevention. *Lancet.* 2006;367:1618–1625.

LeResche L. Defining gender disparities in pain management. *Clin Orthop Relat Res.* 2011;469:1871–1877.

McCarthy MM, Arnold AP, Ball GF, et al. Sex differences in the brain: the not so inconvenient truth. *J Neurosci.* 2012;32:2241–2247.

Mogil JS. Sex differences in pain and pain inhibition: multiple explanations of a controversial phenomenon. *Nat Rev Neurosci.* 2012;13:859–866.

Mogil JS, Wilson SG, Chesler EJ, et al. The melanocortin-1 receptor gene mediates female-specific mechanisms of analgesia in mice and humans. *Proc Natl Acad Sci U S A.* 2003;100:4867–4762.

Niesters M, Dahan A, Kest B, et al. Do sex differences exist in opioid analgesia? A systematic review and meta-analysis of human experimental and clinical studies. *Pain.* 2010;151:61–68.

Olsen MB, Jacobsen LM, Schistad EI, et al. Pain intensity the first year after lumbar disc herniation is associated with the A118G polymorphism in the opioid receptor Mu 1 gene: evidence of a sex and genotype interaction. *J Neurosci.* 2012;32:9831–9834.

Popescu A, LeResche L, Truelove EL, Drangsholt MT. Gender differences in pain modulation by diffuse noxious inhibitory controls: a systematic review. *Pain.* 2010;150:309–318.

Riley JL III, Hastie BA, Glover TL, et al. Cognitive-affective and somatic side effects of morphine and pentazocine: side-effect profiles in healthy adults. *Pain Med.* 2010;11:195–206.

Ruau D, Liu LY, Clark JD, et al. Sex differences in reported pain across 11,000 patients captured in electronic medical records. *J Pain.* 2012;13:228–234.

Smith YR, Stohler CS, Nichols TE, et al. Pronociceptive and antinociceptive effects of estradiol through endogenous opioid neurotransmission in women. *J Neurosci.* 2006;26:5777–5785.

Walton DM, Macdermid JC, Giorgianni AA, et al. Risk factors for persistent problems following acute whiplash injury: update of a systematic review and meta-analysis. *J Orthop Sports Phys Ther.* 2013;43:31–43.

Wizemann TM, Pardue MLe. *Exploring the Biological Contributions to Human Health: Does Sex Matter?* Washington, DC: National Academy Press; 2001.

Zubieta JK, Smith YR, Bueller JA, et al. mu-opioid receptor-mediated antinociceptive responses differ in men and women. *J Neurosci.* 2002;22:5100–5107.

5 PLACEBO RESPONSE

Gregory R. Polston, MD

HISTORIC ASPECTS OF PLACEBO

- Placebo in Latin translates to "I shall please." Psalm 114:9 *"placebo Domino in regione vivorum"* or "I will please the Lord in the land of the living" was sung at funerals in the eighth century, at a time when the term placebo came to mean a person who attended funerals for a fee or to enjoy the free food and drinks. Chaucer, in Canterbury Tales, modified this slightly by naming his sycophant character Placebo.
- In Motherby's *A New Medical Dictionary*, published in 1785, placebo was first used medically as "a commonplace method or medicine."

- Quincy's *Lexicon-Medicum A New Medical Dictionary* from 1811, defined it more specifically as "an epithet given to any medicine adapted more to please than to benefit the patient."
- On March 12, 1782, King Louis XIV of France appointed a scientific commission to investigate the validity of Franz Anton Mesmer's "animal magnetism."
  - Participants included Benjamin Franklin, Antoine-Laurent Lavoisier, and Joseph-Ignace Guillotin.
  - This commission is credited with using placebos for the first time in scientific experiments.
  - In one of its studies, a woman fainted after drinking a glass of normal water that she was led to believe was "magnetized."
  - These experiments are credited with being among the first to identify the power of suggestion, led to the use of hypnosis, and played a role in the development of modern psychology.
- Another early study conducted in 1801 by John Haygarth examined "Perkins tractors," a device thought to "draw out disease." He showed that patients responded just as well to rods made out of wood rather than the real device. He concluded "… what powerful influence upon diseases is produced by mere imagination."
- In America, the first conference on placebos was held at Cornell University in 1946. It outlined the importance of placebo controls in clinical trials, debated the use of placebo in patients, and pointed to the need for further research.
- The first true placebo-controlled, blinded trial was conducted in 1948 when streptomycin was studied in tuberculosis patients.
- In 1954, the Conference on Therapy formally defined the role of placebos in modern clinical trials.
- Finally, in the aftermath of Nazi atrocities, the World Medical Association in the Declaration of Helsinki adopted a set of ethical principles for medical research involving human subjects. It acknowledged the need for placebos and nontreatment groups when there is a compelling scientific reason to use them. The Declaration further states that extreme caution must be exercised and the safety of subjects receiving placebos should not be jeopardized.

PLACEBO AND PAIN

PLACEBO: DEFINITION AND INCIDENCE

- Placebos have often been discounted as something given to a patient with no inherent benefit and without the backing of sound science.
- Before health and disease were well understood, a physician's role was more to watch and palliate than

to diagnose and treat. Placebos were frequently used in lieu of a better alternative.

- As the science of medicine grew more sophisticated, the use of placebos fell out of favor and their role was limited to research.
- Placebos are still defined as an inert substance or procedure that, while not thought to have a physiologic effect, still causes a change in a patient's condition through the context in which it is given. With continuing research, this phenomenon has become much better understood and many are considering an expanded role for placebos in medicine. In fact, in the future, it may be possible to manipulate placebos to better evaluate new drugs and therapies and also employ placebos to personalize therapies.

SPONTANEOUS IMPROVEMENT

- Before placebos can be understood, it is important to remember how illness or disease can improve.
- Improvement can occur because a specific intervention alters the course of the disease. Without this treatment the condition would not improve or change.
- Improvement can also occur because the natural history of the illness is self-limited and requires no treatment. An improvement that occurs not as a result of the actual treatment, but rather from
  - unrecognized disease-modifying therapy that is not understood to be the treatment.
  - Spontaneous changes in illness or complaints can also occur. These can be perceived as response to therapy but actually have no relationship to the treatment being offered.
  - Regression to the mean. Care is often sought when symptoms are the greatest, especially in pain or chronic conditions and, over time, reported symptoms can improve. It is well recognized in research that reports of pain or other symptoms at the start of a study are higher than in subsequent encounters, regardless of treatment.
- Placebo responses are the changes in individuals and the placebo effect is the average difference between a placebo group and the nontreatment group.
- Henry K. Beecher in "The Powerful Placebo" was first to state that the mean effect was 35% (15%–52%) in 15 uncontrolled observational studies. This paper is still one of the most cited in placebo literature but many have questioned it for "both conceptual and methodological mistakes."
- Currently, the placebo effect is believed to be between 5% and 65%. Some studies, however, have demonstrated that with attempted manipulation, 100% of subjects may be responsive to the placebo effect.

- The magnitude of response averages 2 out of 10 on a visual analog scale but in placebo responders, it has been shown to be as high as 5 out of 10.
- Attempts have been made to identify research subjects and clinical patients who respond to placebos.
  - Eliminating placebo responders in clinical trials would significantly improve validity and eliminate the need for placebo. In clinical settings, being able to knowingly add this response to a treatment would have obvious benefit. Unfortunately, no clear markers or traits have been identified.
  - Initially, traits such as anxiety, histrionic, suggestibility, dependence, and lack of intelligence indicated greater susceptibility to placebo. This did not stand up to research.
  - Although altruistic, resilient, and straightforward individuals are now thought to respond more robustly to analgesic placebos, the likelihood of whether or not an individual will respond remains unpredictable.
  - Increased levels of empathy have also been proposed as increasing the magnitude.
  - Age and compliance with treatment plans have shown slightly increased rates in some studies.
  - The health locus of control or the extent to which a person believes they can control their own well-being may also shape susceptibility.
  - Finally, a prior placebo response does not change the probability of a future response to a placebo, even within the same study.

PLACEBO RESPONSE: MECHANISMS AND INTERPRETATION

- Current theories on the mechanism of placebos include expectation, reward, conditioning and learning, and alteration in the emotional state of the individual.
- When trying to understand how an "inert" substance or intervention has a biological action, one needs to consider cognitive and psychological factors that occur within a clinical context.
  - Many factors, including patients' expectations, behavior conditioning, and associative learning from prior treatments, are thought to trigger a placebo response.
  - A response can also result from the observation of other patients, known as social learning.
  - The relationship and interactions between the provider and patient are also important.
  - Verbal suggestions, anxiety reduction, motivation, and potential reward all affect outcomes.
  - These effects are both conscious and unconscious processes.

○ In addition, placebo effects can be reinforced and habituated with learning.

○ Placebo mechanisms cannot be explained by one pathway.

- Placebo analgesia, which is the most studied and best understood of the placebo responses, is thought to occur through psychological mechanisms of conditioning (including verbal conditioning) and expectancy.

  ○ Learning through direct experience is the most important placebo trigger in the conditioning mechanism while expectancy theory's effectiveness derives from patient expectation and verbal input from the provider.

  ○ Although they are thought to be separate mechanisms, there is a considerable overlap between the two theories (expectations can occur because of conditioning, for example).

  ○ Expectancy is considered more powerful and studies have shown that combining conditioning with expectancy increases response.

- Social observations and/or social learning can also lead to robust placebo analgesia.

  ○ Research has shown that observing what is believed to be a beneficial treatment can lead to pain reduction after receiving the same placebo treatment. In this setting, the subsequent behavior of the observer is learned through the experience of another.

  ○ Social learning is ingrained in culture beliefs and behaviors. This may explain differences in response to therapies and healing across cultural and racial groups. For example, Chinese-Americans have worse prognoses than whites if their disease and birth year horoscopes are considered ominous combinations.

BIOLOGICAL UNDERPINNINGS

- Naloxone, when given covertly, reverses or prevents placebo analgesia in several studies. This implies involvement of endogenous opioids. Conditioning, cognition, and motivation have all been shown to affect concentrations of endogenous opioids, activate descending pathways, and influence nociception at the dorsal horn. These all are similar to opioid-induced analgesia.

- Central nervous system activation may be more important than peripheral changes. Brain imaging studies (both PET and fMRI) show an overlap with opioid and placebo analgesia.

  ○ The dorsolateral prefrontal cortex, the anterior cingulate cortex (ACC), and the orbitofrontal cortex (OFC), along with the amygdale and periaqueductal gray regions play a key role when exposed to a placebo. Activation in these areas is consistent with the gate theory of pain.

- However, naloxone does not reverse all placebo analgesia.

  ○ Opioid-independent placebo analgesia is believed to include dopamine, activation of cannabinoid receptors, and genetic variation of catechol-O-methyltransferase.

  ○ In psychiatric disorders, genetic variants of release of catacholamines and changes in the metabolic activity of the ACC, the OFC, and the amygdala have been proposed to explain placebo responses.

  ○ Changes in respiratory function caused by placebos may occur via an alteration in the balance between bronchodilation and bronchoconstriction and the sensitivity of opioid receptors within respiratory centers.

  ○ Changes in β-adrenergic receptors and higher autonomic centers are explanations for placebo-induced effects on blood pressure and heart rate.

  ○ The immune, gastrointestinal, and endocrine systems also respond to placebos. The responses include suppression of cytokine release, changes in gastric motility, and release of growth hormones and cortisol.

ROLE OF PLACEBO IN CLINICAL TRIALS

- Placebo groups in clinical trials are used as comparison controls.

- A major problem with the use of placebos is that negative study results cannot occur because of lack of efficacy in the studied intervention, but because of a large placebo response. This is thought to occur more commonly in clinical studies in which subjective measures are used. Attempts by researchers to address this include reducing the placebo response and/or maximizing drug placebo differences.

  ○ Enrichment trials or multidosing studies attempt to minimize the placebo response. Unfortunately, this strategy can actually increase placebo responses because, when subjects know they have a greater chance of receiving treatment, placebo responses increase.

  ○ Extending clinical trials to extinguish the effects of placebo responses has been unsuccessful.

  ○ Because a nonresponse to a placebo in one setting does not preclude a response in another, a two-phase study that eliminates placebo responders in the first stage does not eliminate the problem of a placebo response.

  ○ Using objective biomarkers rather than patient or clinician reports may better identify placebo responders but these types of markers are limited, especially in pain studies.

○ Increasing differences between drug and placebo groups would be beneficial. This difference can be maximized with randomized run-in and withdrawal periods.

○ Crossover studies do not assist with placebo concerns because of carry-over effects, possible conditioning if active treatment is received first, and the potential un-blinding when side effects are different in each group.

○ Active placebos, which have similar side effects but no physiologic benefit, are being recommended to better evaluate a drug's efficacy but at the cost of increased placebo response.

○ The Zelen design recruits subjects for an observational group who receive standard treatment. It then selects patients from this group who will receive the studied intervention. This creates a natural history group (unselected group) without requiring randomization to a nontreatment group.

○ A comparative effectiveness research trial avoids the use of a placebo altogether by comparing a new drug or treatment to the standard of care. Recruitment is easier and this design is gaining advocates for both procedural and ethical reasons. One limitation with this type of study is that placebo responses increase because subjects know that the chance of receiving active treatment is 100%.

TABLE 5-1 Placebo and Pain

- Placebos show time–effect curves, peak, and cumulative effects similar to active medications
- Placebo analgesics have been shown to work better for severe pain than mild pain
- Large capsules are viewed as stronger than smaller capsules
- Yellow pills tend to be perceived as stimulants or antidepressants
- White pills are perceived as analgesics
- Blue pills are perceived as sedatives
- Pills that have a "brand name" work better than generic pills
- Placebo response is larger when the intervention is a device rather than a pill
- Injections tend to produce larger effects than pills
- Surgery may be one of the most powerful placebos. Reviewing historically invalidated surgeries and sham surgeries such as cryosurgery for gastric ulcers, knee surgery that consist of only scars, and sham dissections of internal mammary artery for angina have shown robust and sustained efficacy
- One explanation for why a reported successful treatment from one highly regarded physician fails in a multicenter trial is that the placebo response is lost when the investigator does not deliver the therapy
- Placebo responders need less dose adjustment when clinical trials allow dose ranges
- Healthy patients are more likely to report nocebo effects
- Multiple studies with placebo and active treatment arms show that outcome correlates better with what therapy patients think they received than with what group they were randomized to
- Original clinical studies establishing efficacy for a medication show greater clinical effect than when the same study is repeated after the drug is available over the counter

---

ROLE OF PLACEBO AND RESPONSE BIAS

- The validity of placebo changes has been questioned by some experts.
- After reviewing 114 randomized studies with placebos and nontreatment groups, it was argued that a placebo response was not seen in studies with objective outcomes and only minimally in studies with subjective endpoints. It stated that the placebo response disappears when natural history, regression to the mean, and bias are taken into account.
- Bias is defined as a distortion of the truth through systemic factors rather than errors caused by chance. These factors include:
  ○ response bias (study subjects wanting to please researcher by giving correct or socially accepted answers),
  ○ selection bias (research patients with differences in same group),
  ○ cointervention bias (receiving other beneficial treatments during study),
  ○ attrition bias (patients who are not benefiting from the study dropout), and
  ○ publication bias (positive studies are published, negative studies are not).
- The Hawthorne effect or observer's paradox, a change in behavior or reported symptoms induced by the fact that subjects know they are being studied, can also falsely lead to a conclusion of a placebo effect. Subsequent meta-analysis publications from this group have shown more robust placebo responses.
- With the emergence of brain imaging studies and better controlled placebo studies, evidence of the placebo effect is no longer questioned.

ETHICS OF PLACEBO IN CLINICAL TRIALS AND CLINICAL PRACTICE

- Use of placebo treatments in both clinical research and practice has generated much ethical debate.
- Withholding known effective therapy in both clinical and research settings is in clear violation of the Nuremburg Code and the Declaration of Helsinki.
- Further arguments include that even with informed consent, patients will rarely be able to make fully informed decisions, should never be placed in this position, and should always be shielded from avoidable harm.
- Others have proposed dropping placebos from research studies completely. They assert that the essential medical question is not whether a new drug is better than nothing but how does it compare against the standard of care.
- Thus, this perspective would suggest that using placebos is not worth the potential risk.

- Finally, deception violates individual rights and patient autonomy. Even if the placebo is completely "inert," the deception creates greater problems as a patient may lose trust in the provider and in the medical profession.
- Despite this, current surveys have found very high rates of physicians knowingly prescribing placebos in clinical practice (20%–80%). In these practice surveys, the definition of what constitutes use of placebos includes "pure" placebos and "impure" placebos.
  ○ Pure placebos are inert substances that are not thought to have a physiologic action and attempt to mimic the appearance of the actual treatments (pills with the same shape and color).
  ○ Impure placebos are real therapies, medicines, or tests that have a physiologic mechanism of action or clinical value but not for the disease or symptom being treated. Examples of impure placebos include prescribing nutritional supplements without known deficiencies, writing for antibiotics when infections are not likely bacterial, and ordering diagnostic exams or tests with low yield or simply to placate the patient.
- One reason for continuing to use them in clinical practice is that placebos are "The Lie That Heals" with physicians stating that the results are "just too good to pass up."
- Clinical research has shown real and measureable effects to placebo that are as good as or even better than available treatments for active diseases.
- A second claim is that placebos are most often used to treat distressful symptoms such as pain or anxiety. Placebo treatment for these kind of subjective complaints often occur when the validity of complaint is questioned, clinical options are exhausted, or when the physician feels "the need to give something."
- A third side to this ethical debate questions whether placebo response can ever be completely eliminated.
- The placebo response occurs because of the patient's prior experiences and expectations as well as their relationship with their provider.
- One paper has proposed that placebo response results from the "meaning of the intervention" and has no bearing on the placebo at all. This definition is an attempt to focus the examination of this response on how the patient changes as opposed to how an inert substance causes a change. Here, the pejorative aspect of placebo is removed.

OPEN–HIDDEN PARADIGM RESEARCH

- In the open–hidden paradigm, a patient is given an active drug in two different settings. One is an open administration where they knowingly receive the drug, the other is hidden or blinded, and patients do not know they are receiving the drug.
- This allows separation of the physiologic response (hidden paradigm) from the psychosocial context in which medication is given (open paradigm).
- Although no placebo is given, the difference between the two responses is thought to be a measure of the placebo response.
- This research has shown that opioids are much less effective when the patient does not know they are receiving them, compared to when they are informed.
- Other studies have shown that when openly discontinuing opioids or anxiolytics, the patient experiences a return in symptoms more quickly than when they are unaware that medications have ceased.

PLACEBO AS TREATMENT MODALITY

- If the placebo response could be reliably prescribed, outcomes would improve with any treatment.
- Unfortunately, personality traits, genetics, underlying disease, or past medical history do not provide markers that identify susceptibility to placebos. Nevertheless, attempts are being made to harness this phenomenon.
- In one recent study, an openly labeled placebo was given without deception and it showed a surprising reduction in symptom severity.
- Manipulating a patient's expectations also has promise. It has been shown to independently contribute to clinical outcomes in numerous diseases including coronary artery disease, orthopedic injuries, and mood disorders.
- In pain medicine, greater efficacy has been shown when a patient knowingly receives a pain medication than when it is given covertly.
- Analgesia can also be decreased simply by negative suggestions before a treatment.
- This research suggests that expectations should always be discussed, identified, and addressed. Further, realigning expectations will best improve patient outcomes and increase satisfaction.
- Another strategy is to openly pair placebos with medications that treat side effects. Once the placebo response is "conditioned," the active medication can be stopped.
  ○ For example, one can pair an antiemetic for chemotherapy with a placebo. Initially both are given to prevent nausea and vomiting (acquisition phase), but eventually the antiemetic is stopped and the placebo alone prevents the side effect (the neutral stimulus becomes the conditioned response).

- Pairing can occur in any setting and it is possible that the neutral response could simply become taking the medication itself. In this situation, seeing the medication could have more of an effect than its physiologic actions. If true, a dose reduction would not change its efficacy and could be used clinically when concerns of tolerance and misuse are present.
- Results from open–hidden studies suggest the use of positive actions (open paradigm) when starting pain therapies and minimizing negative outcomes (hidden paradigm) when ending treatments.
- Promoting social learning, reducing anxiety, and improving patient–physician relationships are always important, but their benefit may actually be, in part, due to the placebo response.

NOCEBO EFFECT

- Nocebos are defined as negative effects that result after a treatment and are not related to known mechanisms of the intervention. They can also reduce efficacy even if the overall outcome is positive. Nocebos are placebos that cause a change for the worse.
- When placebos are used in healthy controls, more nocebo effects are reported than in clinical studies.
- Reported nocebo effects tend to correlate with the experimental drug studied. For example, when a placebo is compared to a nonsteroidal anti-inflammatory drug (NSAID), the placebo arm reports more gastrointestinal complaints.
- Weak predictors of nocebo effects include patients who report more side effects with current treatments and express more concern about potential side effects.
- Like placebos, expectation and verbal conditioning is thought to be one of its mechanisms of action.
  - Patients who receive extensive and explicit information about side effects report more side effects than patients given more general warnings.
  - Verbal suggestions have been shown to cause nausea, vomiting, sedation, and headaches in patients who are actually taking medications known to effectively treat these same symptoms. Just like the placebo effect, conditioning, learning, and provider–patient relationship all play a role.
- The nocebos are not simply the opposite of placebos.
  - With nocebos, anxiety and other negative affective states play a more important role in symptoms.
  - Nocebo responses may be activated through anticipatory anxiety and hyperactivity of the hypothalamic-pituitary–adrenal axis.
  - Cholecystokinin that can enhance pain transmission is also triggered by this same anxiety. Further,

proglumide, a cholecystokinin inhibitor, can prevent some nocebo effects.
  - It has also been speculated that nocebo responses are elicited faster and remain longer than placebo responses.
  - A stronger nocebo response may have an evolutionary advantage by minimizing the exposure to dangerous or negative substances.

BIBLIOGRAPHY

Beecher HK. The powerful placebo. *JAMA.* 1955;159:1602–1606.

Benedetti F, Amanzio M, Vighetti S, Asteggiano G. The biochemical and neuroendicrine bases of the hyperalgesic nocebo effect. *J Neurosci.* 2006;26:12014–12022.

Bingel U, Wanigasekra V, Wiech K, et al. The effect of treatment expectation on drug efficacy: imaging the analgesic benefit of the opioid remifentanil. *Sci Transl Med.* 2011;3:70ra14.

Brody H. The lie that heals: the ethics of giving placebos. *Ann Intern Med.* 1982;97:112–118.

Colloca L, Lopiano L, Lanotte M, Benedetti F. Overt versus covert treatment for pain, anxiety, and Parkinson's disease. *Lancet Neurol.* 2004;3:679–684.

Enck P, Bingel U, Schedlowski M, Rief W. The placebo response in medicine: minimize, maximize, or personalize? *Nat Rev Drug Discov.* 2013;12:191–204.

Fässler M, Meissner K, Schneider A, Linde K. Frequency and circumstances of placebo use in clinical practice—a systematic review of empirical studies. *BMC Med.* 2010;8:15.

Haygarth J. *Of the Imagination, as a Cause and as a Cure of Disorders of the Body; Exemplfied by Fictitious Tractors, and Epidemical Convulsions.* Bath: Crutwell; 1801.

Hoffman GA, Harrington A, Fields HL. Pain and the placebo what we have learned. *Persp Biol Med.* 2005;48:248–265.

Howick J, Bishop FL, Heneghan C, et al. Placebo use in the United Kingdom: results of a national survey of primary care practitioners *PLoS ONE.* 2013;8:e58247.

Hrobjartson A, Gotzsche PC. Is the placebo powerless? An analysis of clinical trials comparing placebo with no treatment. *N Engl J Med.* 2001;344:1594–1602.

Hrobjartsson A, Gøtzsche PC. Placebo interventions for all clinical conditions. *Cochrane Database Syst Rev.* 2010;1:CD003974.

Kaptchuk TJ, Friedlander E, Kelley JM, et al. Placebos without deception: a randomized controlled trial in irritable bowel syndrome. *PLoS ONE.* 2010;5:e15591.

Kienle GS, Kiene H. The powerful placebo effect fact or fiction? *J Clin Epidemiol.* 1997;50:1311–1318.

Moerman DE, Jonas WB. Deconstructing the placebo effect and finding the meaning response. *Ann Intern Med.* 2002; 136:471–476.

Price D, Finniss D, Benedetti F. A comprehensive review of the placebo effect: recent advances and current thought. *Annu Rev Psychol.* 2008;59:565–590.

Shapiro AK. A historic and heuristic definition of the placebo. *Psychiatry.* 1964;27:52–58.

Staats PS, Hekmat H, Staats AW. Suggestion/placebo effects on pain: negative as well as positive. *J Pain Symptom Manage.* 1998;15:235–243.

Staats PS, Hekmat H, Staats AW. The psychological behaviorism theory of pain and the placebo: its principles and results of research application. *Adv Psychosom Med.* 2004;25:28–40.

Walach H. Placebo controls: historical, methodological and general aspects. *Philos Trans R Soc Lond B Biol Sci.* 2011 366:1870–1878.

Zubieta JK, Stohler CS. Neurobiological mechanisms of placebo responses. *Ann N Y Acad Sci.* 2009;1156:198–210.

6   PAIN TAXONOMY

John D. Loeser, MD

INTRODUCTION

Taxonomies and definitions are essential in the processes of science; they permit succinct and accurate communication and are an important step in the development of a subject area. This was clearly recognized by John J. Bonica when he organized the meeting in Issaquah, WA in 1973 that led to the formation of the International Association for the Study of Pain (IASP). Once the IASP had been launched, Bonica identified the task of developing a taxonomy for pain and standardized definitions of important terms. He wrote, "The development and widespread adoption of universally accepted definitions of terms and a classification of pain syndromes are among the most important objectives and responsibilities of the IASP." This important project was led by Harold Merskey and a first draft was published in 1979; a revision was published in 1986 that contained not only terminology but also the novel IASP Classification scheme for chronic pain states. In 2010, the IASP Taxonomy Committee produced a revision of some of the terminology and updated the classification scheme in selected subject areas. These changes were published on the IASP website (http://www.iasp-pain.org/).

To my knowledge, no other pain organization has prepared a classification scheme, although the World Health Organization (WHO) has produced many versions of the International Classification of Diseases (ICD) system and is currently working on yet another version (ICD-11). It is widely recognized that the ICD system is not very useful for chronic pain classification, as it is a hodge-podge scheme based upon a mélange of anatomy, imaging studies, symptoms, environmental factors, infectious agents, pathology, psychological

factors, and some hypothetical etiologies to produce a confusing array of potential diagnoses for painful conditions. The IASP Classification of chronic pain syndromes has never achieved wide-spread acceptance and, to my knowledge, has not often been utilized in either research or clinical activities. Every specialty in medicine requires a reliable and efficient classification of the diseases that it addresses; pain medicine has not yet achieved this status. I know that the IASP and other groups are looking at ways to develop a better classification system for chronic pain. Hopefully, such a scheme will be based upon the mechanisms underlying the painful state, but our knowledge has not advanced far enough yet to permit this.

It is important to note that the IASP Definitions of Terms and Taxonomy are not to be considered as fixed; they are both works in progress with the intention to update them as more information becomes available. The terminology and classification were designed for clinical use; the extrapolation to research in infrahuman species has created some issues that are going to need resolution in the future.

IASP CLASSIFICATION OF CHRONIC PAIN SYNDROMES

The IASP Classification of Chronic Pain Syndromes is based upon five axes—the anatomical, system involved, temporal characteristics, intensity and time, and, finally, presumed etiology.[a] Whereas axes I, II, and V are monotonic and easy to comprehend, axes III and IV combine frequency, intensity, and duration in a nonobvious fashion. This is the probable reason why this taxonomy has rarely been utilized.

Axis I: Regions of the Body with Pain

Head, face, and mouth	000
Cervical region	100
Upper shoulder and limb	200
Thoracic region	300
Abdominal region	400
Lower back lumbar spine, sacrum, and coccyx	500
Lower limbs	600
Pelvic region	700
Anal, perianal, and genital region	800
More than three major sites	900

[a]This taxonomy has been reproduced with the permission of the International Association for the Study of Pain®(IASP). The taxonomy may not be reproduced for any other purpose without permission.

Axis II: Systems

Nervous system (central, peripheral, and autonomic) and special senses	00
Nervous system (psychological and social)	10
Respiratory and cardiovascular systems	20
Musculoskeletal system and connective tissue	30
Cutaneous and subcutaneous and associated glands	40
Gastrointestinal system	50
Genitourinary system	60
Other organs or viscera	70
More than one system	80

Axis III: Temporal Characteristics or Patterns of Occurrence

Not recorded applicable or known	0
Single episode, limited duration	1
Continuous or nearly continuous, nonfluctuating	2
Continuous or nearly continuous, fluctuating	3
Recurring irregularly	4
Recurring regularly	5
Paroxysmal	6
Sustained with superimposed paroxysms	7
Other combinations	8
None of the above	9

Axis IV: Patient's Statement of Intensity and Time Since Onset of Pain

Not recorded, applicable or known	0.0
Mild	
1 month or less	0.1
1–6 months	0.2
More than 6 months	0.3
Medium	
1 month or less	0.4
1–6 months	0.5
More than 6 months	0.6
Severe	
One month or less	0.7
1 month to 6 months	0.8
More than 6 months	0.9

Axis V: Etiology

Genetic or congenital	0.00
Trauma, operation, and burns	0.01
Infection and parasitic	0.02
Inflammation (no known infective agent	0.03
Neoplasm	0.04
Toxic and metabolic	0.05
Degenerative, mechanical	0.06
Dysfunctional (including psychophysiological)	0.07
Unknown or other	0.08
Psychological	0.09

Examples of coding utilizing this system:

Postherpetic neuralgia, abdomen, severe, and >9 months: 402.92

Tic douloureux, right face, severe, and 3-month duration: 006.88

Cervical spinal stenosis, moderate, and >6-month duration: 133.66

IASP PAIN TERMINOLOGY

As soon as the original list of terms was published in 1979, pain clinicians and researchers began to use these definitions. Some have been modified over the intervening 30+ years as new information and understanding of pain mechanisms has developed. Problems have been created by the application of some of these terms to experimental animals in which the nature of any sensation is difficult to determine. The most important definition is listed first: pain. Failure to recognize the last phrase of this definition is a major flaw in thinking about pain.

Pain An unpleasant sensory and emotional experience associated with actual or potential tissue damage or described in terms of such damage.

Allodynia Pain due to a stimulus that does not normally provoke pain.

Analgesia Absence of pain in response to stimulation that would normally be painful.

Anesthesia dolorosa Pain in an area or region which is anesthetic.

Dysesthesia An unpleasant abnormal sensation, whether spontaneous or evoked.

Hyperalgesia Increased pain from a stimulus that normally provokes pain.

Hyperesthesia Increased sensitivity to stimulation, excluding the special senses.

Hyperpathia A painful syndrome characterized by increased reaction to a stimulus, especially a repetitive stimulus, as well as increased threshold.

Hypoalgesia Diminished pain in response to a normally painful stimulus.

Hypoesthesia Decreased sensitivity to stimulation, excluding the special senses.

Neuralgia Pain in the distribution of a nerve or nerves.

Neuritis Inflammation of a nerve or nerves.

Neuropathic pain Pain caused by a lesion or disease of the somatosensory nervous system.

Peripheral neuropathic pain Pain caused by a lesion or disease of the peripheral somatosensory nervous system.

Central neuropathic pain Pain caused by a lesion or disease of the central somatosensory nervous system.

Neuropathy A disturbance of function or pathological change in a nerve: if one nerve, mononeuropathy; in several nerves; mononeuropathy multiplex; if diffuse and bilateral, polyneuropathy.

Nociceptor A sensory receptor of the peripheral nervous system that is capable of transducing and encoding noxious stimuli.

Nociceptive neuron A central or peripheral neuron of the somatosensory nervous system that is capable of encoding noxious stimuli.

Nociception The neural process of encoding noxious stimuli.

Nociceptive pain Pain resulting from damage to non-neuronal tissue.

Noxious stimulus A stimulus that is damaging or threatens damage to normal tissues.

Pain threshold The minimal intensity of a stimulus that is perceived as painful.

Pain tolerance level The maximum intensity of a pain-producing stimulus that a subject is willing to tolerate in a given situation.

Sensitization Increased responsiveness of nociceptive neurons to their normal input, and/or, recruitment of a response to normally subthreshold inputs.

Peripheral sensitization Increased responsiveness and reduced threshold of nociceptive neurons in the periphery to stimulation of their receptive fields.

Central sensitization Increased responsiveness of central nociceptive neurons to their normal or subthreshold input.

Paresthesia An abnormal sensation, whether spontaneous or provoked.

CONCLUSION

The development of a classification scheme and terminology has always been a high priority for the IASP. No other pain organization has taken on the issues of terminology and classification. Both are thought to be essential for progress in pain medicine and the sciences that underpin this specialty. The terminology and classification systems have been developed by a multidisciplinary and multinational group of clinicians and researchers over the past 37 years. These projects will continue to evolve as our knowledge of pain increases. Hopefully, a more utilitarian classification scheme will evolve from better understanding of the mechanisms underlying chronic pain. Language is a living, cultural phenomenon and this terminology will evolve in the future.

BIBLIOGRAPHY

Bonica JJ. The need of a taxonomy. *Pain.* 1979;6:247–248.

Merskey H. Pain terms: a list with definitions and notes on usage. *Pain.* 1979;6:249–252.

Merskey H. Classification of chronic pain. *Pain.* 1986;(suppl 3): S1–S225.

7 ETHICS IN PAIN MEDICINE

Michel Y. Dubois, MD

HISTORICAL BACKGROUND

- Ethics is defined in Webster's *New International Dictionary* as "the science of moral duty; more broadly the science of the ideal human character and the ideal ends of human action."
- In the medical field, and especially in Pain Medicine, it is a "road map," which allows physicians to practice in the face of an increasingly complex environment, often confusing and contradictory, protecting patients and physicians against professional malpractice, misconduct, and other potential medical–legal issues.
- Throughout human history, morality has been an integral part of any medical decision.
  - The field of medical ethics, developed chiefly in the last 50 years, is now formally established as an essential part of the teaching and practice of medicine.
  - Guidelines or laws for the practice of morally acceptable medicine have existed for millennia.
  - Almost 4000 years ago, the code of Hammurabi (1727 BC), one of the first systems of written laws, was engraved on a stone in Babylonia. It still exists and describes the doctor–patient relationship according to a structure, which directly rewards positive outcome while penalizing negative results.
    - A monetary award or corporal punishment was dispensed depending on whether the patient was cured, or partially cured, or deceased.
    - The importance of the award/punishment was also related to the social class of the patient, a distinction being made between free men and slaves.
    - The code was also applied to veterinary medicine.
  - Other examples of such rules were the Book of Thoth in Ancient Egypt and, more recently (400 BC), the Hippocratic oath, which focused primarily on the perception of physicians' behavior and is still quoted in academic circles.

○ Modern medical ethics was essentially the product of the Nuremberg military tribunal of World War II, which raised concerns about the ethical treatment of human subjects for research under Nazi Germany and which led to the Nuremberg code of 1947.

○ The initial Declaration of Helsinki followed this in 1964 by the World Medical Association, which has frequently been revised and updated.

○ In the United States, the Belmont Report, published in 1978, was the key document, which prescribed medical ethics, setting forth a national policy for human subject research. This report was rapidly followed by a flurry of federal regulations, which still continue.

• In the second half of the 20th century, medical interventions have multiplied. In part as this is due to the explosion of new technology, creating complex clinical situations with increasingly difficult decisions.

• Because of this increasing complexity and the waning influence of traditional moral authorities (such as religion), medical ethics became an indispensable tool for grappling with the moral and professional issues in clinical practice.

• Pain Medicine, which emerged as a new specialty over the past several decades, brought its own issues to daily practice.

• Surveys show wide interest among medical professionals in ethics applied to pain management, but also underline the need to examine a growing number of unaddressed issues that have become a significant burden for the pain practitioner.

• In response, some Pain Medicine publications started a regular section on medical ethics, and the American Academy of Pain Medicine published an Ethics Charter in 2005.

• As new problems and new attitudes toward patients and patient care evolved, new ethical issues were discussed and older ones revisited.

TABLE 7-1 Caregiver's Moral Principles—The Hippocratic Oath: Then and Now

HIPPOCRATIC OATH, 5TH CENTURY BC	MEDICAL ETHICS, 21ST CENTURY AD
Had religious overtones	Are secular
Moral commitment	Moral automatism
Driven by caregiver's beneficence	Driven by patient's autonomy
Nonmaleficence = love of art	Nonmaleficence = law
Assumes public trust	Distrusting public
Forbids abortion	Allows abortion
Prohibits euthanasia	Permits assisted suicide
Encourages consultation	Need external approval for consult
Assumes a life of virtue	Virtue not a primary goal

• Medical ethics is a dynamic field, requiring continuous feedback and communication between patients, health care professionals, and society at large.

• Moral attitudes changes with time, as is evident, for example, with the traditional Hippocratic Oath, where some rules and ethical concepts have changed significantly (Table 7-1).

BASIS FOR THE ETHICAL PRACTICE OF PAIN MEDICINE

• Most professional medical organizations have ethics guidelines for the benefit of their members

○ The American Medical Association (AMA) has been a leader in the field publishing a Code of Medical Ethics, which is updated regularly and represents a reference document for most professional organizations.

○ Because the management of pain is a fundamental part of the practice of medicine, all physicians have an obligation to address acute and persistent pain.

○ Providing pain relief is an ethical imperative, which requires a precise list of ethical rules.

○ The primary obligations for the entire medical field are summarized in the AMA Principles of Medical Ethics (Appendix 7-1), and the duties of physicians to their patients are contained in the AMA's Declaration of Professional Responsibility (Appendix 7-2). As applied to Pain Medicine, the physician's duties to relieve pain require special attention in the following areas:

▪ Proper assessment of the pain patient as a whole, including all relevant biological, social, psychological, and spiritual dimensions pertaining to the origin and the impact of pain on the individual.

▪ Treatment of the pain patient with competence and compassion.

▪ Education of professional colleagues, patients, the public, and policy makers on the principles and methods used in Pain Medicine.

▪ Support of and participation in basic and clinical pain research.

▪ Advocacy to ensure success in pain care and its continuous improvement.

As a rule, the following are commitments required of Pain Medicine physicians in order to help patients enjoy proper care:

• Facilitate patient's access to Pain Medicine services.
• Encourage medical institutions to assign priority to routine pain assessment and management.

- Encourage a focus on the diagnosis and treatment of underlying conditions that contribute to pain.
- Avoid acting on unwarranted patient claims of disability.
- Encourage professional education on adequate and full assessment of pain in all patients.
- Provide education about adequate assessment of disability arising from chronic pain problems.
- Familiarize members and colleagues with new evidence-based findings and concepts concerning pain assessment and its treatment.
- Provide education in pain treatment–related substance misuse, abuse, addiction, diversion, and dependence— including risk assessment and management.
- Assist in resolving concerns about iatrogenic addiction and its detection, prevention, and management.
- Participate in Pain Medicine–related focus and policy development.

PHYSICIANS' DUTIES TO THE PATIENT

- The assessment and management of complex chronic pain conditions often require an extraordinary amount of skill and knowledge.
- Pain specialists need to recognize, understand, and respect the ethical bounds that exist in the context of their duties to the patient.
- The four cardinal points that constitute the basis of medical ethics are:
  ○ beneficence,
  ○ nonmaleficence,
  ○ respect for patient autonomy, and
  ○ justice.
- These obviously apply to Pain Medicine.

PROFESSIONAL EXPERTISE

- The practice of Pain Medicine requires a level of competence, which is acquired only through special training and experience.
- Although training and certification in Pain Medicine are presently far from comprehensive, a pain physician must, at a minimum, be acquainted with all the diagnoses and treatment modalities that are part of the specialty. This will allow the practitioner to make a specific diagnosis and explain to patients the risks and advantages of a given treatment modality within an interdisciplinary treatment plan.
- Pain specialists must have pharmacological knowledge of all medications used in pain management, and technical experience with interventional or alternative treatments, which are sometimes used without proper

supervision or adequate regulation (herbs or over-the-counter medication).

- Because pain patients have usually seen several physicians before arriving at a pain clinic (eight on average), it is important to recognize that patients may have undergone ineffective or inappropriate treatment.
- If incompetent or unethical professional behavior is suspected, the pain specialist should be aware of the appropriate channels for action, such as state medical societies, peer-review organizations, or licensing boards.
- Because Pain Medicine is a relatively new field of specialization with frequent new findings and treatments, it is imperative that pain specialists maintain professional expertise through Continuing Medical Education (CME) postgraduate education, in order to counter the alarming amount of misinformation and potentially harmful attitudes concerning pain, which adversely affect patient care, and which current research reports among some health care professionals.

TYPE OF PRACTICE

- Good medical practice should be uniform in all clinical settings. However, there may be subtle differences in the problems that present to the private practice physician and those that are observed by the physician practicing in an academic environment.
  ○ The private practitioner as well as the academician may have undue economic pressure. When faced with economic pressures, physicians who are reimbursed for productivity may sometimes be tempted to perform evaluation and treatment procedures that are outside the scope of his/her expertise or to over-treat patients—a major and relatively frequent occurrence in Pain Medicine.
    ▪ Overtreatment could consist of excessive or inappropriate nerve blocks, excessive prescription habits, and excessive physical therapy among other.
    ▪ It is unethical for a health care professional to provide treatment that exceeds the training and the scope of practice or to recommend interventions that are not purely in the best interest of the patient.
    ▪ Financial pressures and other ethical dilemmas may present themselves to the physician practicing in an academic environment.
      □ For instance, because of the training needs of medical students, residents, and fellows, the care of patients may sometimes be jeopardized.
      □ Enrollment in clinical trials brings academic pressures as well.

▫ The ethical principles of nonmaleficence and beneficence demand adequate support and supervision for all trainees.

▫ Decisions must be made in the best interests of the patient and not the trainees' experience. It is essential to inform the patient of the roles and duties of everyone in the care team.

▫ It is also important to remember that patients have the autonomous right to choose whomever they want to treat them.

REFERRALS

- Pain Medicine specialists often work as consultants to other physicians.
- Regardless of the referral source, their primary duty is toward their patient. This duty is compromised when, for instance, they are asked by the referral source to perform a procedure, such as a nerve block, that the pain specialist does not believe follows the standard of care, is indicated or when the pain specialist is asked to depart from his/her normal practice, for example, a specific request not to consult a pain psychologist.
- Ethical practice requires an independent judgment to determine indications for any diagnostic test or therapeutic intervention, and this determination can only derive from personal evaluation and examination of the patient prior to the provision of treatment.
- Referrals from third-party sources, such as attorneys or workman's compensation boards, require the pain specialist to exercise his/her best judgment and not accede to any unreasonable demands or third-party pressures that might deviate from the standard of care, be contrary to the patient's best interest, or not following ethical standards.
- Economic pressures and incentives and the desire to maintain strong professional relationships with referral sources should never compromise the pain specialist's primary responsibility to the patient and ethical treatment.
- It is not unusual for doctors to have some financial interest in health-related industries (such as rehabilitation facilities, gyms, pharmacies, MRI, and surgery center).
  ○ The AMA's Code of Medical Ethics is clear on this topic: "Physicians should not refer patients to a health care facility, which is outside their office practice and at which they do not directly provide care or service when they have an investment interest in that facility."

  ○ "The physician needs to have personal involvement with the provision of care on-site."
  ○ In general, financial arrangements between patients and physicians, including those that pose potential conflicts of interest, should be clearly described and transparent to all parties.

RELATIONSHIPS WITH PHARMACISTS

- A Pain Medicine physician should obtain information from a pharmacist regarding prescriptions and filling patterns when it is in the best interest of the patient.
- In most states, now, there are databanks, which provide an inventory of all controlled substances dispensed to patients.
  ○ Pharmacists generally maintain these databanks.
- Because of their role, pharmacists can find themselves in conflict with patients and physicians over the prescribing and dispensing of medications.
  ○ It is important that a pharmacist be able to question a prescription's validity without affecting the physician's judgment or the patient's right to have a prescription filled.
  ○ Inquiries from a pharmacist seeking to validate the legality or medical necessity of a prescription are important and should be addressed promptly.
  ○ In keeping with the bioethical principle of justice, all essential and commonly used drugs in Pain Medicine should be available to all patients at all pharmacies regardless of geographic location.
  ○ The reality, however, is a disparity in prescription practice and the stocking of medications, especially controlled substances, such as opioids, which is often based on racial, ethnic, or socioeconomic demographics.
  ○ When promoting safe and effective prescribing, a physician may insist, whenever possible, that a patient use only one pharmacy, with the patient being free to choose the pharmacy, in order to ensure compliance and safety in treatment.

SOCIETAL RESPONSIBILITIES

- Human health does not depend exclusively on the physician–patient relationship through treatment.
  ○ Social and political circumstances can also influence health and well-being, and ill health can be rooted in harmful social practices and unjust political arrangements.

○ For instance, adequate food, clean water, and safe housing directly affect health.

○ Medical ethics acknowledge the connection between human health and the social environment.

○ The AMA recognizes social responsibility as an important factor for human health: "a physician shall recognize the responsibility to participate in activities contributing to the improvement of the community and the betterment of public health."

- This social responsibility is summarized in the core AMA declaration of professional responsibility (see Appendix 7-2).

○ A number of social obstacles preclude that improvement in both the theory and the practice of Pain Medicine.

- Inadequate training and education in the management of pain.
- Barriers limiting the use of pain medications (opioids).
- Inadequate research in pain control due to poor funding.

○ Disparities in pain care exist for all types of pain (acute and chronic) and across all pain-care settings, primarily as a result of patients' sociodemographic factors such as race, ethnicity, socioeconomic status, age, and gender.

- Overall, across the age continuum, minorities report significantly more psychological and physical morbidity, such as posttraumatic stress disorder and disability, than non-Hispanic whites.
- The AMA Code of Ethics is clear that such situations have ethical implications that must be addressed in order to optimize pain care for those at particular risk for substandard pain care:
- "Whether such disparities in health care are caused by treatment decisions, difference in income and education, sociocultural factors, or failures by the medical profession, they are unjustifiable and must be eliminated."
- Physicians should examine their own practices to ensure that racial prejudice does not affect clinical judgment and medical care.

SOCIOECONOMIC DISPARITIES

- Access to health care is strongly influenced by financial status.
- The ethical principle of distributive justice would dictate that all patients under similar clinical circumstances should receive equal access to all necessary treatment modalities.

○ However, low socioeconomic status is broadly associated with poor access to pain care, fewer community health resources, and higher overall morbidity and mortality rates.

○ Minority individuals without insurance are half as likely to have a regular physician when compared with insured African Americans—limiting their access to specialty care, such as Pain Medicine.

GEOGRAPHIC DISPARITIES

- The patient's place of residence strongly influences access to health-related services.

○ Because there are not enough pain specialists, primary care physicians often provide the necessary care, even for patients with complex pain management needs and especially in rural settings.

○ The availability of essential medication or other treatment interventions is highly dependent on where the patient resides.

○ Attempts are being made to improve pain care for the inhabitants of areas of low health-care density.

RACIAL AND ETHNIC DISPARITIES

- In 2003, the Institute of Medicine published a comprehensive review of racial and ethnic disparities in health care, showing that these disparities arise from a complex interplay of economic, social, and cultural factors.

○ It clearly documents the disparities in providing pain care for acute pain problems in the emergency room and for cancer pain.

- Further reviews have demonstrated that this discrimination also occurs in in-patient and nursing homes and in certain pain conditions that are not properly recognized.
- Physicians often handle pain complaints from racial and ethnic minorities, the elderly, and women less aggressively than those of non-Hispanic white men leading to a high risk of undertreatment for those groups.
- There is a twofold increase in the amount of analgesics given to white patients with acute pain who have long bone fractures, when compared with analgesics supplied to racial minorities with similar injuries.
- Studies of elderly nursing home residents with cancer pain show that African Americans were less likely to have their pain evaluated and were 63% more likely than Caucasians to receive no pain medication.
- Even for end-of-life hospice care, services are more available to well-heeled white sectors of society than others.

ACCESS TO PAIN CARE

- Minority patients have been shown to be more likely to refuse recommended treatment, to poorly adhere to recommended treatment regimen, and to delay seeking medical care.
  - This happens because patients mistrust physicians, have had negative experiences with the health care system in the past, or have limited health literacy.
- Also, physicians may suffer from bias or prejudice, stereotyping, poor communication skills, and greater clinical uncertainty when treating minority patients.
- It is therefore essential that Pain Medicine physicians focus on cross-cultural competence and advocate for cultural education and training programs in postgraduate conferences.
- Pain Medicine physicians have a duty to educate the public and their colleagues about advances in the field, through teaching, writing, and lecturing on the subject. Individual and professional organizations' advocacy can bring about major changes in regulations and laws that will improve the ethical practice of Pain Medicine as well as the behavior of physicians and the general public.

ETHICAL OPINIONS IN PAIN MEDICINE PRACTICE

CLINICAL PROBLEMS

Patients in Pain and Decision-Making Capacity

- As previously mentioned, many pain patient subpopulations can be vulnerable because of ethnicity, race, cultural barriers, etc.
- Pain itself can alter the decision-making capacity of patients, who are also often taking medication that may alter their judgment.
- In keeping with the ethical principle of patient autonomy, it is crucial that the patient's decision to proceed with any course of pain treatment be voluntary and expresses the patient's genuine desires.
- When getting consent from the patient in pain, physicians should diligently strive to ensure that the individual understands all the information and consequences of the treatment and demonstrates some ability to discuss and articulate a preference with no external coercion.
- If the physician believes that the patient cannot make a decision for him/herself, the next step is to ascertain whether the patient has identified a surrogate decision maker.
  - Ethical dilemmas may then arise if the physician believes that the surrogate's decision is contrary to the patient's best interest as articulated in the AMA Code of Ethics: "… When a physician believes that a decision is clearly not what a patient would have decided or could not be reasonably judged to be within the patient's best interest, the dispute should be referred to an ethics committee before resorting to the course."

External Barriers to Shared Decisions

- There are many external barriers, which modify the patient–physician communication during pain treatment.
  - One example is the workman's compensation claims and litigation process, which may not represent the best medical interest of the patient.
  - Other sources influencing patients' decisions include ethnocultural beliefs, family, work, and financial pressures, and language comprehension.
  - Pressures from third-party insurance and other payers arising from the cost of the treatment are also routinely encountered.
  - Physicians have an obligation to consider, especially within the context of the new Affordable Care Act, the implication of the cost and availability of treatment when developing a plan of care.
  - Any treatment is doomed if the physician does not facilitate the patient's ability to comply, both financially and socially

Confidentiality and its Limit in Pain Medicine

- Physicians have been ethically bound to protect patient confidentiality and the privacy of patients' medical information for a long time.
  - The Health Insurance Portability and Accountability Act (HIPAA) has raised the legal standard.
  - No information can be given to a third party without a patient's consent, and, even if obtained, only relevant information should be disseminated.
  - Pain Medicine usually includes several different specialists in a treatment plan and exchange of information between professionals is generally thought to improve patient care.
  - Some reports, however, such as those from psychologists—who are frequently involved in the management of chronic pain—may contain sensitive information affording the possibility for ethical conflicts of confidentiality.
  - The patient needs to be fully informed about the limits of confidentiality between all parties.

Pain Undertreatment and Pain Mismanagement

- Mismanagement of pain, especially undertreatment, is a breach of the physician's duty of beneficence, and many awareness campaigns have been directed in the past years, mostly toward primary care physicians and internists, in order to deal with this problem.

- As an indirect consequence, a new kind of drug mismanagement appeared related to the prescription of strong analgesics, and more rules and regulations have appeared—are still appearing—in order to limit the prescription of controlled substances, especially opioids.

Opioids Abuse, Addiction, and Diversion

- The principle of balance was recognized very early in the ethical management of pain.
- When prescribing opioids and controlled substances in general, a balance must be struck between the ability of opioids to relieve pain and suffering, and the fact that opioids are not always successful, can be misused, abused, and potentially diverted for illicit use.
- In the previous decade (2000–2010), as opioids were increasingly prescribed, the rate of drug abuse and death by overdose from their prescriptions more than doubled and created a new ethical obligation for the physician to avoid these major complications.
- The rate of addiction due to prescription opioids ranges from 0% to 50%.
- Opioids are a major treatment modality in the fight against acute and terminal pain and, in some selected cases, in chronic noncancer pain.
- New state and federal regulations intended to combat problems with opioids (ie, abuse, addiction, overdose, and diversion) due to over prescribing controlled substances regularly apply.
- A pain physician who prescribes opioids shares with the patient an ongoing ethical responsibility for the proper use of the drug.
  - This responsibility assumes that the patient's collaboration allows an accurate and ongoing documentation of the titration of dose, changes in level of pain and mood, functional improvement, and adverse events.
  - Continuing follow-up of the patient under opioid treatment—in order to avoid, abuse, misuse, addiction, and diversion—must be performed frequently, and the patient must be made to understand that it is his/her responsibility to safeguard the medication in order to prevent harm to others.
- The ethical principle of autonomy must be interpreted cautiously when using opioids.
  - Because of their complex pharmacology, opioids, taken chronically, create a physical and mental dependence, which may make it very difficult to wean a patient.
    - Associated with treatment-signed agreements, tools designed to recognize misuse of opioids,

either by risk-assessment at the beginning of treatment or urine drug screening during treatment, are particularly useful in monitoring the situation.
  - However, when a clinician judges that a treatment would do more harm than good, there is no obligation to provide or continue that treatment.
  - Nor does the patient have the right to demand it when it is not in their best interest. In other words, denying opioids is ethically justified in this situation.
  - Applying the principle of justice is probably most difficult in the assessment of opioid prescribing, which should be fair and equitable for all patients.
    - An example of injustice might be denying proper pain control to patients labeled "junkies" or "drug seekers."
    - In such instances, rather than dismissing opioid treatment entirely, the patient should be further evaluated and a proper treatment initiated, which may require that the pain specialist work in collaboration with an addictionologist.
- In conclusion, physicians need to ensure that their patients' pain is properly assessed and managed, and reaching optimal pain control might necessitate, for severe pain, prescribing opioids, which remain the most potent systemic painkillers available. However, clinicians who fail to prevent/control misuse and abuse expose themselves to disciplinary action by regulatory authorities. While the freedom to prescribe these drugs is, as of this writing, constrained, physicians should not forget the right of pain patients, who need to receive opioids for appropriate indications. When prescribing laws are in contradiction with a patient's best interest, physicians have a duty to advocate for change in these laws.

PAIN MEDICINE AT THE END OF LIFE

- Pain management at the end of life may present formidable challenges.
- Physicians caring for patients with terminal illnesses are, however, ethically required to manage pain according to the best current clinical science. This may require consultation with colleagues who have special skills and expertise in palliative care.
- Like all other pain treatments, the pain care plan at the end of life requires close communication between the physician and the patient (and often the family), whose wishes must be considered.
- Physicians should help patients develop goal-oriented advance directives, and they should follow patients' directives when implementing treatment choices.

Comfortable Dying and Patient Self-Determination

- Medical organizations, such as the National Hospice and Palliative Care Organization and the American Academy of Hospice and Palliative Care, have written outcome measures for "safe and comfortable dying" and "self-determined life closures" for their members. They pertain to the management of refractory pain, which often occurs in the end stage of some pain-producing illnesses (ie, bone metastases, invasive peritoneal carcinomatosis, etc.).
- All reasonable means to relieve pain should be sought; but the inability of the physician to relieve pain does not justify intentional hastening or causing of death.
  - Euthanasia, which is the intentional administration of a lethal substance by a physician, as a means of relieving pain and suffering by causing death, is still illegal throughout the United States.
  - Assisted suicide, however, is legal in the states of Washington, Oregon, Montana, and Vermont.
  - The key difference between euthanasia and Physician Aid in Dying (PAD), or assisted suicide, is that PAD requires the patient to self-administer the lethal medication and to determine whether and when to do this.
  - The physician and relatives of a patient, who has terminal illness and intractable pain, frequently worry about hastening death, especially through the use of opioids. There is, however, no evidence to demonstrate that titrating opioids to achieve relief of pain causes a foreseeable risk of death. In fact, medical ethics has accepted that pain control is an ethically defensible practice, even if it may have unintended consequences affecting the duration of a patient's life ("double effect").

Palliative Sedation for Intractable Symptoms

- "Palliative sedation" is used in palliative care to induce and maintain sleep and to relieve pain that is refractory to standard care.
- It should be reserved as an intervention of last resort for the management of pain.
- Palliative sedation otherwise has been acknowledged as a medically humane, ethical, and legal alternative to the intentional hastening of death.
- It should be implemented and maintained by physicians who are familiar with, and expert in, this technique.
- A patient who is experiencing profound existential or psychological suffering should receive psychological or spiritual intervention from a specialist trained to relieve end-of-life suffering, in addition or instead of palliative sedation.

THIRD PARTIES, THE PATIENT–PHYSICIAN RELATIONSHIP, AND CONFLICT OF INTEREST

- In the last few decades, third parties (such as government, managed care, and industry) have increasingly played the role of interface between physician and patient, making the traditional, relatively simple patient–physician relationship, increasingly complex.
- All third parties have their own social, economic, and political agendas, which can positively influence both the public and the medical profession. However, conflicts of interest have emerged, requiring intervention, mostly from the government.
- This phenomenon has created new ethical issues for the practitioner, because some of the decisions imposed by *insurance third parties* may not be in the patient's best interests, focusing instead on extraneous factors, such as corporate financial gain or government budget restrictions.
- Interference by managed care (and Medicare) has created a difficult situation for many physicians.
- Medical treatment decisions may have to be made according to what these organizations dictate for reimbursement, rather than based on the knowledge, experience, and skills of the physician.
- An important role for Pain Medicine physicians is to educate/lobby/advocate managed care and other third-party agencies and regulators on the proper standards of care required to achieve "state of the art" pain management.
- Physicians must involve these third parties in an active manner in order to ensure the provision of proper pain care, influencing them so that their policy initiatives will benefit patient care.
- There is an ethical obligation for physicians practicing pain care to support advocacy for people in pain, oriented toward public opinion, governmental agencies, and managed care companies, which have a controlling role in therapeutic decisions.
- Traditionally, the collaboration between the *pharmaceutical industry and device manufacturers* and medicine has been both essential and positive in, for instance, clinical research, education, and patient-assistance programs. Recently, however, as a result of industry's sometimes aggressive marketing techniques when dealing with physicians, the image of the physician–patient relationship has been blurred and public trust in physicians eroded.
- The major issue is *"conflict of interest,"* where the pain physician may neglect the primary goal of taking care of patients and protecting patient rights.
  - Conflicts of interest can be *personal or professional*, such as career advancement, competition for funding, or financial or material gain.

- o Mixing professional responsibilities with economic self-interest damages or threatens the objectivity necessary for patient care.
- o Conflict of interest can take the form of straight profit or a salary from work in clinical practice, academics, or research.
- Although industry's progress requires experts to aid in the development and testing of new products and medications, the system may be abused to such a point that consultants, speakers, and investigators receive sham honoraria for minimal services, a practice which may favorably bias the opinion of the consultant for the product under consideration.
- *CME* is another field where conflicts of interest can blossom.
  - o Although it is a physician's life-long duty to participate in CME, this activity must be scientifically sound and clinically relevant. However, external marketing pressures from companies with considerable promotional budgets for their drugs or devices have significantly increased. (Examples of these pressures are listed in Table 7-2.)
  - o It is imperative to minimize the opportunity for influence from industry in CME and to avoid bias in educational materials.
  - o To reduce or prevent the undesirable effect of such an influence, the CME should have educational activities certified by an independent educational body, faculty disclosure of financial agreements or relationships with industry (at the beginning of any presentation or meeting), a financial divestment strategy, and close examination by an independent office of red flags such as consultancy, speakers' bureaus, stock options, and corporate board of director positions.
  - o Gifts or remuneration out of proportion to educational research activities are both inappropriate and unethical.
  - o In order to help physicians, professional organizations—such as the Institute of Medicine (IOM), Accreditation Counsel for Continuing Medical Education (ACCME), Association of American Medical Colleges (AAMC), and American Medical Association (AMA)—have

published guidelines, scrutinized the conflictual relationships, and tried to restore the covenant of trust between patient and physician. The government has approved a "Sunshine Act," which requires industry to publish all honoraria/gifts given to physicians, initiated in September, 2013.
  - o Pain Medicine physicians have special *expertise* and knowledge, which should be used to assume a major role in public education and advocacy for competent and compassionate pain relief and setting the standard of care.
- This expertise can be used in offering *testimony* within the judicial system or expert opinions to oversight and policy-making agencies. In order to make such an activity ethically acceptable, a pain physician should:
  - o keep an exhaustive record of pain care, which includes a valid instrument to measure pain, suffering, and physical and mental impairment, as well as response to treatment in terms of level of function and quality of life;
  - o be prepared to explain the content of the records in a full and objective manner in relation to pain care;
  - o support and inform the judicial system, by providing competent, credible evidence concerning patients' physical and psychological pain and pain-related disorders; and
  - o provide testimony, which is balanced, objective, and consistent with the best current standards of pain care, whether testifying as a factual or expert witness for the plaintiff or the defendant.
- The primary goal of Pain Medicine is to provide the best possible pain care to the patient. The growing importance of third parties intruding between the patient and the physician has created mounting ethical challenges in the daily practice of pain physicians. Ethical practice obliges the pain physician to be the best advocate for the pain patient. Conflicts are inevitable, and all physicians can be subject to unconscious biases; however, if they try to divest themselves of any activities that may be contrary to the patient's interest, they will have met this ethical requirement.

CONCLUSION

- The pathophysiology of pain is complex, and the diagnosis and management of pain patients can be highly demanding.
- Deciding what is best for the pain patient can be a major challenge in the current economic, legal, and social environment.
- What is morally right today may be wrong tomorrow. (See for instance, the original version and the modern interpretation of the Hippocratic oath in Table 7-1.)

TABLE 7-2 Reasons Why CME Activities Need to be Freed from Industry Marketing Pressures

- Direct marketing [TV, newspapers, radio, representatives, exhibits, free samples, small gifts, speaker's diners/lunches, etc.]
- 40% CME revenues come from Industry [grants, honoraria, advertisement, etc.]
- Alternative sources of revenue are drying up [nonindustry grants, medical school, hospital support, increasing overhead costs, etc.]
- End result: Increasing risk of biases toward sponsoring products, leading at times to *control part or whole CME educational program.*

TABLE 7-3 Representative Duties and Rules of a Normative Ethics of Pain Medicine

1. Entering the practice of Pain Medicine is discretionary and must reflect personal acknowledgement and adherence to a philosophy of Pain Medicine.
2. A core ethic of pain care reflects the belief that pain is "real."
3. This core ethic is based upon unselfishness: the experiences of the moral patient are always of greater moral importance than the motives of the moral agent.
4. Pain and suffering are profound harms.
5. There is a moral objective and obligation to reduce the pain of patients: this moral standard applies equally to all individuals in pain.
6. Whatever benefits. it is wrong to deliberately produce or allow pain that is prolonged or severe.
7. As a general rule, we should adopt the precautionary principle that whenever the potential for pain is uncertain in a living being, it should be assumed.
8. There is a duty upon those caring for pain patients to acknowledge the facts and realities of pain as physiological and psychological event (and recognize comorbid syndromes and conditions).
9. There is a duty for those caring for pain patients to acknowledge the subjectivity of pain.
10. There is a duty for those who profess to be pain clinicians to accept the difficulties, burdens, and responsibilities of caring for those in pain.

Source: Reproduced, with permission, from Giordano J, Schatman ME. A crisis in chronic pain care: an ethical analysis—part two: proposed structure and function of an ethics of pain medicine. *Pain Phys.* 2008;11:591.

- One of the primary goals of medical ethics is the preservation of patient trust in the physician.
- Pain Medicine is obviously an example of a field of medicine where this trust is critical for the success of the treatment.
- Medical ethics is a dynamic field.
- Continuing evaluation of what has been achieved and accepted in Pain Medicine and the social, political, economic, and financial factors is essential.
- A summary of representative duties and rules, imperative for defining the profession and creating guidelines for the future of the specialty, has been proposed as normative ethics of Pain Medicine (Table 7-3).

APPENDIX 7-1

AMA CODE OF ETHICS—PRINCIPLES OF MEDICAL ETHICS

   I. A physician shall be dedicated to providing competent medical care, with compassion and respect for human dignity and rights.
  II. A physician shall uphold the standards of professionalism, be honest in all professional interactions, and strive to report physicians deficient in character or competence, or engaging in fraud or deception, to appropriate entities.
 III. A physician shall respect the law and also recognize a responsibility to seek changes in those requirements which are contrary to the best interests of the patient.
  IV. A physician shall respect the rights of patients, colleagues, and other health professionals, and shall safeguard patient confidences and privacy within the constraints of the law.
   V. A physician shall continue to study, apply, and advance scientific knowledge, maintain a commitment to medical education, make relevant information available to patients, colleagues, and the public, obtain consultation, and use the talents of other health professionals when indicated.
  VI. A physician shall, in the provision of appropriate patient care, except in emergencies, be free to choose whom to serve, with whom to associate, and the environment in which to provide medical care.
 VII. A physician shall recognize a responsibility to participate in activities contributing to the improvement of the community and the betterment of public health.
VIII. A physician shall, while caring for a patient, regard responsibility to the patient as paramount.
  IX. A physician shall support access to medical care for all people.

Adopted June 1957; revised June 1980; revised June 2001

APPENDIX 7-2

DECLARATION OF PROFESSIONAL RESPONSIBILITY—MEDICINE'S SOCIAL CONTRACT WITH HUMANITY

Preamble

Never in the history of human civilization has the well being of each individual been so inextricably linked to that of every other. Plagues and pandemics respect no national borders in a world of global commerce and travel. Wars and acts of terrorism enlist innocents as combatants and mark civilians as targets. Advances in medical science and genetics, while promising great good, may also be harnessed as agents of evil. The unprecedented scope and immediacy of these universal challenges demand concerted action and response by all.

As physicians, we are bound in our response by a common heritage of caring for the sick and the suffering. Through the centuries, individual physicians have fulfilled this obligation by applying their skills and knowledge competently, selflessly and at times heroically. Today, our profession must reaffirm its historical commitment to combat natural and man-made assaults on the health and well being of humankind.

Only by acting together across geographic and ideological divides can we overcome such powerful threats. Humanity is our patient.

Declaration

We, the members of the world community of physicians, solemnly commit ourselves to:

1. Respect human life and the dignity of every individual.
2. Refrain from supporting or committing crimes against humanity and condemn all such acts.
3. Treat the sick and injured with competence and compassion and without prejudice.
4. Apply our knowledge and skills when needed, though doing so may put us at risk.
5. Protect the privacy and confidentiality of those for whom we care and breach that confidence only when keeping it would seriously threaten their health and safety or that of others.
6. Work freely with colleagues to discover, develop, and promote advances in medicine and public health that ameliorate suffering and contribute to human well-being.
7. Educate the public and polity about present and future threats to the health of humanity.
8. Advocate for social, economic, educational, and political changes that ameliorate suffering and contribute to human well-being.
9. Teach and mentor those who follow us for they are the future of our caring profession.

We make these promises solemnly, freely, and upon our personal and professional honor.

Adopted by the House of Delegates of the American Medical Association, December 4, 2001.

BIBLIOGRAPHY

AAPM Council on Ethics American Academy of Pain Medicine. *Ethics Charter*. 2005. Available at: http://www.painmed.org/files/ethics-charter.pdf.

American Medical Association. *Code of Ethics*. 2013. Available at: http://www.ama-assn.org/ama/pub/physician-resources/medical-ethics/code-medical-ethics.page.

Ballantyne JC, Fleisher LA. Ethical issues in opioid prescribing for chronic pain. *Pain*. 2010;148:365–367.

Banja J, Burgess FW, Kulick RJ, et al. On being a legal expert. *Pain Med*. 2003;4:295–297.

Bernabei R, Gambassi G, Lapane K, et al. Management of pain in elderly patients with cancer. SAGE study group. Systematic assessment of geriatric drug use via epidemiology. *JAMA*. 1998;279:1877–1882.

Charlton JE. Ethical standards in pain management and research. *Core Curriculum for Professional Education in Pain*. 3rd ed. Seattle, Wash: IASP Press; 2005.

Chong SM, Bajwa ZH. Diagnostic and treatment of neuropathic pain. *J Pain Symptom Manage*. 2003;25:S4–S11.

Collins KS, Hughes DL, Doty MM, et al. *Diverse Communities, Common Concerns: Assessing Health Care Quality for Minority Americans*. New York, NY: Commonwealth Fund; 2002.

Ferrell BR, Novy D, Sullivan MD, et al. Ethical dilemmas in pain management. *J Pain*. 2001;2:171–180.

Fine PG. The ethical imperative to relieve pain at life's end. *J Pain Symptom Manage*. 2002;23:273–277.

Fohr SA. The double effect of pain medication: separating myth from reality. *J Palliat Med*. 1998;1:315–328.

Giordano J, Schatman ME. A crisis in chronic pain care: an ethical analysis—part two: proposed structure and function of an ethics of pain medicine. *Pain Phys*. 2008;11:591.

Green C, Todd KH, Lebovits AH, et al. Disparities in pain: ethical issues. *Pain Med*. 2006;7:530–533.

Højsted J, Sjøgren P. Addiction to opioids in chronic pain patients: a literature review. *Eur J Pain*. 2007;11:490–518.

Institute of Medicine. *Unequal Treatment, Confronting Racial and Ethnic Disparities in Health Care*. 2002. Available at: http://www.iom.edu/Reports/2002/Unequal-Treatment-Confronting-Racial-and-Ethnic-Disparities-in-Health-Care.aspx.

Lebovits AH, Florence I, Bthina R, et al. Pain knowledge and attitudes of health care professional: practice characteristic differences. *Clin J Pain*. 1997;13:237–243.

Livovich J. Ethics in managed care and pain medicine. *Pain Med*. 2001;2:155–161.

Orr RD. Pain medicine rather than assisted suicide: the ethical high ground. *Pain Med*. 2001;2:131–137.

Quill TE, Byock JR. Responding to intractable suffering: the role of terminal sedation and voluntary refusal of food and fluids. ACP-ASIM end-of-life care consensus panel. *Ann Intern Med*. 2000;132:408–414.

Sedlis SP, Fisher VJ, Tice D, et al. Racial differences in performance of invasive cardiac procedures in a department of veterans affairs medical center. *J Clin Epidemiol*. 1997;50:899–901.

Schofferman J, Banja J. Conflicts of interest in pain medicine: practice patterns and relationship with industry. *Pain*. 2008;139:494–497.

Schofferman J. The medical-industrial complex, professional medical associations, and continuing medical education. *Pain Med*. 2011;12;1713–1719.

Todd KH, Samaroo N, Hoffman J. Ethnicity as a risk factor in inadequate emergency department analgesia. *JAMA*. 1993;269:1537–1539.

Webster's New International Dictionary of the English Language Unabridged. 2nd ed. Springfield, Mass: G.&C. Merriam Company; 1953.

8 CHRONIC PAIN ASSESSMENT AND MEASUREMENT

Elizabeth J. Dansie, PhD
Dennis C. Turk, PhD

EPIDEMIOLOGY

- Chronic pain is extremely prevalent and a great public health concern. The Institute of Medicine (IOM) recently estimated that more than 100 million adults in the United States experience some form of chronic pain. Experiencing symptoms of pain is the most common reason people report consulting a physician.
- Chronic pain causes moderate to severe degradation in physical, psychological, and social functioning in 40% of individuals experiencing chronic pain, as reported by the United States National Center for Health Statistics. The problem is amplified because chronic pain affects not just the individual, but also his or her significant others (eg, partners, relatives, employers, and co-workers).
- Pain is exceedingly costly to the individual with chronic pain, his or her significant others, and society. The expenses for chronic pain involve not only traditional health care, but also indirect costs such as lost productivity at work, lost tax revenue, legal services, and disability payments. The total annual costs of chronic pain in the United States are estimated to range from $550 to $625 billion per year.
- Multiple factors contribute to the chronic pain experience (eg, symptoms, emotional distress, and functional limitations), including biomedical, psychosocial, and behavioral factors.
- Although substantial advances have been made in the understanding of the neurophysiology of pain, along with the development of potent analgesic medications and innovative medical and surgical interventions, the multidimensional nature of chronic pain has made it difficult to adequately treat. The average amount of pain reduction by various procedures is only 30%–40% and occurs in less than one-half of treated patients.

COMPREHENSIVE ASSESSMENT OF THE PERSON WITH CHRONIC PAIN

- No one instrument or assessment can objectively quantify the severity or extent of a person's chronic pain experience, it is a subjective perception. Oftentimes, a biological basis for pain is difficult or impossible to ascertain, and this difficulty is compounded by psychosocial problems that can influence, amplify, maintain the experience of pain, or be caused by the presence of pain.
- A comprehensive assessment process should be performed to identify how the set of biomedical, psychosocial, and behavioral factors interact to influence the nature, magnitude, and persistence of pain and disability, and the patient's response to treatment.
- A comprehensive assessment should include:

  1. specific pain history,
  2. comprehensive medical evaluation,
  3. brief psychosocial evaluation through interviewing, and
  4. more structured assessment using self-report inventories.

- Turk and Meichenbaum suggested that three central questions should guide assessment of people who report pain:

  5. What is the extent of the patient's disease or injury (physical impairment)?

43

6. What is the magnitude of the illness? That is, to what extent is the patient suffering, disabled, and unable to enjoy usual activities?
7. Does the individual's behavior seem appropriate to the disease or injury, or is there any evidence of symptom amplification for any of a variety of psychological or social reasons?

HISTORY AND MEDICAL EXAMINATION

- The goals of the history and medical evaluation are to:

  1. determine/confirm a diagnosis,
  2. guide decisions regarding the necessity of additional diagnostic testing,
  3. determine whether biological data can explain the patient's symptoms, symptom severity, and functional limitations,
  4. establish the objectives of treatment,
  5. determine the availability of appropriate treatment, and
  6. determine the appropriate course for symptom management and longitudinal monitoring if a complete cure is not possible.

- It is insufficient to rely exclusively on a medical examination to diagnose any form of chronic pain, because agreement among physicians in interpretation of data and on the appropriate diagnosis is low, even when trained physicians are using standard mechanical devices. In addition, laboratory findings often only modestly correlate with a patient's subjective report of pain and functional limitations. When using objective measures, the presence or amount of detectable pathology is not linearly related to increases in the patient's rating of pain severity. Moreover, many patients who report persistent pain demonstrate NO physical pathology when examined using technologies such as computed axial tomography scans, magnetic resonance imaging, or electromyography.

INTERVIEW

- An essential component of a comprehensive assessment of patients with chronic pain includes a psychosocial evaluation. Research has demonstrated that preexisting psychological dysfunction may *underlie* mechanisms that maintain chronic pain symptoms, while other investigations have shown that disabling emotional symptoms have been observed in as many as 59% of people *following* initial pain onset. It is likely that the enduring nature of chronic pain is influenced by many factors, including preexisting psychological

experiences and problems, the immediate emotional reaction and subsequent coping with the initial pain onset, social and economic factors, and further medical complications that arise once chronic pain has been initiated.

- In conjunction with a detailed history and medical examination, interviewing (typically semi-structured) can be used as a tool for the psychosocial evaluation to identify potential psychosocial and behavioral factors that influence the patient's subjective reporting of pain.

- Table 8-1 summarizes key components to a brief screening interview that clinicians can use to identify important details about how the patient's pain experience in influencing their functioning (eg, physical, social, and mental) and outlook on their future pain experiences. This interviewing technique is summarized with the acronym "ACT-UP" (*Activity, Coping, Think, Upset, People's responses*). Pending the findings from this brief screening interview, patients can be referred to a mental health specialist if necessary.

- During the screening interview, clinicians should also observe the patient's nonverbal behaviors, how they interact with significant others, and how significant others may reinforce or ignore their pain behaviors, in addition to the patient's verbal responses. The emotional state of the patient, their beliefs about the cause of their pain and the implications of symptoms, and their social support system can greatly influence the extent that a patient adheres to their therapeutic pain management plan. Thus, the interviewer should become aware if there is any dissonance between the beliefs of the patient and those in their social support system and the symptoms, responses, and treatments being recommended.

- Many chronic pain patients consume various medications to help manage their symptoms that can cause side effects including fatigue, impaired sleep, and emotional distress. The interviewer should discuss the current medication regimen with the patient, and be aware of the side effects of various pain medications to help determine the origin of behaviors exhibited by the patient (eg, if side effects of the medication are mimicking depression or if mood difficulties are resultant from depression that must be treated).

TABLE 8-1   Brief Psychosocial Screening: ACT-UP

1. **Activities:** How is your pain affecting your life (ie, sleep, appetite, physical activities, and relationships)?
2. **Coping:** How do you deal/cope with your pain (what makes it better/worse)?
3. **Think:** Do you think your pain will ever get better?
4. **Upset:** Have you been feeling worried (anxious)/depressed (down, blue)?
5. **People:** How do people respond when you have pain?

STANDARDIZED SELF-REPORT INVENTORIES

- Standardized self-report measures have become the gold standard for the assessment of chronic pain, as well as many concomitant symptoms or contributing factors (eg, patients' attitudes, beliefs, symptoms, emotions, quality of life, and expectancies about themselves and the health care system). Table 8-2 provides a sample of standardized assessment tools that can be utilized for a comprehensive pain assessment.

- Standardized measures should not replace an interview, but rather be used as a complement to a thorough examination. Information from self-report measures may guide the clinician to areas that should be discussed in greater detail during interviewing or with subsequent assessment instruments.

- There are numerous advantages to standardized instruments:

  1. They are easy, efficient, and inexpensive to administer.
  2. They can be used to quickly assess a wide range of behaviors.
  3. The clinician can obtain information about behaviors that patients may feel uncomfortable discussing verbally (sexual relations) or are unobservable (thoughts, emotional arousal, etc.).
  4. The clinimetrics (ie, reliability and validity) of the instrument can be assessed.

- There are also some limitations to standardized measures to note:

  1. Patient burden when a set of excessively long measures are selected.
  2. Scoring and interpreting information obtained can be cumbersome and availability of relative comparative groups may not be existent.
  3. Entry into electronic records (although there are procedures that permit patients to directly enter data into their electronic medical records).

Pain Intensity and Quality

- Unidimensional self-report measures are often administered as a means to quickly quantify the patient's pain intensity or severity by using a single, general rating.

- When asking patients to complete a unidimensional pain rating, consideration should be given to potentially important contextual factors that can affect the rating provided by the patient, including:

  1. the level of pain severity the patient is asked to rate (eg, least pain, pain on average, and most severe pain),
  2. the specific area in which the patient is experiencing pain (eg, lower back vs. whole body pain),

TABLE 8-2 Sample of Standardized Tools for Chronic Pain Assessment

MEASURE	NO. OF ITEMS	DOMAIN ASSESSED
Unidimensional Pain Measures		
NRS	1	Pain intensity using a numbered scale
VRS	1	Pain intensity using verbal descriptors
Visual Analog Scale (VAS)	1	Pain intensity using 10 or 100 mm line, anchored by no pain and worst possible pain.
Pain Quality and Location		
Short-form McGill Pain Questionnaire-2 (SF-MPQ)	22	Pain quality, location, exacerbating, and ameliorating factors
Pain Interference and Function: General		
Pain Disability Index (PDI)	7	Pain disability and interference of pain in functional, family, and social domains
Brief Pain Index (BPI)	32	Pain intensity and interference of pain with functional activities
PROMIS Pain Interference and Pain Behaviors item banks	Interference Bank = 41; Behaviors Bank = 39	Pain interference and behaviors related to the impact of pain
Pain Interference and Function: Disease Specific		
Western Ontario MacMaster Osteoarthritis Index (WOMAC)	24	Pain and function in people with osteoarthritis
Roland-Morris Disability Questionnaire (RDQ)	24	Pain and disability for people with back pain
HRQOL		
Medical Outcomes Study Short Form Health Survey (SF-36)	36	Mental and physical health
West Haven-Yale Multidimensional Pain Inventory (MPI)	60	Pain severity, interference, responses by others, activities
Psychosocial Measures		
Beck Depression Inventory (BDI)	21	Depression
GAD-7	7	Generalized anxiety
Pain Catastrophizing Scale (PCS)	13	Catastrophic thoughts related to pain
Coping Strategies Questionnaire (CSQ)	10	Coping strategies for chronic pain

  3. the time frame that patients are asked to recall upon when reporting their pain (eg, pain at that moment or pain over the past 7 days), and
  4. context (eg, at rest, time of day, and response to specific activities).

- The most commonly used unidimensional pain intensity scales are numerical rating scales (NRS) that ask the patient to "Rate your typical pain on a scale from 0 to 10 where 0 equals no pain and 10 is the worst pain you can imagine," and verbal rating scales (VRS) that use verbal descriptors and ask the patient to report "Is your usual level of pain 'mild', 'moderate', or 'severe?'" Both types of measures demonstrate acceptable reliability, validity, and responsivity to detecting change in pain intensity due to treatment.

- Concern has been expressed that retrospective reports may not be valid and suffer from recall bias, as they may reflect current pain severity that serves as an anchor for recall of pain severity over some interval. To overcome the potential biases inherent in single, one-time ratings of pain intensity, patients may be asked to maintain diaries of pain intensity with ratings recorded several times each day (eg, meals and bed time) for several days or weeks, with multiple pain ratings averaged across time. Daily paper-and-pencil diaries are not without their limitations, because patients may not follow the instructions to provide ratings at specified intervals and instead may complete diaries in advance ("fill forward") or shortly before seeing a clinician ("fill backward"). Electronic diaries (eg, smart phone applications and internet accessed) that provide time-stamped data are gaining interest but at this time are primarily used for research.

- Pain severity varies for many people who experience chronic pain and is modified by various factors. Clinicians should determine if, when, and what factors may lead to worsening and reductions in pain intensity, by asking questions such as:

  5. Are there specific times when your pain is worse (eg, morning)?
  6. Are there specific activities that lead to an increase in pain symptoms?
  7. Are their certain circumstances that contribute to exacerbation of pain, such as stress (including interpersonal conflicts and specific activities)?
  8. Do certain medications, prolonged rest or activity, or heat or cold lead to increase or decrease in pain?

- Pain is known to have different sensory and affective qualities. Understanding the quality and characteristics (eg, aching and stabbing) of a patient's pain through assessment can identify treatments that are effective for certain types of pain independent of pain severity. For example, the Short-form McGill Pain Questionnaire-2 assesses word descriptors of pain qualities—sensory, affective, and evaluative—that have been associated with different types of pain (eg, neuropathic, musculoskeletal pain, and visceral).

Pain Interference with Function and Quality of Life

- Focus groups of people with persistent pain indicate that they view their overall physical functioning as degraded due to their pain, supporting the recommendation that an assessment of functioning should accompany pain assessment. The ability (or inability) to perform necessary and desired functions, in turn, can significantly affect overall health-related quality of life (HRQOL). The impact of chronic pain on function can be subdivided into assessments of:

  1. *Physical capacity.* The physical capacities of pain patients are typically assessed using evaluation protocols by a physical therapist in a clinical setting working with the clinician, and this information is typically used to plan a rehabilitative treatment program. Briefly, the clinician can ask about limitations in functional activities (eg, sitting, standing, walking, bending, lying down; specific household chores, work, or recreational activities).

  2. *Ability to function in important roles like work.* Ideally, a vocational rehabilitation counselor would perform a comprehensive evaluation to assess vocational disability, but this responsibility typically falls upon the clinician. Clinicians should determine whether the patient is currently working, and if so, what activities are required by the job. If the patient is not working, the clinician should determine whether this is due to a health-related disability, how long the person has been unemployed, and whether the patient is receiving work disability benefits. If the patient is retired, the clinician should inquire about the impact of pain on routine home-making activities.

  3. *Ability to perform activities of daily living.* Various self-report functional status measures have been developed to assess patients' reports of their abilities to engage in a range of functional activities (eg, walk up stairs, to sit for specific periods of time, lift specific weights, and performance of activities of daily living), as well as the severity of the pain experienced after performing these activities. In addition, multiple well-established, psychometrically supported general and disease-specific HRQOL measures have been developed to assess quality of life and the impact of disability on quality of life.

Emotional Distress and Coping

- Multiple studies have demonstrated that chronic pain is strongly associated with emotional distress, particularly depression, anxiety, anger, and fear of future pain. A challenge arises with assessing chronic pain patients who present with symptoms of emotional distress like fatigue, reduced physical activity, decreased libido, appetite change, sleep disturbance, weight gain or loss, and memory and concentration deficits, because these indications are also symptoms of pain conditions or side effects of treatment medications prescribed to relieve pain.

- Many patients with chronic pain, especially those who attribute their symptoms to trauma, are fearful of engaging in activities they believe may contribute to further injury or exacerbate their symptoms. Avoidance of activities may, in the short term, lead to symptom reduction, but over time, activity restriction is likely to lead to muscle deconditioning, foreshortening, and bone demineralization with a resultant decreased functional capacities.
- Self-report instruments have been developed specifically for pain patients to assess psychological distress, the impact of pain on patients' lives, feeling of control, fear of activity, coping behaviors, and attitudes about disease and pain. For example, the Patient Health Questionnaire-9 (PHQ-9) and Generalized Anxiety Disorder-7 (GAD-7) scales are psychometrically sound for assessing symptoms of depression or anxiety.

OVERT EXPRESSIONS OF PAIN

- Patients display a broad range of controllable and uncontrollable nonverbal responses that communicate to others that they are experiencing pain, distress, and suffering. Using these behaviors, patients are capable of eliciting responses from significant others (including health care providers), and these responses can contribute to the maintenance of behaviors when they receive attention and are reinforced in other ways (eg, cues to take medication and avoid activity).
- A clinician can informally observe a patient's behaviors during interviews and examinations, but should also examine the patient in other contexts whenever possible. When patients know they are being observed and are presenting information to a health care provider, they may use nonverbal behaviors to convey information in ways most likely to support the impact of their symptoms. For example, they may feel a need to convince the health care provider of the severity of their symptoms, functional limitations, and distress. Thus, observing the patient in the waiting room or when ambulating to the examination room may allow the clinician to establish the stability and consistency of pain behaviors.
- Investigation into the patient's health care and medication usage patterns can be used to assess pain behaviors, where diaries can be completed to track the frequency and quantity of medications, as well as

antecedent and consequent events of medication use (eg, stress and activity) that may be associated with factors other than pain.

ASSESSING RISK FOR OPIOID MISUSE AND ABUSE

- The rates of opioid abuse and misuse have increased dramatically since the mid-1990s, in conjunction with increasing rates of opioid prescribing for the management of chronic noncancer pain. Thus, it is essential that health care providers assess a patient's risk for addiction and aberrant medication-related behaviors before placing a patient on long-term opioid therapy.
- The self-report measure known as the Screener and Opioid Assessment for Patients with Pain (SOAPP) was developed to enable providers to identify chronic pain patients who may develop problems with opioid misuse and abuse. Once at-risk patients are identified, it may be necessary for the provider to devise a plan to closely monitor such patients while undergoing long-term opioid therapy or refer the patient to a pain specialist.

BIBLIOGRAPHY

Amtmann D, Cook KF, Jensen MP, et al. Development of a PROMIS item bank to measure pain interference. *Pain.* 2010;150:173–182.

Bellamy N, Buchanan WW, Goldsmith CH, Campbell J, Stitt LW. Validation study of WOMAC: a health status instrument for measuring clinically important patient relevant outcomes to antirheumatic drug therapy in patients with osteoarthritis of the hip or knee. *J Rheumatol.* 1988;15:1833–1840.

Butler SF, Budman SH, Fernandez K, Jamison RN. Validation of a screener and opioid assessment measure for patients with chronic pain. *Pain.* 2004;112:65–75.

Cleeland CS, Ryan KM. Pain assessment: global use of the Brief Pain Inventory. *Ann Acad Med Singapore.* 1994;23:129–138.

de Winter AF, Heemskerk MA, Terwee CB, et al. Inter-observer reproducibility of measurements of range of motion in patients with shoulder pain using a digital inclinometer. *BMC Musculoskelet Disord.* 2004;5:18.

Dworkin RH, Turk DC, Revicki DA, et al. Development and initial validation of an expanded and revised version of the Short-form McGill Pain Questionnaire (SF-MPQ-2). *Pain.* 2009;144:35–42.

Fordyce WE. *Behavioral Methods for Chronic Pain and Illness.* St. Louis, Mo: Mosby; 1976.

Gay JR, Abbott KH. Common whiplash injuries of the neck. *J Am Med Assoc.* 1953;152:1698–1704.

Gendreau M, Hufford MR, Stone AA. Measuring clinical pain in chronic widespread pain: selected methodological issues. *Best Pract Res Clin Rheumatol.* 2003;17:575–592.

Hing E, Hall MJ, Xu J. National Hospital Ambulatory Medical Care Survey: 2006 outpatient department summary. *Natl Health Stat Rep.* 2008:1–31.

Hurst NP, Kind P, Ruta D, Hunter M, Stubbings A. Measuring health-related quality of life in rheumatoid arthritis: validity, responsiveness and reliability of EuroQol (EQ-5D). *Br J Rheumatol.* 1997;36:551–559.

Institute of Medicine, Commitee on Advancing Pain Research Care, and Education. *Relieving Pain in America: A Blueprint for Transforming Prevention, Care, Education, and Research.* Washington, DC: National Academy Press; 2011.

Jensen MP, Karoly P, Braver S. The measurement of clinical pain intensity: a comparison of six methods. *Pain.* 1986;27:117–126.

Jensen MP, Karoly P. Self-report scales and procedures for assessing pain in adults. *Handbook of Pain Assessment.* 3rd ed. New York, NY: Guildford Press; 2011:19–41.

Kroenke K, Price RK. Symptoms in the community. Prevalence, classification, and psychiatric comorbidity. *Arch Intern Med.* 1993;153:2474–2480.

Kroenke K, Spitzer RL, Williams JB. The PHQ-9: validity of a brief depression severity measure. *J Gen Intern Med.* 2001;16:606–613.

National Center for Health Statistics. *Health, United States, 2006 with Chartbook on Trends in the Health of Americans.* Hyattsville, MD: National Center for Health Statistics; 2006.

Pollard CA. Preliminary validity study of the Pain Disability Index. *Percept Mot Skills.* 1984;59:974.

Price DD, Bush FM, Long S, Harkins SW. A comparison of pain measurement characteristics of mechanical visual analogue and simple numerical rating scales. *Pain.* 1994;56:217–226.

Revicki DA, Chen WH, Harnam N, et al. Development and psychometric analysis of the PROMIS pain behavior item bank. *Pain.* 2009;146:158–169.

Roland M, Morris R. A study of the natural history of back pain. Part I: development of a reliable and sensitive measure of disability in low-back pain. *Spine.* 1983;8:141–144.

Rosenstiel AK, Keefe FJ. The use of coping strategies in chronic low-back-pain patients—relationship to patient characteristics and current adjustment. *Pain.* 1983;17:33–44.

Spitzer RL, Kroenke K, Williams JB, Lowe B. A brief measure for assessing generalized anxiety disorder: the GAD-7. *Arch Intern Med.* 2006;166:1092–1097.

Sullivan MJL, Bishop SR, Pivik J. The Pain Catastrophizing Scale: development and validation. *Psychol Assessment.* 1995;7:524–532.

Turk DC, Dworkin RH, Revicki D, et al. Identifying important outcome domains for chronic pain clinical trials: an IMMPACT survey of people with pain. *Pain.* 2008;137:276–285.

Turk DC, Meichenbaum D. A cognitive-behavioral approach to pain management. Textbook of Pain. New York, NY: Churchill-Livingstone; 1984:787–794.

Turk DC, Melzack R. *Handbook of Pain Assessment.* 3rd ed. New York, NY: Guilford Press; 2011.

Turk DC, Okifuji A. Psychological factors in chronic pain: evolution and revolution. *J Consult Clin Psychol.* 2002;70:678–690.

Turk DC, Rudy TE. Toward a comprehensive assessment of chronic pain patients: a multiaxial approach. *Behav Res Ther.* 1987;25:237–249.

Turk DC, Wilson HD, Cahana A. Treatment of chronic non-cancer pain. *Lancet.* 2011;377:2226–2235.

Ware JE Jr., Sherbourne CD. The MOS 36-item short-form health survey (SF-36). I. Conceptual framework and item selection. *Med Care.* 1992;30:473–483.

9 HISTORY AND PHYSICAL EXAMINATION

Zahid Bajwa, MD

INITIAL EVALUATION

- The importance of initial evaluation in improving outcomes in pain management cannot be overstated. This evaluation is a golden opportunity to become acquainted with a patient and develop an understanding of their condition.
- By eliciting useful information and examining the patient in an orderly and logical manner, the diagnosis or a short differential list can usually be made, leading to effective management plan.
- In Western countries, the prevalence of chronic pain in the adult population ranges from 2% to 40%.
- The estimated cost of chronic back pain exceeds $33.6 billion for health care, $11 to $43 billion for disability compensation, $4.6 billion for lost productivity, and $5 billion in legal costs.

HISTORY

CHIEF COMPLAINT

- Transcribe the chief complaint succinctly using the patient's own words.
- Include the patient's expectations and goals.

HISTORY OF PRESENT ILLNESS

- A thorough history should document and characterize all potential pain symptoms.
- Date of onset: atraumatic versus traumatic, acute versus insidious.
- Character and severity of the pain: achy, allodynic (non-noxious stimuli become painful), burning, dull, dysesthesia (unpleasant abnormal sensation), hyperalgesia (increased response to a painful stimuli), lancinating, sharp, shooting, electric (Neuralgic), paresthesia (abnormal sensation), and neuralgia/mononeuropathy (pain in a distribution of a nerve).

- Location of pain in its entirety.
- Associated features, including other neurologic symptoms, such as weakness, numbness, motor control, and balance problems.
- Aggravating and alleviating factors (what makes this pain better or worse).
- Chronicity.
- Previous diagnostic tests and therapeutic treatments, including results and responses.
- Document litigation or secondary gain issues. The current U.S. compensation system can promote pain behavior patterns in the injured worker, which is why an early and accurate diagnosis with appropriate intervention is essential.
- Document functional losses resulting from the pain or injury and the use of assistive devices. Include changes in mobility, cognition, and activities of daily living: household arrangements, community, and vocational activities.
- Explore the history in detail and document inconsistencies in the patient's reported mechanism of injury or complaints.
- Rule out potential surgical emergencies, such as unstable fractures and aggressively progressing neurologic symptoms that may be associated with cauda equina syndrome.

MEDICAL AND SURGICAL HISTORY

- Sometimes the etiology of pain may be uncovered by a thorough review of prior medical illnesses and its treatment, trauma, and surgical interventions, including subsequent outcomes.

PSYCHOSOCIAL HISTORY

- The psychosocial history provides vital information necessary for understanding how pain is affecting the patient and his or her family. Roles may change and new stressors may alter family dynamics, which may influence the outcome of any treatment program.
- A history of substance abuse (alcohol, tobacco, or illegal drugs) may raise the suspicion of drug-seeking behavior and secondary gain. Early identification of actual or potential substance abuse issues allows for the appropriate treatment of pain and associated symptoms.
- Identify a primary caregiver, when appropriate, and family and friends who are able and willing to provide support.
- Identify housing or other living conditions that may exacerbate the pain for modification as appropriate.

- Restrictions in the ability to participate in previous hobbies and social activities can be stressful to a patient. Return to these activities should be a goal of an interdisciplinary treatment program. Feasible substitute hobbies should be identified in the interim.
- Psychiatric problems, such as depression, anxiety, and sleep disorders, can have a major negative influence on an individual's motivation and ability to participate in a treatment program. The stress of a new pain condition or injury can trigger a recurrence of a previous psychiatric problem. Supportive psychotherapy and the appropriate use of psychiatric medications can prevent or treat problems that could interfere with successful pain management.
- Loss of income due to a new pain condition or injury can precipitate a psychiatric crisis. Early identification of any number of such issues should trigger a behavioral medicine referral.

VOCATIONAL HISTORY AND BACK PAIN

- In a study by Suter, the risk of back injury was greater in those below the age of 25 years, but the greatest number of compensation claims occurred in workers between 30 and 40 years of age.
- Handling materials, especially lifting associated with bending or twisting, is the most common work activity associated with back injuries.
- In a study of sewage workers with low back pain, work disability increased with age, the weekly duration of stooping and lifting in the previous 5 years, and high illness–behavior scores.
- Occupations with the largest incidences of back injuries for which the workers receive compensation include machine operation, truck driving, and nursing.
- Factors in the work environment that are associated with the potential for delayed recovery include job satisfaction; monotonous, boring, or repetitious work; new employment; and recent poor job rating by a supervisor.

MEDICATIONS AND ALLERGIES

- Obtain a complete list of prescribed and over-the-counter medications and "home remedies" that are being taken or were taken to manage the pain symptoms. (A recent study revealed that 14% of the U.S. population uses herbal treatments, and 26% of Americans use vitamins regularly.)
- Review this list for each medication's indication, dosage, duration, effectiveness, and side effects.
- Reduction or avoidance of medications with unwanted cognitive and physical side effects is recommended.

FAMILY HISTORY

- Always review the medical history of family members and relatives so as not to miss genetic diseases, some of which include pain in their symptom complex.

REVIEW OF SYSTEMS

- A comprehensive review of systems may uncover problems not previously noted that may be related to the pain condition or can affect the clinical outcome. Follow history-taking format to inquire about problems in all systems of the body including psychiatric, cardiovascular, pulmonary, gastrointestinal, neurologic, rheumatologic, genitourinary, endocrine, and musculoskeletal symptoms.
- Constitutional symptoms, such as unexpected weight loss, low-grade fever, and night sweats, require further investigation.

PAIN SCALES

- Pain diagrams (Figure 9-1) are helpful in visualizing the patient's symptoms.
- Other pain and functional scales include the visual analog scale (VAS; Figure 9-2), the Oswestry Disability Questionnaire, and the Short Form-36 Quality of Life Scale.

Please draw the location of your pain on the diagram below. Mark painful areas as follows:

000 = pins and needles   /// = "lightning" or "shooting" pain   TTT = throbbing
xxx = sharp pain   AAA = aching pain

Feel free to use other symbols or words as necessary.

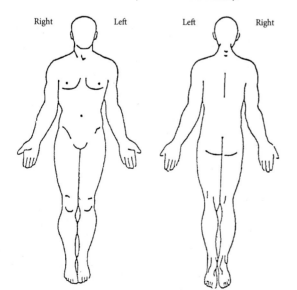

FIG. 9-1. Pain diagram.

Please rate the intensity of your pain by making a mark on this scale

NO PAIN ——————————————————— WORST
                                                          PAIN
                                                          IMAGINABLE

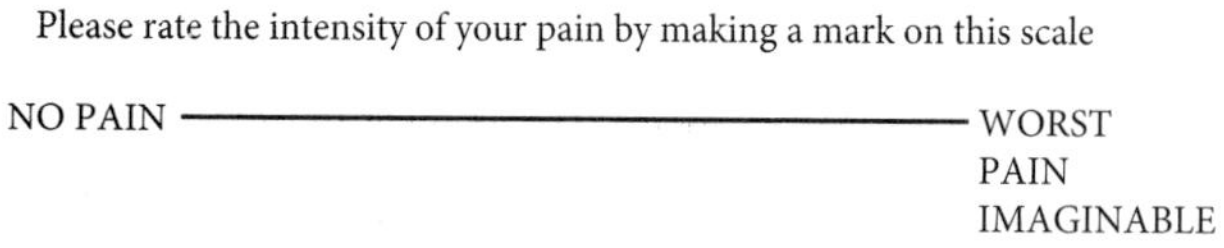

FIG. 9-2. Visual analog scale.

PHYSICAL EXAMINATION

GENERAL

- The patient should be appropriately gowned to allow proper visualization of any pertinent areas during the examination. Use a chaperone as appropriate.
- Record the patient's temperature, blood pressure, pulse, height, and weight during each evaluation. Remember pain is considered the fifth vital sign, and should be recorded.
- Examine the patient's entire body for any skin lesions, such as surgical scars, hyperpigmentation, ulcerations, and needle marks. In addition, look for bony malalignments or areas of muscle atrophy, fasciculations, discoloration, and edema.

MENTAL STATUS

- A thorough mental status evaluation should include a mini-mental examination to assess the patient's orientation; immediate, short, and long-term memory; comprehension; and cognition.
- Assess the patient's emotional well-being, including concurrent signs of depression, hopelessness, or anxiety.

JOINT EXAMINATION

- Always examine both sides of the patient to detect any asymmetries.
- Record the active motion of all joints, noting any obvious limitations, dyskinesis, grimacing, or asymmetry.
- Record the passive range of pertinent joints or joints that appear abnormal during active testing, once again noting limitations, grimacing, or asymmetry.
- Palpate each joint to assess for specific areas of pain and tenderness.
- Joint stability testing identifies underlying ligamentous injuries.

MOTOR EXAMINATION

- Document manual muscle testing as outlined below, noting any give-away pain. Be sure to test all myotomal levels to help distinguish peripheral nerve lesion from plexus or root injuries (Tables 9-1 and 9-2).

GRADE	DEFINITION
5	Complete joint range of motion against gravity with full resistance
4	Complete joint range of motion against gravity with moderate resistance
3	Full joint range of motion against gravity
2	Full joint range of motion with gravity eliminated
1	Visible or palpable muscle contraction; no joint motion produced
0	No visible or palpable muscle contraction

TABLE 9-1   Upper Extremity Muscles and Nerve Innervation

MUSCLE	NERVE	ROOT	TRUNK	DIVISION	CORD
Trapezius	Spinal accessory	C2,C3,C4			
Rhomboid	Dorsal scapular	C4,C5			
Serratus anterior	Long thoracic	C5,C6,C7,C8			
Supraspinatus	Suprascapular	C4,C5,C6	Upper		
Infraspinatus	Suprascapular	C5,C6	Upper		
Pectoralis major	Medial/lateral pectoral	C5–T1	U/M/L	Anterior	Medial/lateral
Pectoralis minor	Medial pectoral	C7,C8,T1	U/M/L	Anterior	Medial/lateral
Latissmus dorsi	Thoracodorsal	C6,C7,C8	U/M/L	Posterior	Posterior
Teres major	Lower subscapular	C5,C6,C7	Upper	Posterior	Posterior
Teres minor	Axillary	C5,C6	Upper	Posterior	Posterior
Deltoid	Axillary	C5,C6	Upper	Posterior	Posterior
Biceps	Musculocutaneous	C5,C6	Upper	Anterior	Lateral
Triceps	Radial	C6,C7,C8,T1	Middle/lower	Posterior	Posterior
Anconeus	Radial	C7,C8	Middle/lower	Posterior	Posterior
Brachioradialis	Radial	C5,C6	Upper	Posterior	Posterior
Supinator	Radial (post. inter.)	C5,C6	Upper	Posterior	Posterior
ECR	Radial (post. inter.)	C5,C6,C7,C8	Upper/middle	Posterior	Posterior
EDC	Radial (post. inter.)	C6,C7,C8	Middle/lower	Posterior	Posterior
EIP	Radial (post. inter.)	C6,C7,C8	Middle/lower	Posterior	Posterior
Pronator teres	Median	C6,C7	Middle/lower	Anterior	Lateral
FCR	Median	C6,C7,C8	U/M/L	Anterior	Medial/lateral
FPL	Median (ant. inter.)	C7,C8,T1	Middle/lower	Anterior	Medial/lateral
FDS	Median	C7,C8,T1	Middle/lower	Anterior	Medial/lateral
FDP (Nos. 1,2)	Median (ant. inter.)	C7,C8,T1	Middle/lower	Anterior	Medial
Pronator quadratus	Median (ant. inter.)	C7,C8,T1	Middle/lower	Anterior	Medial/lateral
APB	Median	C6,C7,C8,T1	Lower	Anterior	Medial
Opponens pollicis	Median	C6,C7,C8,T1	Lower	Anterior	Medial
FPB (sup.)	Median	C6,C7,C8,T1	Lower	Anterior	Medial
FCU	Ulnar	C7,C8,T1	Lower	Anterior	Medial
FDP (Nos. 3,4)	Ulnar	C8,T1	Middle/lower	Anterior	Medial
AbDM	Ulnar	C8,T1	Lower	Anterior	Medial
Interossei	Ulnar	C8,T1	Lower	Anterior	Medial
FPB (deep)	Ulnar	C8,T1	Lower	Anterior	Medial

ECR, extensor carpi radialis; EDC, extensor digitorum communis; EIP, extensor indicis proprius; FCR, flexor carpi radialis; FPL, flexor policis longus; FDS, flexor digitorum superficialis; FDP, flexor digitorum profundus; APB, abductor policis brevis; FPB, flexor policis brevis; FCU, flexor carpiulnaris; AbBM, abductor digiti minimi; sup., superior; post., posterior; ant., anterior; inter., interosseous.

TABLE 9-2   Lower Extremity Muscles and Nerve Innervation

MUSCLE	NERVE	ROOT
Psoas major	Ventral primary rami	L2,L3,L4
Iliacus	Femoral	L2,L3,L4
Sartorius	Femoral	L2,L3,L4
Quadriceps femoris	Femoral	L2,L3,L4
Hip adductors	Obturator	L2,L3,L4
Adductor magnus	Sciatic (tibial)	L2,L3,L4,L5,S1
	Obturator	
Piriformis	Nerve to piriformis	S1,S2
Gluteus minimus	Superior gluteal	L4,L5,S1
Gluteus medius	Superior gluteal	L4,L5,S1
Gluteus maximus	Inferior gluteal	L5,S1,S2
Hamstrings	Sciatic (tibial)	L4,L5,S1,S2
Biceps femoris (SH)	Sciatic (peroneal)	L5,S1,S2
Peroneii	Superficial peroneal	L4,L5,S1
Tibialis anterior	Deep peroneal	L4,L5,S1
Extensor hallucis longus	Deep peroneal	L4,L5,S1
Extensor digitorum brevis	Deep peroneal	L4,L5,S1
Tibialis posterior	Tibial	L5,S1
Soleus	Tibial	L5,S1,S2
Gastrocnemius	Tibial	S1,S2
Abductor halluces	Tibial (medial plantar)	L4,L5,S1
Flexor digitorum brevis	Tibial (medial plantar)	L4,L5,S1
Flexor hallucis brevis	Tibial (medial plantar)	L4,L5,S1
Abductor digiti minimi	Tibial (lateral plantar)	S1,S2
Interossei	Tibial (lateral plantar)	S1,S2

SENSORY EXAMINATION

- A thorough sensory examination requires testing light touch, pin prick, vibration, and joint position, as certain fibers or columns may be preferentially affected. Be sure to test all dermatomal levels (Figure 9-3).

OTHER NEUROLOGIC EXAMINATIONS

- Evaluate cranial nerves II through XII, especially in the setting of headache, cervical, and facial pain.
- Check muscle stretch reflexes commonly known as deep tendon reflexes (Table 9-3), noting asymmetry and clonus. Clonus is defined by more than four muscle contractions following a stimulus.
- Check for the presence of Babinski plantar reflex and Hoffman thumb reflex, both of which may be present in an upper motor neuron syndrome. Cervical spondylosis may show a negative Hoffman sign and

a positive Babinski sign depending on the location of the signature lesion.

- Assess the patient's gait and identify cerebellar deficits by asking the patient to do dysmetric tests (finger-to-nose motion and heel-to-shin motion), rapid alternating movement of the fingers and hand (dysdiadochokinesia), and balance tests with the eyes open and closed.

Romberg test can be used to determine whether ataxia is due to sensory versus cerebellar disturbances. Ataxia with a positive Romberg test suggests a sensory disturbance (ie, loss of proprioception or dorsal column injury). Ataxia with a negative Romberg test suggests a cerebellar disturbance. Romberg test is performed by asking the patient to stand and close their eyes. Loss of balance is a positive Romberg test.

SPECIAL TESTS

- Wadell et al. described five nonorganic signs that help identify patients with physical symptoms without clear anatomic etiology. They identified a constellation of hypochondriasis, hysteria, and depression in patients with three of the five signs. These five signs help indicate when factors other than anatomic concerns should be addressed:
- superficial or nonanatomic distribution of tenderness,
- nonanatomic (regional) motor or sensory impairment,
- excessive verbalization of pain or gesturing (overreaction),
- production of pain complaints by tests that simulate only a specific movement (simulation), and
- inconsistent reports of pain when the same movement is carried out in different positions (distraction).

CONCLUSION

- A detailed history, and physical examination with emphasis on neurologic and musculoskeletal examination, provides foundation for the proper diagnosis of pain patients.
- Such an evaluation must include physical, emotional, and psychosocial factors.
- When developing a treatment plan, a physician should understand the patient's goals.

ACKNOWLEDGMENTS

The authors would like to thank Tania H. Bajwa for editorial assistance on this chapter.

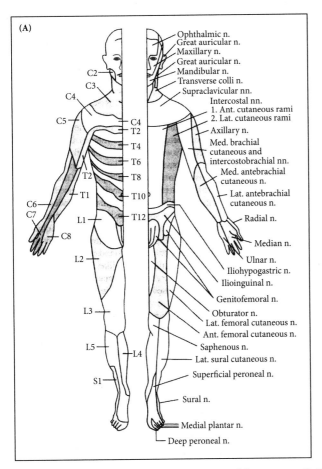
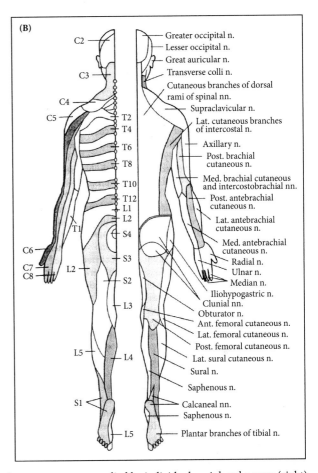

FIG. 9-3. Anterior (A) and Posterior (B) view of dermatomes (left) and cutaneous areas supplied by individual peripheral nerves (right). Modified, with permission, from Carpenter MB, Sutin J. Human Neuroanatomy. 8th ed. Baltimore, Md: Williams & Wilkins; 1983.

TABLE 9-3   Muscle Stretch Reflexes

MUSCLE STRETCH REFLEX	SPINAL SEGMENT
Biceps	C5
Brachioradialis	C6
Triceps	C7
Patella tendon	L4
Medial hamstring	L5
Achilles	S1

BIBLIOGRAPHY

Adapted from Members of the Department of Neurology, Mayo Clinic and Mayo Clinic Foundation for Medical Education and Research. *Clinical Examination in Neurology*. 6th ed. Philadelphia, Pa: Saunders; 1991.

Bigos SJ, Spengler DM, Martin NA, et al. Back injuries in industry: a retrospective study. III. Employee-related factors. *Spine*. 1986;11:252.

Carpenter MB, Sutin J. *Human Neuroanatomy*. 8th ed Baltimore, MD: Williams & Wilkins; 1983.

Friedrich M, Cermak T, Heiller I. Spinal troubles in sewage workers: epidemiological data and work disability due to low back pain. *Int Arch Occup Environ Health*. 2000;73:245.

Frymoyer J, Durett C. The economics of spinal disorders. In: Frymoyer J, ed. *The Adult Spine*. Philadelphia, Pa: Lippincott–Raven; 1997:143.

Kaufman DW, Kelly, JP, Rosenberg L, et al. Recent patterns of medication use in the ambulatory adult population of the United States: the Slone survey. *JAMA*. 2002;287:337.

Linton SJ. A review of psychological risk factors in back and neck pain. *Spine*. 2000;25:1148.

Suter PB. Employment and litigation: improved by work, assisted by verdict. *Pain*. 2002;100:249.

Verhaak PFM, Kerssens JJ, Dekker J, et al. Prevalence of chronic benign pain disorder among adults: a review of the literature. *Pain*. 1998;77:231.

Wadell G, McCulloh JA, Kummel E, et al. Nonorganic physical signs in low-back pain. *Spine*. 1980;5:117.

Walker WC, Cifu DX, Gardner M, et al. Functional assessment in patients with chronic pain: can physicians predict performance? *Am J Phys Med Rehabil*. 2001;80:162.

10 ELECTROMYOGRAPHY AND NERVE CONDUCTION STUDIES*

Nathan J. Rudin, MD, MA

OBJECTIVES

This article is intended to:

- Familiarize the reader with the basic principles of electrodiagnostic testing.
- Provide the basic knowledge necessary to interpret an electrodiagnostic report.
- Teach when and how to utilize electrodiagnostic testing in patients with pain.

GLOSSARY

- *Action potential.* The electrical phenomenon generated by threshold or suprathreshold depolarization of a nerve cell or muscle cell.
- *Antidromic.* Moving in the opposite direction from normal physiologic function.
- *Compound muscle action potential* (CMAP). The potential generated by a muscle when its supplying motor nerve is stimulated; formed by the summation of multiple motor unit action potentials (see below).
- *Fibrillation potential.* A type of spontaneous activity.
- *Insertional activity.* The brief burst of electrical activity following movement of a needle electrode within muscle; may be increased in irritable or damaged muscle and decreased in fibrotic muscle.
- *Motor unit.* A motor neuron and the group of muscle fibers it supplies.
- *Motor unit action potential* (MUAP). The potential generated by the firing of a single motor unit.
- *Nerve conduction velocity* (NCV). Speed of nerve conduction in meters per second; can be calculated during nerve conduction studies (NCS).
- *Orthodromic.* Moving in the direction typical of normal physiologic function.
- *Phase.* The portion of a (MUAP) waveform existing between departure from and return to baseline.
- *Positive sharp wave.* A type of spontaneous activity.
- *Recruitment.* Characteristic firing pattern of motor units during voluntary muscle contraction; units are added in a predictable fashion as the strength of contraction increases.

---

*Dr. Rudin has no financial affiliations or conflicts of interests to disclose.

- *Sensory nerve action potential* (SNAP). The potential generated in a sensory nerve when it is stimulated.
- *Spontaneous activity.* Electrical potentials occurring in a skeletal muscle in the absence of voluntary effort; almost always an indicator of abnormality.

ELECTRODIAGNOSTIC TESTING

- Electrodiagnostic testing is an extension of the history interview and physical examination.
  - o It can help explain the causes of acute or chronic pain.
  - o It can identify focal or diffuse areas of nerve and muscle injury.
  - o It can identify or rule out processes amenable to rehabilitation, injection therapy, surgery, or drug therapy.
  - o It can significantly narrow a differential diagnosis or confirm a diagnosis.
  - o It supplements information gleaned from imaging studies.
  - o By defining the type and extent of injury, it can provide prognostic information.
  - o Serial examinations can be useful in monitoring recovery and therapeutic outcome.
- The two basic components of electrodiagnostic testing are *NCS* and *needle electromyography* (EMG).

NERVE CONDUCTION STUDIES

NCSs permit the noninvasive assessment of nerve physiology and function.

- Slowed conduction velocity or delayed response latency may reflect injury to myelin.
- Diminished response amplitude or temporally dispersed waveforms may reflect axonal injury or loss.
- The distribution of abnormalities can differentiate between focal and diffuse neuropathic processes.

INDICATIONS

- Suspected nerve entrapments or other mononeuropathies.
- Suspected polyneuropathies.
- Suspected radiculopathy or plexopathy.
- Suspected neuromuscular junction disease.

CONTRAINDICATIONS/CAUTIONS

- Avoid electrical stimulation over or near a pacemaker, automatic implantable cardioverter/defibrillator (AICD), spinal cord stimulator, intrathecal drug delivery pump, or other electrosensitive implant. Stimulation distant from the implant does not usually pose a problem for the patient. If needed, check with the device manufacturer before testing.

- Marked edema, morbid obesity, or skin damage may impede both nerve stimulation and signal pickup.

GENERAL PRINCIPLES

- A pickup electrode is placed over the desired recording area, and a reference electrode is placed nearby. A ground electrode is also affixed to the patient.
- The nerve is electrically stimulated to generate an action potential, which is propagated down the nerve and detected at the pickup electrode.
- Electrical stimulation is delivered as a short-duration shock (generally 0.1–0.2 ms), usually perceived as mildly uncomfortable. Transcutaneous stimulation is most often used. The practitioner can also use a fine needle to stimulate deeper nerves. Stimulation is performed at a standard distance from the active electrode.
- Stimulation may be repeated at a different point along the nerve to measure conduction characteristics along a particular nerve segment. This may help to identify focal lesions.
- Potentials are recorded, visually displayed, and analyzed.
- Action potential latency (time for stimulus-generated potential to reach the active electrode) and amplitude are measured. NCV is calculated.
- Each laboratory should consistently use the same techniques and compare results against the same preestablished norms, permitting meaningful data interpretation and comparison.

STUDY TYPES

- Motor NCSs (MNCS; Figure 10-1) measure the CMAP produced by depolarization of muscle fibers in response to electrical stimulation. CMAP is recorded using electrodes positioned over the muscle of interest.
- Sensory nerve conduction studies (SNCS; Figure 10-2) measure the SNAP produced as depolarization propagates along nerve. SNAP is recorded using electrodes positioned directly over the nerve, at a point distal or proximal to the stimulation site.

LIMITATIONS

- NCSs measure only the fastest-conducting fibers; injury to the smallest (unmyelinated or lightly myelinated) fibers, such as those mediating pain and temperature sensation, may go undetected. It is therefore possible

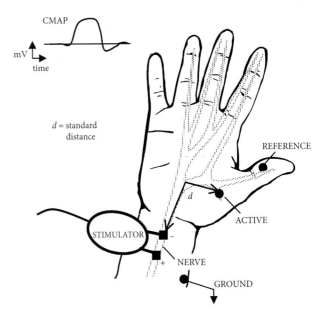

FIG. 10-1. Median motor nerve conduction study. The active electrode is placed over the belly of the muscle to be studied. The reference electrode is placed over an electrically neutral landmark, in this case the Interphalangeal joint of the thumb. Transcutaneous electrical stimulation is applied over the nerve at a standard distance (*d*) from the active electrode. CMAP is detected at the active electrode, amplified, and displayed (upper left). CMAP amplitude and onset latency are recorded and compared with laboratory norms. NCV cannot be calculated over this most distal segment of the nerve because it includes the time for transmission at the neuromuscular junction. One can calculate the NCV over more proximal segments by stimulating proximally to the wrist, measuring inter-stimulus distance, and subtracting distal from proximal latency.

to miss a small-fiber neuropathy using standard NCSs. Small-fiber neuropathy may be evaluated more sensitively using quantitative sensory testing (QST) or skin punch biopsy with stain for peripheral nerve fibers.

- NCS results, particularly for SNCSs, are sensitive to temperature. If the skin and underlying nerves are too cool, conduction velocity and response latency may be slowed, but amplitude may paradoxically increase. Skin should be warmed (to at least 32°C for upper limbs, 30°C for lower limbs) prior to testing.
- SNCSs assess the function of primary afferent neurons, that is, the pathway distal to the dorsal root ganglion (DRG). In radiculopathies, where injury often occurs proximal to the DRG, the SNCS may be normal.

F WAVE

- The F wave is a special NCS that assesses motor conduction along the most proximal segment of the nerve. Antidromic stimulation of a peripheral nerve

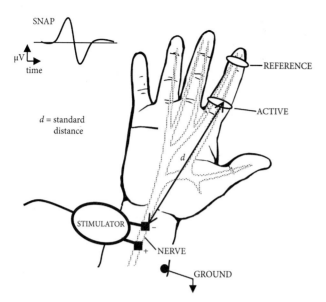

FIG. 10-2. Median sensory nerve conduction study. Active and reference electrodes are placed along the course of the nerve to be studied. Transcutaneous electrical stimulation is applied over the nerve at a standard distance (*d*) from the active electrode. SNAP is detected at the active electrode, amplified, and displayed (upper left). SNAP amplitude and latency are recorded and compared with laboratory norms. NCV (m/s) is calculated by dividing *d* (in mm) by peak latency (in ms).

sends an action potential to the spinal cord, where it activates a small number of anterior horn cells. The resultant action potential is transmitted orthodromically and triggers a small motor response (F wave) in the same peripheral nerve territory.

- F-wave latencies are length-dependent, and normal values must be adjusted for patient height or limb length.
- F waves are frequently abnormal (delayed or absent) in polyneuropathies, entrapment neuropathies, radiculopathies, and motor neuron disease (eg, amyotrophic lateral sclerosis).

H REFLEX

- The H reflex (Figure 10-3) is the electrical equivalent of a muscle stretch reflex elicited by tendon tap. It is examined using a modified MNCS technique.
- In adults, the H reflex is most often present in the soleus muscle and, at times, in the forearm flexor muscles. It may be more widespread in hyperreflexic conditions (eg, myelopathy) and in children.
- H reflex latencies are length-dependent, and normal values must be adjusted for patient height or limb length.
- The soleus H reflex is the most frequently studied. It may be delayed or absent in S1 radiculopathy.

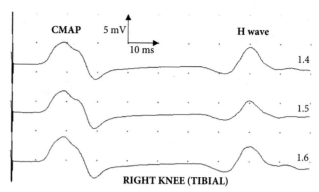

RIGHT KNEE (TIBIAL)

FIG. 10-3. Right tibial H-reflex study. The tibial nerve is stimulated in the popliteal fossa with the cathode directed proximally. The electrical stimulus proceeds bidirectionally along the nerve. Distal spread produces a CMAP in the soleus muscle. Proximal spread reaches the spinal cord and triggers a spinal reflex, which sends a motor signal distally and produces an H wave. Delay or absence of the tibial H wave may reflect S1 radiculopathy or another neuropathic process.

REPETITIVE NERVE STIMULATION

- Repetitive nerve stimulation (RNS) is an invaluable technique for assessing neuromuscular junction physiology.
- Two main factors affect neurotransmitter release at the normal neuromuscular junction: the amount of acetylcholine (Ach) available for release and the amount of available calcium (Ca^{2+}), which affects the probability of transmitter release.
- When MNCS is performed using rapid RNS (usually 2–3 Hz), the amplitude of the CMAP normally does not change.
- In some types of neuromuscular disease, repetitive stimulation can deplete available Ach to the point where a decrement is seen in CMAP amplitude with successive stimuli. Depending on the disease, a brief period of sustained muscle contraction, which increases the availability of Ca^{2+}, may reverse the decrement (eg, myasthenia gravis) or cause an increment in baseline amplitude (eg, Lambert–Eaton myasthenic syndrome).

NEEDLE ELECTROMYOGRAPHY

- Needle EMG uses needle electrodes to evaluate the electrical activity of muscle fibers. It provides copious information about the integrity, function, and innervation of motor units and (using special techniques) individual muscle fibers. The wealth of information is such that EMG has been called "the electrophysiologic biopsy."
- The skilled electromyographer can identify processes causing muscle denervation (neuropathies), muscle

destruction (myopathies), and failure of neuromuscular transmission (eg, myasthenia gravis).

- EMG can provide information about the extent of injury. Serial examinations allow monitoring of recovery or disease progression.

INDICATIONS

- Suspected mononeuropathy or polyneuropathy.
- Suspected radiculopathy or plexopathy.
- Suspected myopathy.
- Suspected neuromuscular junction disease.
- Suspected motor neuron disease.

CONTRAINDICATIONS

- Anticoagulant therapy (depends on planned test location and degree of anticoagulation).
- Coagulopathy.
- Implanted hardware at or near desired exam site.
- Muscle to be biopsied as the exam may introduce abnormalities.

GENERAL PRINCIPLES

- Surface landmarks and physical examination are used to isolate the desired muscle(s). After skin sterilization, a needle electrode is advanced into the muscle. Muscle potentials are monitored visually and audibly (Figure 10-4).

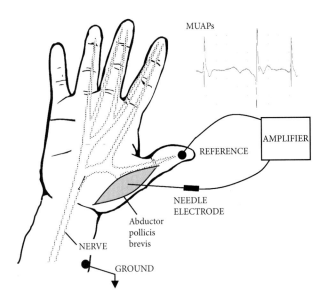

FIG. 10-4. Needle EMG of abductor pollicis brevis. The reference electrode is placed over an electrically neutral landmark. The needle (active electrode) is inserted into the resting muscle and moved in small increments to assess for spontaneous activity. The subject then performs graded muscle contraction to assess MUAP morphology and recruitment.

- The needle is moved through the muscle in small increments. This elicits spontaneous activity in abnormal muscle.
- The patient then voluntarily activates the muscle at mild and strong levels of contraction. MUAP morphology, number, and recruitment are assessed.

SPONTANEOUS ACTIVITY

- A normal muscle produces short bursts of insertional activity when the needle is moved, with electrical silence between insertions.
- A denervated or damaged muscle produces spontaneous activity, which may persist after the needle is moved. Different potentials have characteristic appearances (Figure 10-5) and sounds. Spontaneous

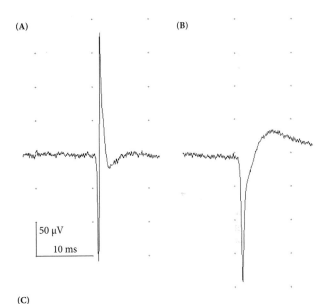

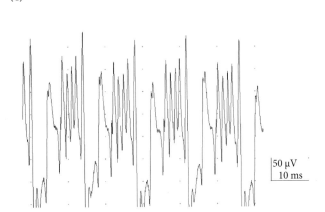

FIG. 10-5. Examples of spontaneous activity. Fibrillation potentials (A) are short-duration potentials occurring in a regular pattern. Positive sharp waves (B) are similar to fibrillation potentials but have no negative spike component. Complex repetitive discharges (C) may be the result of ephaptic transmission causing repetitive, rhythmic firing of irritable muscle fibers. Their rhythmic "buzzsaw" sound is easily recognizable.

TABLE 10-1 **Clinical Significance of EMG Parameters Commonly Mentioned in Electrodiagnostic Reports***

EMG PARAMETER	DECREASED	INCREASED
Amplitude	Loss or denervation of muscle fibers, eg, myopathy, axonal neuropathy, and motor neuron disease	Reinnervation after injury, with spatially larger motor units; hypertrophied muscle fibers (eg, recovery from myopathy or neuropathy)
Duration	Loss or atrophy of muscle fibers, as in myopathy	Reinnervation after injury, with spatially dispersed muscle fibers (myopathy or neuropathy)
Number of phases	Normal units have three or four phases; fewer phases are not generally seen	Increased variability of fiber diameter (myopathy); increased width of Motor Unit Potential endplate zone (neuropathy)
Recruitment	Usually reflects muscle denervation (loss of motor units); initial units fire very rapidly before the next unit is recruited, characteristic of neuropathic processes	Usually reflects muscle damage (fewer motor units per muscle); more units are needed to achieve a given strength of contraction, characteristic of myopathic processes
Spontaneous activity	No spontaneous activity seen in normal muscle	May be caused by myopathy, neuropathy, direct trauma (including surgery)

*This table is provided as a guide to interpretation. The list is incomplete; interested readers are referred to more comprehensive texts.

potentials may include fibrillation potentials, positive sharp waves, and complex repetitive discharges.

- The amount and frequency of spontaneous activity provide information about the severity or acuity of a disease process. Spontaneous activity is graded using this scale:
  0 = none;
  1 + = transient but reproducible discharges after moving needle;
  2 + = occasional discharges at rest in more than two different sites;
  3 + = spontaneous activity at rest regardless of needle position; and
  4 + = abundant, constant spontaneous activity.

EMG ANALYSIS

- A normal MUAP has a characteristic amplitude, duration, and number of phases. The EMG signal as a whole has a characteristic appearance and recruitment pattern. Abnormalities in any of these parameters help to diagnose the type and chronicity of disease (Table 10-1).
- The skilled electromyographer tailors the choice of muscles to the patient's situation. By carefully selecting muscles and observing the distribution of abnormalities, the electromyographer can distinguish among radiculopathy, plexopathy, myopathy, and many other conditions.

USING ELECTRODIAGNOSIS IN PAIN MEDICINE

- Electrodiagnosis is useful when pain is thought to originate from neurologic, intrinsic muscular, or neuromuscular junction disease.

- Before ordering electrodiagnostic testing, identify the specific question you want to answer. Remember that electrodiagnostic testing is uncomfortable. As with all medical interventions, before ordering, ask yourself: Will the test be of practical value? Will an accurate diagnosis change any aspect of the treatment plan or provide other benefits?
- State the question clearly on the referral. If you wish to look for or rule out particular conditions, mention them.
- Be sure that you are comfortable with your chosen electrodiagnostic laboratory and its practices. A well-run electrodiagnostic laboratory should:
  o ensure the most comfortable experience possible for the patient;
  o control for skin temperature during NCS, and record temperatures in the report;
  o have a consistent set of norms for NCS data, and present these norms in the report for comparison; abnormal data should be clearly marked;
  o compare abnormal results against the contralateral side wherever possible;
  o present the findings clearly; and
  o make sure the referring provider receives the results quickly.

SELECTED CLINICAL CONDITIONS

CARPAL TUNNEL SYNDROME

- Median MNCS and SNCS confirm a clinical diagnosis of carpal tunnel syndrome (CTS) with high sensitivity (>85%) and specificity (95%).
- Needle EMG of the thenar muscles can document axonal loss. However, it is painful and its value in CTS diagnosis is controversial. Many practitioners

reserve it for presentations where other neuropathic lesions are suspected; thenar EMG may provide critical diagnostic information. Patients with thenar muscle atrophy or weakness, or those with low-amplitude thenar CMAP, may benefit from thenar EMG.

- When abnormalities are found on one limb, the contralateral limb should also be studied.
- While NCS is helpful diagnostically, the final decision to proceed with surgery versus conservative treatment should be based primarily on symptoms and functional impact.
- Median nerve ultrasonography has been proposed as an alternative to NCSs, but sensitivity and specificity are too low to justify its routine use, and NCSs remain the "gold standard."

COMPLEX REGIONAL PAIN SYNDROME

- By identifying a specific nerve injury, electrodiagnostic testing can distinguish between complex regional pain syndrome (CRPS) subtypes I (no specific nerve injury identified) and II (causalgia, specific nerve injury identified). CRPS-II may be difficult to distinguish from CRPS-I by history and examination alone. Treatment of the underlying nerve injury, where possible, may provide some relief for the CRPS-II patient.
- Cases of CRPS-II have been linked to radiculopathy, brachial plexitis, and many other neuropathic conditions.
- Reserve electrodiagnostic testing for patients with a suspected definable nerve injury. EMG and NCS may be extremely painful in the CRPS patient; additional analgesics and/or anxiolytics may be required.

RADICULOPATHY

- It is essential to tailor the EMG exam to the patient's presentation and physical findings.
- The needle EMG examination is the most useful for identifying radiculopathy. Screening six or more muscles optimizes identification of radiculopathies. Specificity is excellent if appropriate diagnostic criteria are used.
- SNCSs are frequently normal, as spinal lesions causing radiculopathy often spare the DRG.
- MNCSs may be abnormal, particularly in advanced cases.
- EMG findings can help target the site for diagnostic/therapeutic image-guided spinal injection.

- When performed before and after decompressive surgery, EMG and NCS can monitor recovery and provide prognostic information.
- Neither EMG nor MRI is superior in the diagnosis of radiculopathy; they remain complementary diagnostic tools.

GENERALIZED NEUROMUSCULAR DISEASE

- Electrodiagnostic testing remains an important tool for diagnosing muscular dystrophies, inflammatory myopathies, neuromuscular junction disease, hereditary neuropathies, and other generalized neuromuscular disorders.
- To be helpful, testing must be conducted in the context of the patient's physical exam and clinical situation.

MYOFASCIAL PAIN AND FIBROMYALGIA SYNDROME

- Electrodiagnosis is normal in these musculoskeletal pain syndromes unless there are comorbid conditions, such as CTS.
- Generalized neuromuscular disorders such as myopathies, myasthenia gravis, and peripheral neuropathies may mimic fibromyalgia or myofascial pain.
- If the exam and other workup raise concern about neuromuscular disease, electrodiagnosis can provide valuable information.

PAINFUL NEUROPATHY

- When neuropathy is suspected as a cause of pain, NCS and EMG can help confirm the diagnosis and identify the type and bodily distribution of neuropathy (eg, axonal, demyelinating, mixed; sensory, motor, mixed, uniform, and segmental).
- Electrodiagnostic testing can help identify treatable neuropathies (eg, metabolic, toxic, vitamin deficiency, and nerve transections).
- Electrodiagnostic testing provides valuable prognostic information, and serial examinations can document disease progression or recovery.
- When polyneuropathy is suspected, complete examination requires both MNCS and SNCS, preferably on multiple nerves in both upper and lower limbs.
- When abnormalities are observed, the same nerve on the contralateral side should be examined to differentiate between symmetric and asymmetric processes.
- Normal EMG and NCS do not exclude the presence of a purely small-fiber peripheral neuropathy.

BIBLIOGRAPHY

Barkhaus PE, Nandedkar SD. EMG evaluation of the motor unit: the electrophysiologic biopsy. eMedicine.com; 2003.

Bruehl S, Harden RN, Galer BS, et al. External validation of IASP diagnostic criteria for complex regional pain syndrome and proposed research diagnostic criteria. International Association for the Study of Pain. *Pain.* 1999;81:147–154.

Daube JR. AAEM Minimonograph #11: needle examination in clinical electromyography. *Muscle Nerve.* 1991;14:685.

Dillingham TR. Electrodiagnostic approach to patients with suspected generalized neuromuscular disorders. *Phys Med Rehabil Clin North Am.* 2001;12:253.

Dillingham TR. Electrodiagnostic approach to patients with suspected radiculopathy. *Phys Med Rehabil Clin North Am.* 2002;13:567.

Donofrio PD, Albers JW. AAEM Minimonograph #34: polyneuropathy: classification by nerve conduction studies and electromyography. *Muscle Nerve.* 1990;13:889.

Gierthmühlen J, Maier C, Baron R, et al. Sensory signs in complex regional pain syndrome and peripheral nerve injury. *Pain.* 2012;153:765–774.

Jablecki CK, Andary MT, Floeter MK, et al. Practice parameter for electrodiagnostic studies in carpal tunnel syndrome: summary statement. *Muscle Nerve.* 2002;25:918.

Karlsson P, Porretta-Serapiglia C, Lombardi R, et al. Dermal innervation in healthy subjects and small fiber neuropathy patients: a stereological reappraisal. *J Peripher Nerv Syst.* 2013; 18:48–53.

Keesey JC. AAEM Minimonograph #33: electrodiagnostic approach to defects of neuromuscular transmission. *Muscle Nerve.* 1989;12:613.

Kimura J. *Electrodiagnosis in Diseases of Nerve and Muscle: Principles and Practice.* 2nd ed. Philadelphia, Pa: Davis; 1989.

Kimura J. Kugelberg lecture: principles and pitfalls of nerve conduction studies. *Electroencephalogr Clin Neurophysiol.* 1998;106:470.

Kraft GH. An approach to electrodiagnostic medicine: the power of needle electromyography. *Phys Med Rehabil Clin North Am.* 1994;5:495.

Mazur A. Role of thenar electromyography in the evaluation of carpal tunnel syndrome. *Phys Med Rehabil Clin North Am.* 1998;9:755.

Nardin RA, Patel MR, Gudas TF, et al. Electromyography and magnetic resonance imaging in the evaluation of radiculopathy. *Muscle Nerve.* 1999;22:151.

Tong HC. Specificity of needle electromyography for lumbar radiculopathy in 55- to 79-yr-old subjects with low back pain and sciatica without stenosis. *Am J Phys Med Rehabil.* 2011;90:233–242.

Walk D, Sehgal N, Moeller-Bertram T, et al. Quantitative sensory testing and mapping: a review of nonautomated quantitative methods for examination of the patient with neuropathic pain. *Clin J Pain.* 2009;25:632–640.

Wang SH, Robinson LR. Considerations in reference values for nerve conduction studies. *Phys Med Rehabil Clin North Am.* 1998;9:907.

Werner RA, Andary M. Electrodiagnostic evaluation of carpal tunnel syndrome. *Muscle Nerve.* 2011;44:597–607.

Yazdchi M, Tarzemani MK, Mikaeili H, et al. Sensitivity and specificity of median nerve ultrasonography in diagnosis of carpal tunnel syndrome. *Intl J Gen Med.* 2012;5:99–103.

11 QUANTITATIVE SENSORY TESTING

Mark S. Wallace, MD
Miroslav "Misha" Bačkonja, MD

- Quantitative sensory testing (QST) is a psychophysical testing method used to evaluate the function of specific sensory nerve fibers, such as large myelinated—Aβ, small myelinated—Aδ, and small unmyelinated—C fibers. (Table 11-1)
- The correlation between sensation and nerve fiber activity has been extensively studied and there are strong indications that subsets of nerve fibers correlate with specific sensations, for example, warming and burning sensations are mediated by TRPV1 receptors and C fibers, whereas cooling and cold sensations are transduced by TRPM8 receptors and transmitted by Aδ fibers. On the other hand, in case of injury and diseases affecting sensory nerve fibers, the specificity of this function is less clear. Despite these uncertainties, the only way to assess functional status of sensory nervous system, including positive sensory phenomena such as allodynia and negative sensory phenomena such as sensory deficits, is with QST.

TABLE 11-1 Summary of QST

Thermal thresholds
  Cool—Aδ
  Warm—C fiber
  Cold pain—interaction between Aδ and C fiber
  Heat pain (at threshold)—C fiber
  Heat pain (supramaximal)—Aδ

Mechanical pain
  Single stimuli—Aδ and C fiber
  Repetitive stimuli—C fiber

Mechanical nonpainful
  Vibratory—Aβ
  von Frey—Aβ

Current perception monitor
  5 Hz—C
  250 Hz—Aδ
  2000 Hz—Aβ

- Methods used for QST include mechanical nonpainful sensation (vibratory and von Frey hair), mechanical painful sensation (pinch and pressure), thermal sensation, and current perception sensation.
- Although used primarily as the research tool, QST standards are so well developed and published that it could be used in clinical practice.

MECHANICAL NONPAINFUL SENSATION

- Used to measure large myelinated (Aβ) fiber function.
- Of all the sensations, mechanical nonpainful sensation is the most vulnerable to nerve ischemia and will decrease within minutes of nerve ischemia.
- Large myelinated fiber function is often the most decreased after peripheral nerve injury leading to loss of sensation, that is, sensory deficits.
- Vibratory thresholds are most often tested using a C tuning fork but this method is crude and unreliable. More reliable is Seifert-Rydel tuning fork useful for detecting deficits across many neuropathies. More sophisticated computer-driven equipment is reliable but expensive.
- von Frey hairs are a good, inexpensive method of measuring large myelinated fiber function. Calibrated von Frey hairs are monofilaments of varying size. The filaments are applied perpendicular to the testing area starting from smallest, and after three successive stimuli are applied for 2 seconds at 5-second intervals per filament applied in an ascending pattern of thickness of the hair fiber. The testing is applied so that patient is not able to witness the hair fiber being applied and is asked to report when a stimulus from monofilament is felt. Thresholds are expressed in millinewton (mN) and measured as positive if the patient felt any one of the three successive stimuli. At the stimulus intensity evoking a report of sensation, the next hair fiber stimulus used is one unit smaller. This stimulus reversal is repeated twice, and the average reversal intensity defined as the threshold.

MECHANICAL PAINFUL SENSATION

- Single stimulus measures small myelinated (Aδ) and small unmyelinated (C) fiber function. Repetitive stimulus measures C-fiber function.
- Pinch algometer is most often used. A pinch algometer consists of a pistol-shaped handle and a shaft with two circular probes facing each other (area = 1 cm²). A fold of skin is placed between the two probes and one is displaced slowly and evenly (rate 30 kPa/s) toward the other, pinching the skin. A transducer in one of the probes provides constant feedback of the pressure exerted. The subject is instructed to press a switch at the very instant of pain experience. The trial is then terminated.

- Pressure algometer measures lbs or kilograms of pressure, measured either by mechanical or electronic devices, expressed with 5-mm circular rubberized probe while pressure is steadily applied and subject is instructed to report when pain is felt and at that moment trial is terminated.
- Mechanical pain threshold is defined as the mean pressure for three trials. Stimuli are given at 1-minute intervals.

THERMAL SENSATION

- Used to measure small myelinated (Aδ) and small unmyelinated (C) fiber function.
- *Cool sensation.* Measures Aδ-fiber function. Of all the thermal sensation, (1) it is the first thermal sensation to decrease after peripheral nerve injury, (2) depends mostly on spatial summation, so small probes will falsely decrease the sensation, and (3) is the most vulnerable to nerve ischemia. Normal detection occurs with about a minus 2°C change in temperature.
- *Warm sensation.* Measures C-fiber function. It is the second thermal sensation to decrease after peripheral nerve injury. Is less dependent on spatial summation than cool sensation but more dependent than heat pain. And is less vulnerable to nerve ischemia than cool sensation but more vulnerable than heat pain. Normal detection occurs with about a plus 2°C change in temperature.
- *Cold pain sensation.* Results from an interaction between Aδ and C-fiber function. Of all the thermal stimuli, it is the least reproducible between subjects. Evidence suggests that Aδ fibers transmit the cool portion and C fibers transmit the pain portion of the sensation. In peripheral nerve injury, cold pain thresholds can approach cool sensation thresholds resulting in *cold allodynia*. Normal cold pain temperature is around 10°C.
- *Heat pain sensation.* Just painful thresholds measure C-fiber function. Supramaximal painful thresholds measure Aδ-fiber function. In early stages of complex regional pain syndrome, heat pain thresholds approach warm sensation thresholds resulting in *heat hyperalgesia*. As disease progresses, heat pain sensation normalizes. Normal heat pain temperature is around 45°C.

ELECTRICAL STIMULATION—CURRENT PERCEPTION THRESHOLD

- Recent technological advances allow quantitative measurement of the functional integrity of both large- and small-diameter sensory nerve fibers using the

Current Perception Threshold (CPT) sensory testing device. The CPT evaluation is a noninvasive, painless, QST, which provides a functional assessment of the sensory nervous system. The CPT is the minimum amount of a transcutaneously applied current that an individual perceives as evoking a sensation. The CPT evaluation is performed using the NEUROMETER CPT/C (Neurotron, Inc., Baltimore) neuroselective diagnostic stimulator, which uses a microprocessor-controlled constant current sine-wave stimulus to obtain CPT measures. The constant current feature compensates for alterations in skin resistance and standardizes the stimulus between skin thickness and degree of skin moisture. The CPT uses three frequencies, 5, 250, and 2000 Hz, specific for each of the following nerve fibers, respectively, C fiber, Aδ fiber, and Aβ fiber.

PRINCIPLES OF CONDUCTING QST

- For a QST to be conducted four elements are necessary: stimulus, instruction, subject, and the examiner.
- Stimulus that consists of prespecified stimulus characteristics including physical device, intensity, duration, and frequency of application and the method of order by which stimuli are applied.
- Instruction to the subject needs to convey the requirements of QST and each specific step in simple and unambiguous manner.
- As subject needs to be able to participate in psychophysical study, so subject needs to understand each step of testing and be able and willing to participate for the entire duration of the study.
- Examiner needs to be familiar with the concepts of the procedure and each specific step of the procedure. Examiner has to monitor participation of the subject and to record all of the responses.
- Interpretation—QST has to be interpreted within the context of the clinical scenario for each individual patient.

BIBLIOGRAPHY

Gruener G, Dyck PJ. Quantitative sensory testing: methodology, applications, and future directions. *J Clin Neurophys.* 1994; 11:568–583.

Katims JJ. Neuroselective current perception threshold quantitative sensory test. *Muscle Nerve.* 1997;20(11):1468–1469.

Konietzney F. Peripheral neural correlates of temperature sensation in man. *Human Neurobiol.* 1984;3:21–32.

Nordin, N. Low-threshold mechanoreceptive and nociceptive units with unmyelinated C fibers in the human supraorbital nerve. *J Physiol.* 1990;426:229–240.

Ochoa JL, Torebjork E. Sensations evoked by intraneural microstimulation of C nociceptor fibers in human skin nerves. *J Physiol.* 1989;415:583–599.

Ochoa JL, Torebjork E. Sensations evoked by intraneural microstimulation of single mechanoreceptor units innervating the human hand. *J Physiol Lond.* 1993;342:465–472.

Olmos PR, Cataland S, O'Dorisio TM, Casey CA, Smead WL, Simon SR. The Semmes-Weistein monofilament as a potential predictor of foot ulceration in patients with noninsulin-dependent diabetes. *Am J Med Sci.* 1995;309:76–82.

Torebjork HE, Vallbo AB, Ochoa JL. Intraneural microstimulation in man. Its relation to specificity of tactile sensations. *Brain.* 1987;110:1509–1529.

Verdugo R, Ochoa JL. Quantitative somatosensory thermotest: a key method for functional evaluation of small calibre afferent channels. *Brain.* 1992;115:893–913.

Yarnitsky D, Ochoa JL. Release of cold-induced burning pain by block of cold-specific afferent input. *Brain.* 1990;113:893–902.

Yarnitsky D, Ochoa JL. Differential effect of compression-ischemia block on warm sensation and heat-induced pain. *Brain.* 1991a;114:907–913.

Yarnitsky D, Ochoa JL. Warm and cold specific somatosensory systems, psychophysical thresholds, reaction times and peripheral conduction velocities. *Brain.* 1991b;114:1819–1826.

12 RADIOLOGIC EVALUATION

Laura MacNeil
Kieran J. Murphy, MD

INTRODUCTION

- Establishing a diagnosis for a patient with chronic pain requires an advanced evaluation of the patient with chronic pain. It may include an appropriate history and physical exam, the use of electrodiagnostic studies, and the use of diagnostic radiologic tools. Thus, this chapter focuses on the radiologic evaluation of pain resulting from degenerative diseases of the spine.

INDICATIONS FOR THE USE OF IMAGING

- Most cases of back pain do not require imaging. In patients with typical, uncomplicated back pain, imaging studies should only follow failure of a 4-week trial of conservative management, as symptoms usually resolve in 90% of cases after this time period.

- It is important to rule out nondegenerative causes, including neoplasm, infection, inflammatory disease, and vascular causes. A history consistent with these pathologic processes and/or unremitting pain should prompt a thorough laboratory and radiologic workup.
- Radiologic studies are also advisable for patients with motor, bowel, bladder, or sexual neurologic deficits; previous spinal fusion surgery; or symptoms persisting.
- If a patient has nerve root compression symptoms that indicate a possible surgically treatable cause, consult with a surgeon to determine the type of study needed.
- It is critical to remember that radiologic studies cannot image pain and that asymptomatic lesions can mislead physicians. A magnetic resonance imaging (MRI) study of asymptomatic patients found disc bulges in 52%, disc protrusions in 27%, and disc extrusions in 1% of cases.
- The choice of imaging study is guided by the location and type of suspected tissue injury.

PLAIN RADIOGRAPHY

- Plain radiography is an inexpensive, rapid, readily available technique for initial screening of the spine for fractures, misalignment of vertebrae, spondylolisthesis and spondylolysis, and other bone pathologies. It may also detect an underlying infection or neoplastic process.
- The usefulness of plain films is limited due to the low sensitivity, nonspecificity of findings, lack of detail, and poor imaging of soft tissue.
- Plain films should be obtained to rule out fractures in patients presenting with back pain and recent trauma or a history suggesting osteoporosis and compression fractures. Such patients usually also require computed tomography (CT) and MRI if spinal cord damage is suspected.
- Flexion-extension views may provide additional information in patients with spondylolisthesis or a prior spinal fusion surgery.

MAGNETIC RESONANCE IMAGING

- MRI is the most useful tool in the evaluation of the spine.
- The advantages of MRI are that it is noninvasive, can image in sagittal and axial planes, can be used in patients allergic to iodinated contrast, uses no ionizing radiation, produces no beam-hardening artifact, and provides the best soft tissue contrast and visualization of the spinal ligaments.
- Limitations of MRI are the expense, long procedure times, limited availability in some localities, inability to detect calcification, and inability to visualize cortical bone directly.
- Contraindications to the use of MRI include the presence of cardiac pacemakers, ferromagnetic aneurysm clips, ferromagnetic cochlear implants, and intraocular metallic foreign bodies.
- Claustrophobic patients may be unable to tolerate the procedure unmedicated but administration of 5 mg diazepam before leaving for the MRI and 5 mg in the MRI suite usually controls symptoms. Open MRI may also be available for these patients but image quality is inferior.
- MRI is equal to CT in evaluation of a herniated disc and spinal stenosis. The reported sensitivity and specificity are 0.6–1.0 for MRI and 0.43–0.97 for CT for a herniated disc and 0.9 for MRI and 0.72–1.0 for CT for spinal stenosis.
- MRI is more sensitive and specific than other techniques in detecting osteomyelitis, disc space infection, or malignancy. It is also very useful in evaluating arachnoiditis and is the best method of assessing spinal cord compression and damage.
- T1-weighted images provide good anatomic detail in the imaging of end-plate reactive changes, osteophytic narrowing, lateral disc herniation, postoperative scarring, spondylolisthesis, and infiltrative disease.
- T2-weighted images are more time-consuming to obtain but are useful in intramedullary disease, infection, and inflammation because of the increased sensitivity to the higher water content in these conditions.
- Gadolinium–DTPA contrast should be used in postoperative patients to differentiate scarring from the intervertebral discs and also in patients with infection, inflammation, or cancer.
- In the cervical region, thin-section axial images (1.5 mm) should be obtained, but 3- to 5-mm sections usually suffice in the lumbar spine.

COMPUTED TOMOGRAPHY

- Compared with MRI, CT is more rapid, more available, less expensive, and provides superior bone detail.
- Standard CT is well-suited for the evaluation of spinal trauma: CT can clearly establish the extent of fractures seen on plain film, detect subtle fractures not previously seen, and determine the degree to which bony fragments impinge on the spinal canal. The neural damage in as many as half of patients with cervical spine bone injuries, however, requires MRI for accurate evaluation.
- CT can be used in patients with ferromagnetic devices, which preclude the use of MRI.

- CT can also be combined with myelography for increased sensitivity in certain situations (see later).
- As mentioned previously, CT is equivalent to MRI in facilitating diagnosis of disc herniation and spinal stenosis. CT can also accurately depict nerve root impingement but is inferior to MRI in detecting infection and neoplasm.
- Thin CT sections from pedicle to pedicle should be obtained in the region of suspected spinal damage.

MYELOGRAPHY

- Myelography involves the intrathecal injection of a contrast agent followed by plain film or, more often, CT imaging.
- Although relatively safe, myelography is an invasive procedure with risks and side effects. The most common side effect is a postprocedure headache. The incidence of headache can be reduced to 10% of patients by using a 26-gauge needle and having the patient remain prone for 4–8 hours following the procedure.
- Postmyelography CT has a high sensitivity in detecting cervical radiculopathy, osteophytic impingement, disc herniation, and can also identify subarachnoid tumor spread and arachnoiditis.
- CT without intrathecal contrast agent should be used for the lumbar spine because the natural contrast of fat with bone and disc is sufficient in this region.
- Myelography may be indicated in patients with ambiguous diagnoses from MRI and standard CT as well as in those unable to undergo MRI.

RADIONUCLIDE SCANNING

- Radionuclide scans are useful in the detection of early osteomyelitis, compression and small stress fractures, primary malignancy, and skeletal metastasis in patients with back pain of unknown origin.
- Injection of technetium-99m–labeled phosphate complexes followed by a whole-body bone scan is a very sensitive method of detecting regional changes in bone metabolism.
- Plain films are negative in 10%–40% of metastases identified using bone scans, while a bone scan is falsely negative in 5% of spinal metastases identified by plain film.
- The disadvantages of nuclear bone scans are poor detail and specificity. Usually a positive result necessitates further studies to confirm the cause. MRI is more sensitive as well as the test of choice in patients with a strong suspicion of spinal metastases or infection.
- Combining radionuclide imaging with single-proton emission CT improves spatial resolution.

DISCOGRAPHY

- Discography is the injection of a contrast agent under fluoroscopic guidance into the center of the nucleus pulposus of an intervertebral disc.
- The appearance of contrast accumulation and the pain response to a given force of injection are used to determine whether a particular disc is causing the patient's pain.
- This technique can be combined with CT.
- Discography is the only imaging study that seeks to establish a causal relationship between anatomic abnormalities and pain.

ARTERIOGRAPHY

- Spinal arteriography is the intra-arterial injection of iodinated contrast into spinal arteries.
- This test is typically only used to improve preoperative or preembolization visualization or to identify the cause when MRI reveals a possible vascular tumor or malformation.
- Arteriography carries the risks of spinal stroke causing neurologic deficits as well as the non-neurologic complications associated with an invasive procedure.

BIBLIOGRAPHY

Alazraki N. Radionuclide techniques. *Bone Joint Imaging*. 1989; 16:185.

Avrahami E, Tadmor R, Dally O, et al. Early MR demonstration of spinal metastases in patients with normal radiographs and CT and radionuclide bone scans. *J Comput Assist Tomogr*. 1989;13:598.

Bigos S, Bowyer O, Braen G, et al. *Clinical Practice Guideline Number 14: Acute Low Back Problems in Adults*. Rockville, MD: Agency for Health Care Policy and Research, Public Health Service, US Department of Health and Human Services; 1994. AHCPR publication 95-0642.

Jarvik J, Deyo R. Diagnostic evaluation of low back pain with emphasis on imaging. *Ann Intern Med*. 2002;137:586.

Jensen M, Brant-Zawadzki M, Obuchowski N, et al. Magnetic resonance imaging of the lumbar spine in people without back pain. *N Engl J Med*. 1994;331:69.

Riggins RJ, Krause JF. The risk of neurologic damage with fractures of the vertebra. *J Trauma*. 1977;17:126.

Salkever D. Morbidity Cost: National Estimates and Economic Determinants. Report No. (PHS) 86–3343; 1985.

Schroth WS, Schectman JM, Elinsky EG, et al. Utilization of medical services for the treatment of acute low back pain. *J Gen Intern Med*. 1992;7:486–491.

Vezina JL, Fontaine S, Laperriere J. Outpatient myelography with fine-needle technique: an appraisal. *Am J Roentgenol*. 1989;153:383.

13 PSYCHOLOGICAL EVALUATION OF THE PAIN PATIENT

Mohammed A. Issa, MD
Ajay D. Wasan, MD, MSc
Michael T. Smith, PhD
Robert R. Edwards, PhD

OVERVIEW: BIOPSYCHOSOCIAL MODEL OF CHRONIC PAIN

- The experience of pain is not equivalent to nociception, and tissue damage is only one of the many factors influencing the experience of pain.
- Biological, psychological, and social factors interact in complex and incompletely understood ways to produce the experience of pain and pain-related sequelae.
- A comprehensive assessment of the patient with chronic pain should attend to mood, pain-coping strategies, areas of disability, and the social environment. Additional considerations should be given to secondary gain and patient-provider interactions.

CRITICAL PSYCHOSOCIAL AND BEHAVIORAL FACTORS

MOOD

Fear/Anxiety

- Anxiety in acute pain settings is associated with longer hospital stays, greater acute pain, and increased use of pain medications.
- Fear of pain, particularly activity-related pain, such as low back pain, can lead to a debilitating cycle in which the individual becomes increasingly debilitated and pain becomes chronic.
- Pain-related fear may be more disabling than the pain itself. It is a significant predictor of number of sick or absentee days as a result of low back pain.

Assessment Questions

- What activities do you avoid because of your pain?
- What are you worried will happen if you do [this activity]?
- If you do [this activity], do you become anxious or worried about the pain?

Depression

- Of note, 40%–50% of chronic pain patients suffer from depression. It is still unclear whether depression causes chronic pain or if chronic pain causes depression.

- Symptoms of depression in the context of chronic pain are associated with increased pain intensity, increased pain behavior, lower daily activity levels and function, and greater interference of pain in daily activities.
- Depression is associated with greater chronicity of pain, and depression has been implicated as a risk factor for the development of chronic pain following acute injury.
- Higher levels of depressive symptoms predict poorer outcome from surgical, medical, and psychological treatment of pain.
- Both chronic pain and chronic depression are risk factors for suicide; the presence of these factors together may be especially dangerous.
- Patients who believed that they could continue to function, and that they could maintain some control despite their pain, were less likely to become depressed.

Assessment

- The assessment of depression should focus on questions about interest in previously pleasurable activities (eg, sexual activity, hobbies, and time with family), changes in concentration and memory, and thoughts about dying, as well as the usual assessment of mood, sleep, appetite, and energy.

Assessment Questions

- *Interest.* Have you experienced any change in your interest or pleasure in activities you used to enjoy? (*Note*: Be careful to distinguish between interest and ability.)
- *Concentration/memory.* Have you noticed any change in your memory or concentration? Can you follow news stories in the newspaper or on television?
- *Thoughts of dying.* Have you had thoughts of dying? If yes, what have you thought? How frequently do you have these thoughts? Have you ever acted on these thoughts? Do you feel safe? (*Note*: Regular thoughts of dying, having a plan or intent to kill oneself are signals to obtain immediate formal consultation for assessment of depression.)

Anger

- Most patients with chronic pain acknowledged their feelings of anger when sought.
- Anger is associated with higher pain intensity, unpleasantness of pain, and emotional distress in chronic pain patients and their families. It is significantly correlated with disability and highly associated with depression.

- Chronic pain patients tend to inhibit their anger, which leads to increased aversiveness of their pain experience and overt pain behaviors.

Assessment Questions

- How frequently do you have trouble controlling your temper?
- How often do you argue with others?
- Do you routinely feel frustrated by delays or lack of progress?

Catastrophizing

- The most important dimension of pain coping identified during the past few decades is *catastrophizing*, an emotional, cognitive, and attitudinal response to pain that consistently is associated with greater pain and disability, more pain behavior, negative mood, and worsening depression.
- Pain catastrophizing is one of the most important predictors of pain, accounting for 7%–31% of the variance in pain ratings.
- Patients who catastrophize have higher levels of disability, higher rates of health care usage, longer hospitalizations, increased pain medication usage, and higher levels of motor pain behaviors.
- High catastrophizers may also be at elevated risk for misusing their pain medications.
- Current fear-avoidance models propose that catastrophizing beliefs precipitate pain-related fear, leading to avoidance, followed by disuse, disability, and depression.
- Although experts debate the conceptual details, catastrophizing seems to serve as a coping strategy by activating negative emotions, which may motivate the individual to deal with the pain or, when expressed to others, may elicit social responses to pain such as emotional support.

Assessment

- Key components of catastrophizing include hypervigilance to bodily sensations, helplessness about controlling the pain, fear that the pain cannot be controlled and will get worse, and pessimism that the pain will never go away.

Assessment Questions

- How frequently do you feel that you cannot stand the pain?
- How often do you feel overwhelmed by the pain?
- How frequently do you worry that the pain will never go away?
- How often do you feel that there is nothing you can do to reduce the pain?

COPING

- Much of the pain-coping literature distinguishes between active coping strategies (ie, doing something directly about the pain) and passive coping (eg, responding to the pain by cutting back on activities, resting, or looking to others to control the pain).
- Although frequently debated, in general, active coping strategies are associated with better outcomes and higher function, and passive coping strategies are associated with poorer outcomes and lower function in patients with chronic pain syndromes.

Coping Self-statements

- Coping self-statements are realistic statements individuals make to motivate themselves to deal with pain.
- Some studies have found that the use of coping self-statements is associated with lower pain, less distress, and higher function.
- Training in use of these statements is an integral part of cognitive-behavioral therapy (CBT) for pain management, and these thoughts increase as a result of CBT treatment, although such changes are not consistently associated with better long-term outcomes.

Assessment

- Measuring this coping strategy focuses on the individual's ability to see pain as a challenge that can be dealt with and will improve in the future.

Assessment Questions

- Are there times when you are able to consider the pain as a challenge?
- How often do you think of the pain as something you can deal with?
- How often do you think that the pain will get better in the future?

READINESS TO CHANGE

- Patients need to take an active role in learning to manage their pain.
- Individuals may be in one of five stages in terms of their readiness to change: Precontemplation, not intending to change; Contemplation, intending to change in the foreseeable future; Preparation, intending to change in the immediate future; Action, making overt changes to change; or Maintenance, working to stabilize behavior change.
- Clinicians may help patients move from one stage to another utilizing motivational interviewing techniques.

DISABILITY

General Issues

- Chronic pain is associated with widespread impairment in multiple domains of functioning, ranging from disruption in basic activities of daily living to disruption in psychosocial functioning and work-related activities.
- Physical disability can lead to a debilitating cycle in which the individual becomes increasingly deconditioned and pain is exacerbated.
- A subset of chronic pain patients with high levels of pain, affective distress, and maladaptive coping are at greatest risk for increased disability.

Assessment

- Aside from evaluating the specific domains already addressed, evaluation of pain-related disability should focus on identifying how the pain condition affects multiple dimensions of the patient's life.

Assessment Questions

- Please describe a typical day.
- What aspects of your daily life are disrupted by your pain?
- What activities do you no longer do because of your pain?

Fear-avoidance Models of Pain-related Disability

- Fear-avoidance models of pain-related disability have received substantial empirical support.
- The extent to which individuals believe that engaging in physical activities will increase pain or result in harm or reinjury is independently associated with self-reported disability and physical capacity evaluations.
- Pain self-efficacy beliefs, that is, an individual's confidence in his or her ability to perform a range of specific tasks despite pain, are inversely related to pain and avoidance behaviors.
- Changes in fear-avoidance beliefs during pain treatment are associated with improvements in disability.

Assessment

- Assessment should focus on eliciting *specific* beliefs and avoiding *specific* physical activities.
- An evaluation of the degree of conviction of fear-avoidance beliefs and the reasons patient give for holding these beliefs is essential.
- Leading with open-ended questions and following up with specific closed-ended questions can be helpful.

Assessment Questions

- Which activities do you believe are likely to cause your pain to worsen?
- Have you had some bad experiences trying to do these kinds of activities?
- How certain are you that engaging in these activities will lead to pain and reinjury?
- What are you concerned might happen if you were to engage in [this particular activity]?

Sleep Disturbance

- Sleep disturbance is a highly prevalent and often ignored correlate of chronic pain, and sleep problems are associated with increased disability, pain severity, and psychosocial impairment.
- Often a consequence of pain and mood disturbance, sleep disturbance itself may reciprocally exacerbate pain and negative mood.
- Chronic insomnia is often maintained, in part, by cognitive-behavioral factors in addition to or independent from actual pain.
- Aggressive treatment of sleep disturbance is recommended and often includes a sleep disorder center evaluation, use of sedating tricyclic antidepressants, and/or referral for behavioral treatment for insomnia by a behavioral sleep medicine specialist.

Assessment

- Assessing sleep disturbance associated with chronic pain should include consideration of the many contributing factors, including psychiatric disturbance, intrinsic sleep disorders, medications, substance use, and cognitive-behavioral factors.

Assessment Questions

- Tell me about your sleep. How long does it take you to fall asleep?
- About how long are you awake in the middle of the night or early morning?
- During the daytime, are you often so sleepy that you have to fight to stay awake or do you fall asleep at inappropriate times?
- Are you bothered by intrusive thoughts or worries at night?

Work-related Issues

- Chronic pain conditions often affect a person's ability to work, and work-related factors, such as workers' compensation and disability payments, can sometimes influence pain behavior and motivation for treatment.

- About 10%–25% of patients with low back pain remain absent from work in the long term, resulting in 75% of the costs due to sickness leave and disability.
- Predictors of return to work are multifactorial and involve a combination of pain-related factors, nonclinical factors (such as age and education), patients' goals and beliefs about work, and work-related factors (such as availability of modified work programs and workers' compensation status).
- Modified work programs and integrated graded activity may improve return-to-work rates for workers with work-related injuries.

Assessment

- Determine whether the patient's pain condition is associated with a work-related injury, whether the patient is receiving disability compensation, and whether legal claims or actions are pending.
- Identify intentions, goals, and barriers related to return to work, bearing in mind that such issues can often be an extreme source of stress to patients.

Assessment Questions

- Were you injured on your job?
- Are you receiving any workers' compensation or other disability payments due to your injury?
- Do you have any pending legal action related to your injury?
- Do you think you will be able to return to work?
- If so, in what capacity?
- What kinds of things do you anticipate will make it difficult for you to resume working?

SOCIAL ENVIRONMENT

Family History

- Individuals undergoing chronic pain treatment have a disproportionately high likelihood of having a family history of a similar pain condition. This finding is consistent for headache, abdominal pain, and fibromyalgia.
- Chronic pain patients are more likely than controls without pain to report a family history of at least one psychiatric disorder.
- A family history of pain is associated with poor health, more pain complaints, and enhanced sensitivity to pain compared with controls.
- Longitudinal studies suggest that parental modeling and reinforcement of illness behavior in children are related to increased risk of chronic pain as an adult and to health care–seeking behavior.

Assessment

- A standardized assessment of the patient's family history of pain may yield insight into the contribution of social learning to the patient's pain behavior.

Assessment Questions

- Have others in your family had pain conditions?
- How did they cope with the pain?

Social Support

- Individuals with chronic pain are more likely than controls to report current and past distress related to family relationships.
- Perceived social support is positively related to health and inversely related to pain and disability ratings across a number of chronic pain conditions, and poor social support is associated with greater use of inpatient and outpatient medical services.
- The relationship between distress and pain is strongest in those with minimal social support; a positive social environment may buffer the negative effects of pain-related distress.
- Interventions that enhance social support can reduce pain and disability.

Assessment

- An assessment should take into account the amount and the perceived quality of social relationships as well as the patient's preferences regarding the degree of social contact (eg, "I would like to have other people to talk to").

Assessment Questions

- Who is supportive to you in your life? How are the social and family relationships in your life?
- How has your pain affected those relationships?
- Are the people in your life providing the support you need?

Social Interactions

- Pain behavior is, like all behavior, at least partially under operant control. That is, it is influenced by the response of the environment to the behavior. In fact, researchers have found that chronic back pain patients are more susceptible to operant conditioning than are controls.
- Solicitous behavior (attention to pain and, sometimes, encouragement of disability) on the part of a spouse or significant other is associated with higher ratings of pain among chronic pain patients, and greater marital satisfaction is associated with increased severity of

pain, presumably because it is associated with solicitous behavior.

- Marital conflict and negative responses by a spouse are also associated with higher reports of pain among pain patients (possibly as a result of increased distress).
- In contrast, family members who support a patient's efforts to cope with pain may promote improved adjustment to pain.
- Aspects of the social environment may interact with an individual's coping style; catastrophizing may activate the social environment so the patient gains support from others. It is not known how well these efforts work.

Assessment

- Any interview should include a structured or unstructured assessment of the patient's perception of others' responses to pain behavior.
- If a family member is present for some part of the evaluation, behavioral observation of interactions with the patient, the family member's level of support, and specific actions taken in response to pain behavior can be extremely useful.

Assessment Questions

- How does (the person of interest) react when you are in pain?
- How do others help when you are in pain?
- Are there ways that they make things worse?

Secondary Gain

- *Primary gain* refers to the relief of distress by a bodily symptom, and *secondary gain* refers to the benefits to an individual that arise from the development of one or more symptoms.
- *Sick role* refers to a constellation of behaviors that are frequently assumed to be reinforced by one or more secondary gains.
- Many secondary gains have been identified:
  - Financial compensation associated with injury or disability.
  - Conversion of a socially unacceptable disability (eg, psychiatric disorder) into a socially acceptable disability (eg, chronic physical condition).
  - Elicitation of care and sympathy from family and friends.
  - Avoidance of an unpleasant or unsatisfactory life role or activity (eg, a disliked job and undesirable family responsibilities).
  - Increased ease of access to desired drugs and medications.
  - Increased control over family members.

- There are currently no good estimates of the prevalence of secondary gain factors among chronic pain patients.

Assessment

- Assessment of secondary gain is notoriously difficult, especially in the context of brief contacts in a medical setting.
- The rate of false positives when attempting to identify individuals in whom secondary gain is prominent is probably unacceptably high.

Assessment Questions

- Do you have any litigation pending at this time?
- If so, when do you think this will be resolved?
- What do you hope to get from any settlement?
- What would things be like if you no longer had pain?

Evaluation of Opioid Risk

- There is a 40% prevalence of opioid misuse in chronic noncancer pain patients treated with opioids.
- Clinicians should screen for aberrant drug-related behaviors that may be indicative of opioid misuse. There are three major types of aberrant behaviors: loss of control over the drug, compulsive drug use, and continued use despite harm.
- Screening tools for substance abuse may be beneficial in assessing the risk of addiction to opioids before initiation and during maintenance with opioid therapy. Utilization of prescription drug monitoring programs is another complimentary tool that helps identify patients who "doctor shop."
- Urine toxicology screens are the most widely used and possibly the gold standard for detecting illicit substance use in chronic pain patients treated with opioids. Opioid therapy agreement, signed by both patient and clinician, may be an appealing tool for managing many of the potential difficulties related to chronic noncancer opioid therapy.

Assessment

- Screening for risk of opioid abuse/misuse is directed toward identifying aberrant drug behaviors resulting from adverse consequences (eg, over sedation and sleep or mood problems), impaired control over use and/or preoccupation with use due to craving.
- History of personal and/or family history of addiction significantly increases the risk of opioid misuse. It is also important to assess for any implications on work, interpersonal or social function with opioid use.
- Comorbid mood problems, anxiety, and emotional distress significantly increase the risk of misusing prescribed opioids if not appropriately treated.

Assessment Questions

Have you ever taken more pills than prescribed? Did you ever run out of your prescription early? If so, how would you manage your pain?

Do you sometimes take your opioid for other reasons than pain?

Do other family members have chronic pain? If so, have they ever shared their pills with you?

PSYCHOLOGICAL ASPECTS OF PATIENT–PROVIDER INTERACTIONS

- Listening carefully, answering questions, encouraging dialogue, and making clear statements are among the key components of good patient–provider communication. Benefits include improved patient compliance with medical regimens, reduced likelihood of litigation, and improved patient satisfaction with care.
- Research has targeted improving physician–patient relationships as a way of reducing health care utilization. Merely providing patients with a regular source of care does not generally reduce their emergency room usage , although improved communication and patient education seem to be effective.
- Self-management programs, in which patients take an active role in their own health care and focus on adaptive efforts to manage symptoms, improve symptoms, reduce utilization, and improve communication.
- High users of medical services are often characterized by dissonance between themselves and their physician. This dissonance is characterized by such factors as poor patient understanding of the condition, lack of agreement about diagnosis and/or treatment goals, and unclear follow-up plans.
- Relying on patient reports of satisfaction with pain management may lead to overestimates of the quality of care, as many patients report "very good" care even when experiencing inadequate pain relief.
- Patient satisfaction does not correlate with pain ratings at admission or discharge or with change in pain over the course of a hospital stay.

POTENTIAL BIASES ON THE PART OF HEALTH CARE PROVIDERS

- Health care providers often underestimate the pain and disability levels of their patients, and this bias is strongest when the patients are elderly or are members of an ethnic minority group.
- There is little evidence for the validity of expert judgments regarding a chronic pain patient's likely prognosis. For example, among back pain patients followed longitudinally, no relationship was observed between providers' estimates of patients' rehabilitation potential and actual rehabilitation outcomes.
- While some patients may inspire suspicion that their reports of pain are exaggerated or feigned, no accepted methodology exists for detecting malingering. Individuals instructed to simulate or "fake" pain produce higher scores on measures of pain, distress, and impairment than actual pain patients, but cutoff scores with acceptable sensitivity and specificity have not been identified.
- The prevalence of opioid abuse and dependence among patients with chronic pain is consistently overestimated by health care providers.

RECOMMENDATIONS FOR HEALTH CARE PROVIDERS

- Develop standardized assessments of psychosocial factors, such as mood, coping, and social relationships, even if they are as brief as single questions.
- If time and resources are available, assessment of psychosocial factors should include an interview, behavioral observations, and one or more standardized instruments.
- Disability is often not strongly related to pain; assessment of other factors that may contribute to disability (eg, depression) may help with treatment plans.
- Familiarity with local resources, such as support groups and community mental health centers, can facilitate treatment of patients with pain.
- When feasible, involving a spouse or significant other may enhance the effectiveness of behavioral interventions (ie, coping skills training and exercise programs).
- True malingering is probably rare in chronic pain patients, and the impact of secondary gain issues is not well understood; the grounds for disbelieving a patient's report of pain are rarely tenable.
- Patients on chronic opioid therapy should be regularly screened for aberrant drug behaviors, as they are usually indicative of opioid misuse/abuse. Urine toxicology screens, prescription drug monitoring programs, and opioid therapy agreements are helpful tools in assessing and managing many of the potential difficulties related to chronic noncancer opioid therapy.
- To whatever extent possible, encourage patients to be "self-managers" of their pain. That is, provide them with one or more concrete strategies or goals (eg, 5 minutes per day of stretching exercises, simple relaxation techniques, and leaving the house at least once a day) to pursue on their own.
- Assess your communication skills: How well do you educate patients about their condition? How well do

you listen when they speak? How much input do your patients have regarding treatment decisions? How clearly do you describe treatment goals?

BIBLIOGRAPHY

Adams LL, Gatchel RJ, Robinson RC, et al. Development of a self-report screening instrument for assessing potential opioid medication misuse in chronic pain patients. *J Pain Symptom Manage.* 2004;27:440–459.

Alonso C, Coe CL. Disruptions of social relationships accentuate the association between emotional distress and menstrual pain in young women. *Health Psychol.* 2001;20:411.

Asghari A, Nicholas MK. Pain self-efficacy beliefs and pain behaviour: a prospective study. *Pain.* 2001;94:85.

Asmundson G, Norton P, Vlaeyen J. Fear-avoidance models of chronic pain: an overview. In: *Understanding and Treating Fear of Pain.* Oxford, United Kingdom: Oxford University Press; 2004;3–24.

Boersma K, Linton SJ. Screening to identify patients at risk: profiles of psychological risk factors for early intervention. *Clin J Pain.* 2005;21:38–43.

Boushy D, Dubinsky I. Primary care physician and patient factors that result in patients seeking emergency care in a hospital setting: the patient's perspective. *J Emerg Med.* 1999;17:405.

Burchman SL, Pagel PS. Implementation of a formal treatment agreement for outpatient management of chronic nonmalignant pain with opioid analgesics. *J Pain Symptom Manage.* 1995; 10:556–563.

Burke P, Elliott M, Fleissner R. Irritable bowel syndrome and recurrent abdominal pain: a comparative review. *Psychosomatics.* 1999;40:277.

Butler SF, Budman SH, Fernandez K, et al. Validation of a screener and opioid assessment measure for patients with chronic pain. *Pain.* 2004;112:65–75.

Butler SF, Budman SH, Fernandez KC, et al. Development and validation of the current opioid misuse measure. *Pain.* 2007;130:144–156.

Cats-Baril WL, Frymoyer JW. The economics of spinal disorders. In: Frymoyer JW, ed. *The Adult Spine: Principles of Practice.* Raven Press; 1991.

Dersh, J, Gatchel RJ, Mayer TG, et al.. Prevalence of psychiatric disorders in patients with chronic disabling occupational spinal disorders. *Spine.* 2006;31:1156–1162.

Edwards RR, Cahalan C, Mensing G, Smith M, Haythornthwaite JA. Pain, catastrophizing, and depression in the rheumatic diseases. *Nat Rev Rheumatol.* 2011;7:216–224.

Ehde DM, Jensen MP, Engel JM, et al. Chronic pain secondary to disability: a review. *Clin J Pain.* 2003;19:3.

Ferrari R, Kwan O. The no-fault flavor of disability syndromes. *Med Hypotheses.* 2001;56:77.

Fillingim RB, Edwards RR, Powell T. Sex-dependent effects of reported familial pain history on recent pain complaints and experimental pain responses. *Pain.* 2000;86:87.

Flor H, Knost B, Birbaumer N. The role of operant conditioning in chronic pain: an experimental investigation. *Pain.* 2002;95:111.

Flor H, Turk DC, Scholz OB. Impact of chronic pain on the spouse: marital, emotional and physical consequences. *J Psychosom Res.* 1987;31:63–71.

Gatchel RJ, Peng YB, Peters ML, et al. The biopsychosocial approach to chronic pain: scientific advances and future directions. *Psychol Bull.* 2007;133:581–624.

Ives TJ, Chelminski PR, Hammett-Stabler CA, et al. Predictors of opioid misuse in patients with chronic pain: a prospective cohort study. *BMC Health Serv Res.* 2006;6:46.

Jensen IB, Bodin L, Ljungqvist T, et al. Assessing the needs of patients in pain: a matter of opinion? *Spine.* 2000;25:2816.

Jensen JN, Karpatschof B, Labriola M, et al. Do fear-avoidance beliefs play a role on the association between low back pain and sickness absence? A prospective cohort study among female health care workers. *J Occup Environ Med.* 2010;52:85–90.

Jensen MP, Turner JA, Romano JM. Changes in beliefs, catastrophizing, and coping are associated with improvement in multidisciplinary pain treatment. *J Consult Clin Psychol.* 2001; 69:655.

Keefe FJ, Lumley M, Anderson T, et al. Pain and emotion: new research directions. *J Clin Psychol.* 2001;57:587.

Kelly AM. Patient satisfaction with pain management does not correlate with initial or discharge VAS pain score, verbal pain rating at discharge, or change in VAS score in the emergency department. *J Emerg Med.* 2000;19:113.

Kerns RD, Rosenberg R, Jacob M. Anger expression and chronic pain. *J Behav Med.* 1994;17:57–67.

Lambeek LC, Mechelen WV, Knol DL, et al. Randomized controlled trial of integrated care to reduce disability from chronic low back pain in working and private life. *BMJ.* 2010;340:c1035.

Martel MO, Wasan AD, Jamison RN, Edwards RR. Catastrophic thinking and increased risk for prescription opioid misuse in patients with chronic pain. *Drug Alcohol Depend.* 2013.

Michna E, Jamison RN, Pham LD, et al. Urine toxicology screening among chronic pain patients on opioid therapy: frequency and predictability of abnormal findings. *Clin J Pain.* 2007;23:173–179.

Nielson WR, Weir R. Biopsychosocial approaches to the treatment of chronic pain. *Clin J Pain.* 2001;17:S114.

Okifuji A, Turk DC, Curran SL. Anger in chronic pain: investigations of anger targets and intensity. *J Psychosom Res.* 1999;61:771–780.

Picavet HS, Vlaeyen JW, Schouten JS. Pain catastrophizing and kinesophobia: predictors of chronic low back pain. *Am J Epidemiol.* 2002;156:1028.

Portenoy RK. Chronic opioid therapy in non-malignant pain. *J Pain Symptom Manage.* 1990;5:S46–S62.

Portenoy RK. Opioid therapy for chronic nonmalignant pain: a review of the critical issues. *J Pain Symptom Manage.* 1996; 11:127–203.

Prochaska JO, DiClemente CC, Norcross JC. In search of how people change. Applications to addictive behaviors. *Am Psychol.* 1992;47:1102–1111.

Sarver JH, Cydulka RK, Baker DW. Usual source of care and non-urgent emergency department use. *Acad Emerg Med.* 2002;9:916.

Sullivan M, Thorn B, Haythornthwaite J, et al. Theoretical perspectives on the relation between catastrophizing and pain. *Clin J Pain*. 2001;17:52–64.

Trost Z, Vangronsveld K, Linton SJ, Quartana PJ, Sullivan MJ. Cognitive dimensions of anger in chronic pain. *Pain*. 2012; 153:515–517.

Turk DC, Okifuji A. Psychological factors in chronic pain: evolution and revolution. *J Consult Clin Psychol*. 2002;70:678.

Turk DC, Okifuji A, Scharff L. Chronic pain and depression: role of perceived impact and perceived control in different age cohorts. *Pain*. 1995;61:93–101.

Vlaeyen JW, De Jong JR, Onghena P, et al. Can pain-related fear be reduced? The application of cognitive-behavioural exposure in vivo. *Pain Res Manag*. 2002;7:144–153.

Vowles KE, Gross RT. Work-related beliefs about injury and physical capability for work in individuals with chronic pain. *Pain*. 2003;101:291.

Weir R, Nielson WR. Interventions for disability management. *Clin J Pain*. 2001;17:S128.

Whitehead WE, Palsson O, Jones KR. Systematic review of the comorbidity of irritable bowel syndrome with other disorders: what are the causes and implications? *Gastroenterology*. 2002; 122:1140.

Wideman TH, Adams H, Sullivan MJ. A prospective sequential analysis of the fear-avoidance model of pain. *Pain*. 2009; 145:45–51.

Wilson KG, Eriksson MY, D'Eon JL, et al. Major depression and insomnia in chronic pain. *Clin J Pain*. 2002;18:77.

14   URINE DRUG TESTING

Theodore S. Grabow, MD
Brian M. Block, MD, PhD

OVERVIEW OF THE HEALTH PROBLEM

- There is a high prevalence (12%–25%) of chronic pain in the United States and patients are increasingly utilizing the health care system for its treatment. Treatment is driven by patient demand, public policy, physician organizations, and the pharmaceutical industry.
- Despite gaps in scientific evidence, published medical guidelines endorse the use of opioids for chronic non-cancer pain. As a consequence, opioid prescribing has increased dramatically in the past decade.
- Opioid misuse and opioid-related deaths have increased with the better availability of prescription medications. Prescription drug misuse is the fastest growing drug problem in the United States costing $100–200 billion annually.

- Abused opioids typically originate from a valid prescription from a single physician. Urine drug tests (UDT) can detect licit and illicit drug misuse.
- This chapter will focus predominantly on UDTs for screening and compliance monitoring for patients on prescription medications in the clinical setting.

BACKGROUND REQUIRED PRIOR TO ORDERING URINE DRUG TESTS

PRESCRIBING GUIDELINES FOR CONTROLLED SUBSTANCES

- Patients considered for chronic opioid therapy should undergo a comprehensive evaluation including a personal and family history of psychiatric disease and addiction. Patients should be evaluated initially and periodically for aberrant drug-related behaviors and risk for addiction. Patients should receive informed consent for chronic opioid therapy including the risks and benefits and treatment alternatives.
- Chronic opioid therapy is not appropriate for all patients with chronic pain. Furthermore, there should be a high barrier to initiating chronic opioid therapy since high quality long-term (>3 month) studies demonstrating efficacy are lacking.
- Chronic pain, psychiatric disease, and drug addiction are comorbid conditions. Substance abuse disorder and psychiatric disorder are prevalent in the general population and more so in the chronic pain population. Both disorders are associated with greater risk for prescription medication misuse. Chronic pain patients with a history of substance abuse disorder are prescribed opioids more often and at higher doses than their healthy counterparts.
- Physician organizations such as the American Pain Society (APS), the American Academy of Pain Medicine (AAPM), and the American Society of Interventional Pain Physicians (ASIPP) have developed treatment guidelines for chronic opioid therapy (see Chapter 55: Radiation Management for Pain Interventions).

PHARMACOKINETIC PRINCIPLES

- Absorption, distribution, metabolism, and elimination can impact UDTs.
- Drug absorption is influenced by route of administration. Substances with poor bioavailability will have decreased concentrations in the body and in the urine.
- Drug distribution depends on lipid solubility and protein binding. Lipophilic drugs better penetrate adipose tissue, while hydrophilic drugs concentrate

in the urine. Only unbound drug is eliminated in the urine, thus decreased protein binding may lead to increased elimination and shorter urine detection times.

- Drug metabolism is variable and depends on genetics, demographics (gender, age, ethnicity), health (renal and hepatic function), and the environment (diet and concurrent use of other medications).
- Opioids undergo phase I metabolism largely via the cytochrome P450 3A4 (CYP3A4) and 2D6 (CYP2D6) isoenzymes, and phase II metabolism via glucuronidation. CYP2D6 and CYP3A4 are susceptible to drug-drug interactions from inhibitors and inducers that may alter metabolism, influence opioid drug levels, and affect urine drug screens.
- Short elimination opioids have both earlier peak effects and more rapid urine clearance than long half-life opioids. For example, oxycodone (t ½ = 2–3 hours) may generate UDT positive only for oxymorphone (t ½ = 4–12 hours) due to the latter's longer elimination half-life.
- Saturation of any of these pathways via prolonged or elevated drug use can lead to nonlinear pharmacokinetics that may affect measurements during urine drug tests.
- Due to genetic polymorphism, enzymatic activity of CYP3A4 and CYP2D6 are highly variable. CYP3A4 activity can vary 50-fold between individuals and CYP2D6 by 1000-fold. A rapid metabolizer of codeine may test negative for codeine but positive for its metabolite morphine. Conversely, an average or poor metabolizer may test positive for both. Similarly, following hydrocodone or oxycodone use, a poor metabolizer will produce and excrete very little O-demethylated metabolite (eg, hydromorphone or oxymorphone, respectively) in urine.

URINE DRUG TESTING

CLINICAL DRUG TESTING—OVERVIEW

- Drug screening can be done on blood, hair, sweat, saliva, and nails but urine testing is preferred because of ease of use, immediate feedback, limited expense, greater drug concentrations, and longer detection times.
- Initial screening methods are typically office-based immunoassays. Abnormal immunoassay results are considered "presumptive" until confirmatory testing.
- Confirmatory testing generally is performed in an off-site laboratory using single or tandem liquid (LC) and/or gas chromatography (GC) and mass spectrometry (GC-MS).

- The U.S. Federation of State Medical Boards, APS, AAPM, and ASIPP all recommend routine UDTs for patients on chronic opioids. Chronic pain patients not receiving controlled substances can also benefit from random UDT since there are higher rates of drug misuse, abuse, and addiction in this population.
- "Universal precautions" should be adopted for all patients on chronic opioid therapy, including comprehensive evaluation, informed consent, opioid contract, risk stratification, psychiatric assessment, behavioral screening, random UDT, and periodic reassessment. Utilizing a universal set of rules for all patients improves the doctor-patient relationship since patients will not feel targeted.

TYPES OF URINE DRUG TESTS

Immunoassay (Qualitative Testing)

- Immunoassay testing is recommended for initial drug screening and ongoing compliance monitoring.
- It is noninvasive, cost-effective, and convenient to perform and allows for rapid analysis and in-office detection at the time of patient encounter.
- Immunoassay uses a monoclonal antibody that recognizes a structural feature of a drug or its metabolite.
- Accuracy and specificity vary depending on the assay utilized and the substance of detection. False positives may occur when another substance cross-reacts with the immunoassay antibody.
- Class-specific immunoassay panels are common, but drug-specific panels are recommended. Class-specific opioid panels group all testable opioids together whereas a drug-specific panel will distinguish between different opioids and opioid metabolites. Class-specific opioid panels have low or no sensitivity for synthetic (eg, meperidine, methadone, fentanyl) and semisynthetic (eg, hydrocodone, oxycodone, hydromorphone) opioids and a negative immunoassay test for those compounds will require confirmation by GC-MS. Aberrant drug-related behavior within the same drug class will be difficult to detect because positive tests may be nonspecific for the drug of interest and negative tests will miss many commonly used opioids.
- Class-specific panels for benzodiazepines have the same limitations as opioids. In particular, clonazepam cannot be detected by immunoassay.
- Expanded assays (ie, drug-specific panels) for tramadol, oxycodone, and other opioids often are required in the clinical setting. Immunoassay tests have been developed recently for fentanyl, carisoprodol, and meprobamate but are not widely available.

- Clinicians may require tests for other commonly prescribed medications such as antidepressants and even additional illicit substances such as methylene dioxymethamphetamine (MDMA).
- Sensitivity, specificity, accuracy, interferents, and detection thresholds vary by immunoassay and testing laboratory.

Point of Care (POC) Testing

- POC testing uses immunoassay technology without cumbersome instrumentation. Several companies make single-use POC testing devices for routine office use. POC testing devices may be predominantly class-specific unless requested otherwise.
- POC devices are portable, rapid, inexpensive, and require minimal physician training to administer and interpret.
- POC testing has the advantage of providing immediate feedback to the physician at initial or follow-up visits prior to prescribing controlled substances.

Gas/Liquid Chromatography-mass Spectrometry (Confirmatory or Quantitative Testing)

- The gold standard for confirmatory testing is the use of either gas or liquid chromatography with mass spectrometry in various combinations.
- GC-MS breaks down drug molecules into ionized fragments and separates them by mass-to-charge ratio. GC-MS is more accurate, sensitive, and reliable but also more time consuming and expensive compared to immunoassay.
- GC-MS is utilized for confirmatory testing particularly when immunoassay testing demonstrates irregularities. GC-MS can confirm drugs detected in immunoassay tests and identify drugs that are not including in routine screening methods including certain synthetic (eg, methadone, fentanyl) and semi-synthetic (eg, oxycodone, hydrocodone) opioids, certain benzodiazepines (eg, alprazolam, lorazepam, and clonazepam), carisoprodol and its metabolite meprobamate, the barbiturate butalbital, hallucinogens, inhalants, anabolic steroids, opioid normetabolites, designer cannabinoids, synthetic cathinones ("bath salts"), ketamine, and volatile alcohols (eg, ethanol, methanol).
- Opioid normetabolites are not usually included on routine opioid immunoassay but are detected on GC-MS. Testing for these compounds as biomarkers for the parent drug can reduce false-positive results and improve test accuracy.

Cutoff Limits (Limits of Detection)

- Cutoff levels are dependent on the laboratory, assay, specimen, substance being tested, and the reason for the test. GC-MS may fail to identify positive specimens if the threshold for detection is set too high or if the detection method is designed to test only certain substances.
- The United States Department of Health and Human Services (DHSS) established threshold concentrations for marijuana, cocaine, opiates, phencyclidine (PCP), and amphetamines/methamphetamines (the "Federal Five"). Cut off levels for pre-employment screening are set high to avoid false-positive results.
- GC-MS generally is performed to detect the lowest possible drug concentration present. However, clinicians may have to request that samples be evaluated at the more sensitive "limits of detection."

Drug Detection Times

- Commonly reported urinary drug detection times and plasma elimination half-lives are shown in Table 14-1. Drug detection times are determined by: (1) administered dose, (2) preparation and route of administration, (3) duration or chronicity of drug use and time since last use, (4) choice of the matrix, (5) detection threshold and sensitivity of the analytical method, (6) the nature of the molecule or metabolite sought, (7) the pH and concentration of urine, (8) the pharmacokinetic (absorption, distribution metabolism, and elimination) properties of the drug, and (9) individual patient differences (eg, age, body mass and fat content, gender, ethnicity and gene polymorphisms, liver and kidney function, and the coadministration of drugs that alter CYP450 metabolism). Most water-soluble drugs like opioids will be detected in the urine for 1–3 days whereas lipid-soluble drugs such as marijuana, diazepam, and PCP may be detected for more than a week.
- Patients may attempt to mask a given substance in a urine drug screen by increasing fluid consumption that will subsequently produce dilute urine and lower urinary drug concentration below cut off levels leading to a negative result. Conversely, patients who are diverting their medication may restrict fluid intake in order to concentrate urine drug concentration to manufacture a positive result.
- Patients taking low doses of drug, with long intervals between doses, or a long time since their last dose may demonstrate negative results.
- Patients taking drugs for longer periods of time may have longer detection windows than those using drugs for shorter intervals. Consequently, recently discontinued opioids that were used chronically still may be detected in subsequent urine drug screens.
- Environmental factors such as coadministration of drugs that inhibit or induce CYP2D6 or CYP3A4 can influence urine drug detection.

TABLE 14-1 Half-lives and Urine Detection Times for Drugs of Abuse

DRUG	DRUG HALF-LIFE	URINE DETECTION TIME
Alcohol-Ethanol (ETOH)	—	7–12 h
Ethyl Glucuronide (ETOH metabolite)	2–3 h	1–3 days
Amphetamine	7–34 h	48–72 h
Methamphetamine	9–24 h	48 h
Barbiturate		
Short-acting (eg, seco/pentobarbital)	20–30 h	24 h
Long-acting (eg, phenobarbital)	81–117 h	3 wks
Benzodiazepine		
Short-acting (eg, lorazepam)	9–19 h	3 days
Long-acting (eg, diazepam)	21–37 h	30 days
Cocaine (metabolites)	1 hr (15–42 h)	2–4 days
Marijuana (THC & metabolites)	1.6–59 h	
Single use	1–7 h	3 days
Moderate use (4 times/week)		5 days
Heavy Use (daily)	72–96 h	10 days
Chronic heavy use	7 days	30 days
Opioids		
Buprenorphine	3–5 h	<11 days
Codeine	3 h	2–4 days
Fentanyl	3–4 h	2–3 days
Heroin (6-MAM)	2–6 (6–25) h	8–54 h
Hydrocodone	3–9 h	2–4 days
Hydromorphone	2–3 h	2–4 days
Methadone	24 h	<14 days
Meperidine	3–4 h	2–4 days
Morphine	2–3.5 h	2–4 days
Oxycodone	2–3 h	2–4 days
Oxymorphone	4–12	2–4 days
Propoxyphene	12 h	<7 days
Tapentadol	4 h	1–7 days
Tramadol	6 h	2–4 days
Phencyclidine (PCP)	7–50 h	8–30 days
MDMA (ecstasy)	6–10 h	2–4 days
Cotinine (metabolite of nicotine)	20 h	2–4 days
Carisoprodol	1–3 h	

6-MAM, 6-monoacetylmorphine

PRACTICAL APPROACH

DEVELOP A URINE DRUG TESTING PROTOCOL

- Physicians should establish an office protocol prior to urine drug testing. This protocol should include the following provisions: (1) consistent with published opioid prescribing guidelines and State and Federal regulations, (2) selection of an immunoassay laboratory or POC testing device that includes not only class-specific assays but also useful drug-specific tests for the particular patient demographic or geographic region of interest, (3) selection of a GC-MS laboratory that is capable of confirmatory testing at "limits of detection" on a vast array of drugs, able to test for suspected tampering, and available to answer questions involving test interpretation, (4) designation of an appropriate area for random and unobserved specimen collection, (5) formal documentation and in-person discussion of anticipated and unexpected test results, and (6) a specific plan for corrective action to address abnormal results.

WHY TEST?

- Patient self-reports of illicit or unauthorized prescription drug use are often unreliable and physicians are poor at recognizing the signs of medication misuse. Monitoring behavior alone detects less than 50% of patients misusing drugs.
- UDTs can identify undisclosed illicit or prescription drug use and may uncover drug diversion or trafficking. Between 18%–41% of chronic pain patients receiving opioids abuse drugs and the incidence of abnormal UDTs in patients receiving chronic opioid therapy is 9%–50%.
- Drug misuse and aberrant drug-related behavior is a patient and public safety concern. UDT can enhance workplace safety by detecting current drug users. UDT may allow physicians to reduce their office exposure to patients who are engaged in criminal activity.
- UDT may reduce malpractice risk. 17% of closed claims against anesthesiologists were for inappropriate medication management. Of those claims, 94% involved the use of opioids and 57% resulted in death. 59% of the medication claims had evidence of inappropriate management, including the absence of opioid compliance monitoring or use of UDTs.

WHO SHOULD BE TESTED?

- Physicians may elect to UDT all new patients, regardless of intent to initiate or continue opioids, or any patient who is resistant to comprehensive evaluation or who exhibits aberrant behavior.
- Clinicians may also choose to UDT when major medication changes are being considered to avoid potential toxicity from unreported or known substances.

RISK STRATIFICATION

- Guidelines suggest stratifying patients into low-, medium-, and high-risk groups for addiction. Risk stratification tools generally rely on identification of aberrant drug-related behaviors (Table 14-2). Patients who display three or more aberrant behaviors from the Addiction Behaviors Checklist are at higher risk for opioid misuse and may warrant more frequent urine drug screens. Formal psychological evaluation or other psychometric tools such as the Screener and Opioid Assessment for Patients with Pain (SOAPP), SOAPP revised (SOAPP-R), and Common Opioid Misuse Measure (COMM) can assist in risk stratification.
- Risk factors for drug-related aberrant behaviors and addiction include personal or family history of alcoholism or substance abuse, nicotine dependency, age <45 years, depression, impulse control problems (attention deficit disorder, bipolar disease, obsessive-compulsive disorder, schizophrenia, personality disorders), hyper-vigilant states (post-traumatic stress disorder, preadolescent sexual abuse), somatoform disorder, organic mental syndrome, pain after a motor vehicle accident, and pain involving more than three regions of the body.

WHEN AND WHERE TO TEST?

- Random, not scheduled, UDTs are recommended to prevent test altering schemes such as bringing in "clean" urine which can be purchased online.
- UDT is appropriate for all patients prior to initiation of chronic opioid therapy and generally can be done in an office setting with a POC device.
- Some authors recommend testing low-risk patients 1–2 times/year, moderate risk patients 3–4 times/year, and high risk patients either 4 or more times/year including every month, or at every office visit, or at every drug refill.

INTERPRETATION

OVERVIEW

- In general, there are five scenarios that are likely to occur with urine drug testing: (1) the test is positive for the prescribed drug and negative for other drugs including illicit drugs, (2) the test is negative for the prescribed drug, (3) the test is positive for a non-prescribed drug, (4) the test is positive for an illicit drug, and (5) the test is invalid due to tampering or clerical error.

Positive Response

- The physician must determine if the patient actually took the drug in question, had a true false-positive response, or had a pseudo false-positive response due to a metabolite of the prescribed drug.
- The physician must query patients for potential agents that might cause false-positive tests and wait for GC-MS confirmation.

True False-positive Result

- A variety of pharmacologically distinct compounds can cause true false-positive immunoassays including controlled substances, nonprescription over-the-counter (OTC) medications, herbal preparations, and other nonscheduled medications (Table 14-3).

TABLE 14-2 **Aberrant Drug-Related Behaviors and Signs of Misuse/Addiction**

Refusing permission to obtain old medical records or speak with previous doctors

Unwillingness to name regular doctor or previous pain management doctor

Reluctance to undergo comprehensive evaluation including urine drug screen

Requesting a specific drug by name (possibly for higher street value)

Claiming multiple allergies to recommended medications

Refusing or resisting all other therapies and requesting only opioid therapy

Issuing threats, displaying anger, or threatening suicide if opioids are not received

Requesting appointments at the end of the workday or workweek or after hours

Providing excessive flattery to providers

Calling and/or visiting a physician's associates

Repeatedly losing prescriptions or requesting early refills

Use of opioids for non-analgesic reasons

Lack of control over, compulsive use of, or craving of medications

No medical insurance (cash pay)

Telling odd stories regarding need for medication (eg, "just moved to the area")

Reporting vague medical history or textbook symptoms

Requesting frequent dose escalations despite warnings, side effects or harm

New patients presenting for a refill of a chronically prescribed drug

Noncompliance with appointment times, prescription instructions, intake forms

Insistence on being seen urgently or arriving when usual doctor is unavailable

Concurrent misuse of illicit drugs or alcohol; driving under the influence of alcohol

Unauthorized dose escalations or drug hoarding during times of controlled pain

Obtaining drugs from multiple physicians and/or pharmacies

Resistance to change therapy despite low or lack of efficacy

Prescription forgery; selling drugs

Diminished work and home functioning

Obtaining prescription drugs from nonmedical sources; borrowing medications

TABLE 14-3 Compounds that Cause False-Positive Immunoassay Tests

DRUG OR DRUG CLASS	CROSS-REACTANT OR INTERFERING COMPOUND
Cannabinoids	Ibuprofen, naproxen, ketoprofen, piroxicam, clinoril, sulindac, tolmetin, promethazine, dronabinol, pantoprazole, efavirenz, hemp seed
Opioids	Poppy seeds/oil, chlorpromazine, rifampin, buprenorphine, fluoroquinolones, dextromethorphan, papaverine, quinine, diphenhydramine
Amphetamines	Ephedrine, desoxyephedrine, methylphenidate, trazodone, bupropion, desipramine, amantadine, ranitidine, labetolol, fluoxetine, phenylpropanolamine, brompheniramine, chlorpromazine, promethazine, Vicks nasal inhaler, isometheptene, isoxsuprine, phentermine, phenylephrine, phenylpropanolamine, pseudoephedrine, selegiline, thioridazine, trimethobenzamide, trimipramine
Phencyclidine	Chlorpromazine, thioridazine, diphenhydramine, ibuprofen, meperidine, venlafaxine, dextromethorphan, doxylamine, dextroamphetamine, ibuprofen, imipramine, ketamine, tramadol
Benzodiazepine	Oxaprozin, sertraline, some herbal agents
Barbiturates	Ibuprofen, naproxen
Methadone	Verapamil, propoxyphene, diphenhydramine, doxylamine, clomipramine, quetiapine, chlorpromazine, thioridazine, ibuprofen
Alcohol	Asthma inhalers
Cocaine	Topical anesthetics containing cocaine, coca leaf teas, amoxicillin, tonic water
Tricyclic antidepressants	Carbamazepine, cyclobenzaprine, cyproheptadine, diphenhydramine, hydroxyzine, quetiapine
Lyseric acid diethylamine (LSD)	Amitriptyline, dicyclomine, ergotamine, promethazine, sumatriptan

Pseudo False-positive Result

- A pseudo-false positive test is positive for a controlled substance but not through direct ingestion of the identified substance. This is due to either (1) metabolic conversion of an administered drug to another drug (eg, hydrocodone metabolized to hydromorphone), or (2) consumption of a legal substance that contains detectable amounts of the tested for drug (eg, poppy seeds detected as opioid; coca leaf tea detected as cocaine).
- Many commonly prescribed opioids are biotransformed into other pharmaceutically available opioids that independently are subjected to urine drug testing (Table 14-4). Consequently, a positive test for the parent drug and/or its metabolite does not distinguish between exclusive use of the parent drug versus use of the parent drug and concurrent use (or abuse) of one of its metabolites. However, the concentration of the minor metabolite should be less than the concentration of the parent drug.

Negative Response

- There are five scenarios that can lead to a negative test: (1) no drug in the specimen, (2) the concentration of the drug in the specimen is below the level of detection (below the cutoff level), (3) the drug is present in the specimen but the assay antibody reacts only weakly (or not at all) to the particular drug, (4) interference with the assay unintentionally via coadministration of other medications (negative interferents) or intentionally due to the addition of adulterants (tampering), and (5) laboratory error.

True False-negative Result

- A true false-negative test is rare but defined as a negative finding in a sample known to contain the drug of interest in the concentrations normally detected. This situation can result from laboratory or clerical error, or from urine tampering via adulteration or substitution.

Pseudo False-negative Result

- A pseudo false-negative result occurs when the concentration of the suspected drug is below the threshold level at the time of urine collection. This can occur with both appropriate use (eg, low dose, infrequent use, long duration between last dose and test) and inappropriate use (eg, diversion, or running out of drug early due to unauthorized dose escalation) of drugs. It also can occur if the laboratory sets an arbitrarily high cutoff limit for drug detection.
- Due to a variety of genetic (eg, polymorphism), environmental, and pharmacological factors, certain patients may undergo increased metabolism of the drug of interest and will demonstrate a pseudo-false negative test whereby the test correctly fails to demonstrate the drug.

CORRECTIVE ACTION

- When an abnormal UDT is confirmed by GC-MS, physicians have a responsibility to take action. Most physicians have a zero tolerance rule to positive urine drug screens for illicit drugs and many have a zero tolerance for positive screens for certain nonprescribed controlled substances. Policy should be consistent and clearly defined in office procedural manuals and in opioid contracts. In cases of misuse,

TABLE 14-4 **Major Opioid Metabolites**

OPIOID	INACTIVE METABOLITES	ACTIVE METABOLITES IDENTICAL TO PHARMACEUTICAL OPIOIDS	ACTIVE METABOLITES THAT ARE NOT PHARMACEUTICAL OPIOIDS
Morphine	Normorphine	Hydromorphone	Morphine-3-glucuronide, Morphine-6-glucuronide
Hydromorphone	Hydromorphol	None	Hydromorphone-3-glucuronide
Hydrocodone	Norhydrocodone, Hydrocodol, Hydromorphol, Normorphine	Hydromorphone, Dihydrocodeine	None
Codeine	Norcodeine	Hydrocodone, Morphine	None
Oxycodone	Oxycodols Oxymorphols	Oxymorphone	Noroxycodone
Oxymorphone	Oxymorphone-3-glucuronide, oxymorphol	None	6-Hydroxy-oxymorphone
Fentanyl	Norfentanyl	None	None
Tramadol	Nortramadol	None	O-desmethyltramadol
Methadone	2-Ethylidene-1,5-dimethyl-3,3-diphenylpyrrolidine, 2-Ethyl-5-methyl-3,3-diphenylpyrroline	None	None
Heroin	Normorphine	Morphine	6-Monoacetylmorphine
Buprenorphine	None	None	Buprenorphine-3-glucuronide, Norbuprenorphine-3-glucuronide, Norbuprenorphine
Butorphanol	Hydroxybutorphanol	None	Norbutorphanol
Propoxyphene	None	None	Norpropoxyphene

abuse, or addiction, patients should be referred to an addiction medicine specialist.

- Irregular immunoassay tests require confirmatory test results prior to taking definitive action. While awaiting confirmation, physicians may choose to refill the medication, only offer a few days supply, switch to an opioid with a lower abuse potential (eg, BuTrans), or withhold opioids altogether depending on the infraction.
- Corrective action after a confirmed test could include: counseling, more frequent intervals for prescription refills, reduction in the quantity of opioids prescribed, conducting behavioral, psychological, or addiction medicine evaluations, or discontinuation of the opioid altogether. Documentation is key. Physician may choose to diagnose the patient as "noncompliant with the treatment plan" which has its own ICD code (V15.81).

TAMPERING

- Tampering can occur through ingestion of commonly available household chemicals that alter the pH or specific gravity of urine. Other methods of tampering include specimen dilution, specimen substitution with drug-free urine, and specimen adulteration with assay interferents.
- Unobserved specimen collection is the standard for routine office practice. Unfortunately, most forms of tampering will not be detected. If tampering is suspected, an adulteration panel from the laboratory can be requested.
- In the office, tampering may be determined by examining urine appearance and color, measuring urine temperature, specific gravity and pH, and shaking to determine whether soap or other substances have been added. Urine temperature should be between 32°C to 38°C within 4 minutes of collection. Tampering should be suspected if: (1) the urine pH is less than 3 or greater than 10, (2) urine specific gravity is less than 1.001 or greater than 1.020, (3) urinary creatinine concentration <20 mg/dL, (4) urinary nitrite level >500 μg/ml, (5) urine volume <30 ml, and (6) urine temperature <32°C or >38°C.
- Steps to reduce tampering include: removal of any unnecessary outer clothing, removing anything in the collection area that could be used to alter or substitute the urine, requesting the display and removal of any items in the patient's pocket, requiring all other personal belongings to remain outside the testing area, instructing the patient to wash and dry their hands under direct supervision and not to rewash until after delivering the sample, and adding a bluing agent in the commode and turning off the water supply to the testing site.

INTERPRETATION CAVEATS

- Drugs with extremely short half-lives may not show up in urine if the test is performed a long time after taking the drug. Conversely, patients with chronic liver or kidney disease may demonstrate drugs in urine much longer than expected due to impaired metabolism.

- Brand name and generic medications may have significant differences in bioavailability and in theory drug substitution could impact urine drug screens.
- An unexpected positive result does not automatically imply drug misuse, abuse, or addiction, nor does an unexpected negative result necessarily imply criminal intent such as diversion.
- A negative urine drug screen does not rule out casual or even daily drug use depending on the drug, dosing, frequency, and chronicity of use. Urine drug screens are better at detecting moderate and heavy use.
- Any urine that has been tampered with is considered a positive response. Likewise, patient refusal to provide a sample is considered a positive response.
- There currently is insufficient scientific evidence to determine the relationship between the amount of drug detected by a urine drug test and the amount of drug ingested by the patient. Many testing laboratories have developed normalized data based on demographic and other biological variables. However, intra- and inter-individual variations in absorption, distribution, metabolism, and elimination of drug can have a large influence on drug bio-transformation making normalized data unreliable. Urine drug tests cannot tell the physician how much drug was taken, when it was administered, or the source of the drug.

INTERPRETATION PITFALLS

- The anti-Parkinson's medication selegiline is metabolized into *l*-amphetamine and *l*-methylamphetamine. Chiral chromatography may be required to distinguish between routine seligiline use and amphetamine abuse.
- Tests for cocaine and cocaine metabolite benzoylecgonine have low cross-reactivity and thus are highly predictive for cocaine use. Likewise, immunoassays have a high predictive value for marijuana use.
- Tests for amphetamines/methamphetamines have high cross-reactivity particularly to nonprescription sympathomimetic amines (eg, ephedrine, pseudoephedrine) and thus are less predictive of amphetamine use.
- Tests for opioids are very sensitive for the natural alkaloids morphine and codeine but less sensitive for the semisynthetic (eg, hydrocodone, hydromorphone, oxycodone) and synthetic (eg, fentanyl, meperidine, methadone, propoxyphene) opioids. In fact, fentanyl and meperidine are not detected by commercially available opioid immunoassays and require GC-MS identification.

- Codeine may be detected at low concentration in morphine preparations due to manufacturing impurities (high amounts of morphine should be present in these cases).
- Hydrocodone may be detected in oxycodone preparations due to manufacturing impurities (high amounts of oxycodone should be present in these cases).
- Ingestion of poppy seeds or herbal teas containing Papaveris fructus may lead to positive screen for morphine or codeine.
- Oxycodone is metabolized into oxymorphone. It may be difficult to identify an individual who occasionally abuses small amounts of oxymorphone while being prescribed oxydocone.
- Morphine is metabolized in small amounts of hydromorphone. It may be difficult to identify an individual who occasionally abuses small amounts of hydromorphone while being prescribed morphine.
- Hydrocodone is metabolized to hydromorphone and dihydrocodeine. It may be difficult to identify an individual who occasionally abuses small amounts of hydromorphone and/or dihydrocodeine while being prescribed hydrocodone.
- Heroin users will test positive for morphine, which is one of its active metabolites. Heroin itself is unlikely to show up due to its short elimination half-life and detection time of only 8 hours.

POPULAR MISCONCEPTIONS

- Passive marijuana and cocaine inhalation does not cause sufficient urinary concentrations in qualitative or quantitative tests in adults.
- Legally obtained hemp-containing products do not have sufficient tetrahydrocannabinol (THC) concentrations to show up positive on immunoassay tests and thus other sources of THC acquisition should be considered. The synthetic cannabinoids dronabinol (Marinol) and nabiximols (Sativex) will test positive in urine drug screens for THC. A third cannabinoid, nabilone (Cesamet), does not contain THC and therefore will not be detected by immunoassay or GC-MS tests for THC. The synthetic cannabinoids known as "Spice drugs" also will avoid detection by urine drug tests for THC.
- The use of coca leaf teas will cause positive urine drug screens but these products are illegal in the United States according to regulations of the Drug Enforcement Administration and Food and Drug Administration.
- Most bath salts are undetectable by immunoassay and rarely detected by confirmatory drug tests. However

the bath salts mephedrone, methadrone, methylone, butylone, methylenedioxypyrovalerone (MDPV), and naphyrone can be detected by GC-MS.

CONCLUSIONS

- Over the past two decades, there has been in increase in opioid prescribing, opioid dispensing, and opioid related drug misuse and abuse resulting in overdose and death.
- Chronic pain patients have a higher rate of psychiatric disease including substance abuse disorder than their healthy counterparts.
- UDT can assist in both diagnostic and therapeutic decision making and should be part of every comprehensive care plan for patients receiving controlled substances.
- UDTs readily can identify prescription and illicit drug abusers and identify patients who may need more formalized evaluation by an addiction medicine specialist and/or drug detoxification.
- The major criticism of urine drug tests is based on the low level of evidence that these tests actually reduce drug abuse and drug-related behaviors, or affect patient outcomes. In addition, some question the direct economic incentives and health care costs associated with both POC and confirmatory testing.
- Physicians who order and interpret urine drug screens to guide therapy must have a thorough understanding of the types and limitations of drug tests, detection times, the common reasons for false-positive and false-negative results, pharmacokinetics, opioid pharmacogenetics, and opioid metabolism.

BIBLIOGRAPHY

Alturi S, Akbik H, Sudarshan G. Prevention of opioid abuse in chronic non-cancer pain: an algorithmic, evidence based approach. *Pain Physician.* 2012;15(3 Suppl):ES177–ES189.

Brahm NC, Yeager LL, Fox MD, et al. Commonly prescribed medications and potential false-positive urine drug screens. *Am J Health Syst Pharm.* 2010;67:1344–1350.

Chou R, Ballantyne JC, Fanciullo GJ, et al. Research gaps on use of opioids for chronic noncancer pain: findings form a review of the evidence for an American Pain Society and American Academy of Pain Medicine clinical practice guideline. *J Pain.* 2009;10:147–159.

Chou R, Fanciullo GJ, Fine PG, et al. Opioids for chronic noncancer pain: prediction and identification of aberrant drug-related behaviors: a review of the evidence for an American PainSociety and American Academy of Pain Medicine clinical practice guideline. *J Pain.* 2009;10:131–146.

Christo PJ. Manchikanti L, Ruan X, et al. Urine drug testing in chronic pain. *Pain Physician.* 2011;14:123–143.

Fitzgibbon DR, Rathmell JP, Michna E, et al. Malpractice claims associated with medication management for chronic pain. *Anesthesiology.* 2010;112:948–956.

Gourlay DL, Heit HA. Universal precautions revisited: managing the inherited pain patient. *Pain Med.* 2009;10(Suppl 2):S115–S123.

McBane S, Weigle N. Is it time to drug test your chronic pain patient? *J Fam Pract.* 2010;59:628–633.

Moeller KE, Lee KC, Kissack JC. Urine drug screening: practical guide for clinicians. *Mayo Clinic Proc.* 2008;83:66–76.

Morasco BJ, Gritzner S, Lewis L, et al. Systematic review of the prevalence, correlates, and treatment outcomes for chronic noncancer pain in patients with comorbid substance use disorder. *Pain.* 2011;152:488–497.

Owen GT, Burton AW, Schade CM, Passik S. Urine drug testing: current recommendations and best practices. *Pain Physician.* 2012;15(3 Suppl):ES119–ES133.

Reisfield GM, Salazar E, Bertholf RL. Rational use and interpretation of urine drug testing in chronic opioid therapy. *Ann Clin Lab Sci.* 2007;37:301–314.

Smith HS. Opioid Metabolism. *Mayo Clin. Proc.* 2009;84(7):613–624.

Standridge JB, Adams SM, Zotos AP. Urine drug screening: a valuable office procedure. *Am Fam Physician.* 2010;81:635–640.

Starrels JL, Becker WC, Alford DP, et al. Systematic review: treatment agreements and urine drug testing to reduce opioid misuse in patients with chronic pain. *Ann Intern Med.* 2010;152:712–720.

Trescot AM, Datta S, Lee M, Hansen H. Opioid pharmacology. *Pain Physician.* 2008;11(2 Suppl):S133–S153.

Verstraete AG. Detection times of drugs of abuse in blood, urine, and oral fluid. *Ther Drug Monit.* 2004;26:200–205.

Wu SM, Compton P, Bolus R, et al. The addiction behaviors checklist: validation of a new clinician-based measure of inappropriate opioid use in chronic pain. *J Pain Symptom Manage.* 2006;32:342–351.

15 GENETIC TESTING IN PAIN MEDICINE

Andrea M. Trescot, MD
Daniel A. Schwarz, MD

INTRODUCTION

- It has long been recognized that there is a vast interindividual variability in the pain that patients report with seemingly similar painful conditions. In addition, it is well known that there is wide individual variability in analgesic doses required to control pain.
  - The minimum effective dose of opioids also appears to vary widely between patients.

TABLE 15-1   Common Substrates of CYP Enzymes

1A2	2B6	2C9	2C19	2D6	3A4
Amitriptyline	Bupropion	Valproic acid	Barbiturates	Codeine	Alprazolam
Nabumetone	Methadone	Piroxicam	Topiramate	Tramadol	Midazolam
Desipramine	Ketamine	Celecoxib	Diazepam	Meperidine	Cyclosporine
Tizanidine	Testosterone	Ibuprofen	Amitriptyline	Oxycodone	Sildenafil
Imipramine		Warfarin	Imipramine	Hydrocodone	Indinavir
Acetaminophen			Clomipramine	Dextromethorphan	Verapamil
Cyclobenzaprine			Sertraline	Amitriptyline	Atorvastatin
Clozapine			Citalopram	Nortriptyline	Lovastatin
Fluvoxamine			Phenytoin	Doxepin	Digoxin
Theophylline			Carisoprodol	Tamoxifen	Amiodarone
Melatonin			Clopidogrel	Amphetamines	Methadone
Duloxetine				Duloxetine	Erythromyacin
Caffeine				Metoclopramide	Trazodone
Lidocaine				Propranolol	Fentanyl
Warfarin				Venlafaxine	Buprenorphine

Source: Data from Indiana University Web site and Genelex Web site, among others.

○ For many years it has been well established that animals (rats) could be bred to be responsive or nonresponsive to a variety of analgesics.
- At least some of this variability appears to be related to genetic issues, leading to the potential for diagnosis, prediction, and possible therapy based on an individual's genetic profile.
  ○ These processes appear to significantly influence the response to opioids.

BASIC GENETICS

- *SNP*: Single nucleotide polymorphisms
- *Allele*: One of the number of alternative forms of the same gene
- *Haplotypes*: A combination of alleles located at adjacent locations (loci) that tend to be inherited together
- *Wild type*: The "normal" or standard allele, as compared to the "mutant" form
- *Homozygotic*: Identical pairs of genes for a given hereditary characteristic
- *Heterozygotic*: Dissimilar gene pair for a given hereditary characteristic

CYTOCHROME P450 ENZYMES (CYP450)

- There have been 57 CYP450 enzymes identified in humans, and they are divided into family, subfamily, isoenzymes, and allele variants.
- Metabolism of most currently used drugs occurs by about 7 clinically relevant enzymes: CYP1A2, CYP2B6, CYP2C8, CYP2C9, CYP2C19, CYP2D6, and CYP3A4, all of which have different (but partially overlapping) catalytic activities.
- Many common medicines and foods are substrates (Table 15-1), inducers (Table 15-2), or inhibitors (Table 15-3) of medicines used in pain treatments.

TYPES OF METABOLIZERS

Patients can be classified by how effectively they metabolize a medication, which is based on how many copies of normal or abnormal alleles they inherited (Table 15-4). There is a population distribution of these isoenzymes (Table 15-5). There is also an ethnic distribution of this polymorphism.

TABLE 15-2   Common Inducers of CYP Enzymes [Modified from Indiana University Web Site and Genelex Web Site, among Others]

1A2	2C9	2C19	2D6	3A4
Carbamazepine	Rifampin	Carbamazepine	Carbamazepine	Carbamazepine
Griseofulvin	Ritonavir	Rifampin	Phenobarbital	Phenytoin
Lansoprazole	Barbiturates	Ginko	Phenytoin	Nevirapine
Omeprazole	St. John's Wort		Rifampin	Modafinil
Ritonavir			Dexamethasone	Topiramate
Tobacco				Butalbital
St. John's Wort				St. John's Wort

TABLE 15-3   **Common Inhibitors of CYP Enzymes [Modified from Indiana University Web Site and Genelex Web Site, among Others]**

1A2	2B6	2C9	2C19	2D6	3A4
Fluvoxamine	Orphenadrine	Fluvoxamine	Fluoxetine	Duloxine	Ketoconazole
Ciprofloxacin		Paroxetine	Fluvoxamine	Cimetidine	Erythromycin
Mexiletine		Amiodarone	Paroxetine	Sertraline	Mifepristone
Verapamil		Modafinil	Topiramate	Fluoxetine	Nefazodone
Caffeine		Tamoxifen	Modafinil	Haloperidol	Grapefruit
Grapefruit juice			Birth control pill	Methadone	Indinavir
				Paroxetine	Ritonavir
				Quinidine	Verapamil
				Celecoxib	Diltiazem
				Bupropion	Midazolam
				Ritonavir	
				Amiodarone	
				Metoclopramide	
				Chlorpromazine	
				Ropivacaine	
				Methadone	

TABLE 15-4   **Types of Metabolizers**

TYPE OF METABOLIZER	ABBREVIATION	ALLELES	RESPONSE
Extensive metabolizer	EM	2 "wild type"	Normal
Intermediate metabolizer	IM	1 ⇓allele or 2 partially ⇓alleles.	Partially ⇓ response
Poor metabolizer	PM	2 mutant alleles	Poor response
Ultra rapid metabolizer	UM	Multiple copies of functional alleles	Exaggerated response

- Approximately 7%–10% of Caucasians are CYP2D6 deficient (PM).
  - But only 1%–2% of Asians and 2%–4% of African-Americans are PM.
- Approximately 30% of Asians and African-Americans have intermediate metabolism (IM) of CYP2D6.
  - On the other hand, approximately 29% of Ethiopians, 10% of Southern Europeans, and 1%–2% of Northern Europeans are ultra rapid metabolizers (UM) of CYP2D6.

Even EM activity is highly variable, with as much as 10,000 fold difference in activity between individuals.

- In psychiatry, 52% of the psychiatric medication (TCAs, SSRIs, and SNRIs) and 62% of antipsychotic drugs are metabolized by CYP2D6.

SINGLE NUCLEOTIDE POLYMORPHISMS

- Genetic association studies in humans have looked at variability in specific gene sites.

TABLE 15-5   **Population Distribution of Isoenzymes**

GENE	PM	IM	EM	UM
CYP2C9	2%–4%	>35%	60%	NA
CYP2C19	2%–20%	24%–36%	14%–44%	30%
CYP2D6	10%	35%	48%	7%

- These SNPs or haplotypes have been linked to increased or decreased sensitivity to pain, as well as the metabolism of various opioids. Letters or numbers identify SNP variations.
  - For example, normal functional activity alleles of the cytochrome P450 2D6 (CYP2D6) gene are designated CYP2D6*1 and CYP2D6*2, while the most common mutant alleles are CYP2D6*3, CYP2D6*4, CYP2D6*5, and CYP2D6*6.
  - On the other hand, one of the mu opioid receptor gene SNPs called A118 is designated as A118AA, A118AG, or A118GG, depending on the wild type, heterozygotic, or homozygotic mutation, respectively. The inconsistency in how these genes are named is one of the issues that make genetic studies so difficult to follow.

WHY CONSIDER GENETIC TESTING?

- There are a multitude of different types of serious adverse events (SAEs) or adverse drug reactions (ADRs) of medications, such as sudden death, seizures, cardiac arrhythmias, and delirium.
- Knowledge of these polymorphisms *before* beginning a drug therapy could help in choosing the right agent at a safe dosage, especially those drugs with a narrow therapeutic index and a high risk for the development of ADRs.

- Allele-based association studies are expected to shed light on the medical mystery of why pain persists in some patients but not in others, despite seemingly identical traumas. In other words, why do some diabetic patients develop only numbness as the manifestation of their peripheral neuropathy while others with the same blood sugar fluctuations develop a painful peripheral neuropathy? Why do only some shingles patients develop post herpetic neuralgia? Why don't all of the persons in a car accident with the same mechanism of injury develop the same whiplash related pain?

GENOTYPE-BASED DOSE ADJUSTMENTS (GENE-DOSE)

- Standard dose adjustments look at the differences in pharmacokinetic parameters, such as weight, clearance and area under the curve (AUC).
- Genotype-based dose adjustments assess the genetic metabolism to pick a medication dose. For instance:
  - A standard dose of medication X might be 2 tablets for an EM patient
  - A PM patient might need only 1 tablet
  - An IM might need 1.5 tablets
  - An UM might need 3 or more tablets of the same medication to achieve a similar effect
- In a study of antidepressant drugs, it was calculated that, for a CYP2D6 PM patient taking nortriptyline, the therapeutic dose would be 50 mg, while an UM patient would need a dose of 500 mg to obtain the same blood level.

CYP2D6 INFLUENCE ON OPIOIDS

- CYP2D6 activity can have substantial influence on the opioids that are commonly used in pain management.
  - Poor metabolizers (PM) of CYP2D6 will have decreased conversion of inactive to active opioid formulations.
- *Codeine* is an inactive compound (a prodrug), metabolized by CYP2D6 into its active form, *morphine.*
  - It has only a weak affinity for the mu receptor, 300 times less binding than morphine.
  - CYP2D6 PM patients and patients taking CYP2D6 inhibitors (see Table 15-3) who are given acetaminophen with codeine are really then being given only acetaminophen.
  - UM patients may have dangerously high levels of morphine after standard doses.
- *Tramadol* is metabolized by CYP2D6 to its M1 metabolite, which is at least six times more potent than the parent compound.

- *Hydrocodone* displays weak binding capacity for the mu receptor, but the CYP2D6 enzyme demethylates it into *hydromorphone*, which has much stronger mu binding than hydrocodone.
  - The maximal plasma level of hydromorphone was five times higher in EMs than PM or EM pretreated with quinidine (a potent CYP2D6 inhibitor).
  - Otton et al. also found that subjects identified as EM reported more "good opiate effects" and fewer "bad opiate effects" than PM or EM patients pretreated with quinidine. They concluded that activity of CYP2D6 may limit the abuse liability of hydrocodone.
- *Oxycodone* is metabolized by glucuronidation to noroxycodone (which has less than 1% of the analgesia potency of oxycodone), and by CYP2D6 to *oxymorphone.*
  - Oxycodone is an analgesic, not a pro-drug; however, oxymorphone is an active metabolite of oxycodone, and may have significant impact on analgesia.
  - Yang et al. showed that 71% of a group of postoperative patients with acute severe pain were PM for CYP2D6, compared to other metabolizers.
    - They also found that PMs of CYP2D6 who were also smokers had more pain than the nonsmokers.

CYP3A4 INFLUENCE ON OPIOID METABOLISM

- Fentanyl and buprenorphine are excreted via CYP3A4, and blood levels would be expected to rise in PM patients or those receiving CYP3A4 inhibitors.
- Buprenorphine is also metabolized by CYP3A4 to active compounds, and CYP3A4 inhibitors may lead to decreased analgesia.
- Methadone has been widely reported to be metabolized by CYP3A4, and 60%–75% of the formation of 2-ethyl-1,5-dimethyl-3,3,-diphenylpyrrolidine (EDDP), which is not pharmacologically active, comes from this enzyme pathway.

CYP2B6 INFLUENCE ON OPIOID METABOLISM

- Some evidence suggests that methadone is primarily metabolized by CYP2B6.
  - Patients who are homozygous for the variant CYP2B6*6 gene required lower doses of methadone than the heterozotes or noncarriers.
- Both CYP3A4 and CYP2B6 may both have a significant influence on methadone metabolism.

○ CYP2B6 has greater activity toward metabolism of (S)-methadone.
- An imbalance in the response of CYP2B6 and 3A4 during drug interactions may lead to differences between the (R)- and (S)- enantiomers.
○ Increases or decreases in (R)-methadone could cause respiratory depression or withdrawal, while increase in (S)- methadone could increase the QT interval, the risk of arrhythmias.

OTHER PHARMACOGENIC VARIANTS

MU OPIOID RECEPTOR

The gene encoding the mu opioid receptor is OPRM1.

- The analgesic efficacy of mu-acting drugs has been linked to the 118 SNP of OPRM1.
  ○ Studies show that patients carrying the GG (homozygous variant) genotype require much higher opioid doses to achieve pain relief.

KAPPA OPIOID RECEPTOR

The gene OPRK1 encodes the kappa-opioid receptor.

The kappa receptor is involved in the response to addictive drugs, particularly cocaine, but also has been shown to produce aversive states, which may prevent the development of opioid use reinforcement. Accordingly variants of the gene that encode this receptor may alter behavioral response to opiates.

DELTA OPIOID RECEPTOR

The delta opioid receptor gene is called OPRD1.

- Mutations in this gene have been associated with cocaine and opioid addiction.
  ○ A study of more than 1400 heroin addicts found that the delta opioid gene (OPRD1) alleles rs2236857 and rs58111 had a high association with heroin abuse.

CATECHOL-O-METHYLTRANSFERASE

- Catechol-O-methyltransferase (COMT) is both a soluble (S-COMT) and membrane bound, (MB-COMT) gene, which metabolizes catecholamines, including dopamine, epinephrine, and norepinephrine and is important for dopaminergic and adrenergic/noradrenergic neurotransmission.
- COMT is located throughout the body, from the kidneys, liver, and intestine, to the brain, including the prefrontal cortex, where dopamine plays a key role in cognition, reward, memory, etc.
- The relationship of COMT to pain has been found to be complex.
  ○ The most commonly studied COMT SNP has been the wild type Val/Val, the heterozygous Val158Met, and the homozygous Met/Met genotype (which causes a 3-4 fold reduction in COMT activity).
    - In a study of whiplash patients, the Met/Met patients described more intense acute pain and overall symptoms, and required a longer time for resolution of symptoms, despite no significant difference in quality or mechanism of injury.
- COMT is also associated with depression and the response to antidepressant medications.
  ○ Several alleles are being studied, including Val158Met, to predict response to specific antidepressant medications.
- COMT and addiction
  ○ The common link in all addictions, whether legal or illicit substances, is the mesolimbic system, with activation of neurons in the Ventral Tegmental Area (VTA) of the midbrain, converging on the Nucleus Accumbens (NAc) in the limbic forebrain, with activation of dopaminergic transmission within the NAc.
  ○ Even other drugs, like alcohol and nicotine, stimulate our natural opioid and cannibinoid receptors directly within the VTA-NAc dopaminergic releasing pathway.
  ○ Nicotine Dependence (ND) is primarily a dopamine regulated disorder, and thus would be regulated by COMT variability.

GAMMA-AMINOBUTYRIC ACID

- Gamma-aminobutyric acid (GABA) is the main inhibitory neurotransmitter in the human brain, which plays a role in regulating neuronal excitability.
  ○ The 1519T>C GABA (A) alpha 6 gene is associated with:
    - alcohol dependence
    - methamphetamine dependence

UDP-GLUCURONO-SYLTRANSFERASES

- Uridine diphosphate glucuronosyltransferase (UGT) is involved in the metabolism of many drugs (such as morphine and acetaminophen) as well as the biotransformation of important endogenous substrates (e.g. bilirubin, ethinylestradiol).
  ○ Morphine is metabolized by UGT2B7 to morphine-6-glucuronide (M6G) and morphine-3-glucuronide

(M3G) in a usual ratio of 1:6, while approximately 5% of the medication is demethylated by CYP3A4 to normorphine.

- M6G adds to the analgesia of morphine, while M3G appears to be hyperalgic, causing pain.
- UGT2B7 inhibition can influence the levels of M3G compared to M6G.
- Tamoxifen, diclofenac, naloxone, carbamazepine, TCAs, and benzodiapines are all inhibitors of UGT2B7, potentially leading to opioid hyperalgia.

D2 DOPAMINE RECEPTOR

The D2 dopamine receptor (DRD2) plays a critical role in reward and reinforcement behavior.

- Interestingly, there was strong evidence that this gene is associated with heroin dependence in Chinese patients but carries a low risk of heroin dependence in German patients.

DNA TESTING

Since the price has decreased dramatically, the use of oral samples or buccal swabs for specific genetic testing has recently become economically feasible.

- Several SNPs are readily available, providing information on CYP enzymes 2D6, 2C9, 2C19 as well as VKORC1 (reflecting the metabolism of warfarin).
- Other companies provide genetic testing that includes 2B6 (for methadone metabolism) and 2B15 (for benzodiazepine metabolism).
  - However, intriguing information regarding potential risk of addiction and misuse may also be available through genetic testing.

WHAT SHOULD THE CLINICIAN DO?

- Take a medication history of prior adverse effects or inadequate effects ("What has worked well for you in the past?" "What hasn't helped?" "Are you sensitive to medications or do you need larger than normal doses of medications?")
- Check for common potential interactions with opioids, especially CYP2D6 inhibitors.
- When starting new medications, check the metabolic pathway for activation or excretion issues.
- Be aware of potential drug-drug interactions when adding new medications.
- Consider formal genetic testing to evaluate appropriate opioid choices and potentially to predict opioid risks.

CONCLUSION

- Patient care may be improved by genotyping and following drug concentration levels.
- Pharmacogenetics and therapeutic drug monitoring can potentially minimize adverse events, while maximizing efficacy.
- Integration of genetic analysis in clinical studies will increase the likelihood of identifying clinical and genetic factors that can be used to predict opioid responses.
- With knowledge of a patient's potential for beneficial response to a given opioid, a physician is armed with critical information that can guide therapeutic decisions.

BIBLIOGRAPHY

Ahmed I, Dagincourt PG, Miller LG, Shader RI. Possible interaction between fluoxetine and pimozide causing sinus bradycardia. *Can J Psychiatry.* 1993;38:62–63.

Armstrong SC, Cozza KL. Pharmacokinetic drug interactions of morphine, codeine, and their derivatives: theory and clinical reality, Part II. *Psychosomatics.* 2003;44:515–520.

Bertilsson L, Dahl ML, Ekqvist B, Llerena A. Disposition of the neuroleptics perphenazine, zuclopenthixol, and haloperidol cosegregates with polymorphic debrisoquine hydroxylation. *Psychopharmacol Ser.* 1993;10:230–237.

Bradford LD. CYP2D6 allele frequency in European Caucasians, Asians, Africans and their decendants. *Pharmacogenomics.* 2002;3:229–243.

Brown SM, Holtzman M, Kim T, Kharasch ED. Buprenorphine metabolites, buprenorphine-3-glucuronide and norbuprenorphine-3-glucuronide, are biologically active. *Anesthesiology.* 2011;115:1251–1260.

Chang Y, Fang WB, Lin SN, Moody DE. Stereo-selective metabolism of methadone by human liver microsomes and cDNA-expressed cytochrome P450s: a reconciliation. *Basic Clin Pharmacol Toxicol.* 2011;108:55–62.

Crist RC, Ambrose-Lanci LM, Vaswani M, et al. Case-control association analysis of polymorphisms in the delta-opioid receptor, OPRD1, with cocaine and opioid addicted populations. *Drug Alcohol Depend.* 2012;127:122–128.

de Wildt SN, Kearns GL, Leeder JS, van den Anker JN. Glucuronidation in humans. Pharmacogenetic and developmental aspects. *Clin Pharmacokinet.* 1999;36:439–452.

Donato MT, Montero S, Castell JV, Gomez-Lechon MJ, Lahoz A. Validated assay for studying activity profiles of human liver UGTs after drug exposure: inhibition and induction studies. *Anal Bioanal Chem.* 2010;396:2251–2263.

Drug Interaction Table: Abbreviated "Clinically Relevant" Table. http://medicine.iupui.edu/clinpharm/DDIs/ClinicalTable.aspx. Accessed September 21, 2012.

Grond S, Sablotzki A. Clinical pharmacology of tramadol. *Clin Pharmacokinet.* 2004;43:879–923.

Han DH, Bolo N, Daniels MA, et al. Craving for alcohol and food during treatment for alcohol dependence: modulation by T allele of 1519T>C GABA Aalpha 6. *Alcohol Clin Exp Res.* 2008;32:1593–1599.

Hara Y, Nakajima M, Miyamoto K, Yokoi T. Morphine glucuronosyltransferase activity in human liver microsomes is inhibited by a variety of drugs that are co-administered with morphine. *Drug Metab Pharmacokinet.* 2007;22:103–112.

Iribarne C, Berthou F, Baird S, et al. Involvement of cytochrome P450 3A4 enzyme in the N-demethylation of methadone in human liver microsomes. *Chem Res Toxicol.* 1996;9:365–373.

Kadiev E, Patel V, Rad P, et al. Role of pharmacogenetics in variable response to drugs: focus on opioids. *Expert Opin Drug Metab Toxicol.* 2008;4:77–91.

Kaplan HL, Busto UE, Baylon GJ, et al. Inhibition of cytochrome P450 2D6 metabolism of hydrocodone to hydromorphone does not importantly affect abuse liability. *J Pharmacol Exp Ther.* 1997;281:103–108.

Kirchheiner J, Nickchen K, Bauer M, et al. Pharmacogenetics of antidepressants and antipsychotics: the contribution of allelic variations to the phenotype of drug response. *Mol Psychiatry.* 2004;9:442–473.

Kirchheiner J, Schmidt H, Tzvetkov M, et al. Pharmacokinetics of codeine and its metabolite morphine in ultra-rapid metabolizers due to CYP2D6 duplication. *Pharmacogenomics J.* 2007;7:257–265.

Kocabas NA. Catechol-O-methyltransferase (COMT) pharmacogenetics in the treatment response phenotypes of major depressive disorder (MDD). *CNS Neurol Disord Drug Targets.* 2012;11:264–272.

Levran O, Peles E, Hamon S, Randesi M, Adelson M, Kreek MJ. CYP2B6 SNPs are associated with methadone dose required for effective treatment of opioid addiction. *Addict Biol.* 2013;18(4):709–716.

Linder MW, Valdes R. Fundamentals and applications of pharmacogenetics for the clinical laboratory. *Ann Clin Lab Sci.* 1999;29:140–149.

Ling W, Shoptaw S, Hillhouse M, et al. Double-blind placebo-controlled evaluation of the PROMETA protocol for methamphetamine dependence. *Addiction.* 2011;107:361–369.

Marcucci C, Sandson NB, Thorn EM, Bourke DL. Unrecognized drug-drug interactions: a cause of intraoperative cardiac arrest? *Anesth Analg.* 2006;102:1569–1572.

McLean SA, Diatchenko L, Lee YM, et al. Catechol O-methyltransferase haplotype predicts immediate musculoskeletal neck pain and psychological symptoms after motor vehicle collision. *J Pain.* 2010;12:101–107.

Mulder H, Heerdink ER, van Iersel EE, Wilmink FW, Egberts AC. Prevalence of patients using drugs metabolized by cytochrome P450 2D6 in different populations: a cross-sectional study. *Ann Pharmacother.* 2007;41:408–413.

Nelson EC, Lynskey MT, Heath AC, et al. Association of OPRD1 polymorphisms with heroin dependence in a large case-control series. *Addict Biol.* 2014;19(1):111–121.

Oda Y, Kharasch ED. Metabolism of methadone and levo-alpha-acetylmethadol (LAAM) by human intestinal cytochrome P450 3A4 (CYP3A4): potential contribution of intestinal metabolism to presystemic clearance and bioactivation. *J Pharmacol Exp Ther.* 2001;298:1021–1032.

Oesterheld J. Cytochrome P-450 (CYP) Metabolism Reference Table. http://youscript.com/healthcare-professionals/why-youscript/cytochrome-p450-drug-table/. Accessed February 21, 2013.

Otton SV, Schadel M, Cheung SW, Kaplan HL, Busto UE, Sellers EM. CYP2D6 phenotype determines the metabolic conversion of hydrocodone to hydromorphone. *Clin Pharmacol Ther.* 1993;54:463–472.

Preskorn SH, Baker B. Fatality associated with combined fluoxetine-amitriptyline therapy. *JAMA.* 1997;277:1682.

Spigset O, Hedenmalm K, Dahl ML, Wiholm BE, Dahlqvist R. Seizures and myoclonus associated with antidepressant treatment: assessment of potential risk factors, including CYP2D6 and CYP2C19 polymorphisms, and treatment with CYP2D6 inhibitors. *Acta Psychiatr Scand.* 1997;96:379–384.

Stanford BJ, Stanford SC. Postoperative delirium indicating an adverse drug interaction involving the selective serotonin reuptake inhibitor, paroxetine? *J Psychopharmacol.* 1999;13:313–317.

Totah RA, Sheffels P, Roberts T, Whittington D, Thummel K, Kharasch ED. Role of CYP2B6 in stereoselective human methadone metabolism. *Anesthesiology.* 2008;108:363–374.

Xu K, Lichtermann D, Lipsky RH, et al. Association of specific haplotypes of D2 dopamine receptor gene with vulnerability to heroin dependence in 2 distinct populations. *Arch Gen Psychiatry.* 2004;61:597–606.

Yang Z, Arheart KL, Morris R, et al. CYP2D6 poor metabolizer genotype and smoking predict severe postoperative pain in female patients on arrival to the recovery room. *Pain Med.* 2012;13:604–609.

Zhang Y, Wang D, Johnson AD, Papp AC, Sadee W. Allelic expression imbalance of human mu opioid receptor (OPRM1) caused by variant A118G. *J Biol Chem.* 2005;280: 32618–32624.

ANALGESIC PHARMACOLOGY

16   TOPICAL AGENTS

Arnold R. Gammaitoni, PharmD
Bradley S. Galer, MD

RATIONALE FOR USE

- Peripheral mechanisms of pain are inherent in most chronic pain states including peripheral neuropathies, rheumatologic conditions, and musculoskeletal conditions. These mechanisms are believed to be clinically relevant sources of pain and, thus, appropriate targets for drug therapy.
- Targeted peripheral (or topically applied) analgesics (TPAs), by definition, produce their pharmacologic action primarily by local activity in the peripheral tissues, including nerves and/or soft tissues, without producing clinically significant serum drug levels. Unlike transdermal agents, which are specifically formulated to produce a systemic effect (eg, the fentanyl patch), TPAs have a reduced risk of producing systemic side effects or drug–drug interactions. This is particularly advantageous in patients with chronic pain conditions who are often receiving numerous systemic medications for multiple medical conditions.
- Nine prescription TPAs are currently available in the United States and fall under three categories of treatments:
  1. Topical Local Anesthetics:
     - Heated lidocaine/tetracaine topical patch (Synera®, Zars Pharmaceuticals, Inc., Salt Lake City, UT)
     - Lidocaine/tetracaine cream 7%/7% (Pliaglis®, Galderma USA, Fort Worth, TX)
     - Lidocaine patch 5% (Lidoderm®, Endo Pharmaceuticals Inc., Malvern, Pa)
     - Eutectic mixture of lidocaine 2.5% and prilocaine 2.5% (EMLA®, AstraZeneca Pharmaceuticals LP, Wilmington, Del)
  2. Topical Nonsteroidal Anti-inflammatory Drugs (NSAIDs):
     - Diclofenac topical solution 1.5% (Pennsaid® and[a] Pennsaid 2%, Mallinckrodt Pharmaceuticals, Hazelwood, MO)
     - Diclofenac sodium gel 1% (Voltaren® Gel, Endo Pharmaceuticals, Malvern, PA)
     - Diclofenac epolamine patch 1.3% (Flector®, Pfizer, New York, NY)
  3. Topical Capsaicin
     - Capsaicin cream or lotion (Zostrix®, GenDerm, Scottsdale, Ariz)
     - Capsaicin Patch 8% (Qutenza®, NeurogesX, San Mateo, CA)

TOPICAL LOCAL ANESTHETICS: HEATED LIDOCAINE/TETRACAINE TOPICAL PATCH (SYNERA)

FORMULATION

- Synera consists of a thin, uniform layer of local anesthetic formulation with an integrated, oxygen-activated heating component that is intended to enhance delivery of the local anesthetic. The drug formulation is a mixture of two local anesthetics, lidocaine 70 mg and tetracaine 70 mg.

MECHANISM OF ACTION

- Synera applied to intact skin provides local dermal analgesia by the release of lidocaine and tetracaine

---

[a](at time of writing, Pennsaid 2% was under review by the Food and Drug Administration (FDA) for marketing approval)

from the patch into the skin. The novel heating element heats the skin up to 39°C for approximately two hours, enhancing skin penetration of lidocaine and tetracaine. Lidocaine is an amide-type local anesthetic agent and tetracaine is an ester-type local anesthetic agent. Both lidocaine and tetracaine block sodium ion channels required for the initiation and conduction of neuronal impulses, resulting in local anesthesia. Tetracaine, compared with other local anesthetics, is also the most potent NMDA channel blocker of the class.

- In inflammatory conditions, such as osteoarthritis, animal studies have reported clinically active abnormal sodium channels, which, when antagonized, reduce spontaneous nociceptive activity and alleviate pain behaviors of the rodent and, therefore, provide a novel target for the heated lidocaine/tetracaine patch.

- Lidocaine has also been shown to inhibit the expression of nitric oxide and subsequent release of proinflammatory cytokines from T cells and, thus, provides another potential analgesic mechanism for the heated lidocaine/tetracaine patch in the treatment of inflammatory pain conditions.

EFFICACY

- Table 16-1 summarizes clinical studies of the Synera Patch.

TABLE 16-1   Heated Lidocaine/Tetracaine (Synera) Topical Patch Evidence Base

POPULATION	DESIGN	RESULTS
Adult—VA	Randomized, double-blind, placebo-controlled, crossover clinical study-blind: $N = 79$; subjects received simultaneous applications of the Synera patch and a placebo patch 20 minutes before undergoing vascular access procedures. The application sites were randomized 1:1 between the right and left antecubital surfaces.	The median VAS score for procedural pain with S-Caine treatment was 5 mm versus 28 mm for placebo treatment ($P < 0.001$). 73% of subjects reported elimination of pain following S-Caine treatment compared with 31% of subjects following placebo treatment.
Children—VA	Randomized, double-blind, placebo-controlled clinical study evaluating: $N = 60$; patients were randomized (2:1) to receive a 20-minute application of either the Synera patch or a placebo patch before undergoing a vascular access procedure.	The Synera patch was more effective than placebo in younger children (0.0 vs. 80.0, $P < 0.001$). Median Oucher scores for older patients were 7.5 for Synera patch and 50 for placebo ($P = 0.159$).
Adult—MDP	Randomized, double-blind, placebo-controlled study: $N = 94$; patients were randomized to receive a 30-minute application of either the Synera or placebo patch immediately before undergoing the dermatologic procedure.	Median VAS scores were 5 mm for the S-Caine group and 31 mm for the placebo group ($P < 0.001$). 73% of patients who received S-Caine reported adequate anesthesia compared with 37% of patients who received placebo ($P < 0.001$).
Child—MDP	Randomized, double-blind, placebo-controlled study: $N = 60$; Synera or a placebo patch applied for 60 minutes before undergoing a minor dermatologic procedure	Adequate anesthesia was achieved in 87% of S-Caine-treated patients versus 17% of the placebo group ($P < 0.001$),
Adult—VA vs. EMLA	Randomized, double-blind, paired study. Subjects randomized to a 10-, 20-, 30- or 60-minute application group of Synera Patch and EMLA Cream.	Synera Patch more effective than EMLA at 10 minutes ($P = 0.01$), 20 minutes ($P = .042$), and 30 minutes ($P = 0.001$). Both treatments equal at 60 minutes.
Adult—Healthy volunteer depth & duration of anesthesia	Randomized, double-blind, placebo-controlled, 2-period crossover study: $N = 25$; Synera Patch or placebo patch applied for 30 minutes	Pain and sensory depths with the Synera patch were greater than with placebo ($P < 0.001$) at all postdose time points. Maximum mean pain depth achieved with the active patch was 8.22 mm; anesthesia lasted at least 100 minutes after patch removal.
Adult—SIS	2-week, Open-label, pilot study: $N = 20$; Synera patch to shoulder for 2–4 hours, twice daily (~12 hours apart) for 14 days.	Mean NPRS average pain score decreased from 5.6 ± 1.1 to 3.3 ± 2.4 at Day 14. 65% of patients experienced a >30% reduction in average pain
Adult—SIS	6-week, Open-label, pilot study: $N = 60$; patients randomized to treatment with Synera patch for 4 hours twice daily or to a single subacromial corticosteroid injection.	Synera patch provided comparable improvements after 6 weeks in pain (−54 ± 29% and −56 ± 36%), pain interference, and range of motion.
Adult—MTP	2-week, Open-label, pilot study: $N = 20$; Synera patch over a myofascial trigger point for 4 hours, twice daily(~12 hours apart).	Mean NPRS average pain score decreased from 6.3 ± 1.6 to 4.4 ± 2.2 at Day 14. 35% of patients experienced a >30% reduction in average pain.
Adult—PT	2-week, Open-label, pilot study: $N = 13$; Synera patch to a painful patellar tendon for 2 to 4 hours, twice daily for 14 days.	After 14 days of treatment, the mean (±SD) 24-hour average pain score had declined from 5.5 ± 1.3 (range, 4–8) to 3.7 ± 2.5. 60% of patients experienced a >30% reduction in average pain.
Adult—CTS	2-week, Open-label, pilot study: $N = 20$; Synera patch applied to the painful wrist for 2 hours, twice daily for 14 days.	Baseline average pain score decreased from 5.1 ± 1.5 to 2.5 ± 1.6 after 2 weeks of treatment. Two-thirds of patients experienced a >30% reduction in average pain.

VA, Vascular Access; MDP, Minor Dermatologic Procedures; MTP, Myofascial Trigger Points; PT, Patellar Tendinopathy; CTS, Carpal Tunnel Syndrome.

Prevention of Needle Based Procedure Pain

Local Dermal Analgesia for Superficial Venous Access

- In randomized, double-blind, placebo-controlled clinical trials adults and the elderly patients who were administered a 20-minute treatment with Synera reported lower pain intensity with subsequent venipuncture (measured by a 100-mm visual analog scale [VAS]) than patients treated with a heated placebo patch.
- In pediatric patients 3–6 years old, a 20-minute treatment with Synera before venipuncture or intravenous cannulations in the antecubital fossa or dorsum of the hand reduced patient reported pain intensity (rated using a 6-point Oucher pain scale with faces) compared with a placebo patch. In children 7–17 years of age, pain intensity (rated using an 11-point Oucher pain scale with faces and numbers) was not significantly different between the treatment and placebo groups.

Local Dermal Analgesia for Superficial Dermatologic Procedures

- In a randomized, double-blind, placebo-controlled study, adults treated with Synera for 30 minutes before a superficial dermatologic procedure (eg, excision, electrodesiccation, or shave biopsy of skin lesions) reported lower VAS scores than patients administered a placebo patch.
- Treating children 3–6 years old with Synera 30 minutes before a lidocaine injection resulted in lower pain intensity, as reported with a 6-point Oucher pain scale with faces, compared with treatment with a placebo patch.

Versus EMLA

- In a study of adult patients undergoing superficial venous access, subjects were randomized to receive either Synera or EMLA for 10-, 20-, 30-, and 60-minute applications. The Synera patch was more effective in reducing the median VAS score than EMLA cream for 10- and 20-minute applications, but the most highly significant difference was seen for 30-minute application. 95% of patients in the Synera group reported "no pain" after a 30-minute application compared to 64% of the patients in the EMLA group.

Depth and Duration of Analgesia

- Application of the heated lidocaine/tetracaine topical patch has been shown to provide analgesic efficacy to an average depth of 8.22 mm from the skin's surface and duration of effect lasting at least 2 hours, suggesting that this patch may have benefit for acute musculoskeletal pain conditions, such as tendinopathies and shoulder impingement syndrome.

Acute Musculoskeletal Pain[b]

Shoulder Impingement Syndrome (SIS)

- Patients ≥18 years old with moderate-severe pain (numerical pain rating scale, NPRS, average pain intensity score of ≥4 at the screening/baseline visit) associated with SIS in a single shoulder (minimum of 2-weeks duration) were eligible to enroll in this 2-week, open-label, pilot study. Mean NPRS average pain score decreased from 5.6 ± 1.1 (mean ± SD) to 3.3 ± 2.4 at Day 14. About 65% of patients (12 of 19) had a clinically meaningful reduction in pain (≥30%), and greater than 45% of patients (9 of 19) demonstrated a ≥50% decrease from baseline in NPRS average pain score.
- 60 patients ≥18 years old with unilateral pain associated with SIS of at least 2 weeks' duration participated in this 6-week, open-label, randomized study comparing Synera to subacromial corticosteroid injection. On Day 42, 83% of patients in the HLT patch group demonstrated a clinically meaningful reduction (≥30% reduction in average pain score) compared with 74% of patients in the Injection group. Three times more patients in the Injection group were withdrawn due to acetaminophen rescue usage (2 patients in HLT group versus six patients in the Injection group).

Myofascial Trigger Point Pain

- 20 patients ≥18 years old that had a clinical diagnosis of pain associated with up to three myofascial trigger points participated in this 2-week open-label pilot study. The NPRS average pain score decreased from 6.3 ± 1.6 (mean ± SD) at baseline to 4.4 ± 2.2 at Day 14 and 35% of patients experienced a clinically meaningful reduction (>/= 30%) in pain.

Patellar Tendinopathy

- 13 patients ≥14 years old with patellar tendinopathy of a minimum 2-week duration and with an average pain intensity score of ≥4 (on a 0–10 scale) over the past 24 hours participated in this 2-week open-label pilot study. After 14 days of treatment, the mean (±SD) 24-hour average pain score had declined from 5.5 ± 1.3 (range, 4–8) to 3.7 ± 2.5 (range, 0–8). More than 60% of patients demonstrated a clinically meaningful (≥30%) reduction in pain.

---

[b][Synera is not currently FDA approved for this indication.]

Neuropathic Pain[c]

Carpal Tunnel Syndrome

- Twenty patients ≥18 years old and had pain associated with mild-to-moderate carpal tunnel syndrome in a single wrist participated in this 2-week open-label pilot study. Reductions in scores for average pain, worst pain, and pain now were −37%, −41%, and −34%, respectively.
- Additional randomized, controlled trials are needed to further validate the efficacy and safety of the heated lidocaine/tetracaine patch for other indications other than use prior to superficial venous access and superficial dermatologic procedures.

SIDE EFFECTS

- In clinical studies, the most common skin reactions occurred at the application site, including redness, blanching, and swelling. These reactions were generally mild and went away by themselves.
- SYNERA® should also not beused in patients who have a para-aminobenzoic acid (PABA) hypersensitivity.
- Even a used patch contains a large amount of lidocaine and tetracaine. A child or pet could suffer adverse effects from chewing or swallowing a new or used SYNERA® patch. Store and dispose patches out of their reach.

DOSAGE AND ADMINISTRATION

- Synera should only be applied to intact skin and should be used immediately after opening the pouch. The FDA approved dosing of Synera for adults and children 3 years of age and older is:
  - Venipuncture or intravenous cannulation: Prior to venipuncture or intravenous cannulation:
    - Apply Synera to intact skin for 20–30 minutes.
  - Superficial dermatological procedures:
    - For superficial dermatological procedures such as superficial excision or shave biopsy, apply Synera to intact skin for 30 minutes prior to the procedure.
- In the pilot studies for myofascial trigger points, patellar tendinopathy, carpal tunnel syndrome, and shoulder impingement syndrome the patch was applied for 2–4 hours twice daily separated by approximately 12 hours.
- A recently published pharmacokinetic study evaluated the plasma concentrations and tolerability of 2-hour, 4-hour, and 12-hour application of four patches. In the study the maximum plasma concentration of lidocaine

observed in any subject (43.0 ng/mL) was approximately 1/50 of that expected to cause ECG effects and 1/100 of those typically associated with CNS toxicity. No serious AE's were reported and the most common observed AE was local skin reactions (ie, erythema).

LIDOCAINE/TETRACAINE TOPICAL CREAM 7%/7% (PLIAGLIS)

FORMULATION

- PLIAGLIS (lidocaine and tetracaine) Cream 7%/7% is a topical local anesthetic cream that forms a pliable peel on the skin when exposed to air. The drug formulation is an emulsion in which the oil phase is a 1:1 eutectic mixture of lidocaine 7% and tetracaine 7%.18 PLIAGLIS when initially applied is a spreadable cream that becomes a peelable patch after 20–60 minutes of application.

MECHANISM OF ACTION

- Lidocaine is an amide-type local anesthetic agent and tetracaine is an ester-type local anesthetic agent. Both lidocaine and tetracaine block sodium ion channels required for the initiation and conduction of neuronal impulses which, in certain instances, results in local anesthesia. When applied to intact skin, PLIAGLIS provides local dermal analgesia by the release of lidocaine and tetracaine from the peel into the skin.
- In inflammatory conditions, such as osteoarthritis, animal studies have reported clinically active abnormal sodium channels, which, when antagonized, reduce spontaneous nociceptive activity and alleviate pain behaviors of the rodent and, therefore, provide a novel target for the lidocaine/tetracaine cream 7%/7%.
- Lidocaine has also been shown to inhibit the expression of nitric oxide and subsequent release of proinflammatory cytokines from T cells and, thus, provides another potential analgesic mechanism for the lidocaine/tetracaine cream 7%/7% patch in the treatment of inflammatory pain conditions.

EFFICACY

- Table 16-2 summarizes clinical studies of the Pliaglis cream.

Prevention of Pain Associate with Laser Therapy

- Two, double-blind, placebo controlled trials evaluated 30-, 60-, and 90-minute applications of lidocaine/tetracaine 7%/7% phase changing cream in adult

---

[c][Synera is not currently FDA approved for this indication.]

TABLE 16-2   Lidocaine/Tetracaine Topical Cream (Pliaglis) 7%/7% Evidence Base

POPULATION	DESIGN	RESULTS
LTLV	Two randomized, double-blinded, placebo-controlled trials: Study 1($N = 60$) and Study 2 ($N = 40$); Study 1 Pliaglis or placebo applied for 30 or 60 minutes; Study 2 Pliaglis or placebo applied for 60 or 90 minutes.	In Study 1, the 30- and 60-minute application times were grouped: Patients had adequate pain relief in 48% of Pliaglis sites versus 23% of placebo sites ($P < 0.001$). In study 2, adequate anesthesia in 70% and 85% of 60 and 90 minutes of active sites versus 25% and 20% of placebo sites ($P = 0.029$ and $P = 0.001$, respectively).
LATR	Randomized, double-blind, placebo-controlled study: $N = 30$; each subject received both the Pliaglis and placebo simultaneously for 60 minutes.	Mean VAS scores were 42 mm for the Pliaglis and 66 mm for placebo treatment sites ($p = .001$). Patients received adequate pain relief in 50% of Pliaglis sites versus 7% of placebo sites ($p = .002$)

LTLV, laser therapy for leg veins; LATR, laser-assisted tattoo removal.

patients scheduled to undergo YAG laser therapy for leg veins demonstrated it provided safe and highly effective local anesthesia when applied for at least 60 minutes for laser therapy of leg veins.

○ In Study 1, patients had adequate pain relief in 48% of S-Caine sites versus 23% of placebo sites ($P < 0.001$).

○ In study 2, patients reported adequate anesthesia in 70% and 85% of 60 and 90 minutes of active sites versus 25% and 20% of placebo sites ($P = 0.029$ and $P = 0.001$, respectively).

• One double-blind, placebo controlled trial evaluated a 60-minute application of lidocaine/tetracaine 7%/7% phase changing cream in adult patients scheduled for laser-assisted tattoo removal.

○ Patients received adequate pain relief in 50% of S-Caine Peel sites versus 7% of placebo sites ($p = .002$). The percentage of those who would like to use the S-Caine Peel again were 43% for the S-Caine Peel compared with 7% for placebo ($p = .005$).

SIDE EFFECTS

• In clinical studies, the most common local reactions were erythema (47%), skin discoloration (eg, blanching, ecchymosis, and purpura) (16%), and edema (14%). These reactions were generally mild and transient, resolving spontaneously soon after treatment. There were no serious adverse events.

• Across all trials, 19 subjects experienced a systemic adverse event, 15 of who were treated with PLIAGLIS and 4 with placebo. The most common systemic adverse events were headache, vomiting, dizziness, and fever, all of which occurred with a frequency of <1%.

DOSAGE AND ADMINISTRATION

• The amount (length) of PLIAGLIS that should be dispensed is determined by the size of the area to be treated. It should be evenly and thinly (approximately 1 mm or the thickness of a dime) across the treatment area using a flat-surfaced tool such as a metal spatula or tongue depressor.

• For superficial minor dermatological procedures such as dermal filler injection or facial laser ablation, apply PLIAGLIS to intact skin for 20–30 minutes prior to the procedure.

• For superficial major dermatological procedures such as laser-assisted tattoo removal, apply PLIAGLIS to intact skin for 60 minutes prior to the procedure.

LIDOCAINE PATCH 5% (LIDODERM)

FORMULATION

• The lidocaine patch 5% is a 10 × 14-cm topical patch composed of an adhesive material containing 5% lidocaine (700 mg) in an aqueous base, which is applied to a nonwoven polyester felt backing and covered with a polyethylene terephthalate film-release liner. The release liner is removed prior to application.

MECHANISM OF ACTION

• Lidocaine blocks abnormal activity in neuronal sodium channels, which are believed to play a critical role in the etiology of many types of pain, in both its initiation and its maintenance.

• In neuropathic pain, animal models have demonstrated an upregulation of abnormal sodium channels on the damaged sensory peripheral nerve.

• In inflammatory conditions, such as osteoarthritis, animal studies have reported clinically active abnormal sodium channels, which, when antagonized, reduce spontaneous nociceptive activity and alleviate pain behaviors of the rodent and, therefore, provide a novel target for the lidocaine patch 5%.

• Lidocaine has also been shown to inhibit the expression of nitric oxide and subsequent release of proinflammatory cytokines from T cells and, thus, provides another potential analgesic mechanism for the lidocaine patch in the treatment of inflammatory pain conditions.

- In addition to its sodium channel-blocking activity, the lidocaine patch acts as a protective barrier against cutaneous stimuli for patients with allodynia.
- Importantly and uniquely, the novel formulation of the lidocaine patch delivers sufficient levels of lidocaine to the local tissues to produce an analgesic effect (pain relief) without anesthesia (sensory deficits, ie, "numbness").

EFFICACY

- Table 16-3 summarizes clinical studies of the lidocaine patch 5%.

Neuropathic Pain

Postherpetic Neuralgia

- The lidocaine patch is the first drug ever approved by the FDA for a neuropathic pain disorder, that is, postherpetic neuralgia (PHN).
- The lidocaine patch has been confirmed in several randomized controlled studies to be of benefit in PHN.
- In patients with PHN and moderate allodynia, the lidocaine patch significantly reduces pain intensity compared with observation or a vehicle patch. Most patients experience at least moderate pain relief. In one study of refractory PHN, 24 of 35 patients reported slight or better pain relief (averaging scores at 4 and 6 hours), and 10 patients reported moderate or better relief.

TABLE 16-3 **Lidocaine Patch 5% (Lidoderm) Evidence Base**

POPULATION	DESIGN	RESULTS
PHN	Randomized, double-blind, crossover controlled study: $N = 35$; four single sessions (12 hours): two with lidocaine patch, one with vehicle patch (double-blind), and one with observation only	Reduced pain intensity significantly versus vehicle (at 4, 6, 9, and 12 hours; $P < 0.05$) and observation (at all time points from 30 minutes to 12 hours; $P < 0.05$)
PHN (responders to lidocaine patch >1 mo before trial)	Randomized, double-blind, placebo-controlled, enriched enrollment study: $N = 32$; patients randomized to lidocaine patch or vehicle, then switched to other Tx after maximum of 14 days or when pain relief worsened by ≥2 categories on two consecutive days	Median time to exit >14 days vs. 3.8 days with vehicle ($P < 0.001$)
PHN	Randomized, double-blind, parallel-design study: $N = 96$; 3-week duration	Significant improvement in all common neuropathic pain qualities ($P < 0.05$); potential benefit for nonallodynic pain states
PHN	Open-label, nonrandomized, effectiveness study: $N = 332$; 28-day duration	Statistically significant reductions in pain intensity and pain interference with quality of life ($P = 0.001$); approximately 60% of patients reported moderate to complete pain relief
Peripheral neuropathic pain conditions	Randomized, double-blind, controlled trial: $N = 40$; 1-week duration	Significant reduction in pain versus placebo ($P < 0.05$)
Refractory neuropathic pain with allodynia	Open-label prospective study: $N = 16$; mean duration 6.2 week for 15 patients (one patient dropped out after 4 days due to lack of relief)	13 patients (87%) experienced moderate or better pain relief with lidocaine patch
Diabetic neuropathy	Nonrandomized, open-label, pilot study: $N = 56$; 3-week therapy	Significant reductions in overall pain intensity ($P < 0.001$), and improvements in common pain qualities ($P < 0.05$) and functional outcomes ($P < 0.005$)
Idiopathic sensory polyneuropathy	Open-label, flexible dosing, 3-week study period with a 5-week extension: $N = 20$	Subjects with and without impaired glucose tolerance showed significant improvements in pain and quality of life over a 3-week treatment period. Improvements were maintained in a subgroup of patients treated for an additional 5 weeks and permitted a taper of concomitant analgesics in 25% of subjects
HIV peripheral neuropathy	Nonrandomized, open-label, pilot study: $N = 16$; 4-week therapy	Significant reductions in pain intensity ($P < 0.05$), and improvements in common pain qualities ($P \leq 0.001$) and functional outcomes ($P < 0.05$)
Carpal tunnel syndrome	6-week, randomized, parallel-group, open-label, multicenter study; $N = 100$; Lidoderm versus Naproxen	Significant reductions in average pain scores were observed between baseline and Week 6 for both lidocaine patch 5% ($P < .0001$) and naproxen 500 mg twice daily ($P = .0004$); there were no statistically significant differences between treatments ($P = .083$).

(Continued)

TABLE 16-3   Lidocaine Patch 5% (Lidoderm) Evidence Base (*Continued*)

POPULATION	DESIGN	RESULTS
Carpal tunnel syndrome	Randomized, parallel-group, open-label, single-center, active-controlled, prospective pilot study; $N = 40$; Lidoderm versus Depo-Medrol, 4-week treatment period	Both groups reported significant changes ($P < .05$) in worst pain, average pain, and pain "right now." Eighty percent of patients in the lidocaine patch group and 59% of patients who received the injection reported being "satisfied" or "very satisfied."
Low back pain of varying duration from acute through chronic	Nonrandomized, open-label, pilot study: $N = 129$; 2-week therapy	Significant reductions in overall pain intensity, and improvements in common pain qualities and functional outcomes ($P < 0.0001$)
Low back pain	Randomized, double-blind, placebo-controlled, 2-week study with fMRI brain imaging: $N = 30$	No significant difference between the treatment groups in either pain intensity, sensory and affective qualities of pain or in pain related brain activation at any time point.
Myofascial pain, moderate to severe intensity, with identifiable trigger points; 66.6% had low-back pain	Nonrandomized, open-label study: $N = 27$; 28-day duration	Significant improvements in average pain intensity, walking, ability to work, and sleep ($P < 0.05$); 30% of patients experienced moderate/better relief
Myofascial pain syndrome	Prospective, randomized, double-blind, placebo-controlled study; $N = 60$; Lidoderm or placebo for 4-week treatment period.	No significant difference between the two groups in the VRS, the Pressure Pain Threshold, the ranges of motion, and the Neck Disability Index
Osteoarthritis pain of one or both knees	Nonrandomized, open-label, pilot study: $N = 167$; 135 patients with lidocaine patch as add-on therapy and 32 as monotherapy; 2-week duration	Significant reductions in overall pain intensity and improvements in functional outcomes and QOL ($P < 0.0001$)
Osteoarthritis of the knee	12-week, prospective, randomized, active-controlled, open-label, parallel-group trial: $N = 143$; Lidoderm versus Celecoxib for 12-week treatment period	Change in WOMAC OA pain subscale scores was not significantly different between the 2 groups. Improvement in additional WOMAC subscales and in several BPI measures were not significantly different between the two groups.
Post-op pain	Prospective cohort study (53 patients treated with Lidoderm, 22 controls); 11-day treatment period following total knee arthroplasty	Concurrent use of lidocaine patch 5% in treating the postoperative pain of patients after TKA does not provide significant additional pain relief compared with control subjects

QOL, quality of life.

- In an enriched enrollment study of 32 patients with PHN who were known responders to the lidocaine patch, the lidocaine patch provided significantly more pain relief than a vehicle patch, using "time to exit" as the primary endpoint.
- The lidocaine patch was superior to a vehicle patch in reducing all common pain qualities associated with neuropathic pain (eg, "burning," "dull," "deep," "superficial," and "sharp" pains) in a 3-week, prospective, randomized, controlled trial of 96 patients with PHN.
- Statistically significant reductions in pain interference with quality of life were noted with the lidocaine patch in a large ($N = 332$), open-label, effectiveness study.

Peripheral Neuropathic Pain (Other than PHN)[d]

- A randomized, controlled trial demonstrated significant benefit of the lidocaine patch over placebo in patients with diverse peripheral neuropathic pain conditions (ie, PHN, diabetic neuropathy,

stump neuralgia, postsurgical neuralgia, meralgia paresthetica).
- In an open-label trial, the lidocaine patch improved pain in patients with a variety of refractory neuropathic conditions with allodynia, including post-thoracotomy pain, stump neuroma pain, intercostal neuralgia, painful diabetic polyneuropathy, meralgia paresthetica, complex regional pain syndrome, radiculopathy, and postmastectomy pain: 13 of 16 patients reported moderate or better pain relief with the lidocaine patch.

Painful Diabetic Neuropathy[e]

- The lidocaine patch may have clinical utility in the treatment of painful diabetic neuropathy. Data from a multicenter, open-label, pilot study indicate that the lidocaine patch significantly reduces overall pain intensity, improves commonly reported pain qualities, and results in improved functional outcomes in patients with painful diabetic neuropathy with and without allodynia.

---

[d][Lidoderm is not currently FDA approved for this indication.]

[e][Lidoderm is not currently FDA approved for this indication.]

Idiopathic Sensory Polyneuropathy[f]

- A prospective open-label, flexible dosing, 3-week study period with a 5-week extension to assess the safety, tolerability, and effectiveness study of the lidocaine patch 5% in painful idiopathic distal sensory polyneuropathy. Subjects with idiopathic distal sensory polyneuropathy, both with and without impaired glucose tolerance, showed significant improvements in pain and quality of life outcome measures over a 3-week treatment period. These improvements were maintained in a subgroup of patients treated for an additional 5 weeks and permitted a taper of concomitant analgesics in 25% of subjects. The lidocaine patch 5% was well tolerated.

HIV-Associated Neuropathy[g]

- In a multicenter, open-label, pilot study reported the lidocaine patch significantly reduced overall pain intensity, improved common pain qualities, and resulted in improved functional outcomes in patients with painful HIV-associated neuropathy.

Carpal Tunnel Syndrome[h]

- Two randomized, open-label, active comparator trials compared the lidocaine patch 5% to naproxen and corticosteroid injection for the treatment of pain associated with carpal tunnel syndrome. In both trials the lidocaine patch 5% provided comparable degrees of improvement in pain, pain interference, and satisfaction to both oral naproxen and a corticosteroid injection.

Erythromelalgia[i]

- According to a recently published case report, the lidocaine patch significantly relieved the pain of erythromelalgia of the feet in a 15-year-old girl.

Other Pain States

Low Back Pain[j]

- Several clinical reports have described successful treatment of chronic low back pain patients with the addition of the lidocaine patch to analgesic regimens, with patches applied directly over the painful back region.

- In a multicenter, prospective, open-label study, the lidocaine patch significantly improved all common pain qualities and functionality in 129 patients with acute, subacute, and chronic low back pain.
- A prospective, double-blind, placebo-controlled, brain imaging study examined the effectiveness of the 5% Lidocaine patch was compared with placebo in 30 CBP patients in a randomized double-blind study where 15 patients received 5% Lidocaine patches and the remaining patients received placebo patches. Functional MRI was used to identify brain activity for fluctuations of spontaneous pain, at baseline and at two time points after start of treatment (6 hours and 2 weeks). There was no significant difference between the treatment groups in either pain intensity, sensory and affective qualities of pain or in pain related brain activation at any time point. These findings suggest that although the 5% Lidocaine is not better than placebo in its effectiveness for treating pain, the patch itself induces a potent placebo effect in a significant proportion of CBP patients.

Myofascial Pain[k]

- A prospective, single-site, open-label trial has reported successful treatment of regional, chronic, refractory, myofascial pain with the lidocaine patch. Statistically significant mean improvements were noted for average daily pain intensity and pain interference with general activity, walking, ability to work, relationships, sleep, and enjoyment of life.
- A prospective, double-blind, placebo controlled study in 60 patients with myofascial pain syndrome of the upper trapezius. There was no significant difference between the two groups in the VRS, the Pressure Pain Threshold, the ranges of motion, and the Neck Disability Index. At Day 14, the experimental group continued to improve in the VRS (1.06), but the pain of the placebo group aggravated (VRS, 1.5). The difference is significant ($P = 0.03$). In addition, the Neck Disability Index in the lidocaine patch group decreased significantly as compared to that in the placebo group. The pain-relieving effect of the lidocaine patch attenuated, and it was not significantly different between the two groups at Day 28 in the VRS and the Neck Disability Index. Neither the Pressure Pain Threshold nor the ranges of motion were significantly different through the periods of this study.

Osteoarthritis[l]

- A large, multicenter, prospective, open-label trial, brief report, and a Letter to the Editor from a

---

[f][Lidoderm is not currently FDA approved for this indication.]
[g][Lidoderm is not currently FDA approved for this indication.]
[h][Lidoderm is not currently FDA approved for this indication.]
[i][Lidoderm is not currently FDA approved for this indication.]
[j][Lidoderm is not currently FDA approved for this indication.]

---

[k][Lidoderm is not currently FDA approved for this indication.]
[l][Lidoderm is not currently FDA approved for this indication.]

practicing rheumatologist have reported significant clinical benefit from the lidocaine patch in the treatment of osteoarthritis (OA).

- A large prospective trial of 167 patients with osteoarthritis demonstrated that placing the lidocaine patch directly on the skin of an osteoarthritic knee results in statistically significant improvements in the pain, stiffness, physical function, and composite indices measured by the validated Western Ontario and McMaster Universities Osteoarthritis Index.
- Authors of a randomized, open-label, active controlled study compared the effectiveness of the lidocaine patch 5% with that of celecoxib 200 mg/d in the treatment of OA-related knee pain presented a post hoc analysis of a trial which was terminated early due to the withdrawal of rofecoxib at the time of the study and uncertainty of the safety surrounding the cox-2 inhibitor class at the time. A total of 143 patients were randomized to treatment (69 lidocaine patch, 74 celecoxib). Both treatments provided comparable improvements in WOMAC pain and functional outcomes.

Post-op Pain[m]

- A prospective, cohort study investigated the potential benefits of the lidocaine patch 5% for pain control during the postoperative period after a total knee arthroplasty (TKA). A statistically significant difference in VAS was found on Day 3 ($P = .05$) between the two groups, with the control group demonstrating better pain relief. However, both groups reported similar pain improvements by the end of their hospital stay. The authors concluded that, overall, the concurrent use of lidocaine patch 5% in treating the postoperative pain of patients after TKA does not provide significant additional pain relief compared with control subjects.
- Additional randomized, controlled trials are needed to further validate the efficacy and safety of the lidocaine patch in conditions other than PHN.

SIDE EFFECTS

- A major clinical advantage to all TPAs, such as the lidocaine patch 5%, is their lack of clinically significant systemic activity.
- Only a small amount (ie, 3 ± 2%) of lidocaine has been found to be absorbed in healthy subjects treated with the lidocaine patch.

- Side effects appear to be limited to mild skin irritation at the lidocaine patch application site.
- The most common adverse reactions are local, in the skin region directly underlying the patch, and generally tend to be mild, resolving without the need for intervention.
  - Application site burning: 1.8%
  - Dermatitis: 1.8%
  - Pruritis: 1.1%
  - Rash: <1%
- No serious systemic adverse events have been related to treatment with the lidocaine patch in six recent clinical trials to date. Of the 450 patients studied in these trials, the most frequently reported systemic adverse event was mild to moderate headache (1.8%). Other less common systemic adverse events included dizziness and somnolence (<1%).

DOSAGE AND ADMINISTRATION

- The current FDA-approved labeling recommends that patients apply up to three lidocaine patches to the most painful areas of intact skin and wear them no longer than 12 hours in a 24-hour period. Patients should be instructed to cover as much of the painful area as possible.
- Increasing the dosage to four lidocaine patches applied either once daily for 24 hours or twice daily every 12 hours for three consecutive days was shown to be safe and well-tolerated in a pharmacokinetic study of 20 normal subjects. Plasma lidocaine levels were approximately 14.3% of those associated with cardiac activity and 4% of those typically associated with toxicity. Continuous 24-hour application of up to four lidocaine patches was safe and well tolerated in recent studies of patients with low back pain and osteoarthritis.
- A regimen of four lidocaine patches worn 18 hours/day for three consecutive days also was shown to be well-tolerated in 20 normal subjects. This "18-hours-on, 6-hours-off" regimen with a maximum of four lidocaine patches was used successfully in a trial of patients with diabetic neuropathy ($N = 56$).
- The lidocaine patch 5% should be used with caution in patients with severe hepatic disease and in those receiving antiarrhythmic or local anesthetic drugs.
- One to two weeks of therapy with the lidocaine patch may be required to determine whether a patient will experience satisfactory relief. However, one study reported that a small subgroup of patients with PHN required up to 4 weeks of treatment with the lidocaine patch to obtain maximal benefit. No dose escalation is necessary and tolerance does not develop with the lidocaine patch.

---

[m][Lidoderm is not currently FDA approved for this indication.]

EUTECTIC MIXTURE OF LOCAL ANESTHETICS (EMLA)

FORMULATION

- Eutectic mixture of local anesthetics (EMLA) cream (lidocaine 2.5% and prilocaine 2.5%) generally is applied to intact skin under an occlusive dressing.
- EMLA is indicated as a topical anesthetic for use on normal intact skin for local analgesia and on genital mucous membranes for superficial minor surgery and as pretreatment for infiltration anesthesia.

MECHANISM OF ACTION

- EMLA causes an anesthetic effect (sensory loss) in the skin area to which it is applied by producing an absolute sodium channel blockade of sensory nerves, resulting in a dense anesthesia. (Note: This is in contradistinction to the lidocaine patch 5%, which does not produce anesthesia, but only analgesia.).
- The onset of skin anesthesia depends primarily on the amount of cream applied. Skin anesthesia increases for 2–3 hours under an occlusive dressing and persists for 1–2 hours after removal. EMLA should be used with caution in patients receiving class 1 antiarrhythmic agents.

EFFICACY

- Table 16-4 summarizes clinical studies of EMLA cream.

Postoperative Pain Skin Anesthesia[n]

- Multiple randomized controlled studies have demonstrated the clinical efficacy of EMLA for its approved skin anesthetic indication.

Postherpetic Neuralgia[o]

- In one small study ($N = 12$), EMLA cream 5% applied for 24-hour periods significantly improved mean pain intensity 6 hours after application as measured by a visual analog scale.
- In another small study ($N = 11$), 5% EMLA cream applied daily under an adhesive occlusive dressing for 5 hours/day for 6 days had no significant effect on mean ongoing pain intensity as measured by a visual analog scale. However, eight patients reported that the number of painful attacks decreased by $\geq 50\%$. EMLA had significant benefit in a subset of eight patients with tactile allodynia.

Acute and Chronic Postsurgical Pain[p]

- In one double-blind, randomized study of women undergoing breast surgery for cancer ($N = 45$), EMLA cream 5% or placebo was applied 5 minutes prior to surgery and daily for 4 days during the postsurgical period. Acute pain at rest and with movement in the chest wall, axilla, and/or medial upper arm was assessed by visual analog scale. Acute pain at rest and with movement did not differ between the EMLA and control groups, and the analgesics consumed during the first 24 hours were the same. However, time to the first analgesia requirement was longer and analgesic consumption during the second to fifth days was less in the EMLA group. Three months postoperatively, pain in the chest wall and axilla and total incidence and intensity of chronic pain were significantly less in the EMLA group than the control group. Use of analgesics at home and abnormal sensations did not differ between the two groups.
- Additional randomized, controlled trials are needed to further validate the efficacy and safety of the EMLA in conditions other than use on normal intact skin for local analgesia and on genital mucous membranes for superficial minor surgery and as pretreatment for infiltration anesthesia.

SIDE EFFECTS

- A major clinical advantage to all TPAs, such as EMLA, is their lack of clinically significant systemic activity. Thus, minimal systemic side effects or drug–drug interactions have been noted with appropriate use of EMLA.
- The peak blood levels of lidocaine and prilocaine absorbed with the application of EMLA 60 g to 400 cm^2 are well below systemic toxicity levels.
- Treatment with EMLA results in localized reactions in 56% of patients. These reactions are usually mild and transient, resolving spontaneously within 1–2 hours.
- The most commonly reported local adverse reactions include:
  - Pallor/blanching: 37%
  - Erythema: 30%
  - Temperature sensation alteration: 7%
  - Edema: 6%

[n][EMLA is not currently FDA approved for this indication.]
[o][EMLA is not currently FDA approved for this indication.]

[p][EMLA is not currently FDA approved for this indication.]

TABLE 16-4 **EMLA Evidence Base**

POPULATION	DESIGN	RESULTS
Refractory PHN	Open-label study: $N = 12$; EMLA cream 5% applied for 24-hours periods	Significant decrease in pain intensity after 6 hours ($P < 0.05$)
PHN, spontaneous and evoked pain	Open-label study: $N = 11$; EMLA cream 5% applied daily for 5 hours/day for 6 days	No significant reduction in ongoing pain intensity and mechanical allodynia, but repeated applications significantly reduced paroxysmal pain ($P < 0.05$) and dynamic and static mechanical hyperalgesia ($P < 0.01$); significant improvements in spontaneous ongoing pain were seen only in patients with mechanical allodynia
Postoperative pain (acute/chronic)	Double-blind, randomized, placebo-controlled study: $N = 45$; EMLA cream 5% or placebo applied preoperatively and then daily for 4 days postoperatively	No significant reduction in acute pain at rest or with movement; time to first analgesic requirement ($P = 0.04$) and analgesic consumption on Days 2–5 ($P < 0.01$) significantly better for EMLA versus placebo; 3 mo postoperatively, pain in chest wall and axilla, and total incidence and intensity of chronic pain were significantly less in EMLA group ($P = 0.004$, $P = 0.025$, $P = 0.002$, and $P = 0.003$, respectively)

PHN, postherpetic neuralgia.

- ○ Itching: 2%
- ○ Rash: <1%
- EMLA should not be used in patients with congenital or idiopathic methemoglobinemia or in those taking drugs associated with drug-induced methemoglobinemia.

DOSAGE AND ADMINISTRATION

- A thick layer of EMLA should be applied to intact skin and covered with an occlusive dressing.
- Dermal analgesia can be expected to increase for up to 3 hours and continue for 1–2 hours after removal of EMLA.
- Although the incidence of systemic adverse events with EMLA is very low, caution should be used, especially when applying it over large areas of skin and leaving it on longer than >3 hours.

TOPICAL NONSTEROIDAL ANTIINFLAMMATORY DRUGS (NSAIDS): DICLOFENAC 1.5% TOPICAL SOLUTION (PENNSAID)

FORMULATION

- PENNSAID is a nonsteroidal anti-inflammatory drug (NSAID) indicated for the treatment of signs and symptoms of osteoarthritis of the knee(s). Pennsaid is a 1.5% w/w topical solution containing diclofenac sodium combined with DMSO to enhance penetration of the NSAID into the local tissues and joint.

MECHANISM OF ACTION

- The mechanism of action of diclofenac is similar to other nonsteroidal anti-inflammatory drugs. Diclofenac inhibits the enzyme, cyclooxygenase (COX), an early component of the arachidonic acid cascade, resulting in reduced formation of prostaglandins, thromboxanes, and prostacyclin. It is not completely understood how reduced synthesis of these compounds results in therapeutic efficacy.

EFFICACY

- Table 16-5 summarizes clinical studies of Pennsaid 1.5% topical solution.

Osteoarthritis of the Knee

- The use of PENNSAID for the treatment of the signs and symptoms of osteoarthritis of the knee was evaluated in five double-blind placebo controlled trials. The two pivotal 12-week, double-blind, placebo controlled trials were conducted in the US and Canada, involving patients treated with PENNSAID at a dose of 40 drops four times a day.
- PENNSAID treatment resulted in statistically significant clinical improvement compared to placebo and/or vehicle, in all three primary efficacy variables—pain, physical function (Western Ontario and McMaster Universities LK3.1 OA Index (WOMAC) pain and physical function dimensions) and Patient Overall Health Assessment (POHA)/Patient Global Assessment (PGA).
  - ○ The 1st Phase III trial was a 12-week double-blind, placebo-controlled study in which topical diclofenac solution was significantly more effective than the vehicle-control solution for all outcome measures; pain, $P = .001$; physical function, $P = .002$; patient global assessment, $P = .003$; stiffness, $P = .005$; and pain on walking, $P = .004$.

TABLE 16-5   Diclofenac 1.5% Topical Solution (Pennsaid) Evidence Base

POPULATION	DESIGN	RESULTS
OA of knee	Randomized, double-blind, vehicle-controlled study: $N = 326$; Pennsaid or vehicle 40 drops applied four times daily for 12 weeks.	Topical diclofenac solution was significantly more effective than the vehicle-control solution for all outcome measures; pain, $P = .001$; physical function, $P = .002$; patient global assessment, $P = .003$; stiffness, $P = .005$; and pain on walking, $P = .004$.
OA of knee	12-week, double-blind, double-dummy, randomized controlled trial: $N = 775$; Subjects randomized to 1 of 5 treatments (TDiclo, placebo solution, DMSO vehicle, oral diclofenac (ODiclo) and the combination) applied 40 drops of study solution and took one study tablet daily for 12 weeks.	TDiclo was superior to placebo for pain (-6.0 vs. -4.7, $P = 0.015$), physical function (-15.8 vs. -12.3, $P = 0.034$), overall health (-0.95 vs. -0.37, $P < 0.0001$), and PGA (-1.36 vs. -1.01, $P = 0.016$), and was superior to DMSO vehicle for all efficacy variables. No significant difference was observed between DMSO vehicle and placebo or between TDiclo and ODiclo.
Cochrane review—Topical NSAIDs	To examine the efficacy of topical NSAIDs in chronic musculoskeletal pain in longer duration studies of at least 8 weeks. 7688 participants in 34 studies from 32 publications; 23 studies compared a topical NSAID with placebo.	The best data were for topical diclofenac in osteoarthritis, where the NNT for at least 50% pain relief over 8–12 weeks compared with placebo was 6.4 for Pennsaid versus 11 for Voltaren Gel.

OA, osteoarthritis; TDiclo, topical diclofenac solution; DMSO, dimethylsulfoxide; ODiclo, oral diclofenac; NSAIDs, nonsteroidal anti-inflammatory drugs.

○ The 2nd Phase III trial was a 12-week, 5-arm, double-blind, double-dummy, randomized controlled trail in which TDiclo was superior to placebo for pain ($P = 0.015$), physical function ($P = 0.034$), overall health ($P < 0.0001$), and PGA ($P = 0.016$), and was superior to DMSO vehicle for all efficacy variables.

Cochrane Review

- In the fall of 2012 the Cochrane Collaboration published a systematic review of topical NSAIDs for the treatment of chronic musculoskeletal pain. The objective of the review was to examine the use of topical NSAIDs in chronic musculoskeletal pain, focusing on studies of high methodological quality, and examining the measured effect of the preparations according to study duration. The principal aim was to estimate treatment efficacy in longer duration studies of at least 8 weeks.
- Information was available from 7688 participants in 34 studies from 32 publications; 23 studies compared a topical NSAID with placebo. Topical NSAIDs were significantly more effective than placebo for reducing pain due to chronic musculoskeletal conditions.
- The best data were for topical diclofenac in osteoarthritis, where the NNT for at least 50% pain relief over 8–12 weeks compared with placebo was 6.4 for Pennsaid versus 11 for Voltaren Gel, the other US FDA approved topical NSAID approved for osteoarthritis, underscoring one conclusion reached by the authors that formulation, not just active medication, is critically important with regards to efficacy.

SIDE EFFECTS

- Systemic exposure, as measured by maximum plasma concentration of diclofenac, after use of Pennsaid is approximately 1/25th to 1/75th of that observed with various oral formulations of diclofenac.
- The most frequent of these reactions were dry skin (32%), contact dermatitis characterized by skin erythema and induration (9%), contact dermatitis with vesicles (2%) and pruritus (4%).

DOSAGE AND ADMINISTRATION

- Apply PENNSAID to clean, dry skin by dispensing 10 drops at a time either directly onto the knee or first into the hand and then onto the knee. Spread PENNSAID evenly around front, back and sides of the knee. Repeat this procedure until 40 drops have been applied and the knee is completely covered with solution.
- Wash hands completely after administering the product and wait until the area is completely dry before covering with clothing or applying sunscreen, insect repellent, cosmetics, topical medications, or other substances.
- Do not get PENNSAID in your eyes, nose, or mouth.

DICLOFENAC GEL 1% (VOLTAREN GEL)

FORMULATION

- Voltaren® Gel is a nonsteroidal anti-inflammatory drug containing 1% diclofenac that is indicated for the relief of the pain of osteoarthritis of joints amenable to topical treatment, such as the knees and those of the hands.

MECHANISM OF ACTION

- The mechanism of action of diclofenac is similar to that of other nonsteroidal anti-inflammatory drugs. Diclofenac inhibits the enzyme, cyclooxygenase (COX), an early component of the arachidonic acid cascade, resulting in the reduced formation of prostaglandins, thromboxanes and prostacyclin. It is not completely understood how reduced synthesis of these compounds results in therapeutic efficacy.

EFFICACY

- Table 16-6 summarizes clinical studies of Voltaren Gel 1%.

Osteoarthritis

- The first pivotal Phase III study evaluated the efficacy of Voltaren® Gel for the treatment of osteoarthritis of the knee in a 12-week, randomized, double-blind, multicenter, placebo-controlled, parallel-group trial. Voltaren® Gel was administered at a dose of 4 g, four times daily, on one knee (16 g per day). Pain as assessed by the patients at Week 12 using the WOMAC (Western Ontario and McMaster Universities Osteoarthritis Index) Pain Subindex was lower in the Voltaren® Gel group than the placebo group.
- The second Phase III study evaluated the efficacy of Voltaren® Gel for the treatment of osteoarthritis in subjects with osteoarthritis of the hand in an 8-week, randomized, double-blind, multicenter, placebo-controlled, parallel-group study. Voltaren® Gel was administered at a dose of 2 g per hand, four times daily, on both hands (16 g per day). Pain in the target hand as assessed by the patients at Weeks 4 and 6 on a visual analog scale from 0 to 100 was lower in the Voltaren® Gel group than the placebo group.

- Voltaren Gel did not reach statistical significance on all three endpoints (WOMAC Pain, Physical Function, and global assessment) and therefore only received an indication for pain of OA (unlike Pennsaid which was positive on all three WOMAC endpoints for both Phase III studies and hence received the indication of "treatment of signs and symptoms of OA.").

SIDE EFFECTS

- Nonserious adverse reactions that were reported during the short-term placebo-controlled studies comparing Voltaren® Gel and placebo (vehicle gel) over study periods of 8–12 weeks (16 g per day), were application site reactions. These were the only adverse reactions that occurred in >1% of treated patients with a greater frequency in the Voltaren® Gel group (7%) than the placebo group (2%).

DOSAGE AND ADMINISTRATION

- The proper amount of Voltaren® Gel should be measured using the dosing card supplied in the drug product carton. The gel should be applied within the oblong area of the dosing card up to the 2 or 4 g line (2 g for each elbow, wrist, or hand, and 4 g for each knee, ankle, or foot). The dosing card containing Voltaren® Gel can be used to apply the gel. The hands should then be used to gently rub the gel into the skin. After using the dosing card, hold with fingertips, rinse, and dry. If treatment site is the hands, patients should wait at least one (1) hour to wash their hands.
- Apply the gel four times daily:
  - (4 g) to the affected foot or knee or ankle
  - (2 g) to the affected hand or elbow or wrist, four times daily.
- Total dose should not exceed 32 g per day, over all affected joints.

TABLE 16-6 **Diclofenac Gel 1% (Voltaren Gel) Evidence Base**

POPULATION	DESIGN	RESULTS
OA of knee	12-week, randomized, double-blind, multicenter, placebo-controlled, parallel-group trial; Voltaren Gel or placebo administered at a dose of 4 g, four times daily, on one knee (16 g per day).	Pain as assessed by the patients at Week 12 using the WOMAC Pain Subindex was significantly lower in the Voltaren® Gel group than the placebo group. Voltaren Gel did not reach statistical significance on all 3 endpoints (WOMAC Pain, Physical Function, and global assessment)
OA of knee	8-week, randomized, double-blind, multicenter, placebo-controlled, parallel-group study; Voltaren Gel or placebo administered at a dose of 2 g per hand, four times daily, on both hands (16 g per day)	Pain in the target hand as assessed by the patients at Weeks 4 and 6 on a visual analog scale from 0 to 100 was significantly lower in the Voltaren Gel group than the placebo group

OA, osteoarthritis; WOMAC, Western Ontario and McMaster Universities Osteoarthritis Index.

DICLOFENAC PATCH 1.3% (FLECTOR)

FORMULATION

- Flector Patch contains diclofenac epolamine 1.3%, an NSAID and is indicated for the topical treatment of acute pain due to minor strains, sprains, and contusions.

MECHANISM OF ACTION

- In pharmacologic studies, diclofenac has shown anti-inflammatory, analgesic, and antipyretic activity. As with other NSAIDs, its mode of action is not known; its ability to inhibit prostaglandin synthesis, however, may be involved in its anti-inflammatory activity, as well as contribute to its efficacy in relieving pain associated with inflammation.

EFFICACY

- Table 16-7 summarizes clinical studies of Flector Patch 1.3%.

Acute Pain—Ankle Sprain

- Efficacy of Flector Patch was demonstrated in two of four studies of patients with minor sprains, strains, and contusions.

- The first study was a 7-day ankle sprain study in which Flector patch was superior to placebo patch from 4 hours after the first application ($P < 0.02$), with pain relief maintained to the end of the 7-day study ($P < 0.01$ at Day 7) and led to significant improvements in all secondary criteria (pain at rest, pain on passive stretch, pain on pressure, pain on the single foot leaning) from Day 3.
- The second study was a 14-day evaluation of Flector patch versus placebo for minor sprains, strains, and contusions. Flector was more effective than placebo in reducing pain on 0–10 scale on Day 14.

Acute Pain—Minor Soft Tissue Injury

- A randomized, double-blind, placebo-controlled study evaluated the safety and efficacy of the diclofenac epolamine topical patch for the treatment of acute pain due to minor soft tissue injury (mild or moderate sprain, strain, or contusion) in patients 18–65 years of age.
  - Twice-daily treatment with diclofenac epolamine topical patch produced a statistically significant reduction in mean pain score relative to baseline by an additional 18.2% in the diclofenac epolamine topical patch group (0.435 ± 0.268) compared with the placebo group (0.532 ± 0.293) ($P = 0.002$; overall) beginning after application of the second patch.
  - The most common adverse events were treatment site related ($n = 16$, 7.9% diclofenac epolamine topical patch; $n = 12$, 5.8% placebo patch).
- A multicenter, randomized, placebo-controlled, parallel design study assessed the efficacy and safety of

---

TABLE 16-7   Diclofenac Patch 1.3% (Flector) Evidence Base

POPULATION	DESIGN	RESULTS
Acute pain—Sprains, strains	Randomized, double-blind, placebo-controlled trial: 14-day evaluation of Flector Patch or placebo applied twice daily	Flector was more effective than placebo in reducing pain on 0–10 scale on Day 14.
Acute pain—Ankle sprain	Randomized, double-blind, placebo-controlled 7-day trial evaluating twice daily application of Flector Patch or placebo.	Flector patch was superior to placebo patch from 4 hours after the first application ($p < 0.02$), with pain relief maintained to the end of the 7-day study ($p < 0.01$ at Day 7) and led to significant improvements in all secondary criteria (pain at rest, pain on passive stretch, pain on pressure, pain on the single foot leaning) from Day 3.
Acute pain—Minor soft tissue injury	Randomized, double-blind, placebo-controlled study; $N = 418$; Flector Patch or placebo applied twice daily for 14 days or until pain resolution.	Flector patch provided statistically significant reduction in mean pain score by an additional 18.2% compared with the placebo group ($p = 0.002$; overall) beginning after application of the second patch. Median time to pain resolution was shortened by 2 days in the Flector patch group relative to the placebo group ($p = 0.007$).
Acute pain—Minor sports injury	Randomized, double-blind, placebo-controlled, parallel design study: $N = 222$; twice daily application of Flector Patch or placebo for 2 weeks	Flector patch was superior to placebo patch in relieving pain. Statistical significance was seen on clinic Days 3 ($P = 0.036$) and 14 ($P = 0.048$), as well as the daily diary pain ratings at Days 3, 7, and 14 ($P <$ or $= 0.044$).
Acute pain—Back strain	Open-label study: $N = 123$; 7–14 days treatment with twice daily application of Flector Patch	Baseline mean $\pm$ standard deviation average pain score was 6.5 ± 1.3, which decreased to 2.5 ± 2.4 ($P < 0.0001$) at end of treatment. Similarly, least, worst, and current pain scores were also reduced ($P < 0.0001$). Sixty-three percent of patients achieved $\geq$50% pain reduction from baseline.

topical diclofenac (NSAID) patch applied directly to the painful injury site for the treatment of acute minor sports injury pain in adult subjects ($N = 222$). Diclofenac epolamine or placebo topical patch was applied directly to the skin overlying the painful injured site twice daily for 2 weeks.

- Diclofenac patch was superior to placebo patch in relieving pain. Statistical significance was seen on clinic days 3 ($P = 0.036$) and 14 ($P = 0.048$), as well as the daily diary pain ratings at Days 3, 7, and 14 ($P <$ or $= 0.044$).
- No statistically significant differences were seen in any safety or side-effect measures with the diclofenac patch as compared to the placebo patch.

Other Pain States

Acute Pain—Due to Back Strain

- A multicenter, open-label study evaluated effectiveness and safety of DETP in patients with acute pain due to back strain in patients aged ≥18 years with acute pain due to nonradicular back strain with an average pain intensity of ≥4 (0 = no pain, 10 = pain as bad as you can imagine).
  - In 123 enrolled patients, baseline mean ± standard deviation average pain score was 6.5 ± 1.3, which decreased to 2.5 ± 2.4 ($P < 0.0001$) at end of treatment. Sixty-three percent of patients achieved ≥50% pain reduction from baseline.
  - Fifteen patients experienced a total of 19 adverse events (AEs), 17 of which were mild to moderate, and 2 of which were severe. Three AEs were treatment related (application site rash, nausea, and tachycardia); 1 patient had a serious AE (noncardiac chest pain) considered unrelated to DETP.

SIDE EFFECTS

- Overall, the most common adverse events associated with Flector Patch treatment were skin reactions at the site of treatment occurring in 11% of patients during the development program.

DOSAGE AND ADMINISTRATION

- The recommended dose of Flector Patch is one (1) patch to the most painful area twice a day.
- Do not apply Flector Patch to non-intact or damaged skin resulting from any etiology, eg, exudative dermatitis, eczema, infected lesion, burns, or wounds.
- Do not wear a Flector Patch when bathing or showering.

TOPICAL CAPSAICIN: TOPICAL CAPSAICIN CREAM/LOTION 0.025% AND 0.075%. (ZOSTRIX)[q]

FORMULATION

- Capsaicin (*trans*-8-methyl-*N*-vanillyl-6-nonenamide), a naturally occurring substance, is a component of the red chili pepper.
- For many centuries, even prior to the advent of clinical study, the contents of the chili pepper have been compounded into topical mixtures for the treatment of a variety of pains.
- Capsaicin is available in the United States without prescription as a cream or lotion in strengths of 0.025% and 0.075%.
- Medicinally available capsaicin is a natural mixture of several different active chemicals and has not actually obtained a full FDA new drug application approval.

MECHANISM OF ACTION

- Several different potential analgesic mechanisms of action have been postulated for topically applied capsaicin.

Substance P Depletion

- One theory of the analgesic effect of capsaicin is the depletion of substance P from presynaptic terminals, which depresses the function of type C nociceptive fibers (substance P is one of the principal mediators of pain).

Neurodegeneration

- Animal and human studies have demonstrated that topical application of capsaicin to the skin results in damage to the underlying nociceptive peripheral nerves. One study found that application of capsaicin cream 0.075% to human skin four times daily for 3 weeks results in a reduction in the average number of epidermal nerve fibers by 82% compared with pretreatment values. Epidermal innervation recovered gradually to nearly 83% of normal at 6 weeks after discontinuing capsaicin usage. The investigators concluded that neurodegeneration may account for the pain relief associated with capsaicin.

EFFICACY

- Table 16-8 summarizes clinical trials of capsaicin cream.

---

[q][Note: At these doses capsaicin is considered a "natural product," therefore FDA approval was not required for marketing.]

TABLE 16-8   Topical Capsaicin Cream/Lotion 0.025% & 0.075% (Zostrix) Evidence Base

POPULATION	DESIGN	RESULTS
PHN >12 mo	Randomized, double-blind, vehicle-controlled: $N = 32$; capsaicin cream 0.075% or vehicle applied three to four times/day for 6 week	Significant decrease in pain with capsaicin versus control ($P < 0.05$)
PHN >6 mo	Randomized, double-blind, vehicle-controlled: $N = 131$; capsaicin cream 0.075% or vehicle applied four times/day for 6 week	Significant improvements in pain with capsaicin versus vehicle ($P < 0.05$)
Chronic neuropathic pain	Randomized, double-blind, placebo-controlled: $N = 200$; placebo cream, doxepin 3.3%/capsaicin 0.025% cream, or doxepin 3.3%/capsaicin 0.025% cream three times/day for 4 week	Significant reductions in overall pain scores in all 3 treatment groups ($P < 0.001$); overall pain relief was similar among groups
Postmastectomy pain >5 mo	Randomized, parallel, double-blind, vehicle-controlled trial: $N = 25$; capsaicin cream 0.075% or vehicle applied four times/day for 6 week	Significantly greater improvement in jabbing pain and pain relief with capsaicin than with vehicle ($P < 0.05$)
Diabetic neuropathy and radiculopathy	Randomized, double-blind, vehicle-controlled trial: $N = 252$; capsaicin cream 0.075% or vehicle applied four times/day for 8 week	Significantly greater pain relief and improvement in pain intensity ($P < 0.05$)
Diabetic neuropathy	Randomized, double-blind, vehicle-controlled trial: $N = 22$; capsaicin cream 0.075% or vehicle applied four times/day for 8 week	Significantly more capsaicin patients had overall improvement ($P < 0.05$)
Variety of painful polyneuropathies	Randomized, double-blind, placebo-controlled study	No improvement versus placebo
HIV-associated peripheral neuropathy	Randomized, double-masked, controlled, multicenter trial: $N = 26$; capsaicin cream 0.075% or vehicle applied four times/day for 4 week	Current pain scores were worse at 1 week with capsaicin patients versus vehicle ($P < 0.05$); no other statistically significant differences in pain measures; dropout rate was significantly higher with capsaicin
OA and RA, moderate to very severe knee pain	Randomized, double-blind, vehicle-controlled: $N = 70$ (OA) and $N = 31$ (RA); capsaicin cream 0.025% or vehicle applied	Significantly greater reduction in pain scores versus placebo (OA: $P < 0.05$; RA: $P = 0.003$) four times/day for 4 week
OA	Randomized, double-blind, vehicle-controlled: $N = 200$; patients randomized to vehicle, capsaicin cream 0.025%, glyceryl trinitrate 1.33%, or capsaicin cream 0.025% + glyceryl trinitrate cream 1.33% for 6 week	Capsaicin+glyceryl trinitrate was more effective than either agent alone in reducing pain scores ($P < 0.05$); each agent alone and combination significantly reduced pain versus baseline ($P < 0.05$)

OA, osteoarthritis; PHN, postherpetic neuralgia; RA, rheumatoid arthritis.

Neuropathic Pain

Postherpetic Neuralgia

- Two randomized, controlled studies reported statistically significant pain reduction with capsaicin in patients with PHN. In one trial, 54% of patients treated with capsaicin and 6% of control subjects reported ≥40% pain relief after 6 weeks of therapy ($P = 0.02$); however, it should be noted that this trial failed to use an intent-to-treat efficacy analysis.

Chronic Neuropathic Pain

- One randomized, controlled study demonstrated the efficacy of capsaicin compared with placebo for the treatment of a variety of neuropathic conditions.

Postmastectomy Pain

- A randomized, controlled study found capsaicin to be efficacious compared with placebo in the treatment of postmastectomy pain: 46% of patients receiving capsaicin were satisfied with the pain relief and tolerability of this agent.

Painful Diabetic Neuropathy

- Two randomized trials reported that capsaicin produced significant pain relief in patients with painful diabetic neuropathy.

Painful Polyneuropathy

- A randomized, double-blind, placebo-controlled study from the Mayo Clinic reported negative results in patients with chronic distal painful polyneuropathy treated with capsaicin cream.

HIV-Associated Neuropathy

- Capsaicin failed to demonstrate benefit in HIV-associated peripheral neuropathy.

Other Pain States

Osteoarthritis and Rheumatoid Arthritis

- In a randomized, double-blind, controlled trial, capsaicin was significantly superior to vehicle in reducing pain scores compared with baseline for patients with osteoarthritis or rheumatoid arthritis.

- In another randomized, double-blind, controlled trial, the combination of glyceryl trinitrate cream 1.33% and topical capsaicin 0.025% was more effective in osteoarthritis than either agent alone. Because pain relief was not immediate, it was concluded that capsaicin cream is more appropriate treatment for background pain than for acute flares.

Periocular and Facial Pain

- Case reports have indicated that capsaicin has some benefit in periocular or facial pain (if patients can describe a trigger point and have a history of nerve damage).

Neurogenic Residual Limb Pain

- Case reports have described relief in neurogenic residual limb pain with capsaicin treatment.

SIDE EFFECTS

- A major clinical advantage to all TPAs, such as capsaicin, is their lack of clinically significant systemic activity. Thus, minimal systemic side effects or drug–drug interactions have been demonstrated with appropriate use of capsaicin.

Burning Sensation at Application Site

- A major clinically significant side effect associated with topical capsaicin is a burning or stinging sensation at the application site.
- From 30%–92% of patients experience a burning or stinging sensation after application of capsaicin. This reaction usually diminishes with time (after 3 days to 2 weeks of regular use), but also seriously limits patient compliance with treatment. Capsaicin cream 0.025% may be more tolerable than the 0.075% preparation.
- Combining capsaicin with topical doxepin 3.3%, a tri-cyclic antidepressant, or glyceryl trinitrate cream 1.33% has been reported to attenuate the burning effect of capsaicin.
- The burning sensation associated with capsaicin complicates the blinding of clinical trials.

Burning Sensation in Other Bodily Regions

- Patients must be instructed to wash their hands immediately following capsaicin application. Failure to do so with subsequent touching of sensitive bodily regions (eg, eyes, mucous membranes, broken or irritated skin, genitalia) can result in an immediate severe burning sensation.

Sneezing and Coughing

- If inhaled, capsaicin can be an irritant to the nose and lungs. Sneezing and coughing, therefore, are observed occasionally with capsaicin treatment.

DOSAGE AND ADMINISTRATION

- Topical capsaicin cream generally is applied three or four times daily.
- Topical capsaicin should be applied in a well-ventilated area and thinly enough to prevent formation of a layered or caked residue. Patients should consider wearing a plastic glove or using a cotton applicator to apply the medication.
- The treated area should not be washed for at least 1 hour after application.
- Pain relief usually is noted within 2–6 weeks, although one trial in patients with osteoarthritis or rheumatoid arthritis recorded significant relief at 1 week.

TOPICAL CAPSAICIN PATCH 8% (QUTENZA)

FORMULATION

- Qutenza (capsaicin) 8% patch contains capsaicin in a localized dermal delivery system. The capsaicin in Qutenza is a synthetic equivalent of the naturally occurring compound found in chili peppers.
- Each Qutenza patch is 14 cm × 20 cm (280 cm²) and consists of a polyester backing film coated with a drug-containing silicone adhesive mixture, and covered with a removable polyester release liner.

MECHANISM OF ACTION

- Capsaicin is an agonist for the transient receptor potential vanilloid 1 receptor (TRPV1), which is an ion channel-receptor complex expressed on nociceptive nerve fibers in the skin.
- Topical administration of capsaicin causes an initial enhanced stimulation of the TRPV1-expressing cutaneous nociceptors that may be associated with painful sensations followed by pain relief thought to be mediated by a reduction in TRPV1-expressing nociceptive nerve endings.

Neurodegeneration

- Recent animal and human studies have demonstrated that topical application of capsaicin to the skin results in damage to the underlying nociceptive peripheral nerves. One study found that application of capsaicin cream 0.075% to human skin four times daily for 3 weeks results in a reduction in the average number of epidermal nerve fibers by 82% compared with pretreatment values. Epidermal innervation recovered gradually to nearly 83% of normal at 6 weeks after discontinuing capsaicin usage. The investigators concluded that neurodegeneration may account for the pain relief associated with capsaicin.

- Over the course of several months, there may be a gradual reemergence of painful neuropathy thought to be due to TRPV1 nerve fiber reinnervation of the treated area.

EFFICACY

- Table 16-9 summarizes clinical trials of capsaicin patch.

Neuropathic Pain

Postherpetic Neuralgia

- The efficacy of Qutenza was established in two 12-week, double blind, randomized, dose-controlled, multicenter studies.
- PHN Study 1: In this 12-week study, the Qutenza group demonstrated a greater reduction in pain compared to the Control group during the primary assessment at Week 8. The percent change in average pain from baseline to Week 8 was −18% (±2%) for the low-dose control and −29% (±2%) for Qutenza.
- PHN Study 2: In this 12-week study the Qutenza group demonstrated a greater reduction in pain compared to the Control group during the primary assessment at Week 8. The percent change in average pain from baseline to Week 8 was −26% (±2%) for the low-dose control and −33% (±2%) for Qutenza.
- Another double-blind, placebo-controlled 12-week study, randomized 155 patients 2:1 to receive either NGX-4010 or a 0.04% capsaicin control patch. The mean percent reduction in "average pain for the past 24 hours" NPRS scores from baseline to Weeks 2–8 was greater in the NGX-4010 group (36.5%) compared with control (29.9%) although the difference was not significant ($p = 0.296$).

HIV Polyneuropathy[r]

- This double-blind multicenter study randomized 307 patients with painful HIV-DSP to receive NGX-4010 or control, a low-concentration capsaicin patch.

After application of a topical anesthetic, NGX-4010 or control was applied once for 30, 60, or 90 minutes to painful areas on the feet. The primary efficacy endpoint was percent change in Numeric Pain Rating Scale (NPRS) from baseline in mean "average pain for past 24 hours" scores from Weeks 2–12.

- A single NGX-4010 application resulted in a mean pain reduction of 22.8% during Weeks 2–12 as compared to a 10.7% reduction for controls ($p = 0.0026$).
- In this randomized, double-blind, controlled study, patients with pain due to HIV-associated distal sensory polyneuropathy received a single 30-minute or 60-minute application of NGX-4010—a capsaicin 8% patch ($n = 332$)—or a low-dose capsaicin (0.04%) control patch ($n = 162$). The primary endpoint was the mean percent change from baseline in Numeric Pain Rating Scale score to Weeks 2–12. Secondary endpoints included patient global impression of change at Week 12.
- Pain reduction was not significantly different between the total NGX-4010 group (−29.5%) and the total control group (−24.5%; $P = 0.097$).

Painful Peripheral Neuropathy (DN, HIV, PHN)[s]

- An open-label, uncontrolled, 12-week study enrolled 25 patients with postherpetic neuralgia (PHN), one with HIV-distal sensory polyneuropathy, and 91 with painful diabetic neuropathy (PDN). Patients received pretreatment with one of three 4% lidocaine topical anesthetics (L.M.X.4[1], Topicaine Gel[2], or Betacaine Enhanced Gel 4[3]) followed by a single 60- or 90-minute NGX-4010 application. The primary efficacy variable was the percentage change in Numeric Pain Rating Scale scores from baseline to Weeks 2–12.
- PDN and PHN patients achieved a 31% and 28% mean pain decrease from baseline during Weeks 2–12, respectively, and 47% and 44%, respectively, were responders (≥30% pain decrease).

SIDE EFFECTS

- Adverse reactions observed in clinical trials occurring in ≥5% of patients in the Qutenza group and at an incidence greater than in the control group were application site erythema (63%), application site pain (42%), application site pruritus (6%) and application site papules (6%). The majority of application site reactions were transient and self-limited.
- Transient increases in pain were commonly observed on the day of treatment in patients treated with

---

[r][QUTENZA is not currently FDA approved for this indication.]

[s][QUTENZA is not FDA approved for this indication.]

TABLE 16-9   Topical Capsaicin Patch 8% (Qutenza) Evidence Base

POPULATION	DESIGN	RESULTS
PHN	Randomized, double-blind, placebo-controlled trial: $N = 402$; one 60-minute application of Qutenza patch or a low-concentration capsaicin control patch.	Quntenza group had a significantly greater reduction in pain during Weeks 2–8. Mean changes in NPRS score were −29.6% vs. −19.9% ($p = 0.001$). 87 (42%) patients who received Qutenza and 63 (32%) controls had a 30% or greater reduction in mean NPRS score.
PHN	Randomized, double-blind, controlled study: $N = 418$; a single 60-minute application of Qutenza patch or a 0.04% capsaicin control patch	Qutenza group had a significantly greater mean reduction from baseline in pain during Weeks 2–8 compared with the control group ($P = 0.011$). A ≥30% reduction in mean NPRS scores was achieved in 46% of Qutenza recipients compared with 34% of controls ($P = 0.02$).
PHN	Randomized, double-blind, controlled study: $N = 155$; single 60-minute application or a 0.04% capsaicin control patch.	The mean percent reduction in "average pain for the past 24 hours" NPRS scores from baseline to Weeks 2–8 was greater in the Qutenza group (36.5%) compared with control (29.9%) the difference was not significant ($p = 0.296$).
HIV polyneuropathy	Randomized, double-blind, controlled study: $N = 307$; Qutenza or control was applied once for 30, 60, or 90 minutes to painful areas on the feet.	A single Qutenza application resulted in a mean pain reduction of 22.8% during Weeks 2–12 as compared to a 10.7% reduction for controls ($p = 0.0026$). Mean pain reductions in the Qutenza 30-, 60- and 90-minute groups were 27.7%, 15.9%, and 24.7% ($p = 0.0007, 0.287$, and 0.0046 vs. control).
HIV polyneuropathy	Randomized, double-blind, controlled study: $N = 495$; a single 30- or 60-minute application of Qutenza or capsaicin (0.04%) control patch.	Pain reduction was not significantly different between the total Qutenza group (−29.5%) and the total control group (−24.5%; $P = 0.097$).
PN	Open-label, uncontrolled, 12-week study: $N = 117$; a single 60- or 90-minute Qutenza application.	PDN and PHN patients achieved a 31% and 28% mean pain decrease from baseline during Weeks 2–12, respectively, and 47% and 44%, respectively, were responders (≥30% pain decrease).

PHN, postherpetic neuralgia; HIV, human immunodeficiency virus; PN, peripheral neuropathy.

Qutenza. Pain increases occurring during patch application usually began to resolve after patch removal. On average, pain scores returned to baseline by the end of the treatment day and then remained at or below baseline levels.

- The majority of Qutenza treated patients in clinical studies had adverse reactions with a maximum intensity of "mild" or "moderate."

DOSAGE AND ADMINISTRATION

- The recommended dose of Qutenza is a single, 60-minute application of up to four patches.
- Treatment with Qutenza may be repeated every three months or as warranted by the return of pain (not more frequently than every three months).
- Pre-treat with a topical anesthetic to reduce discomfort associated with the application of Qutenza.
- Use Qutenza only on dry, intact (unbroken) skin.
- Apply the Qutenza patch within 2 hours of opening the pouch.

BIBLIOGRAHPY

Argoff CE. New analgesics for neuropathic pain: The lidocaine patch. *Clin J Pain.* 2000;16(2, suppl):S62–S66.

Attal N, Brasseur L, Chauvin M, Bouhassira D. Effects of single and repeated applications of a eutectic mixture of local anesthetic (EMLA) cream on spontaneous and evoked pain in postherpetic neuralgia. *Pain.* 1999;81:203–209.

Backonja M, Wallace MS, Blonsky ER, et al. NGX-4010 C116 Study Group. NGX-4010, a high-concentration capsaicin patch, for the treatment of postherpetic neuralgia: a randomised, double-blind study. *Lancet Neurol.* 2008;7:1106–1112.

Barbano RL, Herrmann DN, Hart-Gouleau S, Pennella-Vaughan J, Lodewick PA, Dworkin RH. Effectiveness, tolerability, and impact on quality of life of the 5% lidocaine patch in diabetic polyneuropathy. *Arch Neurol.* 2004;61:914–918.

Berman B, Flores J, Pariser D, Pariser R, de Araujo T, Ramirez CC. Self-warming lidocaine/tetracaine patch effectively and safely induces local anesthesia during minor dermatologic procedures. *Dermatol Surg.* 2005;31:135–138.

Berman SM, Justis JC, Ho MI, Ing M, Eldridge D, Gammaitoni AR. Lidocaine patch 5% (Lidoderm®) improves common pain qualities reported by patients with HIV-associated painful peripheral neuropathy: an open-label pilot study using the Neuropathic Pain Scale. In: Proceedings of the 10th World Congress of Pain; August 17–22, 2002; San Diego, Calif.

Bernstein JE, Korman NJ, Bickers DR, Dahl MV, Millikan LE. Topical capsaicin treatment of chronic postherpetic neuralgia. *J Am Acad Dermatol.* 1989;21: 265–270.

Burch F, Codding C, Patel N, et al. Lidocaine patch 5% improves pain, stiffness, and physical function in osteoarthritis pain patients. *OsteoArthritis and Cartilage.* 2004;12:253–255.

Cannon DT, Wu Y. Topical capsaicin as an adjuvant analgesic for the treatment of traumatic amputee neurogenic residual limb pain. *Arch Phys Med Rehabil.* 1998;79:591–593.

Cataflam® (diclofenac potassium immediate-release tablets) [package insert]. East Hanover, NJ: Novartis; 2009.

Chen JZ, Alexiades-Armenakas MR, Bernstein LJ, Jacobson LG, Friedman PM, Geronemus RG. Two randomized, double-blind, placebo-controlled studies evaluating the S-Caine Peel for induction of local anesthesia before long-pulsed Nd:YAG laser therapy for leg veins. *Dermatol Surg.* 2003;29(10):1012–1018.

Chen JZ, Jacobson LG, Bakus AD, et al. Evaluation of the S-Caine Peel for induction of local anesthesia for laser-assisted tattoo removal: randomized, double-blind, placebo-controlled, multicenter study. *Dermatol Surg.* 2005;31:281–286.

Clifford DB, Simpson DM, Brown S, et al. A randomized, double-blind, controlled study of NGX-4010, a capsaicin 8% dermal patch, for the treatment of painful HIV-associated distal sensory polyneuropathy. *J Acquir Immune Defic Syndr.* 2012;59:126–133.

Comer AM, Lamb HM. Lidocaine patch 5%. *Drugs.* 2000;59:245–249.

Curry SE, Finkelx JC. Use of the Synera patch for local anesthesia before vascular access procedures: a randomized, double-blind, placebo-controlled study. *Pain Med.* 2007;8:497–502.

Dalpiaz AS, Lordon SP Lipman AG. Topical lidocaine patch therapy for myfascial pain. *J Pain Palliat Care Pharmacother.* 2004;18:15–34.

Davis MD, Sandroni P. Lidocaine patch for pain of erythromelalgia. *Arch Dermatol.* 2002;138:17–19.

Deal CL, Schnitzer TJ, Lipstein E, et al. Treatment of arthritis with topical capsaicin: A double-blind trial. *Clin Ther.* 1991;13:383–395.

Derry S, Moore RA, Rabbie R. Topical NSAIDs for chronic musculoskeletal pain in adults. *Cochrane Database of Syst. Rev.* 2012, 9: CD007400.

Devers A, Galer BS. Topical lidocaine patch relieves a variety of neuropathic pain conditions: an open-label study. *Clin J Pain.* 2000;16:205–208.

Drug Facts and Comparisons 2002. 56th ed. St. Louis, Mo: Wolters Kluwer; 2002:1792.

EMLA® Cream (lidocaine 2.5% and prilocaine 2.5%) [package insert]. Wilmington, Del: AstraZeneca LP; 2002.

Fassoulaki A, Sarantopoulos C, Melemeni A, Hogan Q. EMLA reduces acute and chronic pain after breast surgery for cancer. *Reg Anesth Pain Med.* 2000;25: 350–355.

FLECTOR PATCH® (diclofenac epolamine patch) 1.3% [package insert]. Bristol, TN: King Pharmaceuticals. 2011.

Galer BS. Topical drugs for the treatment of pain. In: Loeser JD, ed. *Bonica's Managment of Pain.* 3rd ed. Hagerstown, Md: Lippincott Williams & Wilkins; 2001:2.

Galer BS, Jensen MP, Ma T, Davies PS, Rowbotham MC. The lidocaine patch 5% effectively treats all neuropathic pain qualities: results of a randomized, double-blind, vehicle-controlled, 3-week efficacy study with use of the neuropathic pain scale. *Clin J Pain.* 2002;18:297–301.

Galer BS, Rowbotham M, Perander J, Devers A, Friedman E. Topical diclofenac patch relieves minor sports injury pain: results of a multicenter controlled clinical trial. *J Pain Symptom Manage.* 2000;19:287–294.

Galer BS, Rowbotham MC, Perander J, Friedman E. Topical lidocaine patch relieves postherpetic neuralgia more effectively than a vehicle topical patch: results of an enriched enrollment study. *Pain.* 1999;80:533–538.

Galer BS, Sheldon E, Patel N, Codding C, Burch F, Gammaioni A. Topical lidocaine patch 5% may target a novel underlying pain mechanism in osteoarthritis. *CMRO.* 2004;20:1455–1458.

Gammaitoni AR, Davis MW. Pharmacokinetics and tolerability of lidocaine patch 5% with extended dosing. *Ann Pharmacother.* 2002;36:236–240.

Gammaitoni AR, Goitz HT, Marsh S, Marriott TB, Galer BS. Heated lidocaine/tetracaine patch for treatment of patellar tendinopathy pain. *J Pain Research.* 2013;6:565–570.

Gimbel J, Jacobs D, Pixton G, Paterson C. Effectiveness and safety of diclofenac epolamine topical patch 1.3% for the treatment of acute pain due to back strain: an open-label, uncontrolled study. *Phys Sportsmed.* 2011;39:11–18.

Gimbel J, Linn R, Hale M, Nicholson B. Lidocaine patch treatment in patients with low back pain: results of an open-label nonrandomized pilot study. *Am J Ther.* 2005;12:311–319.

Hashmi JA, Baliki MN, Huang L, et al. Lidocaine patch (5%) is no more potent than placebo in treating chronic back pain when tested in a randomised double blind placebo controlled brain imaging study. *Mol Pain.* 2012;8:29.

Herrmann DN, Barbano RL, Hart-Gouleau S, Pennella-Vaughan J, Dworkin RH. An open-label study of the lidocaine patch 5% in painful idiopathic sensory polyneuropathy. *Pain Med.* 2005;6:379–384.

Hines R, Keaney D, Moskowitz MH, Prakken S. Use of lidocaine patch 5% for chronic low back pain: a report of four cases. *Pain Med.* 2002;4:361–365.

Irving GA, Backonja MM, Dunteman E, et al. NGX-4010 C117 Study Group. A multicenter, randomized, double-blind, controlled study of NGX-4010, a high-concentration capsaicin patch, for the treatment of postherpetic neuralgia. *Pain Med.* 2011;12:99–109.

Jousssellin E. Flector Tissugel in the treatment of painful ankle sprain. *J Traumatol Sport.* 2003;20:1S5–1S9.

Kanazi GE, Johnson RW, Dworkin RH. Treatment of postherpetic neuralgia: an update. *Drugs.* 2000;59:1113–1126.

Katz NP, Gammaitoni AR, Davis MW, Dworkin RH, and the Lidoderm Patch Study Group. Lidocaine patch 5% reduces pain intensity and interference with quality of life in patients with postherpetic neuralgia: an effectiveness trial. *Pain Med.* 2002;4:324–332.

Khanna M, Peters C, Singh JR. Treating pain with the lidocaine patch 5% after total knee arthroplasty. *PMR.* 2012;4:642–646.

Khasar SG, Gold MS, Levine JD. A tetrodotoxin-resistant sodium current mediates inflammatory pain in the rat. *Neurosci Lett.* 1998;256:17–20.

Kivitz A, Fairfax M, Sheldon EA, et al. Comparison of the effectiveness and tolerability of lidocaine patch 5% versus celecoxib for osteoarthritis-related knee pain: post hoc analysis of a 12 week, prospective, randomized, active-controlled, open-label, parallel-group trial in adults. *Clin Ther.* 2008;30:2366–2377.

Kuehl K, Carr W, Yanchick J, Magelli M, Rovati S. Analgesic efficacy and safety of the diclofenac epolamine topical patch 1.3% (DETP) in minor soft tissue injury. *Int J Sports Med.* 2011;32:635–643.

Low PA, Opfer-Gehrking TL, Dyck PJ, Litchy WJ, O'Brien PC. Double-blind, placebo-controlled study of the application of capsaicin cream in chronic distal painful polyneuropathy. *Pain.* 1995;62:163–168.

Lidoderm® (Lidocaine Patch 5%) [package insert]. Chadds Ford, Penn: Endo Pharmaceuticals Inc; 2002.

Lin YC, Kuan TS, Hsieh PC, Yen WJ, Chang WC, Chen SM. Therapeutic effects of lidocaine patch on myofascial pain syndrome of the upper trapezius: a randomized, double-blind, placebo-controlled study. *Am J Phys Med Rehabil.* 2012;91: 871–882.

Lincoff NS, Rath PP, Hirano M. The treatment of periocular and facial pain with topical capsaicin. *J Neuro-ophthalmol.* 1998;18:17–20.

Louis J. EMLA Cream. International Center for the Control of Pain in Children and Adults. Available at: http://www.nursing .uiowa.edu/sites/adultpain/Topicals/emlatt.htm. Accessed July 3, 2002.

Mannion RJ, Doubell TP, Coggeshall RE, Woolf CJ. Collateral sprouting of uninjured primary afferent A-fibers into the superficial dorsal horn of the adult rat spinal cord after topical capsaicin treatment to the sciatic nerve. *J Neurosci.* 1996;16: 5189–5195.

Marriott TB, Charney MR, Stanworth S. Effects of application durations and heat on the pharmacokinetic properties of drug delivered by a lidocaine/tetracaine patch: a randomized, open-label, controlled study in healthy volunteers. *Clin Ther.* 2012;34:2174–2183.

McCleane G. Topical capsaicin of doxepin hydrochloride, capsaicin and a combination of both produces analgesia in chronic human neuropathic pain: A randomized, double-blind, placebo-controlled study. *Br J Clin Pharmacol.* 2000;49: 574–579.

McCleane G. The analgesic efficacy of topical capsaicin is enhanced by glyceryl trinitrate in painful osteoarthritis: a randomized, double blind, placebo controlled study. *Eur J Pain.* 2000;4:355–360.

Meier T, Baron R, Faust M, et al. Efficacy of the lidocaine patch 5% in the treatment of focal peripheral neuropathic pain syndromes: A randomized, double-blind, placebo-controlled study. *Pain.* 2003;106:151–158.

Nalamachu S, Crockett RS, Gammaitoni AR, Gould EM. A comparison of the lidocaine patch 5% vs naproxen 500 mg twice daily for the relief of pain associated with carpal tunnel syndrome: a 6-week, randomized, parallel-group study. *MedGenMed.* 2006;8:33.

Nalamachu S, Crockett RS, Mathur D. Lidocaine patch 5 for carpal tunnel syndrome: how it compares with injections: a pilot study. *J Fam Pract.* 2006;55:209–214.

Nalamachu S, Nalamasu R, Jenkins J, Smith M, Heusner J, Marriott T. A open-label pilot study evaluating heated lidocaine/tetracaine patches in the treatment of patients with carpal tunnel syndrome. Presented at PAINWeek: The National Conference on Pain for Frontline Practitioners, September 8–11, 2010, Las Vegas, Nevada. Abstract 66.

Nolano M, Simone DA, Wendelschafer-Crabb G, Johnson T, Hazen E, Kennedy WR. Topical capsaicin in humans: parallel loss of epidermal nerve fibers and pain sensation. *Pain.* 1999;81:135–145.

Paice JA, Ferrans CE, Lashley FR, Shott S, Vizgirda V, Pitrak D. Topical capsaicin in the management of HIV-associated peripheral neuropathy. *J Pain Symptom Manage.* 2000;19:45–52.

PENNSAID® (diclofenac sodium topical solution) 1.5% w/w [package insert]. Hazelwood, MO: Mallinckrodt.

PLIAGLIS® (lidocaine and tetracaine) Cream 7% / 7% [package insert]. Fort Worth, Tx: Galderma Laboratories LP. 2012.

QUTENZA® (capsaicin) 8% patch [package insert]. San Mateo, CA. NeurogesX, Inc. 2009.

Radnovich R, Gammaitoni A, Trudeau J, Marriott T. Comparison of Heated Lidocaine/Tetracaine Patch and Corticosteroid Injection for Treatment of Shoulder Impingement Syndrome Pain. Presented at the American College of Sports Medicine Annual Meeting, May 29–31, 2013, Indianapolis, IN. Abstract #1244

Radnovich R, Marriott M. Utility of the heated lidocaine/tetracaine patch in the treatment of pain associated with shoulder impingement syndrome: a pilot study. *Int J General Medicine.* 2013;6:641–646.

Rauck R, Busch M, Marriott T, et.al. Effectiveness of a heated lidocaine/tetracaine topical patch for pain associated with myofascial trigger points: results of an open label pilot study. *Pain Pract.* 2013;13(7):533–538.

Roth SH, Shainhouse JZ. Efficacy and safety of a topical diclofenac solution (Pennsaid) in the treatment of primary osteoarthritis of the knee: a randomized, double-blind, vehicle-controlled clinical trial. *Arch Intern Med.* 2004;164:2017–2023.

Rowbotham MC, Davies PS, Verkempinck C, Galer BS. Lidocaine patch: double-blind controlled study of a new treatment method for post-herpetic neuralgia. *Pain.* 1996;65:39–44.

Saito I, Koshino T, Nakashima K, Uesugi M, Saito T. Increased cellular infiltrate in inflammatory synovia of osteoarthritic knees. *Osteoarthritis Cartilage.* 2002;10:156–162.

Sawyer J, Febbraro S, Masud S, Ashburn MA, Campbell JC. Heated lidocaine/tetracaine patch (Synera, Rapydan) compared with lidocaine/prilocaine cream (EMLA) for topical anaesthesia before vascular access. *Br J Anaesth.* 2009;102:210–215.

Sethna NF, Verghese ST, Hannallah RS, Solodiuk JC, Zurakowski D, Berde CB. A randomized controlled trial to evaluate S-Caine patch for reducing pain associated with vascular access in children. *Anesthesiology.* 2005;102:403–408.

SC-04-99. Data on file. Zars Pharma Inc.

Simon LS, Grierson LM, Naseer Z, Bookman AAM, Shainhouse JZ. Efficacy and safety of topical diclofenac containing dimethyl sulfoxide (DMSO) compared with those of topical placebo, DMSO vehicle and oral diclofenac for knee osteoarthritis. *Pain.* 2009;143:238–245.

Simpson DM, Brown S, Tobias J, NGX-4010 C107 Study Group. Controlled trial of high-concentration capsaicin patch for treatment of painful HIV neuropathy. *Neurology.* 2008;70:2305–2313.

Sugimoto M, Uchida I, Mashimo T. Local anaesthetics have different mechanisms and sites of action at the recombinant N-methyl-D-aspartate (NMDA) receptors. *Br J Pharmacol.* 2003;138:876–882.

Stow PJ, Glynn CJ, Minor B. EMLA cream in the treatment of post-herpetic neuralgia: efficacy and pharmacokinetic profile. *Pain.* 1989;39:301–305.

Synera® (Lidocaine 70 mg/Tetracaine 70 mg Topical Patch) [package insert]. Salt Lake City, UT: Zars Pharma Inc.; 2009.

Tandan R, Lewis GA, Krusinski PB, Badger GB, Fries TJ. Topical capsaicin in painful diabetic neuropathy: Controlled study with long-term follow-up. *Diabetes Care.* 1992;15:8–14.

The Capsaicin Study Group. Treatment of painful diabetic neuropathy with topical capsaicin: A multicenter, double-blind, vehicle-controlled study. *Arch Intern Med.* 1991;151:2225–2229.

Voltaren® Gel (diclofenac sodium topical gel) 1% [package insert]. Chadds Ford, Penn: Endo Pharmaceuticals Inc.; 2009.

Wallace MS, Kopecky EA, Ma T, et al. Evaluation of the depth and duration of anesthesia from heated lidocaine/tetracaine (Synera) patches compared with placebo patches applied to healthy adult volunteers. *Reg Anesth Pain Med.* 2010;35:507–513.

Watson CP. Topical capsaicin as an adjuvant analgesic. *J Pain Symptom Manage.* 1994;9:425–433.

Watson CP, Evans RJ. The postmastectomy pain syndrome and topical capsaicin: a randomized trial. *Pain.* 1992;51:375–379.

Watson CP, Tyler KI, Bickers DR, Millikan LE, Smith S, Coleman E. A randomized vehicle-controlled trial of topical capsaicin in the treatment of postherpetic neuralgia. *Clin Ther.* 1993;15:510–526.

Waxman SG. The molecular pathophysiology of pain: abnormal expression of sodium channel genes and its contribution to hyperexcitability of primary sensory neurons. *Pain.* 1999;6: S133–S140.

Webster LR, Peppin JF, Murphy FT, Lu B, Tobias JK, Vanhove GF. Efficacy, safety, and tolerability of NGX-4010, capsaicin 8% patch, in an open-label study of patients with peripheral neuropathic pain. *Diabetes Res Clin Pract.* 2011;93:187–197.

Webster LR, Tark M, Rauck R, Tobias JK, Vanhove GF. Effect of duration of postherpetic neuralgia on efficacy analyses in a multicenter, randomized, controlled study of NGX-4010, an 8% capsaicin patch evaluated for the treatment of postherpetic neuralgia. *BMC Neurol.* 2010;10:92.

17 ACETAMINOPHEN AND NONSTEROIDAL ANTI-INFLAMMATORY DRUGS

Michael W. Loes, MD
Jennifer Schneider, PhD, MD

ACETAMINOPHEN

- Acetaminophen is a synthetic, short-centrally acting analgesic derived from p-aminophenol; the full chemical name is N-acetyl-p-aminophenol.
- It also has antipyretic and mild anti-inflammatory properties.
- The plasma half-life is 2–3 hours.
- The absorption rate is rapid, usually exceeding 95%.
- Its major metabolite is phenacetin, an analgesic widely used in Europe but banned in the United States because of an association with analgesic nephropathy typically presenting as either acute papillary necrosis or interstitial nephritis.

- Acetaminophen is metabolized by the microsomal enzyme system of the liver as are many other analgesics, anticonvulsants, antibiotics, antifungal agents, and other drugs.
- Acetaminophen is listed as paracetamol in the British pharmacopeia but is the same drug.
  - As paracetamol, it is widely available as an oral medication, an intravenous and intramuscular preparation.
  - Parental usage of acetaminophen is not widely used in the United States.
- The analgesic mechanism of acetaminophen is central, both through the spinal cord and cerebral cortex.
- It also causes a weak central inhibition of prostaglandin synthetase.
- It also raises pain threshold through complex mechanisms involving the inhibition of the nitric oxide pathway which is mediated by a variety of neurotransmitter receptors including N-methyl-D-aspartate and substance P, a tachykinin neuropeptide.
- Acetaminophen is arguably the most commonly used analgesic and is considered first-step pharmacotherapy for controlling the pain of osteoarthritis in doses up to 4000 mg/d.
- The drug is frequently used in combination with opioid analgesics, such as codeine, dihydrocodeine, hydrocodone, oxycodone and pentazocine.
- A combination product with tramadol is available as are many products that contain aspirin, diphenhydramine (an antihistamine) and/or dextromethorphan (a cough suppressant).
- Acetaminophen is also an effective antipyretic.
  - Because of its ability to lower fever, it is extensively used in preparations to treat upper respiratory infections, kidney and bladder problems, and any other clinical state where fever or pain may be present.
- Combination products for flu, sinus congestion, menstrual cramps, and insomnia are abundant on the shelves of pharmacies and grocery stores.
- It behooves physicians to question their patients regarding these products, especially when prescribing 3 or 4 g/d for arthritis, because many patients are taking products that they do not realize contain acetaminophen. The result can be inadvertent overdose and toxicity.
- For analgesia, the conventional dose for older children or adults is 325–650 mg every 4–6 hours until pain is relieved.
- For younger children, a single dose should not exceed 60–12 mg depending on age and weight and should not be administered for more than 10 days. (See Chapter 44 for more information on pediatric pain management.)

- Extended-release tablets are available that release 325 mg immediately from the outer shell, with a matrix core releasing an additional 325 mg during an 8-hour period.
- In equal doses, the degree of analgesia and antipyresis is similar to that produced by aspirin.
- Although traditionally 4000 mg/kg has been considered the maximum safe dose, over a third of healthy adults prescribed this dose for up to 14 days were found to develop more than a threefold elevation in the liver enzyme ALT. These changes resolved after acetaminophen treatment was stopped.
  - Especially for chronic use, it may be wise to limit daily dose to less than 4 gm.
  - As for patients with liver disease, although no consensus has been reached, a limit of 2 mg/d is advisable.
- In 2011, the FDA asked drug manufacturers to limit the strength of acetaminophen to 325 mg per tablet in prescription drug products, as well as to include a boxed warning about the risk of severe liver injury. (http://www.fda.gov/Drugs/DrugSafety/ucm 239821.htm)
- Acute toxicity is common with acetaminophen overdoses.
  - This occurs either singularly or in combination with other available drugs.
  - Because the acetaminophen is rapidly absorbed intervention gastric lavage followed by activated charcoal is recommended.
  - There are protocols for using acetylcysteine.

NONSTEROIDAL ANTI-INFLAMMATORY DRUGS (NSAIDS)

ASPIRIN: A BALANCED VIEW

- Aspirin, a nonsteroidal anti-inflammatory drug (NSAID), is a tried and tested analgesic, anti-inflammatory agent and antipyretic.
- It is also called acetylsalicylic acid.
- Aspirin was first isolated by Felix Hoffmann, a chemist with the German company, Bayer, in 1897.
  - It was extracted from willow bark, an herb which is still widely used for pain and inflammation.
- Aspirin is a broad-spectrum inhibitor of prostaglandins, a family of fatty acids so ubiquitous in the human body they are detected in almost every tissue and body fluid.
  - Prostaglandins produce a wide range of effects, notably the sensitization of nociceptors.
- It is rapid acting and extremely effective for short-term pain problems, especially headaches, aspirin competes with acetaminophen for being the most frequently purchased over-the-counter pain reliever worldwide and with good reason; it works.
- Yet aspirin therapy is not without significant risks.
  - A select group of patients—those with asthma, nasal polyps, and/or urticaria (known as Franklin's triad)—are at significant risk of anaphylaxis leading to rapid bronchial constriction, laryngeal edema, hypotension, and, often, death.
  - Cross-reacting aspirin sensitivity is rare in asthmatic patients under age 10 in the absence of Franklin's triad.
  - In adults, cross-reactivity is estimated at about 20% among those who are sensitive to aspirin. In patients with Franklin's triad, cross-reactivity is extremely high (approximately 85%).
  - Another important precaution regarding aspirin is that it should not be given to children under the age of 2 years who are suffering from a cold, flu, or chicken pox because there is a small risk of Reye's syndrome, a potentially fatal pediatric illness.
  - When an individual is sensitive or allergic to aspirin or to a particular class of NSAID, usually another NSAID from another class will be tolerated though caution advised; the reactions are more structurally related that functionally related at least as related to a true allergy.
  - Often individuals complain of a sensitive stomach or nausea with NSAIDS but this is not a true allergy and may be attenuated with change of diet or the concurrent use of an H2 blocker or a proton pump inhibitor.
    - If this occurs, celecoxib might be used but is contraindicated in patients with allergy to sulfa drugs.
    - Other structurally different NSAIDs are usually tolerated.
  - A rash can develop which resolves when the agent is stopped.
  - Unlike other NSAIDs aspirin irreversibly bind to platelets and effects on bleeding time will last up to 3 weeks.
  - Also seen frequently is a mild reduction in glomerular filtration which can be more than mild in sensitive individuals.
  - And, often seen is the bothersome occurrence of tinnitus.
  - And, when aspirin is in the system post operatively in the plastic surgery setting, there is a general consensus that bleeding is more frequent and healing is not optimal.
- While aspirin is recognized as preventive therapy for heart attacks and strokes and approved by the FDA for this usage, the data supporting this widespread usage is thin and reading the insert that can be found in a box of Bayer Aspirin® is worth the time.

○ The specific recommendation is more for those who have actually suffered a heart attack or an ischemic stroke or who are at high risk for other reasons; the recommendation is not universal.

○ A 2012 meta-analysis of the effect of aspirin for primary prevention of vascular (stroke and heart attack) or nonvascular (cancer) deaths found that aspirin was not effective for any of these.

■ Moreover, any benefits were offset by the increased risk of bleeding events.

■ The study concluded that routine use of aspirin for primary prevention is not warranted, so that treatment decisions need to be made on a case-by-case basis.

■ The FDA also advises that taking ibuprofen (for pain relief) and aspirin at the same time may interfere with the benefits of aspirin for the heart (fda.gov/Drugs/DrugSafety/PostmarketDrugSafetyInformation forPatientsandProviders/ucm110510.htm

○ Aspirin has also seen increasing usage for to prevent clot formation in those individuals that go in and out of atrial fibrillation.

■ It is also used for those who have thromboemboli from various hypercoagulability states.

■ Notably, there are many therapeutic agents in the class called blood thinners or anti-clot drugs.

■ The disease state must be balanced against the individual risks in each case and cautious choices need to be made within a cooperative guidance model of care.

■ Sometimes the obvious—quit smoking—is the best advice to prevent the hypercoagulability state.

• A 6-year randomized trial conducted among 5139 apparently healthy male doctors found that those taking 500 mg aspirin daily had significantly fewer migraines than the nonaspirin users.

• For any or all of these conditions, evidence-based data is limited.

• When it is supportive, it is usually not overwhelming and needs to be assessed against the increased incidences of other problems such as bleeding states from unintended gastro-intestinal problems.

• Bottom line: Aspirin prophylaxis is not a universal recommendation for aging individuals. The risks are significant and the benefits may be overstated. The interest of the individual patient is the only interest to be considered.

NONSTEROIDAL AND OTHER ANTI-INFLAMMATORY DRUGS

• NSAIDs, aspirin inclusive, are an important component in balanced analgesia in the management of acute and chronic pain.

TABLE 17-1 Conservative Adult Starting Doses of NSAIDs for Pain

NSAID	STARTING DOSE
Celecoxib (Celebrex)	100 mg qd
Choline magnesium salicylate (Trilisate)	750 mg bid
Diclofenac sodium (Voltaren)	50 mg bid
Diclofenac potassium: immediate release	50 mg tid
Diflunisal (Dolobid)	500 mg bid
Etodolac (Lodine)	400 mg bid
Fenoprofen (Nalfon)	200 mg qid
Ibuprofen (Motrin, Advil, Nuprin)	200 mg qid
Indomethacin (Indocin)	25 mg bid
Ketorolac (Toradol)	10 mg bid
Ketoprofen tromethamine (Orudis, Oruvail)	75 mg bid
Meclofenamate (Meclofen)	50 mg tid
Mefenamic acid (Ponstel)	250 mg qd
Meloxicam (Mobic)	7.5 mg qd
Nabumetone (Relafen)	1000 mg qd
Naproxen (Naprosyn)	50 mg qd
Naproxen sodium (Anaprox)	275 mg tid
Oxaprozin (Daypro)	600 mg qd
Piroxicam (Feldene)	20 mg qd
Rofecoxib (Vioxx)	12.5 mg qd
Salsalate (Disalcid)	750 mg bid
Sulindac (Clinoril)	150 mg bid
Tolmetin (Tolectin)	400 mg tid
Valdecoxib (Bextra)	10 mg qd

• The starting doses of available NSAIDs are listed in Table 17-1, and the elimination half-lives in Table 17-2.
• All NSAIDs are highly protein bound.
• NSAIDs are contraindicated only in individuals with Franklin's triad. This is the syndrome of nasal polyps, angioedema, and urticaria. In this group, anaphylactoid reactions have occurred.
• The use of NSAIDs concurrent with warfarin (Coumadin) or other blood thinning agents is not advisable.
• Unless contraindicated, NSAIDs should be considered as standard therapy for pain and fever reduction in the inpatient and outpatient settings.

TABLE 17-2 Elimination Half-Lives of NSAIDs

NSAID	ELIMINATION HALF-LIFE (h)
Celecoxib	8
Diclofenac	1–2
Fenoprofen	3
Ibuprofen	1–2
Ketoprofen	2
Ketorolac	4–6
Nabumetone (6NMA)	24
Naproxen	14
Oxaprozin	40
Rofecoxib	17
Piroxicam	50
Tolmetin	5
Valdecoxib	8–11

- NSAIDs have a direct action on spinal nociceptive processing with a relative order of potency that correlates with their capacity to inhibit cyclooxygenase (COX) activity.
- The two isoforms of cyclooxygenase, COX-1 and COX-2, are genetically distinct, with COX-1 located on chromosome 7 and COX-2 on chromosome 1.
- COX-1 is considered constitutive or part of the basic constitutional homeostasis, while COX-2 is inducible; that is, it responds to specific insult.
- Various NSAIDs inhibit the isoforms differentially.
  - The goal is to inhibit COX-2 while preserving COX-1 because gastric problems are reduced by protecting the constitutional homeostasis of the COX-1 system.
  - Quantification tables exist for the relative inhibition of COX-1/COX-2 by various NSAIDs, but introduction of the relatively selective agents (celecoxib and less so meloxicam) render this kind of data less useful.
- Two popular coxibs, valdecoxib and rofecoxib were voluntarily removed from the market by the manufacturer: rofecoxib (Vioxx®) in 2004 and valdecoxib (Bextra) in 2005.
  - The reason related to unforeseen cardiovascular complications in some of their extended studies—an increased incidence of congestive heart failure and unexpected coronary infarcts.
  - This was opined to have occurred particularly in those individuals who were taken off aspirin when initiated on coxib therapy.
  - Celecoxib (Celebrex®) survived these inquiries primarily because of extended high dose trials in mixed populations that did not show a similar incidence. And, because additional long term trials had been completed that showed a reduced incidence of colon cancer in familial polyposis.
- The potential ulceration sparing effect of selective COX-2 inhibitors may be rendered insignificant by concurrent low dose aspirin therapy for prevention of cardiovascular or cerebral vascular disease.
- Etodolac (Lodine), nabumetone (Relafen), and meloxicam (Mobic) remain in use because they are relatively more selective than the first NSAIDs produced and less expensive than the coxibs.
- Although NSAIDs act primarily through their effects on peripheral prostaglandin synthetase, additional central mechanisms for their action have also been discussed.
- Clinically, NSAIDs have an important role as adjuvants to other analgesics and have an opioid-sparing effect in the range of 20%–35%.
  - Although it has been generally accepted that NSAIDs are synergistic with opioids, a 2011 Cochrane review of studies of the efficacy of either

or both for the treatment of cancer pain concluded that, for short term use, there is not a significant clinical difference between using either medication alone or combining them.
  - As for long-term use, there have not been enough studies to draw conclusions. (http://summaries.cochrane .org/CD005180/non-steroidal-anti-inflammatory -drugs-nsaids-or-paracetamol-alone-or-combined -with-opioids-for-the-treatment-of-cancer-pain)
- Clinically NSAIDs do not produce any form of temporal tolerance like has been seen in opioids and some muscle relaxants such as carisoprodol (Soma), diazepam (Valium), and clonazepam (Klonopin).
  - Notably, these specific muscle relaxants are more appropriated labeled as central nervous system tranquilizers and best avoided in the treatment of pain problems because of dependency issues or in some cases addiction; they are hard to get off once a patient is started on one of these medications.
- Elimination kinetics and degree of protein binding vary widely among NSAIDs.
  - Hence, drug displacement occurs when NSAIDs are combined with other highly protein-bound drugs, including warfarin (Coumadin) and lithium salts (Eskalith); caution is advised in such cases because the increased levels affect clotting time and the potential for lithium toxicity.
  - The protein binding of all NSAIDs except aspirin to platelet cyclooxygenase is reversible.
    - Thus, coagulation is affected by aspirin as long as that platelet is alive and circulating, approximately 3 weeks.
    - If a patient is on daily aspirin and is scheduled for major surgery, especially cardiovascular surgery, it is prudent to substitute a shorter-acting NSAID with an equally short effect on coagulation, such as ibuprofen (Advil, Motrin), 2–3 weeks prior to surgery.
- Only ketorolac (Toradol) and more recently ibuprofen is available in both oral and parenteral formulations.
  - The parenteral form of ketorolac (Toradol) has been successfully used to manage postoperative pain either by intermittent intravenous boluses or by patient-controlled devices. In Europe, diclofenac is widely available as intramuscular analgesia.
- Indomethacin (Indocin) and aspirin are available in oral form and also as suppositories.
- Choline magnesium trisalicylate (Trilisate) and ibuprofen (Motrin) come in liquid forms.
- The rapidly dissolving NSAID formulations are useful for acute pain but are not optimally indicated for the treatment of osteoarthritis or rheumatoid arthritis. These include naprosyn sodium (Anaprox), and ketorolac (Toradol).

- The following nonsteroidal agents with anti-inflammatory effects are not considered NSAIDs. The major mechanisms for these agents are immunologic:
  - acetaminophen
  - tramadol (Ultram®)
  - colchicine
    - Colchicine is not an analgesic and is generally effective only when used to treat acute gouty arthritis, although some investigators have found it effective in low back pain syndromes.
  - methotrexate (Immunex)
  - hydroxychloroquine (Plaquenil)
  - penicillamine (Cuprimine, Depen)
  - gold salts (Thiomalate)
  - etanercept (Enbrel)
  - infliximab (Remicade, Centocor)
  - leflunomide (Arava)
  - mycophenolate mofetil (Cell Cept)
  - cyclosporin (Neoral)
- There are options for inflammation and pain that are more herbal or naturopathic.
  - In surveys, as many as one-third of patients are using these options on a regular basis.
  - These include various proteolytic enzyme formulae such as Wobenzym®, Rotazyme®, or Medizyme® T.
  - Here is evidence based research supporting the usage of these formulae (see The Aspirin Alternative, ©2011 The Healing Response ©2003 Healing Sports Injuries Naturally ©2003 by MW Loes).
  - Other herbals such as turmeric, aescin (horse chestnut) and willow bark are in common usage.
  - And there are homeopathic formulae that also have evidence to support their usage such as arnica, ruta, and rhus tox. (see E book by Dr. D Ullman)

STRUCTURE AND FUNCTION

- Chemical structure determines metabolism, absorption, volume of distribution, protein binding, and elimination pathways.
- NSAIDs have varying chemical structures and are in different classes.
  - Some clinicians have advocated trying an agent from another class if the first choice does not work. Although this view has not been well supported, switching classes may be of value in patients who experience problematic side effects.
- Drug interactions and effects on platelet function may differ among specific NSAIDs.
- Receptor affinity differs, and there may be other subtle differences in pharmacodynamics.
- Table 17-3 displays the structural classification of NSAIDs.

TABLE 17-3 NSAID Structural Classification

Propionic acid derivatives
  Fenoprofen calcium (Nalfon)
  Flurbiprofen (Ansaid)
  Ibuprofen (multiple trade names)
  Ketoprofen (Orudis)
  Naproxen sodium (Naprelan, Naprosyn)
  Naproxen sodium (Aleve, Anaprox)
  Oxaprozin (Daypro)
Fenamates
  Mefenamic acid (Ponstel)
  Meclofenamate sodium (Meclomen)
Indoles
  Indomethacin (Indocin)
  Sulindac (Clinoril)
  Tolmetin sodium (Tolectin)
Phenylacetic acids
  Diclofenac sodium (Voltaren)
  Diclofenac potassium (Cataflam)
Benzylacetic acid
  Bromfenac sodium (Duract)
Pyranocarboxylic acid
  Etodolac (Lodine)
Salicylates
  Acetylsalicylic (aspirin)
  Salsalate (various)
  Magnesium salicylate
  Diflunisal (Dolobid)
Naphthylalkanone
  Nabumetone (Relafen)
Oxicam
  Piroxicam (Feldene)
Pyrazole derivatives
  Phenylbutazone (Butazolidin)
  Oxyphenbutazone (Tandearil)
Pyrrolo
  Ketorolac tromethamine
(Toradol)
Coxibs
  Celecoxib (Celebrex)
  Rofecoxib (Vioxx)
  Valdecoxib (Bextra)

PAIN

Pain is "what the patient says it is" but the generators may not be inflammatory; they may be neuropathic or even mental emotional.

- In the American Pain Society's March 2002 guidelines for the management of pain in osteoarthritis, rheumatoid arthritis, and juvenile chronic arthritis, acetaminophen was recommended for mild pain associated with osteoarthritis and a selective COX-2 inhibitor for moderate to severe pain and inflammation.
- For arthritis of either type, the maximum daily dose is disputed.
  - Whereas, it was felt for a number of years that up to 4000 mg of acetaminophen was tolerated and safe, this number is now generally judged as too high.
  - It is best not to exceed 3000 mg a day and even this dose needs to be reevaluated.

- Unrecognized renal dysfunction is common and sometimes the patient just forgets to tell you that they only have one kidney.
- In combinations, high dose NSAIDs and acetaminophen have been associated with both liver problems and both acute and chronic renal failure.
- In patients with only one functioning kidney, further consideration of NSAIDs or acetaminophen dosage is warranted. Reducing by half and following kidney function is advisable.
- These guidelines have now been updated in 2008 and continue to recommend the use of acetaminophen but that nonselective coxibs such as Celecoxib (Celebrex®) be used rarely and only in highly selected individuals.
- Because of primarily cardiovascular concerns, they now recommend that "all patients with moderate to severe pain, pain-related functional impairment or diminished quality of life due to pain be considered for opioid therapy."
- The prolonged use of NSAIDs and/or acetaminophen for pain needs to be an individual decision and certain laboratory parameters should be periodically followed such as hemoglobin, liver, and kidney panels.
- Notably, there have been several high profile sports figures that have had kidney transplants and had their professional careers shortened because of long term combination NSAID and acetaminophen toxicities.
- Although COX-2 inhibitors are worthwhile analgesics and have both an improved gastrointestinal side effect profile and reduced or absent platelet inhibition activity compared with nonselective NSAIDs, the consensus of the International COX-2 Study Group was that the rates of hypertension and edema with coxibs are similar to those observed with nonselective NSAIDs.
- Because NSAIDs and acetaminophen are not without potential problems, other options for pain management should be considered.
- Certain herbals have anti-inflammatory effects and may allow home remedies at a lower cost.
  - Turmeric
  - Certain anti-inflammatory enzyme formulae, most of which contain variations of the German formula (Wobenzym®—bromelain, papain, trypsin, chymotrypsin, rutacid).
  - Some proteolytic formulas contain serratiopeptidase and some add quercetin.
  - Aescin (horse chestnut),
  - Common homeopathic single agents such as arnica, rhus tox, and ruta.
  - An open awareness and positive reception toward these alternatives is increasing important because they are largely safe and many patients are already taking them on a regular basis. Asking will allow options to be developed and in some cases, cautionary advice to be given.
- There are injectable formulae such as Hyalgan® and Synvisc® used to lubricate joints.

INFLUENCE IN TRAUMATIC, OPERATIVE, AND POSTOPERATIVE SETTINGS

- In that NSAIDs affect the arachidonic pathway involved in the response to injury, they affect the surgical stress response.
  - In the acute postoperative model, most of these effects are favorable and have led to increased usage.
- NSAIDS reduce opioid requirements, fevers, and, perhaps, reduce fluid loss.
- On the negative side is the concern regarding the effect of NSAIDs on platelet adhesion and the potential of NSAIDs to cause postoperative bleeding, a concern that ended with the introduction of selective COX-2 agents that do not appreciably affect bleeding times.
- And, in that NSAIDs block inflammation and fever, both components of natural healing, there is concern, especially in sports medicine doctors and also expressed by plastic surgeons that complete natural healing is compromised by NSAIDs.
  - There is concern that the block in the arachidonic pathway is prior to optimal fibrin deposition reducing the stability of healing sprains.
- And, likely because of their analgesic, antipyretic, and sodium-retaining effects, NSAIDs attenuate endocrine metabolic effects.
- Parameters under dispute are those concerning post-traumatic immunosuppression, nitrogen balance, and acute-phase reactant proteins.
- With the controversy still current, evidence of fewer or more infectious complications is lacking.

NSAID SUMMARY ADVICE

- Use NSAIDs; they work.
- Don't use them brazenly.
- Use reduced dosages when able and shorter periods of use.
- Use alternative when there are risks to using NSAIDs in individual patients.
- Take into consideration cost in that they vary enormously and are often tier II or III on some health plans.
- Don't assume that over-the-counter drugs are any safer than prescription drugs.
- If on chronic therapy, check basic renal and hepatic chemistries twice a year or even quarterly if there are complex combinations of drugs being given.

- A routine urine analysis may pick up protein or cellular casts in the urine and these need to be investigated.
- Beware of the staggering polypharmacy that is so present in patient populations, both licit and illicit.

CAUTIONS AND ADVERSE EFFECTS

The following represents the kind of computer generated list a person receiving NSAIDs might be given at the pharmacy. Because we would like our patients to actually take what is prescribed and not be too fearful to do so, some discussion is prudent when initiating NSAID therapy.

Gastrointestinal

- Gastrointestinal (GI) tract complications associated with NSAIDs are the most common and are often serious.
- Endoscopic studies have shown that within 1 week of starting NSAID therapy, more than 30% of patients develop gastric erosions or ulcers, and within 1 year, approximately 3%–6% have significant GI bleeding.
- NSAID-associated gastropathy accounts for at least 2600 deaths and 20,000 hospitalizations each year in the United States in patients with rheumatoid arthritis alone.
- Across-the-board data show that 200,000–400,000 hospitalizations are caused by GI complications (bleeding and perforation).
  - The cost of these hospitalizations is $0.8–$1.6 billion per year.
- A prospective study of the rate of GI complications in patients with rheumatoid arthritis demonstrated that approximately 6% per year experience a significant GI side effect from NSAIDs, and approximately 1.3% of these require hospitalization.
- The duration of NSAID therapy appears to be the single most important factor predicting GI bleeding.
  - Patients on NSAIDs for 5 years have a five times greater risk of GI bleeding than those on NSAIDs for 1 year, and the risk at 1 year is four times greater than it is at 3 months.
  - Most of these patients did not have preceding GI problems, and prophylactic treatment with antacids and H2 blockers was of marginal value for duodenal ulcers and of no value for gastric ulcers.
- The relative risk of a GI-provoked hospitalization was more than five times greater in patients taking NSAIDs.
- A toxicity index in patients with rheumatoid arthritis revealed that salsalate and ibuprofen are the least toxic and tolmetin sodium, meclofenamate, and

TABLE 17-4 Comparative NSAID Toxicity Scores*

Salsalate	1.00
Ibuprofen	1.25
Diclofenac	3.57
Fenoprofen	3.57
Sulindac	4.75
Naproxen	5.20
Ketoprofen	6.00
Indomethacin	6.25
Piroxicam	8.00
Tolmetin	8.73
Meclofenamate	9.00

*Serious reactions per million prescriptions; based on data from (1) the Committee on Safety of Medicine: *Br Med J.* 1986;292:614 and 1986; 292:1190; (2) Griffin MR, et al. *Ann Intern Med.* 1991;114:257; and (3) Fries, et al. *Arthritis Rheum.* 1991;34:1353.

indomethacin the most toxic (see Table 17-4 for comparative NSAID toxicity scores).

- Most serious GI bleeds during NSAID use occur without prior GI symptoms.
- Risk factors include a history of duodenal or gastric ulceration, age, smoking ethanol use, concomitant use of corticosteroid.
- The use of NSAIDs concurrent with warfarin (Coumadin) or other blood thinning agents is not advisable. When combined, additive effects toward decreasing coagulation, lengthening bleeding times, or displacing bound warfarin can and does occur.
- Aspirin is likely the worst offender because it irreversibly binds to platelets for up to 3 weeks, the usual life of a platelet.
  - Because the use of prophylactic 81 mg aspirin is widespread in the prevention of heart disease, combination warfarin and 81 mg aspirin is often seen.
  - This should be openly discussed with cardiology to assess its advisability.
- The use of ibuprofen with warfarin is also frequently seen.
  - While this also should be discussed with cardiology or vascular surgery if it is to be continue, ibuprofen is less problematic because it has a short half liver (2–3 hours) and because it does not irreversibly bind with platelets.
- A synthetic prostaglandin E analog, misoprostol, decreases the risk of NSAID induced ulceration but may cause diarrhea and is an abortifacient.
- Alternatives recommended include famotidine 40 mg po bid or omeprazole 20 mg po daily.

Renal

- NSAID-associated kidney problems are common because more than 17 million Americans take these drugs.

- The most common renal problem associated with NSAID usage is reversible depression of renal function.
- Fenoprofen and indomethacin are associated with the highest incidence of renal dysfunction, and nonacetylated salicylates with the lowest.
- Fenoprofen has been implicated in the development of interstitial nephritis. Specific risk factors for renal toxicity include congestive heart failure, coexistent liver failure, and consumption of diuretics.
- Renal problems are most common in patients taking aspirin and ibuprofen, not because these drugs are the most toxic, but because so many people take them. It has been estimated that aspirin and ibuprofen cause renal dysfunction in 13%–18% of users.
- The elderly are at highest risk because, by age 65, they have usually already lost 25%–40% of normal renal function.
  - In a sensitive individual, significant adverse changes in kidney function can occur within 3–7 days.
  - The result can be acute renal failure, dialysis, and/or death if the complication is not recognized.
  - Subtle alternations in creatinine clearance are common and frequently overlooked.
  - In one study, aspirin reduced creatinine clearance by as much as 58% in patients with lupus nephritis.
- Another renal adverse event is "analgesic nephropathy," which occurs when large quantities of combination over-the-counter analgesics, most often acetaminophen, aspirin, and caffeine, are consumed.
- Phenacetin, which is also associated with renal failure, remains in wide use from international sources.

Hepatic

- The most common hepatic problem with NSAIDs is mild elevations of hepatic enzymes, estimated at 2%–5%.
- This elevation is higher in patients with rheumatoid arthritis, congestive heart failure, renal failure, and concurrent acetaminophen use and in those who are alcohol drinkers or of advanced age.
- Diclofenac (Voltaren) has been associated with more hepatic problems than other agents.
- In 1998, bromfenac sodium (Duract) was pulled off the market because of hepatic toxicity.
- Acute NSAID-associated hepatic injury, primarily cholestatic injury, leads to 5 in 100,000 Medicare hospitalizations.
- Liver toxicity is more likely to be dose-related than idiosyncratic. For diclofenac (Voltaren) or diclofenac potassium (Cataflam), the base incidence doubles for every doubling of dose.
- Because elevations in liver function tests are the first warning of more problems to come, checking and following liver profiles when patients are on NSAIDs is advisable.

Cardiac

- The elderly taking NSAIDs daily have an increased risk of heart problems, especially in the presence of congestive heart failure. NSAIDs inhibit prostaglandins in the kidney and, in doing so, often cause salt retention and edema.
- The 2%–4% incidence of edema from NSAIDs has not appreciably changed with the introduction of the coxibs.
- Patients with a history of congestive heart failure have a twofold increase in exacerbation of this condition, resulting in hospitalization when they are placed on an NSAID.
- The Warfarin Aspirin Study of Heart Failure (WASH) randomized 279 congestive heart failure patients to receive either aspirin 300 mg/d, warfarin to a target international ratio of 2.5, or no antithrombotic therapy.
  - During a mean follow-up of 27 months, 64% in the aspirin group required hospitalization compared with 47% in the warfarin group and 48% in the control group.
  - The increased incidence of hospitalization in the aspirin group was for worsening heart failure.
  - The combined endpoint of death, nonfatal myocardial infarction, or stroke occurred in 32% of the aspirin patients compared with 26% in the other two groups.
- NSAIDs, especially indomethacin, piroxicam, and naproxen, also cause an average increase in mean blood pressure of 10 mm Hg.

Cutaneous

- Between 5% and 10% of patients on NSAIDs develop a rash or pruritus.
  - This most commonly occurs with use of piroxicam, sulindac, or meclofenamate.
- Urticaria alone most commonly occurs with aspirin, indomethacin, and ibuprofen, while photosensitivity is most often seen with piroxicam.

Central Nervous System

- Severe headache is the most frequent central nervous system (CNS) toxic effect reported, though others include cognitive dysfunction, dizziness, sleeplessness, irritability, syncope, and, rarely, seizures. Indomethacin (Indocin) is the worst offender here, with 10%–25% of patients reporting headache.

- Elderly patients using NSAIDs, especially naproxen and ibuprofen, are the most likely to report confusion.
  - Elderly patients, in general, do not tolerate long term NSAID usage. There may be a poorly described irritability, a low-grade nausea. In elderly patients who could not tolerate NSAIDs, several longitudinal studies alternatively using tramadol were carried out with favorable results, better tolerability and prolonged pain relief.

Miscellaneous Toxic Effects

- Tinnitus is most commonly seen with aspirin use, although nonacetylated salicylates can also cause this condition.
- Anaphylactoid reactions are more common with tolmetin and aspirin than with other NSAIDs.
- Hematologic effects are common with all NSAIDs because these pharmaceuticals decrease platelet adhesiveness.
  - The most serious hematologic adverse event, aplastic anemia, has been reported with use of phenylbutazone, which is no longer available in the United States but is still available internationally.
  - Indomethacin and diclofenac have also been associated with anemia more often than other NSAIDs.
- Aspirin is associated with Reye's syndrome and not advised in children with febrile viral syndromes.
- The single doses and maximal daily doses of NSAIDs for children are listed in Table 17-5.

Platelets

- NSAIDs prevent platelet aggregation.
  - Only salsalate (Disalcid) and choline magnesium trisalicylate (Trilisate) lack this property.
- Because NSAIDs are highly protein bound, all have the potential of displacing warfarin (Coumadin) and potentiating its anticoagulant effect.
- Aspirin should be stopped at least 7 days prior to surgery.

Drug Interactions

- See Table 17-6.

TABLE 17-5   NSAIDs in the Pediatric Population

	SINGLE DOSE (mg/kg)	MAXIMAL DAILY DOSE (mg/kg)
Aspirin	10–15	60
Diclofenac	1.0–2.0	No information
Ibuprofen	10	40
Indomethacin	1	3
Ketoprofen	2.5	5
Naproxen	7	15

TABLE 17-6   Interactions of Other Pharmaceuticals with NSAIDs

Antacids	May decrease the absorption of NSAIDs.
Anticoagulants	NSAIDs are highly protein bound (99%), and, when given with anticoagulants, some displacement of Coumadin will potentiate the effect of warfarin. NSAIDs also reversibly inhibit platelet aggregation (except for aspirin where the effect is irreversible). The effect parallels the drug elimination time. Hence, for drugs with long elimination times (piroxicam and oxaprozin) the effect lasts days. Giving NSAIDs to patients who are anticoagulated is not contraindicated but caution is advised! Because nonacetylated NSAIDs, such as salsalate and choline magnesium salicylate, do not directly affect platelet function, they are safer but can still potentiate Coumadin by displacing protein-bound drug.
Antirheumatic agents	Many drugs used in rheumatoid arthritis (aza-thioprine [Imuran], penicillamine [Depen, Cuprimine], gold compounds, and methotrexate) can cause bone marrow toxicity, including decreased white blood cells and platelets. NSAIDs may potentiate this toxic effect.
Corticosteroids	Patients who take corticosteroids concurrently are at higher risk for NSAID-induced gastropathy.
Diuretics	The action of diuretics may be potentiated with concurrent use of NSAIDs.
Lithium	The pharmacologic activity of lithium is heightened in patients taking NSAIDs. One proposed mechanism is decreased renal clearance because of decreased renal prostaglandin synthesis.
Oral hypoglycemic agents	Several NSAIDs potentiate oral hypoglycemic agents (fenoprofen, naproxen, and piroxicam) primarily by displacing sulfonylureas from plasma protein binding sites.
Phenytoin	The effect of phenytoin may be potentiated, again because NSAIDs have a high affinity for protein binding sites and can displace it. This effect has been shown with the same agents noted to displace sulfonylureas, most notably fenoprofen, naproxen, and piroxicam.
Probenecid	This agent increases plasma levels of indomethacin, naproxen, ketoprofen, and meclofenamate. Hence, lower dosages of these NSAIDs are advised when given with probenecid.

BIBLIOGRAPHY

Claeys MA, Camu F, Maes V. Prophylactic diclofenac infusions in major orthopedic surgery: Effects of analgesia and acute phase proteins. *Acta Anaesthesiol Scand.* 1992;36:270.

Datar P, Stravastava, S. Coutinho E., Govil G. Substance P: structure, function and therapeutics. *Current Topics in Medicinal Chemistry.* 2004;4:75–103.

Engel C, Dristensen SS, Axel C, et al. Indomethacin and the stress response to hysterectomy. *Acta Anaesthesiol Scand.* 1989;33:540.

Faist E, Ertel W, Cohnert T, et al. Immunoprotective effects of cyclooxygenase inhibition in patients with major surgical trauma. *Trauma.* 1990;30:8.

Guideline for Management of Pain in Osteoarthritis, Rheumatoid Arthritis and Juvenile Chronic Arthritis. Glenview, Ill: American Pain Society; 2002:54.

Haupt MT, Jastremiski MS, Clemmer TP, et al. Effect of ibuprofen in patents with severe sepsis: A randomized double blind multicenter study. *Crit Care Med.* 1991;19:1339.

Hochberg MC, Altman RS, Brandt KD, et al. Guidelines for the medical management of osteoarthritis. *Arthritis Rheum.* 1995;38:1535.

Hulton NR, Johnson DJ, Evans A, et al. Inhibition of prostaglandin synthesis improves postoperative nitrogen balance. *Clin Nutr.* 1988;7:81.

Lalonde C, Knox J, Daryani R, et al. Topical flurbiprofen decreases burn wound induced hypermetabolism and systemic lipid peroxidation. *Surgery.* 1991;109:645.

Malmberg AB, Yaksh TL. Hyperalgesia mediated by spinal glutamate or substance P receptor blocked by spinal cyclooxygenase inhibition. *Science.* 1992;257:1276.

Michie HR, Majzoub JA, O'Dwyer ST, et al. Both cyclooxygenase dependent and cyclooxygenase independent pathways mediate the neuroendocrine response in humans. *Surgery.* 1990;108:54.

Loes MW, Ullmann D. Weiner's 7th Ed of pain management, Chapter 78.

Perneger TV, Whelton PK, Klag MJ. Risk of kidney failure associated with the use of acetaminophen, aspirin and nonsteroidal anti-inflammatory drugs. *N Engl J Med.* 1994;331:1675.

Rahme E, Pilote L, LeLorier J. Association between naproxen use and protection against acute myocardial infarction. *Arch Intern Med.* 2002;162:1111.

Ray WA, Stein CM, Hall K, et al. Non-steroidal anti-inflammatory drugs and the risk of serious coronary heart disease: An observational cohort study. *Lancet.* 2002;359:118.

Schilling A, Corey R, Leonard M, Eghtesad B. 2010. Acetaminophen: Old drug, new warnings. *Cleveland Clinic J Med.* 77:19–27.

Seshasai SRK, Wijesuriya S, Sivakumaren R, et al. Effect of aspirin on vascular and nonvascular outcomes; meta-analysis of randomized controlled trials. *Arch Intern Med.* 2012;172:209–216.

Silverstein FE, Faich G, Goldstein JL, et al. Gastrointestinal toxicity with celecoxib vs nonsteroidal anti-inflammatory drugs for osteoarthritis and rheumatoid arthritis: the CLASS study: A randomized controlled trial of 8059 subjects receiving treatment for six months. Celecoxib Long term Arthritis Safety Study. *JAMA.* 2000; 2841247–1255.

Sneader, W. The discovery of aspirin: a reappraisal. *Br Med J.* 2000;321:1591–1594.

Solomon DH, Glynn RJ, Levin R, et al. Nonsteroidal anti-inflammatory drug use and acute myocardial infarction. *Arch Intern Med.* 2002;162:1099.

Revhaug A, Michie HR, Manson JM, et al. Inhibition of cyclooxygenase attenuates the metabolic response to endotoxin in humans. *Arch Surg.* 1988;123:162.

Varassi G, Panella L, Piroli A, et al. The effects of perioperative ketorolac infusion on postoperative pain an endocrine metabolic response. *Anesth Analg.* 1994;78:514.

Watkins PB, Kaplowitz N, Slattery JT, et al. Aminotransferase elevations in healthy adults receiving 4 grams of acetaminophen daily. *J Americ Med Assn.* 2008;296:87–93.

Watson DJ, Rhodes T, Cai B, et al. Lower risk of thromboembolic cardiovascular events with naproxen among patients with rheumatoid arthritis. *Arch Intern Med.* 2002;162:1105.

18 ANTIDEPRESSANTS

Michael R. Clark, MD, MPH, MBA

INTRODUCTION

ANTIDEPRESSANTS AND PAIN

- Since the first report of imipramine use for trigeminal neuralgia was published in 1960, antidepressants, particularly tricyclic antidepressants (TCAs), have been commonly prescribed for the treatment of many chronic pain syndromes, especially those involving neuropathic pain, including diabetic neuropathy, postherpetic neuralgia, trigeminal neuralgia, chronic radiculopathy, HIV neuropathy, central pain, poststroke pain, tension-type headache, migraine, and orofacial pain.

- The neurobiology of pain and pathophysiology of neuropathic pain suggest that all antidepressants would be potentially effective for the treatment of chronic pain. The analgesic effects of antidepressants are independent of the presence of depression or improvement in mood.

- Antidepressants improve both brief lancinating pain and constant burning pain.

- Analgesia usually occurs at lower doses and with earlier onset of action than expected for the treatment of depression. However, TCAs are woefully underdosed suggesting unrealized potential for incremental analgesia.

- Pharmacological properties of antidepressants include those affecting: monoamine transmission, cholinergic neurotransmission, glutamatergic neurotransmission, opioid receptors, sigma receptors, neurokinin receptors, and corticotrophin-releasing factor receptors.

- Established guidelines for the treatment of neuropathic pain recommend antidepressants, especially SNRIs and TCAs, as first-line medications.

- Evidence is growing for the effectiveness of antidepressants in the treatment of non-neuropathic pain such as chronic low back pain, osteoarthritis and noncardiac chest pain.

- Polyanalgesic therapy combining medications effective for the treatment of pain is likely to improve outcome compared with monotherapy.

CLASSIFICATION SYSTEMS

- Neuropathic pain has been classified according to underlying pathology, such as diabetes mellitus, herpes zoster, and ischemia due to vascular occlusion.

- Linking possible mechanisms of pain [N-methyl-D-aspartate (NMDA) receptor stimulation, alternations in ion channels, activation of microglia, increased production of nerve growth factors, sympathetic hyperactivity, C-fiber mechanosensitivity, spontaneous activity in dorsal root ganglion cells] to specific features of pain phenomenology could improve treatment selection.

PHARMACOLOGIC MECHANISMS OF ANTINOCICEPTION

DESCENDING INHIBITION

- Research suggests that the analgesic effect of antidepressants is mediated primarily by the blockade of reuptake of norepinephrine and serotonin. The resulting increase in the levels of these neurotransmitters enhances the activation of descending inhibitory neurons. Noradrenaline (vs. serontonin) reuptake is proposed as more essential to the antihyperalgesic action of antidepressants.
- However, milnacipran produced prolonged inhibition of c-fiber-evoked field potentials after the establishment of long-term potentiation and in a model of neuropathic pain suggesting novel pharmacological actions for blocking a synaptic mechanism of neuronal hypersensitivity.
- Antidepressants, however, may produce antinociceptive effects through a variety of pharmacologic mechanisms, including other types of monoamine modulation; interactions with opioid receptors; and inhibition of ion channel activity and of N-methyl-D-aspartate (NMDA), histamine, and cholinergic receptors.

MONOAMINE MODULATION

- Investigations have demonstrated differential effects of monoamine receptor subtypes in antidepressant-induced antinociception in the rat formalin test. The effects of antidepressants with varying degrees of norepinephrine and serotonin reuptake inhibition as well as those of their antagonists indicate that α_1 adrenoceptors and several serotonin receptor subtypes (5-HT2, 5-HT3, and 5-HT4) contribute to antinociception.
- The antinociceptive activity of a variety of antidepressants irrespective of the propensity for inhibiting reuptake of norepinephrine and/or serotonin is blocked by an α_2 but not by an α_1 adrenoceptor in the mouse abdominal constriction assay, and β adrenoceptors mediate the analgesic effects of desipramine and nortriptyline.
- In animal models, effects of dopamine reuptake inhibitors suggest analgesic effects.

GLUTAMATERGIC NEUROTRANSMISSION

- The glutamatergic system is involved with both the neurobiology of depression and the central sensitization of neuropathic pain via the NMDA receptor complex.
- Ketamine is an NMDA antagonist under study as a novel therapeutic agent for both Major Depressive Disorder and chronic pain.
- Milnacipran (not desipramine or citalopram) suppressed NMDA activation of thermal hyperalgesia suggesting an antinociceptive action of inhibiting gluatamatergic NMDA receptor activity.

OPIOID INTERACTIONS

Monoamine Receptors

- Because they interact with opioids or their antagonists, antidepressants may interact with opioid receptors or stimulate endogenous opioid peptide release.
- Studies of hot plate analgesia in mice found that the antinociceptive effect of trazodone involves mu-1 and mu-2 opioid receptor subtypes combined with the serotonergic receptor.
- Similar studies with venlafaxine showed that antinociception is partly mediated by mu, kappa-1, kappa-3, and delta opioid receptor subtypes as well as by the α_2 adrenergic receptor.
- In contrast, mirtazapine-induced antinociception involves primarily kappa-3 opioid receptors in conjunction with serotonergic and noradrenergic receptors.

Opioid Utilization

- In patients with diabetic peripheral neuropathic pain treated with duloxetine compared to other antidepressants (TCAs, venlafaxine), measures of opioid use and health care costs were significantly reduced.

Synergistic Effects

- In the rat tail-flick model, the antinociception produced by individual intrathecal administration of serotonin, desipramine, and morphine can be achieved with sub-threshold doses of combinations of these agents.
- In the rat formalin test, the fluoxetine-induced antinociception that potentiates morphine analgesia is blocked by naloxone. Similar results for fluoxetine have been found in mice using acetic acid-induced writhing, tail-flick, and hot plate assays.
- Using the acetic acid-induced abdominal constriction assay in mice, investigators found that naloxone and

naltrindole shift the antidepressant dose–response relationships to the right.

- These data in conjunction with findings that only naloxone displaces morphine antinociception and neither opioid antagonist affects aspirin antinociception support the role of the delta opioid receptor, as well as of endogenous opioids, in antidepressant-induced antinociception.

MISCELLANEOUS MECHANISMS

Adenosine

- Studies of imipramine demonstrated differential hypoalgesic effects depending on the experimental paradigm used to assess pain. For example, TCAs may reduce hyperalgesia but not tactile allodynia because different neuronal mechanisms underlie different manifestations of neuropathic pain.
- The blocking by caffeine of this effect induced with amitriptyline indicates a role for endogenous adenosine systems.

Ion Channels

- The opening of voltage-gated and Ca^{2+}-gated K^+ channels has been implicated in the central antinociception induced by amitriptyline and clomipramine in the mouse hot plate test. Intravenous amitriptyline impairs the function of tetrodotoxin-resistant Na^+ channels in rat dorsal root ganglia, particularly in conditions of repetitive firing and depolarizing

membrane potential, which may reduce firing frequency in ectopic sites of damaged nociceptive fibers.

Relationship to Inflammation

- Amitriptyline and desipramine, but not fluoxetine, have peripheral antinociceptive action in inflammatory and neuropathic rat models. In contrast, systemic and spinal administration of antidepressants produces analgesic effects in the rat formalin model that are not due to anti-inflammatory actions.

CLINICAL APPLICATIONS

SEROTONIN AND NOREPINEPHRINE

- Antidepressants are typically characterized according to the specificity of their neurotransmitter reuptake (Table 18-1).
- The presence of noradrenergic activity is often associated with better analgesic effect than is serotonergic activity alone but the evidence is not conclusive.
- Antidepressants with a 5-HT (serotonin)/NE (norepinephrine) ratio of less than 1 (noradrenergic) include amitriptyline, imipramine, bupropion, doxepin, nortriptyline, desipramine, and maprotiline.
- Antidepressants with a 5-HT/NE ratio of more than 1 (serotonergic) include venlafaxine, nefazodone, trazodone, clomipramine, fluoxetine, fluvoxamine, paroxetine, sertraline, and citalopram.

TABLE 18-1   Commonly Used Antidepressant Medications

GENERIC (BRAND) NAME	DAILY DOSE	PRIMARY MECHANISM
Heterocyclic Tertiary Amines (TCAs)		
Amitriptyline (Elavil)	50–300 mg	Mixed NE and 5-HT reuptake inhibition
Imipramine (Tofranil)	50–300 mg	
Doxepin (Sinequan)	50–300 mg	
Heterocyclic Secondary Amines (TCAs)		
Nortriptyline (Pamelor)	50–150 mg	NE > 5-HT reuptake inhibition
Desipramine (Norpramin)	75–300 mg	
Selective Serotonin Reuptake Inhibitors (SSRIs)		
Fluoxetine (Prozac)	10–80 mg	5-HT >>NE reuptake inhibition
Sertraline (Zoloft)	50–200 mg	
Paroxetine (Paxil)	10–40 mg	
Fluvoxamine (Luvox)	100–300 mg	
Citalopram (Celexa)	20–40 mg	
Atypical Antidepressants		
Venlafaxine (Effexor)	75–450 mg	5-HT > NE >> DA reuptake inhibition (dose dependent)
Nefazodone (Serzone)	100–600 mg	5-HT > NE reuptake
Trazodone (Desyrel)	100–600 mg	inhibition with 5-HT2 receptor blockade
Bupropion (Wellbutrin)	100–450 mg	DA and NE reuptake inhibition
Mirtazapine (Remeron)	15–90 mg	α_2-NE and 5-HT2 presynaptic agonist with 5-HT2/3 receptor blockade

TRICYCLIC ANTIDEPRESSANTS

Utilization

- A study of TCA use found that 25% of patients in a multidisciplinary pain center were prescribed these medications. The fact that 73% of treated patients were prescribed the equivalent of 50 mg or less of amitriptyline, however, suggests there is a potential for additional pain relief with higher doses.
- The cost of TCAs for pain treatment is generally much lower (less than $5.00 per month) than the cost of other antidepressants and medications with analgesic activity.
- The results of investigations to determine drug concentrations needed for pain relief support higher serum levels but are contradictory; thus, no clear guidelines have been established.

Tertiary versus Secondary

- Generally, the tertiary TCAs with balanced effects on 5-HT and NE reuptake (imipramine, amitriptyline, doxepin) are no more effective analgesic agents than the secondary TCAs with more selective NE reuptake inhibition (desipramine, nortriptyline, maprotiline).
- Although tertiary amines have been used most commonly, they are metabolized to secondary amines that are associated with fewer side effects, such as decreased gastrointestinal motility and urinary retention. The fact that desipramine and nortriptyline had significantly fewer side effects led to less frequent discontinuation of the drug than seen with clomipramine, amitriptyline, and doxepin. Nortriptyline, the major metabolite of amitriptyline, causes less sedation, orthostatic hypotension, and falls than does imipramine and is as effective as amitriptyline in treating chronic pain.
- Amitriptyline is considered a first-line treatment for neuropathic pain but comprehensive reviews find strong evidence for a beneficial effect and satisfactory pain relief is lacking.
- Randomized controlled trials, however, have not demonstrated consistent differences among TCAs.

Efficacy

- TCAs have been most effective in relieving neuropathic pain and headache syndromes. The findings in a number of these studies have been challenged, however, because of poor study design and variable protocol criteria.
- Placebo-controlled, double-blind, randomized, clinical trials for chronic low back pain in patients without depression demonstrated significant reduction in pain intensity scores for patients treated with nortriptyline or maprotiline but not paroxetine.
- A review of 59 randomized, placebo-controlled trials concludes that high-quality research supports the TCAs as effective analgesics.
- Newer antidepressants offer different mechanisms of action, fewer side effects, and less toxicity but have not been rigorously studied in the treatment of chronic pain.

SELECTIVE SEROTONIN REUPTAKE INHIBITORS

- Many studies have investigated the potential role of serotonin receptor subtypes in both nociceptive and hyperalgesic mechanisms of pain, but no definitive conclusions have been drawn.
- Selective serotonin reuptake inhibitors (SSRIs) produce weak antinociceptive effects in animal models of acute pain. This antinociception is blocked by serotonin receptor antagonists and enhanced by opioid receptor agonists.
- In human clinical trials, the efficacy of SSRIs in chronic pain syndromes has been variable and inconsistent.
- Desipramine was superior to fluoxetine in the treatment of painful diabetic peripheral neuropathy.
- Paroxetine and citalopram were beneficial in patients with diabetic neuropathy and irritable bowel syndrome.
- Fluoxetine significantly reduced pain in patients with rheumatoid arthritis and was comparable to amitriptyline. A 12-week course of fluoxetine also improved a variety of self-reported outcome measures in women with fibromyalgia.
- The SSRIs were well tolerated and effective in the treatment of headache, especially migraine. Patient satisfaction, compliance and mood are better with SSRIs compared to gabapentin for painful diabetic peripheral neuropathy.
- In a study of chronic tension-type headache, amitriptyline significantly reduced the duration of headache, headache frequency, and the intake of analgesics, but citalopram, an SSRI, did not.
- Until the results with SSRIs are more consistent, they are not recommended as first-choice medications unless a specific contraindication exists for TCAs.

SEROTONIN AND NORADRENALINE REUPTAKE INHIBITORS

Venlafaxine and Desvenlafaxine

- The neurobiology of pain suggests a potential efficacy for all antidepressants, despite their different pharmacologic actions, in the treatment of chronic pain.

- Venlafaxine inhibits the presynaptic reuptake of both serotonin and norepinephrine and, to a lesser extent, of dopamine, with fewer side effects than TCAs and SSRIs.
- In an animal model of neuropathic pain, venlafaxine reversed hyperalgesia and prevented its development. In another study of a diabetic neuropathic pain model, the antihyperalgesic effect of single and repeated administration of venlafaxine was reversed by an adrenergic antagonist and serotonin neurotoxin but not an opioid antagonist.
- In humans, venlafaxine increased thresholds for pain tolerance to single electrical sural nerve stimulation and pain summation but had no effect on thresholds for pain detection to sural nerve stimulation, pressure pain, or pain experienced during a cold pressor test.
- Venlafaxine has shown efficacy in the treatment of neuropathic pain, atypical facial pain, migraine, and tension-type headache.
- Average pain relief and maximum pain intensity were significantly lower with venlafaxine than with placebo in a group of 13 patients with neuropathic pain following treatment of breast cancer. Additional analyses suggested that response improved with higher doses of venlafaxine.
- Higher doses (>150 mg/d) of venlafaxine produced greater percentage reduction in pain (50% vs. 32%) than 75 mg/d in a study of painful diabetic neuropathy.
- Desvenlafaxine, the major metabolite of venlafaxine, may reduce painful physician symptoms.

Duloxetine

- Duloxetine reduces pain associated with diabetic peripheral neuropathy, post-herpetic neuralgia, and fibromyalgia.
- The efficacy of duloxetine in painful diabetic neuropathy increased with increased pain intensity independent of the severity of diabetes or the peripheral neuropathy.
- Duloxetine has recently been approved for the treatment of non-neuropathic conditions including chronic musculoskeletal low back pain and painful osteoarthritis of the knee.

Milnacipran

- Milnacipran reduces the pain of fibromyalgia significantly more than reducing fatigue, sleep problems, and limitations of quality of life. Symptom improvements were independent of effects on depressive symptoms.
- In patients with fibromyalgia treated with duloxetine and dissatisfied with treatment including persistent pain, 33% switched to milnacipran reported significant improvements in Patient Global Impression of Change, pain and disability measures.
- In the treatment of patients with orofacial pain, the decrease in pain was positively correlated with plasma levels of milnacipran.

ATYPICAL ANTIDEPRESSANTS

- Norepinephrine and dopamine reuptake inhibitors, such as bupropion, produced antinociception in studies of thermal nociception. In a randomized, double-blind, placebo-controlled, crossover study of patients with neuropathic pain but without depression, bupropion SR (sustained-release) decreased pain intensity and interference of pain in quality of life.
- Nefazodone possesses the actions of analgesia and the potentiation of opioid analgesia in the mouse hot plate assay. In an open-label trial of diabetic neuropathy in 10 men, nefazodone significantly reduced self-ratings of pain, paresthesias, and numbness.
- Mirtazapine enhances postsynaptic noradrenergic and 5-HT1A-mediated serotonergic neurotransmission through antagonism of central α-auto- and heteroadrenoreceptors. Mirtazapine decreased the duration and intensity of chornic tension-type headache in a controlled trial with treatment-refractory patients.
- Monoamine oxidase inhibitors decrease the frequency and severity of migraine headaches.
- Buspirone is effective in the prophylaxis of chronic tension-type headache; however, buspirone-treated patients used more rescue analgesics for acute treatment of headache than did patients treated with amitriptyline.
- Compared with placebo, protriptyline decreased chronic tension-type headache frequency by 86% in women.
- Trazodone did not decrease pain in a double-blind, placebo-controlled study of patients with chronic low back pain.

COMPARISONS

- Comparing the relative efficacy of antidepressants and other pharmacologic agents used in the treatment of pain is difficult. In patients with MDD, the evidence comparing antidepressants for the effective treatment of comorbid pain finds no difference in four head-to-head trials.
- Several investigators suggest calculating the number needed to treat (NNT) to determine which medications are most likely to improve pain. The NNT is defined as how many patients would need to receive

TABLE 18-2   Numbers Needed to Treat for Antidepressants and Chronic Pain Conditions*

ANTIDEPRESSANT	DIABETIC NEUROPATHY	POSTHERPETIC NEURALGIA	PERIPHERAL NERVE INJURY	CENTRAL PAIN	ALL CONDITIONS
All types	3.0 (2.4–4.0)*	2.3 (1.7–3.3)*	2.5 (1.4–10.6)*	1.7 (1.1–3.0)*	
	3.4 (2.6–4.7)†	2.1 (1.7–3.0)†			2.9 (2.4–3.7)†
TCA (pooled)	2.4 (2.0–3.0)*	2.3 (1.7–3.3)*	2.5 (1.4–10.6)*	1.7 (1.1–3.0)*	2.6 (2.2–3.3)*
					3.5 (2.5–5.6)†
TCA (5-HT/NE)	2.0 (1.7–2.5)*	2.4 (1.8–3.9)*	2.5 (1.4–10.6)*	1.7 (1.1–3.0)*	2.7*
TCA (NE)	3.4 (2.3–6.6)*	1.9 (1.3–3.7)*	No data	No data	2.5*
TCA (5-HT/NE with optimal dosing)	1.4 (1.1–1.9)*	No data	No data	No data	
SSRI	6.7 (3.4–435)*	No data	No data	Inactive*	

*From Sindrup and Jensen.

†From Collins et al.

the specific treatment for one patient to achieve at least 50% pain relief. The formula for NNT is the inverse of the difference between the fractional response in the active treatment group and that in the placebo group. The NNT for the antidepressants used in the treatment of several types of neuropathic pain is approximately 2.5 and improves with higher serum levels (Table 18-2). The NNT varies across studies due to differences in criteria for the calculation and definition of 50% pain relief.

• Only the effectiveness of the TCAs used to treat diabetic neuropathy and postherpetic neuralgia is supported with a variety of experimental studies that include a large number of patients.

• In the treatment of fibromyalgia, a Cochrane review calculated a 30% pain reduction of 42% for SNRIs, 36% for SSRIs, and 48% for TCAs with dropout rates highest for SNRIs and lowest for TCAs.

• Compliance with medications is an important aspect of treatment. Patients taking venlafaxine were found to be most compliant (69%) compared to TCAs (42%) and all antidepressants (42%) with only 21% of patients taking antidepressants meeting criteria for persistence with medication refills.

CONCLUSIONS

• The effectiveness of antidepressants for the treatment of major depression is well documented; however, these medications are underutilized and underdosed suggesting the analgesic properties of this class of medication are underappreciated.

• The complexity of chronic pain requires an extensive knowledge of the potential actions of many pharmacologic agents.

• It is important for the patient to understand the reason an antidepressant is being prescribed.

• It is even more important that the physician understand that one medication may be treating both pain and depression in a patient with chronic pain.

• The physician should always consider the innovative application of medications regardless of how they are traditionally classified.

BIBLIOGRAPHY

Arnold LM, Palmer RH, Gendreau RM, Chen W. Relationships among pain, depressed mood, and global status in fibromyalgia patients: post hoc analyses of a randomized, placebo-controlled trial of milnacipran. *Psychosomatics.* 2012;53: 371–379.

Attl N, Cruccu G, Baron R, et al. EFNS guidelines on the pharmacological treatment of neuropathic pain: 2010 revision. *Eur J Neurol.* 2010;17:e1113–e1188.

Barkin RL, Fawcett J. The management challenges of chronic pain: the role of antidepressants. *Am J Ther.* 2000;7:31.

Bateman L, Palmer RH, Trugman JM, Lin Y. Results of switching to milnacipran in fibromyalgia patients with an inadequate response to duloxetine: a phase IV pilot study. *J Pain Res.* 2013;6:311–318.

Bendtsen L, Jensen R. Mirtazapine is effective in the prophylactic treatment of chronic tension-type headache. *Neurology.* 2004;62:1706–1711.

Berger A, Dukes EM, Edelsberg J, et al. Use of tricyclic antidepressants in older patients with painful neuropathies. *Eur J Clin Pharmacol.* 2006;62:757–764.

Bril V, England J, Franklin GM, et al. Evidence-based guideline: treatment of painful diabetic neuropathy. Report of the American Academy of Neurology, the American Association of Neuromuscular and Electrodiagnostic Medicine, and the American Academy of Physical Medicine and Rehabilitation. *PMR.* 2011;3:345–352.

Cegielska-Perun K, Bujalska-Zadrozny M, Tatarkiewicz J, et al. Venlafaxine and neuropathic pain. *Pharmacology.* 2013;91:69–76.

Connolly KR, Thase ME. Emerging drugs for major depressive disorder. *Expert Opin Emerg Drugs.* 2012;17:105–126.

De Leon-Casasola O. New developments in the treatment algorithm for peripheral neuropathic pain. *Pain Med.* 2011;12(Suppl 3):S100–S108.

Derry S, Gill D, Phillips T, Moore RA. Milnacipran for neuropathic pain and fibromyalgia in adults. *Cochrane Database Syst Rev.* 2012;3:CD008244.

Dick IE, Brochu RM, Purohit Y, et al. Sodium channel blockade may contribute to the analgesic efficacy of antidepressants. *J Pain.* 2007;8:315–324.

Dworkin RH, O'Connor AB, Backonja M, et al. Pharmacologic management of neuropathic pain: evidence-based recommendations. *Pain.* 2007;132:237–251.

Feighner JP. Mechanism of action of antidepressant medications. *J Clin Psychiatry.* 1999;60(suppl 4):4.

Fharmshaktu P, Tayal V, Kalra BS. Efficacy of antidepressants as analgesics: a review. *J Clin Pharmacol.* 2012;52:6–17.

Finnerup NB, Otto M, McQuay HJ, et al. Algorithm for neuropathic pain treatment: an evidence based proposal. *Pain.* 2005;118:289–305.

Forssell H, Tasmuth T, Tenovuo O, et al. Venlafaxine in the treatment of atypical facial pain: a randomized controlled trial. *J Orofac Pain.* 2004;18:131–137.

Gharibian D, Polzin JK, Rho JP. Compliance and persistence of antidepressants versus anticonvulsants in patients with neuropathic pain during the first year of therapy. *Clin J Pain.* 2013;29:377–381.

Gilron I, Bailey J, Weaver DF, et al. Patients' attitudes and prior treatments in neuropathic pain: a pilot study. *Pain Res Manag.* 2002;7:199–203.

Hauser W, Urrutia G, Tort S, Uceyler N, Walitt B. Serotonin and noradrenaline reuptake inhibitors (SNRIs) for fibromyalgia syndrome. *Cochrane Database Syst Rev.* 2013;1:CD010292.

Hauser W, Wolfe F, Tolle T, Uceyler N, Sommer C. The role of antidepressants in the management of fibromyalgia syndrome: a systematic review and meta-analysis. *CNS Drugs.* 2012;26:297–307.

Kimura H, Yoshida K, Ito M, et al. Plasma levels of milnacipran and its effectiveness for the treatment of chronic pain in the orofacial region. *Hum Psychopharmacol.* 2012;27:322–328.

Kohno T, Kimura M, Sasaki M, Obata H, Amaya F, Saito S. Milnacipran inhibits glutamatergic N-methyl-D-aspartate receptor activity in spinal dorsal horn neurons. *Mol Pain.* 2012;8:45.

Kostadinov ID, Delev DP, Kostadinova II. Antinociceptive effect of clomipramine through interaction with serotonin 5-HT2 and 5-HT3 receptor subtypes. *Folia Med.* 2012;54:69–77.

Krymchantowski AV, da Cunha Jevouz C, Bigal ME. Topiramate plus nortriptyline in the preventive treatment of migraine: a controlled study for nonresponders. *J Headache Pain.* 2012;13:53–59.

Lee YC, Chen PP. A review of SSRIs and SNRIs in neuropathic pain. *Expert Opin Pharmacother.* 2010;11:2813–2825.

Lynch ME. Antidepressants as analgesics: a review of randomized controlled trials. *J Psychiatry Neurosci.* 2001;26:30.

Mathews DC, Henter ID, Zarate CA. Targeting the glutamatergic system to treat major depressive disorder: rationale and progress to date. *Drugs.* 2012;72:1313–1333.

McCleane G. Antidepressants as analgesics. *CNS Drugs.* 2008;22:139–156.

Mico JA, Ardid D, Berrocoso E, et al. Antidepressants and pain. *Trends Pharmacol Sci.* 2006;27:348–354.

Moore RA, Derry S, Aldington D, Cole P, Wiffen PJ. Amitriptyline for neuropathic pain and fibromyalgia in adults. *Cochrane Database Syst Rev.* 2012;12:DC008242.

Nakajima K, Obata H, Iriuchijima N, Saito S. An increase in spinal cord noradrenaline is a major contributor to the antihyperalgesic effect of antidepressants after peripheral nerve injury in the rat. *Pain.* 2012;153:990–997.

Nguyen TM, Eslick GD. Systematic review: the treatment of noncardiac chest pain with antidepressants. *Aliment Pharmacol Ther.* 2012;35:493–500.

Ohnami S, Kato A, Ogawa K, Shinohara S, Ono H, Tanabe M. Effects of milnacipran, a 5-HT and noradrenaline reuptake inhibitor, on C-fibre-evoked field potentials in spinal long-term potentiation and neuropathic pain. *Br J Pharmacol.* 2012;167:537–547.

Ozyalcin SN, Talu GK, Kiziltan E, et al. The efficacy and safety of venlafaxine in the prophylaxis of migraine. *Headache.* 2005;45:144–152.

Pae CU, Park MH, Marks DM, Han C, Patkar AA, Masand PS. Desvenlafaxine, a serotonin-norepinephrine uptake inhibitor for major depressive disorder, neuropathic pain and the vasomotor symptoms associated with menopause. *Curr Opin Investig Drugs.* 2009;10:75–90.

Rojas-Corrales MO, Casas J, Moreno-Brea MR, et al. Antinociceptive effects of tricyclic antidepressants and their noradrenergic metabolites. *Eur Neuropsychopharmacol.* 2003;13:355–363.

Rosenberg MB, Carroll FI, Negus SS. Effects of monoamine reuptake inhibitors in assays of acute pain-stimulated and pain-depressed behavior in rats. *J Pain.* 2013;14:246–259.

Rowbotham MC, Goli V, Kunz NR, et al. Venlafaxine extended release in the treatment of painful diabetic neuropathy: a double-blind, placebo-controlled study. *Pain.* 2004;110:697–706.

Saarto T, Wiffen PJ. Antidepressants for neuropathic pain. *Cochrane Database Syst Rev.* 2007;CD005454.

Semenchuk MR, Sherman S, Davis B. Double-blind, randomized trial of bupropion SR for the treatment of neuropathic pain. *Neurology.* 2001;57:1583–1588.

Sindrup SH, Jensen TS. Efficacy of pharmacological treatments of neuropathic pain: an update and effect related to mechanism of drug action. *Pain.* 1999;83:389.

Smitherman TA, Walters AB, Maizels M, Penzien DB. The use of antidepressants for headache prophylaxis. *CNS Neurosci Ther.* 2011;17:462–469.

Tack J, Broekaert D, Fischler B, et al. A controlled crossover study of the selective serotonin reuptake inhibitor citalopram in irritable bowel syndrome. *Gut.* 2006;55:1095–1103.

Thaler KJ, Morgan LC, Van Noord M, et al. Comparative effectiveness of second-generation antidepressants for accompanying anxiety, insomnia, and pain in depressed patients: a systematic review. *Depress Anxiety.* 2012;29:495–505.

Vranken JH. Elucidation of pathophysiology and treatment of neuropathic pain. *Cent Nerv Syst Agents Med Chem.* 2012;12:304–314.

Watson CP, Gilron I, Sawynok J, Lynch ME. Nontricyclic antidepressant analgesics and pain: are serotonin norepinephrine reuptake inhibitors (SNRIs) any better? *Pain.* 2011;152:2206–2210.

Wu N, Chen SY, Hallett LA, et al. Opioid utilization and healthcare costs among patients with diabetic peripheral neuropathic pain treated with duloxetine vs. other therapies. *Pain Pract.* 2011;11:48–56.

Yucel A, Ozyalcin S, Koknel TG, et al. The effect of venlafaxine on ongoing and experimentally induced pain in neuropathic pain patients: a double blind, placebo controlled study. *Eur J Pain.* 2005;9:407–416.

Ziegler D, Pritchett YL, Wang F, et al. Impact of disease characteristics on the efficacy of duloxetine in diabetic peripheral neuropathic pain. *Diabetes Care.* 2007;30:664–669.

19 ANTICONVULSANT DRUGS

Erin Lawson, MD
Miroslav "Misha" Bačkonja, MD

INTRODUCTION

- The involvement of many receptors and neurotransmitter systems offers an opportunity to alleviate various manifestations of neuropathic pain with agents, such as anticonvulsant drugs (ACDs), that act on those mechanisms in specific ways.
- ACDs inhibit neuronal hyperactivity along pain pathways via multiple mechanisms of action including modulation of γ-aminobutyric acid (GABA)ergic and glutamatergic neurotransmission, and alteration of voltage-gated ion channels or intracellular signaling pathways.
- ACDs used to treat neuropathic pain provide relief for the duration of drug administration, during which sensitization processes are presumably modulated, so these drugs may be considered neuromodulators.
- ACDs are often used in combination with other drugs with different mechanisms, referred to as *rational polypharmacy* (although a more appropriate term is combination therapy).
- Though early focus for development of ACDs has been for treatment of neuropathic pain, other pain disorders characterized by sensitization of the nervous system, primarily central sensitization, such as migraine and fibromyalgia, have been a fruitful area where ACDs demonstrated efficacy.
- ACDs are not recommended for use during pregnancy due to risk of varying degrees of teratogenesis (see Chapter 49).

ANTICONVULSANTS: EFFICACY DEMONSTRATED IN RANDOMIZED CLINICAL TRIALS

- Randomized clinical trials have demonstrated the efficacy of carbamazepine and gabapentin for relief of neuropathic pain disorders, pregabalin for neuropathic pain and fibromyalgia, and topiramate for migraine headaches.

CARBAMAZEPINE

- Carbamazepine blocks ionic conductance of frequency-dependent neuronal activity without affecting normal nerve conduction, suppressing spontaneous Aδ and C-fiber activity, which are implicated in the genesis of pain.
- It was the first ACD used in clinical trials to treat a neuropathic painful disorder, trigeminal neuralgia (TN). The American Academy of Neurology and the European Federation of Neurological Societies recommend carbamazepine as a first-line agent for the treatment of pain from TN.
- Common side effects include somnolence, dizziness, and gait disturbance; previous studies raised a concern about hematopoietic effects and hyponatremia, and it is advisable to monitor this possible complication of carbamazepine therapy.
- Despite evidence from randomized clinical trials that carbamazepine is effective, clinically the drug is not consistently effective and is difficult to administer due to the complex monitoring it requires.

GABAPENTIN

- Gabapentin was developed as a structural GABA analog, but it does not have direct effect on GABAergic action and GABA uptake or metabolism; best evidence is that gabapentin acts through modulation of the α2δ subunit of N-type Ca^{2+} channels.
- Recent evidence with clinical trials on intrathecal delivery and animal studies suggest that gabapentin works supraspinally at the locus coeruleus.
- Gabapentin is effective in the treatment of many neuropathic pain conditions including painful diabetic neuropathy and postherpetic neuralgia and is FDA approved for the treatment of postherpetic neuralgia.
- Both gabapentin and pregabalin are recommended among first-line treatment options for postherpetic neuralgia based on Level A, class I and II evidence by the American Academy of Neurology.
- Gabapentin is relatively well tolerated and does not significantly differ from placebo in reference to any

serious adverse effects. With respect to common adverse effects, they are reversible and include dizziness, somnolence, ataxia, and swollen legs.
- Ease of use, good tolerability, lack of significant interaction with other medications, and a safe side effect profile make gabapentin the first choice for most physicians treating patients with any type of neuropathic pain.

PREGABALIN

- Pregabalin reduces neurotransmitter release as a calcium channel–modulating agent by binding at $\alpha 2\delta$ subunit of N-type calcium channels, same as gabapentin.
- It is FDA approved for the treatment of neuropathic pain associated with diabetic peripheral neuropathy, neuropathic pain associated with spinal cord injury, postherpetic neuralgia, and fibromyalgia.
- Pregabalin is more effective in pain reduction in fibromyalgia compared to placebo in randomized, double-blind, placebo-controlled trials. Effective doses used were 300, 450, or 600 mg qd in divided doses.
- Diabetic Peripheral Neuropathic Pain Consensus Treatment Guidelines Advisory Board recommends pregabalin as a first-tier medication for painful diabetic peripheral neuropathy.
- Pregabalin is unique in that it is the only anticonvulsant that is FDA approved for the treatment of neuropathic pain associated with spinal cord injury at doses of 150–600 mg/d.
- The US Department of Health and Human Services Agency for Healthcare Research and Quality guidelines for the treatment of neuropathic pain in adults in nonspecialist settings recommend pregabalin as a first-line treatment.
- Common side effects include dizziness and somnolence, and less commonly peripheral edema and weight gain.

TOPIRAMATE

- Topiramate blocks voltage-dependent sodium channels, increases GABA-A, blocks AMPA/kainite glutamate receptors, and inhibits carbonic anhydrase.
- It is FDA approved for migraine prophylaxis.
- An amount of 100 mg/d showed statistically significant improvements compared with placebo in mean monthly migraine days.
- Common side effects include paresthesias, anorexia, weight loss, fatigue, dizziness, somnolence, nervousness, and difficulty with memory.

SUMMARY

- Evidence supports the use of carbamazepine for treatment of TN, topiramate for migraine prophylaxis, and gabapentin and pregabalin for treatment of neuropathic pain in more general terms with best evidence supporting use for PHN and PDN.
- Randomized clinical trials support ACDs as first choice for treatment of neuropathic pain. Using appropriate doses of these medications is key; for example, doses for gabapentin may require at least 1800 mg/d in three divided doses.
- All of these therapies provide only partial and temporary pain relief only in a subset of patients, so treatment trials in individual patients need to be undertaken to determine optimal therapy for specific patients.
- With their safe side effect profile, newer ACDs have become an important component of combination pharmacotherapy, but this concept needs to be further developed in clinical practice to demonstrate the best way combination therapy could be implemented.
- Most of the newer anticonvulsants have a very wide dosing range, and that property should be explored and used.

BIBLIOGRAPHY

Arnold LM, Russell IJ, Diri EW, et al. A 14-week, randomized, double-blind, placebo-controlled, monotherapy trial of pregabalin in patients with fibromyalgia. *J Pain.* 2008;9:792–805.

Bialer M. Why are antiepileptic drugs used for non-epileptic conditions? *Epilepsia.* 2012;53(suppl 7):26–33.

Bril V, England J, Franklin GM, et al. Evidence-based guideline: treatment of painful diabetic neuropathy: a report of the American Academy of Neurology, the American Association of Neuromuscular and Electrodiagnostic Medicine, and the American Academy of Physical Medicine and Rehabilitation. *Neurology.* 2011;76(20):1758–1765.

Crofford LJ, Mease PJ, Simpson SL, et al. Fibromyalgia relapse evaluation and efficacy for durability of meaningful relief (FREEDOM): a six-month, double-blind, placebo-controlled trial with pregabalin. *Pain.* 2008;136:419–431.

Diener HC, Bussone G, Van Oene JC, Lahaye M, Schwalen S, Goadsby PJ; TOPMAT-MIG-201(TOP-CHROME) Study Group. Topiramate reduces headache days in chronic migraine: a randomized, double-blind, placebo-controlled study. *Cephalalgia.* 2007;27(7):814–823.

Dubinsky RM, Kabbani H, El-Chami Z, Boutwell C, Ali H. Practice parameter: treatment of postherpetic neuralgia: an evidence-based report of the Quality Standards Subcommittee of the American Academy of Neurology. *Neurology.* 2004;63:959.

Finnerup NB, Sindrup SH, Jensen TS. The evidence for pharmacological treatment of neuropathic pain. *Pain.* 2010;150(3): 573–581.

Fujii H, Goel A, Bernard N, et al. Pregnancy outcomes following gabapentin use: results of a prospective comparative cohort study. *Neurology.* 2013;80(17):1565–1570.

Gronseth G, Gruccu G, Alksne J, et al. *Practice Parameter: The Diagnostic Evaluation and Treatment of Trigeminal Neuralgia (An Evidence-Based Review): Report of the Quality Standards Subcommittee of the American Academy of Neurology and the European Federation of Neurological Societies.* April 26, 2010. Available at: http://www.neurology.org/cgi/content/full/71/15/1183).

Hernández-Díaz S, Smith CR, Shen A, et al.; for the North American AED Pregnancy Registry, North American AED Pregnancy Registry. Comparative safety of antiepileptic drugs during pregnancy. *Neurology.* 2012;78(21):1692–1699.

Mølgaard-Nielsen D, Hviid A. Newer-generation antiepileptic drugs and the risk of major birth defects. *JAMA.* 2011;305(19):1996–2002.

Siddall PJ, Cousins MJ, Otte A, et al. Pregabalin in central neuropathic pain associated with spinal cord injury: a placebo-controlled trial. *Neurology.* 2006;67:1792–1800.

Siddall PJ, Murphy TK, Emir B, et al. Pregabalin's efficacy for relieving central neuropathic pain (NeP) and related sleep interference is not influenced by concomitantly-administered medications (poster). Presented at the 10th Congress of the European Federation of Neurological Societies (EFNS); September 2–5, 2006; Glasgow, UK.

Silberstein SD, Lipton RB, Dodick DW, et al.; Topiramate Chronic Migraine Study Group. Efficacy and safety of topiramate for the treatment of chronic migraine: a randomized, double blind, placebo-controlled trial. *Headache.* 2007;47(2):170–180.

Sindrup SH, Jensen TS. Efficacy of pharmacological treatments of neuropathic pain: an update and effect related to mechanism of drug action. *Pain.* 1999;83:389–400.

Tremont-Lukats IW, Megeff C, Backonja MM. Anti-convulsants for neuropathic pain syndromes: mechanisms of action and place in therapy. *Drugs.* 2001;60:1029–1052.

U.S. Department of Health and Human Services Agency for Healthcare Research and Quality National Guideline Clearinghouse. Neuropathic pain. The pharmacological management of neuropathic pain in adults in non-specialist settings. Available at: http://www.guidelines.gov/content.aspx?id=24108.

Wiffen P, McQuay H, Carroll D, et al. Anticonvulsant drugs for acute and chronic pain. *Cochrane Database Syst Rev.* 2000:CD001133.

20 SODIUM AND CALCIUM CHANNEL ANTAGONISTS

Mark S. Wallace, MD

INTRODUCTION

- Several lines of evidence suggest that both spontaneous and evoked pain are mediated in part by voltage-sensitive sodium and calcium channels.

- Sodium and calcium channel antagonists used in clinical practice are of the voltage-dependent type in that the neurons must remain depolarized for a significant period of time for maximal blocking action to occur.
- Both the central and peripheral nervous system has an abundance of sodium and calcium channels.
- Clinically, the calcium channel antagonists have been more widely used than the sodium channel antagonists.
- This chapter will focus on the antagonists. The calcium channel modulators (pregabalin and gabapentin) are discussed in Chapter 19.

SODIUM CHANNEL ANTAGONISTS

MECHANISM OF ACTION

- There are many subtypes of sodium channels expressed throughout the nervous system.
- Blockade of the sodium channel prevents the upstroke of the axonal action potential. If this blockade occurs in pain-sensitive sensory neurons, pain relief may result.
- At least seven different sodium channels have been isolated, all with important biophysical and pharmacological differences resulting in differing sensitivities to sodium channel blockers.
- Sodium channels are classified by their sensitivity to tetrodotoxin (TTX), a potent sodium channel blocker. TTX-sensitive (TTXs) sodium channels are blocked by small concentrations of TTX, whereas TTX-resistant (TTXr) sodium channels are not blocked even when exposed to high concentrations of TTX. The role of TTXs and TTXr sodium channels in nociception is controversial; however, as described above, it is clear that after nerve injury and during inflammation, there are dynamic and expression changes that occur in both TTXs and TTXr sodium channels.
- Proponents for the TTXr sodium channel as being important in nociception argue that because of their different voltage sensitivities of activation and inactivation, TTXr channels are still capable of generating impulses at depolarized potentials (which characterize the chronically damaged nerve fibers), whereas TTXs channels are inactivated and cannot contribute to excitability. For example, PN3 is a subclass of the TTXr sodium channel that is located only in the peripheral nervous system on small neurons in the dorsal root ganglion and is thought to be specific to pain transmission.
- The development of the spontaneous and evoked pain after nervous system injury is thought to be due to not only a change in the number of sodium channels but also a change in the distribution and type of sodium channels. These sodium channels display marked pharmacological differences from the uninjured state.

- It is speculated that in the presence of injury, sodium channels on C fibers display an exaggerated response to sodium channel blockade as opposed to the uninjured state; therefore, it has been suggested that neuropathic pain is more responsive to sodium channel blockade than nociceptive pain.
- The exact site of action of the sodium channel antagonists is unclear. However, systemic lidocaine and mexiletine decrease the flare response after intradermal capsaicin, suggesting a peripheral site of action.

EFFICACY

- Systemic sodium channel antagonists have little to no effect on acute thermal and mechanical thresholds (both painful and nonpainful).
- The systemic delivery of sodium channel antagonists has been shown to decrease postoperative pain and analgesic requirements in limited clinical studies.
- Studies on the systemic delivery of sodium channel antagonists for the treatment of neuropathic pain have had conflicting results. Overall, there appears to be an effect on neuropathic pain but there is a difference in efficacy between agents that may be due to dose-limiting side effects (see below).

INDIVIDUAL DRUGS

Lidocaine

- Lidocaine has been extensively studied in experimental, postoperative, and neuropathic pain states.
- At maximally tolerable doses (3 µg/mL plasma level), intravenous lidocaine has little effect on human experimental pain.
- At doses <3 µg/mL plasma level, intravenous lidocaine reduces postoperative and neuropathic pain.
- When examined in patients reporting significant pain secondary to a variety of neuropathic states, subanesthetic doses of systemic lidocaine produce clinically relevant relief in diabetes, nerve injury pain states, and cancer.
- Lidocaine dose is 2 mg/kg over 20 min followed by 1–3 mg/kg/h titrated to effect.
- The correlation between plasma levels and side effects has been studied the most with intravenous lidocaine (Table 20–1).

Mexiletine

- Mexiletine is an oral bioavailable analog of lidocaine.
- At plasma concentrations of up to 0.5 µg/mL plasma level, there is no effect on human experimental pain.

TABLE 20-1 Intravenous Lidocaine Side Effects Versus Plasma Level

SIDE EFFECT	PLASMA LEVEL (µg/mL)
1. Light-headedness	1–2
2. Periorbital numbness	2
3. Metallic taste	2–3
4. Tinnitus	5–6
5. Blurred vision	6
6. Muscular twitching	8
7. Convulsions	10
8. Cardiac depression	20–25

- Mexiletine has been reported to be effective in a variety of neuropathic pain syndromes including diabetic neuropathy, alcoholic neuropathy, peripheral nerve injury, and thalamic pain. However, later reports question the efficacy of oral mexiletine in neuropathic pain, making it difficult to draw conclusions on efficacy.
- It appears that oral mexiletine is a poor choice for the management of neuropathic pain and is rarely used. The exact therapeutic plasma concentration for analgesia is yet to be determined, but it appears that dose-limiting side effects occur at a lower plasma concentration than analgesia.
- It appears that the maximum tolerable dose of mexiletine is between 800 and 900 mg/d. However, it is questionable if this dose results in analgesic plasma levels. The highest tolerated plasma mexiletine level is about 0.5 µg/mL, which is below the analgesic level.

Lamotrigine

- Lamotrigine is a sodium channel antagonist with activity at glutaminergic sites resulting in anticonvulsant activity.
- It has been shown to decrease acute pain induced by the cold pressor test.
- Lamotrigine significantly reduces the analgesic requirements of postoperative pain.
- Studies on the efficacy of lamotrigine for neuropathic pain have shown conflicting results likely due to differences in total daily doses. Doses <200 mg/d are likely not efficacious. Doses between 200 and 400 mg/d appear to be efficacious in neuropathic pain.
- Lamotrigine appears to be well tolerated with few side effects.

Procaine

- Procaine was one of the first local anesthetics to be used systemically for the treatment of pain.
- An advantage of procaine is the extremely low toxicity when administered systemically. A disadvantage is the extremely short half-life due to ester hydrolysis by plasma pseudocholinesterases and red cell esterases.

- The earliest use of procaine was to supplement general anesthesia and to treat chronic musculoskeletal disorders.
- It has also been shown anecdotally to be effective in the treatment of postherpetic neuralgia.
- There is one controlled study using procaine 4–6.5 mg/kg that shows efficacy in postoperative pain.
- Procaine is currently not clinically used.

Flecainide

- Systemic flecainide has been demonstrated to suppress ectopic nerve discharge in neuropathic rats.
- The clinical use of flecainide has been mixed.
- In postherpetic neuralgia, flecainide was effective in 15/20 patients.
- Flecainide was ineffective in a pilot study in cancer pain.
- Currently, flecainide is rarely used.

CALCIUM CHANNEL ANTAGONISTS

MECHANISM OF ACTION

- There are six unique types of calcium channels expressed throughout the nervous system (designated L, N, P, Q, R, and T).
- Voltage-sensitive calcium channels of the N-type exist in the superficial laminae of the dorsal horn and are thought to modulate nociceptive processing by a central mechanism.
- Blockade of the N-type calcium channel in the superficial dorsal horn modulates membrane excitability and inhibits neurotransmitter release, resulting in pain relief.

EFFICACY

- The N-type calcium channel antagonists have the most analgesic efficacy. L-type antagonists have moderate analgesic efficacy, and the P/Q-type antagonists have minimal analgesic efficacy.
- Unlike the systemic sodium channel antagonists, animal studies suggest that only the N-type calcium channel antagonists have an effect on acute thermal and mechanical thresholds (both painful and non-painful). This suggests a greater analgesic potency than the sodium channel blockers.
- Phase III trials have shown that the epidural and intrathecal delivery of the N-type calcium channel antagonist (ziconotide) decreases postoperative pain.
- Rigorous phase III trials have demonstrated that the intrathecal delivery of the N-type calcium channel antagonist (ziconotide) is effective in the treatment of neuropathic pain.

INDIVIDUAL DRUGS

Ziconotide

- Ziconotide is a 25-amino acid peptide that is a synthetic version of a naturally occurring peptide found in the venom of the marine snail, *Conus magus*.
- It specifically and selectively binds to N-type voltage-sensitive calcium channels.
- It is the first and only intrathecal N-type calcium channel antagonist to enter clinical development.
- Phase II/III clinical trials on intrathecally administered ziconotide for neuropathic pain reported the following side effects: dizziness, nausea, nystagmus, gait imbalance, confusion, constipation, and urinary retention. These side effects are dose related and rapidly reversible on decreasing or stopping the drug. Clinical experience suggests that these side effects can be managed by a slower titration than was used in the clinical trials.
- It appears that spinally delivered ziconotide has a narrow therapeutic window. When this therapeutic window is achieved, analgesia is possible without unacceptable side effects.
- Therapeutic dose is in the range of 1–3 μg/d.
- Ziconotide is more widely used in combination with other intrathecal agents.
- It has no known lethal dose.
- It has no withdrawal syndrome with abrupt cessation. However, it does not prevent opioid withdrawal.

L-type Calcium Channel Antagonists (Nimodipine, Verapamil)

- Nimodipine has been shown to decrease postoperative opioid requirements.
- There are numerous reports on the efficacy of the L-type calcium channel antagonists for the prevention and treatment of migraine and chronic daily headaches.
- Nimodipine has been shown to significantly reduce the morphine requirements in cancer patients requiring morphine dose escalation.

BIBLIOGRAPHY

Ando K, Wallace MS, Schulteis G, Braun J. Neurosensory finding after oral mexiletine in healthy volunteers. *Reg Anesth Pain Med*. 2000;25:468–474.

Atanassoff PG, Hartmannsgruber MW, Thrasher J, et al. Ziconotide, a new N-type calcium channel blocker, administered intrathecally for acute postoperative pain. *Reg Anesth Pain Med*. 2000;25:274–278.

Attal N, Gaude V, Brasseur L, et al. Intravenous lidocaine in central pain: a double-blind, placebo-controlled, psychophysical study. *Neurology*. 2000;54:564–574.

Awerbuch G, Sandyk R. Mexiletine for thalamic pain syndrome. *Int J Neurosci*. 1990;55:129–133.

Bonicalzi V, Canavero S, Cerutti F, Piazza M, Clemente M, Chio A. Lamotrigine reduces total postoperative analgesic requirement: a randomized double-blind placebo-controlled pilot study. *Surgery*. 1997;122:567–570.

Cassuto J, Wallin G, Hogstrom S, Faxen A, Rimback G. Inhibition of postoperative pain by continuous low-dose intravenous infusion of lidocaine. *Anesth Analg*. 1985;64:971–974.

Chaplan SR, Bach FW, Yaksh TL. Systemic use of local anesthetics in pain states. In: Yaksh TL, Lynch C, Zapol WM, et al, eds. *Anesthesia: Biologic Foundations*. Philadelphia, PA: Lippincott-Raven; 1997:977–986.

Chiou-Tan F, Tuel S, Johnson J. Effect of mexiletine on spinal cord injury dysesthetic pain. *Am J Phys Med Rehabil*. 1996;75: 84–87.

Chong SF, Bretscher ME, Maillard JA. Pilot study evaluating local anesthetics administered systemically for treatment of pain in patients with advanced cancer. *J Pain Symptom Manage*. 1997;13:112–117.

Cummins TR, Waxman SG. Down regulation of tetrodotoxin-resistant sodium currents and upregulation of a rapidly repriming tetrodotoxin-sensitive sodium current in small spinal sensory neurons after nerve injury. *Neuroscience*. 1997;17: 3503–3514.

Davis RW. Successful treatment for phantom pain. *Orthopedics*. 1993;16:691–695.

Dunlop R, Davies RJ, Hockley J, Turner P. Analgesic effects of oral flecainide. *Lancet*. 1988;1:420–421.

Edmonds GW, Comer WH, Kennedy JD, Taylor IB. Intravenous use of procaine in general anesthesia. *JAMA*. 1949;141:761–765.

Ichimata M, Ikebe H, Yoshitake S, Hattori S, Iwasaka H, Noguchi T. Analgesic effects of flecainide on postherpetic neuralgia. *Int J Clin Pharmacol Res*. 2001;21:15–19.

Kastrup J, Petersen P, Dejgard A, Angeo HR, Hilsted J. Intravenous lidocaine infusion—a new treatment of chronic painful diabetic neuropathy? *Pain*. 1987;28:69–75.

Keats AS, D'Alessandro GL, Beecher HK. A controlled study of pain relief by intravenous procaine. *JAMA*. 1951;147:1761–1763.

Lehmann KA, Ribbert N, Horrichs-Haermeyer G. Postoperative patient-controlled analgesia with alfentanil: analgesic efficacy and minimum effective concentrations. *J Pain Symptom Manage*. 1990;5:249–258.

Marchettini P, Lacerenza M, Marangoni C, Pellegata G, Sotgiu ML, Smirne S. Lidocaine test in neuralgia. *Pain*. 1992;48:S63–S66.

McCleane G. 200mg daily of lamotrigine has no analgesic effect in neuropathic pain: a randomized, double-blind, placebo controlled trial. *Pain*. 1999;83:105–107.

Micieli D, Piazza D, Sinforiani E, et al. Antimigraine drugs in the management of daily chronic headaches: clinical profiles of responsive patients. *Cephalgia*. 1985;5(suppl 2):219–224.

Nishiyama K, Sakuta M. Mexiletine for painful alcoholic neuropathy. *Int Med*. 1995;34:577–579.

Presley R, Charapata S, Perrar-Brechner T, et al. Chronic, opioid-resistant, neuropathic pain: marked analgesic efficacy of intrathecal ziconotide. Paper presented at: 1998 Annual American Pain Society; 1998; San Diego, CA. Abstract A894.

Rowbotham M, Reisner-Keller L, Fields H. Both intravenous lidocaine and morphine reduce the pain of postherpetic neuralgia. *Neurology*. 1991;41:1024–1028.

Santillán R, Hurlé M, Armijo J, de los Mozos R, Flórez J. Nimodipine-enhanced opiate analgesia in cancer patients requiring morphine dose escalation: a double-blind, placebo-controlled study. *Pain*. 1998;76:17–26.

Shanbrom E. Treatment of herpetic pain and postherpetic neuralgia with intravenous procaine. *JAMA*. 1961;176:1041–1043.

Simpson DM, Olney R, McArthur JC, Khan A, Godbold J, Ebel-Frommer K. A placebo-controlled trial of lamotrigine for painful HIV-associated neuropathy. *Neurology*. 2000;54:2115–2119.

Stracke H, Meyer UE. Mexiletine in the treatment of diabetic neuropathy. *Diabetes Care*. 1992;15:1550–1555.

Tanaka M, Cummins TR, Ishikawa K, et al. SNS sodium channel expression increases in dorsal root ganglion neurons in the carrageenan inflammatory pain model. *Neuroreport*. 1998;9:967–972.

Wallace MS, Laitin S, Licht D, Yaksh TL. Concentration–effect relations for intravenous lidocaine infusions in human volunteers: effect on acute sensory thresholds and capsaicin-evoked hyperpathia. *Anesthesiology*. 1997;86:1262–1272.

Wallace MS, Magnuson S, Ridgeway B. Oral mexiletine in the treatment of neuropathic pain. *Reg Anesth Pain Med*. 2000;25:459–467.

Wright JM, Oki JC, Graves L. Mexiletine in the symptomatic treatment of diabetic peripheral neuropathy. *Ann Pharmacother*. 1997;31:29–34.

Zakrzewska JM, Chaudhry Z, Nurmikko TJ, Patton DW, Mullens EL. Lamotrigine (Lamictal) in refractory trigeminal neuralgia: results from a double-blind placebo controlled crossover trial. *Pain*. 1997;73:223–230.

21 TRAMADOL

Michelle Stern, MD
Kevin Sperber, MD
Marco Pappagallo, MD

INTRODUCTION

- Tramadol was introduced to the US market in 1995 after being widely used throughout the world for approximately 20 years.
- Because it can be used for acute and chronic pain, tramadol was introduced to the United States as an alternative to nonsteroidal anti-inflammatory drugs (NSAIDs) and opioids for moderate–moderately severe pain.

- Tramadol is considered to be a more potent analgesic than oral NSAIDs and to have fewer gastrointestinal, renal, and cardiac side effects. Compared with traditional opioids, tramadol offers analgesia with a reduced risk of abuse, physical dependence, sedation, and constipation.
- Although in other countries it can be administered via the epidural, intravenous, rectal, or oral route (immediate and sustained release), in the United States, tramadol is available only in the immediate-release oral formulation.
- The oral formulation is available in a 50-mg tramadol-only tablet (Ultram®) and a 325/37.5-mg acetaminophen/tramadol combination (Ultracet™).
- An extended-release formulation is undergoing Food and Drug Administration (FDA) trials in doses of 100–400 mg daily.
- The Drug Enforcement Administration (DEA) has classified the drug as a nonscheduled analgesic.

MECHANISM OF ACTION/ PHARMACODYNAMICS

- Tramadol is a synthetic 4-phenyl-piperidine analogue of codeine.
- Tramadol's mode of action is not completely understood, but it is thought to work primarily in the central nervous system (CNS).
- It differs from traditional opioids because tramadol-induced analgesia is only partially blocked by the opiate antagonist naloxone, which suggests an additional nonopioid component for the pain relief.
- Laboratory studies have provided insight about this possible dual mode of action: tramadol binds weakly to the μ-opioid receptor sites and inhibits the reuptake of norepinephrine and serotonin. Its affinity for the μ-opioid receptor is 1/6000 that of morphine and 1/10 that of codeine. The α_2-adrenoceptor antagonist, yohimbine, reduces the analgesic effects of tramadol, further supporting a nonopioid component of pain relief.
- The chemical name is *cis*-2-[(dimethylamino)methyl]-1-(3-methoxyphenyl) cyclohexanol hydrochloride. The parent compound is a racemic drug, and both its (+) and (−) forms play an important role in its mechanism. The (+) enantiomer has a higher affinity for the μ-receptor and increases serotonin levels by inhibiting uptake and enhancing release. The (−) enantiomer increases norepinephrine levels by stimulating the α_2-adrenergic receptors that inhibit norepinephrine reuptake.
- Tramadol is extensively metabolized by the liver, with the major pathways being: N- and O-demethylation (phase 1) and glucuronidation or sulfation.

- The drug and its metabolites are eliminated primarily through the kidneys, with 30% being excreted unchanged.
- Of the 23 identified metabolites, 11 are phase 1 and 12 are conjugates, but only M1 has been shown to play a significant role in tramadol's analgesic properties. The M1 metabolite is the O-demethylated form of tramadol with the (+) form having the greater potential for analgesic effect. An isoenzyme of the cytochrome P450, the CYP2D6, is responsible for conversion to the M1 metabolite. In the 7% of the Caucasian population that lacks this isoenzyme, therefore, tramadol metabolizes poorly and provides decreased analgesia. The analgesic potency of the M1 metabolite is 6 times greater than that of its parent drug, owing to its 200 × greater affinity to the μ-opioid binding site.
- Bioavailability after oral administration is 75%, with only 20% binding to plasma proteins.

DOSAGE

- The average dose for a healthy adult is 50–100 mg every 6 h.
- The peak plasma levels after a single 100-mg dose are 1.6 h for the parent drug and 3 h for the M1 metabolite. The half-life levels after a single 100-mg dose are 6.3 h for the parent drug and 7.4 h for the M1 metabolite.
- The analgesic benefit peaks at 2 h after the initial dose and lasts approximately 6 h, with steady state occurring after 48 h.
- When given with food, the percentage absorbed and peak plasma concentration are unaffected, but the time to peak plasma concentration increases by 35 min.
- Dosage adjustment is recommended in the elderly and in patients with renal and liver disease.
- The maximum dose recommended by the manufacturer is 400 mg in a 24-h period secondary to the increased risk of side effects with higher doses; however, some clinical reports document the use of up to 600 mg/d in carefully selected patients.
- For Ultracet™, the recommended dose is two tablets every 4–6 h as needed for pain, with a duration of use not to exceed five days and a maximum daily dose of eight tablets (300 mg of tramadol and 2.6 g of acetaminophen). Despite the limited use recommended, we have found it efficacious in patients with chronic pain.
- A carbamazepine dose of 800 mg daily increases the metabolism of tramadol and, thus, may necessitate a dosage adjustment.
- Ondansetron, a serotonin 5HT-3 receptor antagonist, also inhibits the analgesic effects of tramadol.
- Tramadol can also have a synergistic effect with other sedating medication, which may necessitate a dosage adjustment.

SPECIAL POPULATIONS

- The elderly and/or patients with liver or renal disease require an adjustment in the usual dosage of tramadol.
- Due to the increased elimination time of the drug in the elderly (75 years and older), the dosage should not exceed 300 mg/d.
- Advanced liver disease prolongs the drug's half-life and requires dosage reduction to 50 mg every 12 h (maximum daily dose 100 mg/d). Ultracet is not recommended for patients with liver disease.
- Since tramadol is primarily excreted through the kidneys, the rate and extent of excretion will be significantly reduced in patients with a creatinine clearance of less than 30 mL/min; thus, they require a dosage adjustment of 50–100 mg every 12 h (maximum daily dose 200 mg/d). For Ultracet, the recommendation in these patients is two tablets every 12 h.
- Only 7% of tramadol and its metabolites is cleared by a 4-h dialysis. Dialysis patients can receive their dose on dialysis day.
- The safety of tramadol in the pediatric population, during pregnancy, and in nursing mothers is not established; therefore, use of the drug in these populations is not recommended in the United States. Multiple studies abroad, however, of the use of tramadol for acute pain in children as young as one-month-old consistently report that a 1–2 mg/kg single dose is safe and effective.
- Tramadol is classified by the FDA as a pregnancy risk factor C because 1% of the drug dose is transferred via the placenta and 0.1% of the dose can be found in breast milk. Studies of the use of tramadol during labor showed that it provides adequate maternal analgesia with no significant respiratory depression in the newborn.
- A single case report signals the potential for neonatal withdrawal after chronic maternal use during pregnancy.

INDICATION FOR USE

- The World Health Organization (WHO) recommends tramadol as a step 2 analgesic agent for a variety of painful conditions.
- It has been used successfully for malignant pain, osteoarthritic pain, low back pain, diabetic neuropathy, fibromyalgia, restless leg syndrome, postherpetic neuralgia, pain from surgical and dental procedures, and with NSAIDs to help control breakthrough pain.

SIDE EFFECT PROFILE

- Intolerable side effects cause 20–30% of patients to discontinue tramadol.
- Dizziness, lethargy, nausea, vomiting, and constipation are common complaints after the first week of usage.
- Complaints of nausea and vomiting may decrease with continued usage, but the incidence of other side effects such as dizziness, lethargy, headache, and constipation may fail to improve significantly.
- The incidence of side effects may appear daunting, but it is similar to that of many opioids.

TITRATION SCHEDULE

- A slow titration schedule improves tolerance for the medication (Table 21–1).
- Although a slow titration is not desirable for treatment of acute pain, it may be useful in the treatment of a

TABLE 21-1   Titration Schedule

TITRATION PROTOCOL	INITIAL DOSE	TITRATION SCHEDULE	RECOMMENDED FOR
10-day titration	50 mg qd for 3 days	50 mg bid for 3 days Then increase to 50 mg tid for 3 days Then continue at 50 mg qid May increase further until analgesic effect or recommended therapeutic dosage is reached	Elderly Fall risks Medication sensitivity
16-day titration	25 mg qd for 3 days	25 mg bid for 3 days Then increase to 25 mg tid for 3 days Then increase to 25 mg qid for 3 days Then increase to 25 mg qid for 3 days Then increase to 50 mg bid and 25 mg bid for 3 days Then increase to 50 mg qid May increase until analgesic effect or recommended therapeutic dosage is achieved	Elderly Fall risks Medication sensitivity
Author's rapid titration recommendation	75 mg daily divided into 25 mg tid with first dose at bedtime or 100 mg daily divided into 50 mg bid with first at bedtime dose	Increase by 50 or 75 mg every 3–5 days until analgesic effect or recommended therapeutic dosage	Medication sensitivity Mild to moderate fall risks

- patient with chronic pain having a history of poor tolerance for medication or who is at increased risk for falls.
- A balance must be struck between maximizing tolerance to the drug and achieving timely pain relief.
- The suggested regimens for a slow titration include a 10-day and a 16-day schedule. In the 10-day titration, 50 mg of tramadol daily is started and increased by 50 mg every 3 days until the target of 200 mg/d is reached. A slower titration schedule for high-risk elderly patients starts with 25 mg of tramadol daily and increases by 25 mg every three days until a dose of 25 mg qid is achieved. Then, the total daily dose is increased by 50 mg every three days until a dosage of 50 mg qid or 200 mg/d is reached. After titration, the dosage can be increased to the maximum recommended dosage for the patient.
- Most patients will tolerate a slightly more aggressive titration schedule. We initiate treatment with 25 mg every 8 h or 50 mg every 12 h. If this dose is adequately tolerated after three days, we increase to 50 mg every 8 h. The dose is titrated upward by 50–75 mg every three to five days until adequate analgesia is obtained or maximum safe dosage is reached. If significant side effects develop, the dose is titrated downward to a previously tolerated dose, and more time is allowed before further titration is attempted. Patients are instructed to take the initial dose and all subsequent increased dosage of this medication in the evening and warned of the potential psychomotor effects of the medication. Written instructions may improve patients' compliance. The recently introduced generic tramadol is a 50-mg tablet that is not scored, unlike Ultram®, and this may complicate the gradual titration schedule using a 25-mg dosage. In this case, the alternate titration schedule starting with 50 mg bid may be preferred.

DRUG–DRUG INTERACTIONS

- Although tramadol has been associated with many possible side effects, the two most striking side effects are seizures and the serotonin syndrome.

SEIZURES

- There have been reports of seizures in patients taking tramadol both alone and in conjunction with other medications, although some studies have suggested that the risk of seizures with tramadol usage alone is comparable to that of other centrally acting analgesics.
- The risk of seizures is increased with tramadol overdosage and as the number and dosage of other psychoactive medications are increased.

- The psychoactive medications most commonly cited as increasing the risk are the antidepressant agents (monoamine oxidase inhibitors [MAOI], tricyclic antidepressants, and selective serotonin reuptake inhibitors [SSRI]), the neuroleptics, and other opioids.
- If it is essential to use these medications in combination, caution is required and the risk–benefit of this treatment plan should be discussed with the patient in advance.
- In one large retrospective study, seizures occurred in less than 1% of tramadol users.
- Patients with spontaneous seizures with tramadol alone may be poor metabolizers of the drug.
- Avoid the coadministration of tramadol with any medication that may lower the seizure threshold.
- Avoid administration of tramadol to patients with a history of seizures/epilepsy, head trauma, alcohol and drug withdrawal, and any other insult to the CNS.
- Any protective effect of coadministration of anticonvulsant medication with tramadol has not been established.
- A seizure associated with tramadol should be treated with benzodiazepines or barbiturates.
- In cases of tramadol overdose, 800 mg was needed to cause coma, and respiratory depression started at 500 mg. The use of naloxone merely reversed some of the cardiorespiratory effects of tramadol and was associated with an increased risk of seizure activity.

SEROTONIN SYNDROME

- A severe complication that may occur is the serotonin syndrome.
- This is associated with the use of tramadol and other agents, such as the SSRI and the MAOI, that can increase CNS serotonin levels.
- Serotonin syndrome should be suspected in any patient who develops an abrupt change in mental status accompanied by autonomic symptoms (eg, fever, shivering, diaphoresis, nausea, vomiting, and diarrhea) and other neurological changes (eg, an increase in muscle tone, myoclonus, tremor, ataxia, agitation, hypomania, and hallucinations).
- Treatment includes cessation of the medication, symptom management, and administration of antiserotonergic drugs such as cyproheptadine.

WHY USE (OR AVOID) TRAMADOL

- The benefits of using tramadol instead of traditional opioids include lower abuse potential and physical dependence as well as reduced side effects, such as constipation, respiratory depression, and sedation.

- The rate of abuse with tramadol has been reported at less than 1/100,000 patients. Of this, 97% had a history of alcohol or drug dependence; therefore, tramadol should be used with caution in this patient population.
- When the drug is withdrawn abruptly, it is possible to develop an abstinence syndrome similar to that seen with other opioid compounds, but the rate is reported at 1 per month per 100,000 cases. The abstinence syndrome of tramadol can be treated by reinstituting tramadol and gradually titrating the dose downward. Methadone is effective in treating abstinence syndrome secondary to abrupt discontinuation of tramadol.
- Patients with a true allergic reaction to codeine or morphine should use tramadol with caution, as there is the potential for cross-reactivity since tramadol is a codeine analogue.

SUMMARY

- Tramadol's mechanism of action is not completely understood. It works both at the μ-opioid receptors and by inhibiting the reuptake of norepinephrine and serotonin in the CNS.
- Tramadol has proven effectiveness for moderate to moderately severe pain.
- It does not affect the prostaglandin cycle as do NSAIDs and has a lower incidence of dependence and physical abuse than traditional opioids.
- Tramadol has been described as one-fifth as potent as oral morphine.
- While the efficacy of morphine and tramadol increases with the size of the dose, dose-related toxicity limits the maximum potential of tramadol.

BIBLIOGRAPHY

Arcioni R, Della Rocca M, Romano S, et al. Ondansetron inhibits the analgesic effects of tramadol: a possible 5-HT(3) spinal receptor involvement in acute pain in humans. *Anesth Analg.* 2002;94(6):1553.

Bamigbade TA, Davidson C, Langford RM, et al. Actions of tramadol, its enantiomers and principal metabolite, O-desmethyltramadol, on serotonin (5-HT) efflux and uptake in the rat dorsal raphe nucleus. *Br J Anaesth.* 1997;79(3):352.

Bamigbade T, Langford R. The clinical use of tramadol hydrochloride. *Pain Rev.* 1998;5:155.

Baraka A, Siddick S, Assaf B. Supplementation of general anaesthesia with tramadol or fentanyl in parturients undergoing elective caesarean section. *Can J Anaesth.* 1998;45(7):631.

Barsoum M. Comparison of the efficacy and tolerability of tramadol, pethidine and nalbuphine in children with post-operative pain. *Clin Drug Invest.* 1995;9:183.

Bertilsson L. Geographical/interracial differences in polymorphic drug oxidation. Current state of knowledge of cytochromes P450(CYP)2D6 and 2C19. *Clin Pharmacokinet.* 1995;29:192.

Biasi G, Manca S, Manganelli S, et al. Tramadol in the fibromyalgia syndrome: a controlled clinical trial versus placebo. *Int J Clin Pharmacol Res.* 1998;18(1):13.

Bosenberg A, Ratcliffe S. The respiratory effects of tramadol in children under halothane anaesthesia. *Anaesthesia.* 1998;53:960.

Cicero T, Adams E, Geller A, et al. A postmarketing surveillance program to monitor Ultram abuse in the United States. *Drug Alcohol Depend.* 1999;57:7.

Cossmann M, Wilsmann KM. Effect and side effects of tramadol. *Therapiewoche.* 1987;37:3475.

Dalgin PH. Use of tramadol in chronic pain. *Clin Geriatr.* 1995;3:1.

Dayer P, Desmeules J, Collart L. Pharmacology of tramadol. *Drugs.* 1997;53(suppl 2):18.

De Witte J, Schoenmaekers B, Sessler D, et al. The analgesic efficacy of tramadol is impaired by concurrent administration of ondansetron. *Anesth Analg.* 2001;92(5):1319.

Desmeules J, Piguet V, Collart L, et al. Yohimbine antagonism as a tool to assess the extent of monoaminergic modulation in analgesic effects experience with tramadol. *Experientia.* 1994;50:A79.

Duggal HS, Fetchko J. Serotonin syndrome and atypical antipsychotics. *Am J Psychiatry.* 2002;159(4):672.

Duthie D. Remifentanil and tramadol. *Br J Anaesth.* 1998;81:51.

Finkel JC, Rose JB, Schmitz ML, et al. An evaluation of the efficacy and tolerability of oral tramadol hydrochloride tablets for the treatment of postsurgical pain in children. *Anesth Analg.* 2002;94(6):1469.

Freye E, Levy J. Acute abstinence syndrome following abrupt cessation of long-term use of tramadol (Ultram): a case study. *Eur J Pain.* 2000;4(3):307.

Gardner JS, Blough D, Drinkard CR, et al. Tramadol and seizures: a surveillance study in a managed care population. *Pharmacotherapy.* 2000;20(12):1423.

Gasse C, Derby L, Vasilakis-Scaramozza C, et al. Incidence of first-time idiopathic seizures in users of tramadol. *Pharmacotherapy.* 2000;20(6):629.

Gibson TP. Pharmacokinetics, efficacy, and safety of analgesia with a focus on tramadol HCl. *Am J Med.* 1996;101(1A):47S.

Grond S, Radbruch L, Meuser T, et al. High-dose tramadol in comparison to low-dose morphine for cancer pain relief. *J Pain Symptom Manage.* 1999;18(3):174.

Harati Y, Gooch C, Swenson M, et al. Double-blind randomized trial of tramadol for the treatment of the pain of diabetic neuropathy. *Neurology.* 1998;50:1842.

Harati Y, Gooch C, Swenson M, et al. Maintenance of the long-term effectiveness of tramadol in treatment of the pain of diabetic neuropathy. *J Diabetes Complications.* 2000;14(2):65.

Hernandez-Diaz S, Garcia-Rodriguez LA. Epidemiologic assessment of the safety of conventional nonsteroidal anti-inflammatory drugs. *Am J Med.* 2001;110(suppl 3A):20S.

Jick H, Derby LE, Vasilakis C, et al. The risk of seizures associated with tramadol. *Pharmacotherapy.* 1998;18(3):607.

Katz WA. Pharmacology and clinical experience with tramadol in osteoarthritis. *Drugs.* 1996;52(suppl 3):39.

Keeley PW, Foster G, Whitelaw L. Hear my song: auditory hallucinations with tramadol hydrochloride. *BMJ.* 2000;321(7276):1608.

Kesavan S, Sobala GM. Serotonin syndrome with fluoxetine plus tramadol. *J R Soc Med.* 1999;92(9):474.

Lange-Asschenfeldt C, Weigmann H, Hiemke C, et al. Serotonin syndrome as a result of fluoxetine in a patient with tramadol abuse: plasma level-correlated symptomatology. *J Clin Psychopharmacol.* 2002;22(4):440.

Lee CR, McTavish D, Sorkin EM. Tramadol. A preliminary review of its pharmacodynamic and pharmacokinetic properties, and therapeutic potential in acute and chronic pain states. *Drugs.* 1993;46:313.

Leo R, Narendran R, DeGuiseppe B. Methadone detoxification of tramadol dependence. *J Subst Abuse Treat.* 2000;19(3):297.

Lewis KS, Han NH. Tramadol: a new centrally acting analgesic. *Am J Health Syst Pharm.* 1997;54(6):643.

Lintz W, Barth H, Osterloh G, et al. Bioavailability of enteral tramadol formulations. First communication: capsules. *Arzeneimittelforschung.* 1986;36:1278.

Liu ZM, Zhou WH, Lian Z, et al. Drug dependence and abuse potential of tramadol. *Zhongguo Yao Li Xue Bao.* 1999; 20(1):52.

Mason BJ, Blackburn KH. Possible serotonin syndrome associated with tramadol and sertraline coadministration. *Ann Pharmacother.* 1997;31(2):175.

Mehlisch DR. The efficacy of combination analgesic therapy in relieving dental pain. *J Am Dent Assoc.* 2002;133(7):861.

Meyer FP, Rimasch H, Blaha B, et al. Tramadol withdrawal in a neonate. *Eur J Clin Pharmacol.* 1997;53(2):159.

Payne K, Roelofse J, Shipton E. Tears at bedtime. *Br J Anaesth.* 1999;83:359.

Payne KA, Roelofse JA. Tramadol drops in children: analgesic efficacy, lack of respiratory effects, and normal recovery times. *Anesth Prog.* 1999;46(3):91.

Petrone D, Kamin M, Olson W. Slowing the titration rate of tramadol HCl reduces the incidence of discontinuation due to nausea and/or vomiting: a double-blind randomized trial. *J Clin Pharm Ther.* 1999;24(2):115.

Portenoy RK. Management of common opioid side effects during long-term therapy of cancer pain. *Ann Acad Med Singapore.* 1994;23(2):160.

Poulsen L, Arendt-Nielsen L, Brosen K, et al. The hypoalgesic effect of tramadol in relation to CYP2D6. *Clin Pharmacol Ther.* 1996;60(6):636.

Product Information. *Ultracet, Tramadol Hydrochloride.* Raritan, NJ: Ortho-McNeil Pharmaceutical; 1998.

Product Information. *Ultracet, Tramadol Hydrochloride/Acetaminophen.* Raritan, NJ: Ortho-McNeil Pharmaceutical; 2001.

Raffa R, Friderichs E, Reimann W. Opioid and nonopiod components independently contribute to the mechanism of action of tramadol, an atypical opioid analgesic. *J Pharmacol Exp Ther.* 1992;260:275.

Rauck R, Ruoff G, McMillen J. Comparison of tramadol and acetaminophen with codeine for long term management in elderly patients. *Curr Ther Res.* 1994;55:1417.

Reig E. Tramadol in musculoskeletal pain—a survey. *Clin Rheumatol.* 2002;21(suppl 1):S9 [discussion S11].

Ripple MG, Pestaner JP, Levine BS, et al. Lethal combination of tramadol and multiple drugs affecting serotonin. *Am J Forensic Med Pathol.* 2000;21(4):370.

Rister M, Paul M. Management of pain in infants with opioid analgesics. In: 7th World Congress on Pain; August 1993; Paris. Seattle: International Association for the Study of Pain; 1994. Abstract.

Rodriguez JC, Albaladejo C, Sanchez A, et al. Withdrawal syndrome after long-term treatment with tramadol. *Br J Gen Pract.* 2000;50(454):406.

Ruoff GE. Slowing the initial titration rate of tramadol improves tolerability. *Pharmacotherapy.* 1999;19(1):88.

Schnitzer T, Gray W, Paster R, et al. Efficacy of tramadol in treatment of chronic low back pain. *J Rheumatol.* 2000;27:772.

Schnitzer TJ, Kamin M, Olson WH. Tramadol allows reduction of naproxen dose among patients with naproxen-responsive osteoarthritis pain: a randomized, double-blind, placebo-controlled study. *Arthritis Rheum.* 1999;42(7):1370.

Shipton E. Tramadol—present and future. *Anaesth Intensive Care.* 2000;28:4.

Silverfield JC, Kamin M, Wu SC, et al. CAPSS-105 Study Group. Tramadol/acetaminophen combination tablets for the treatment of osteoarthritis flare pain: a multicenter, outpatient, randomized, double-blind, placebo-controlled, parallel-group, add-on study. *Clin Ther.* 2002;24(2):282.

Spiller H, Gorman S, Villalobos D, et al. Prospective multicenter evaluation of tramadol exposure. *J Toxicol Clin Toxicol.* 1997;35(4):361.

Sunshine A. New clinical experience with tramadol. *Drugs.* 1994;47(suppl 1):8.

Wall P, Melzack R. *The Textbook of Pain.* 4th ed. Harcourt; 1999:1200.

22 OPIOIDS

Tony L. Yaksh, PhD

Among the remedies which it has pleased Almighty God to give to man to relieve his sufferings, none is so universal and so efficacious as opium.

Sydenham, 1680

INTRODUCTION

- Opioids, originally represented by the extracts of the poppy, have historically been known to produce a powerful and selective reduction in the human and animal response to a strong and otherwise noxious stimulus.
- Work by the German pharmaceutical chemist Frederich Serterner in the 1800s led to the extraction and purification (by crystallization) of an active

sleep-inducing agent, which he named morphine (from the god of dreams: *Morpheus*).

- This purification in conjunction with the development of the hollow needle and syringe, in the mid 1800s, must be considered a landmark in the development of therapeutics in general and pain management in particular.
- By the mid 1800s, it was widely used as a pain-relieving agent in the Civil War of the United States and in the Franco-Prussian War.
- There is little doubt that morphine and its congeners have been among the most important elements in the therapeutic armamentarium employed for the management of pain.
- The issue that concerns this chapter is by what mechanisms does this therapeutically important effect occur.
- The answer consists of four parts: (1) With what membrane structures do these molecules interact? (2) What are the effects of the opiate receptor interactions on neuronal function? (3) With what neuraxial systems are these receptors associated? (4) By what mechanisms does this interaction alter pain behavior?

PHARMACOLOGIC DEFINITION OF THE OPIOID RECEPTOR FAMILY

- Families of agents structurally related to morphine were uniformly observed to have similar physiologic effects: sedation, respiratory depression, block of pain (analgesia), and constipation.
- Importantly, the overall body of data suggested that the ordering of activity of the numerous structural congeners on one end point often reflected that activity on another end point. This structure–activity relationship pointed to a specific pharmacologically defined membrane site, a receptor.
- Further, by the turn of the 20th century, a molecule had been synthesized that, while structurally resembling morphine, had no morphine-like actions but prevented the depressive effects of morphine (but not barbiturates). These results jointly provided the basis for the subsequent notion that opiates acted at a specific site.

MULTIPLE OPIATE RECEPTORS

- In the early 1970s, targeted pharmacologic investigations provided defining data supporting the hypothesis that there were several subtypes of opiate receptors.
- Historic work by William Martin at the Addiction Research Center in Lexington, Kentucky, in large animal models and in humans, using pharmacologic criteria (the activity relationship ranging from

TABLE 22–1 Summary of Opioid Receptor Pharmacology

RECEPTOR	BIOASSAY	AGONISTS	ANTAGONISTS
Mu	Guinea pig ileum	Morphine	Naloxone
		Sufentanil	Naltrexone
		Meperidine	β-Funaltrexamine
		Methadone	
		DAMGO	
Delta	Mouse vas deferens	DPDPE	Naloxone
		Deltorphin	Naltrindole
Kappa	Rabbit vas deferens	Butorphanol	Naloxone
		Bremazocine	Nor-BNI
		Spiradoline	

DAMGO, [D-Ala(2), *N*-MePhe(4), Gly-ol(5)]enkephalin; DPDPE, Tyr-D-Pen-Gly-Phe-D-Pen-OH.

full agonists to antagonists for different structurally related congeners of morphine and differential cross-tolerance), led to the postulation of three receptors, mu, kappa, and sigma, the first two being responsible for the antagonist-reversible analgesia produced by different opioid alkaloids. The sigma receptor was considered to be the antagonist's insensitive site, accounting for the excitatory effects of morphine.

- Subsequent pharmacologic studies by Hans Kosterlitz and colleagues at Aberdeen Scotland carried out after their identification of the endogenous opioid peptides met and leu enkephalin led to the identification of the delta opioid receptor.
- As indicated in Table 22–1, a variety of specific agents are believed to reflect the specific activation of the several respective receptors.

RECEPTOR SUBTYPE SUBCLASSES

- In subsequent years, additional studies on opioid pharmacology suggested the possibility that there were multiple subclasses of each of the receptors.
- It should be stressed that the definition of receptor subclasses may hinge on small differential potencies of the agonists and antagonists.
- Moreover, many studies employ noncompetitive antagonists and the use of such agents in defining multiple receptor subtypes can be misleading. Still, the proposed subtype subclasses based on pharmacology are presented here for completeness.
  - *Mu subclasses*: Pasternak and colleagues proposed the existence of mu1/mu2 sites in the early 1980s based on the differential antagonism by a noncompetitive ligand (naloxonazine). Though still considered relevant by some, no specific agents have in fact been found for the proposed sites.
  - *Delta receptor subclasses*: Porreca and his colleagues have proposed two subtypes ($\partial 1$ and $\partial 2$) based

on the differential effects of several agonists and antagonists.

- *Kappa receptor subclasses*: Based on the effects of the differential pharmacology of several agonists and antagonists, up to five receptor subclasses have been hypothesized.

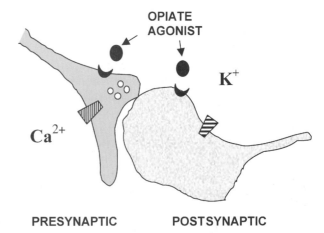

FIG. 22–1. Summary of the effects that presynaptic opiates have on terminal excitability by preventing the opening of voltage-sensitive Ca channels to attenuate transmitter release and a postsynaptic effect that is associated with hyperpolarization through an opening of potassium channels.

CLONING AND DEFINITION OF THE OPIOID RECEPTOR FAMILY

- The mu, delta, and kappa opioid receptors have all been cloned and sequenced.
- For each receptor, a single gene has been identified.
- Multiple splice variants have been identified for several of these receptors.
- Thus, to the degree that there are opioid receptor subclasses (eg, $\mu1/\mu2$; $\partial1/\partial2$), these distinct sites may represent splice variants, products of posttranslational processing, or some membrane combination of distinct receptors (eg, dimerization of a mu and delta binding site).
- Splice variants have indeed been identified for all of these receptors, although their role as receptor subclasses is not known at this time.

STRUCTURAL PROPERTIES OF OPIOID RECEPTORS

- Extensive work characterizing the sequence and functionality of these receptors has revealed that the three receptors are members of the G protein–coupled superfamily of receptors.
- All three opioid receptors largely exert their cellular effects via activation of the heterotrimeric G proteins.
- The principal coupling appears to be mediated though pertussis toxin–sensitive Gi/o proteins.
- These receptors range in length from 371 (delta) to 398 (mu) amino acids and are organized with 7 hydrophobic transmembrane spanning regions.
- A significant degree of sequence homology exists among the receptors, with the mu receptor, for example, having 75% amino acid homology with the delta and kappa opioid receptors.

RECEPTOR PHARMACODYNAMICS

RECEPTOR COUPLING

- Agonist occupancy of opioid receptors typically leads to a wide variety of events that typically serve to inhibit the activation of the neuron.

- These effects are typically blocked by the addition of pertussis toxin, indicating that they are mediated though a G protein.
- When occupied, the mu opiate receptor leads to phosphorylation of the intracellular components of the receptor by G protein–coupled receptor kinases and a variety of second messenger–regulated protein kinases. After phosphorylation, β-arrestin is recruited to the receptor where it initiates uncoupling of G protein from the receptor and facilitates binding to clathrin, which leads to internalization of the receptor complex.
- It should be noted that receptor internalization is a common property of G protein–coupled receptors with agonist occupancy.
- Of the several events initiated by the opioid receptor occupancy, the overall effects on system excitability often appear to be mediated by (1) membrane hyperpolarization through activation of an inwardly rectifying K^+ channel and (2) inhibition of the opening of voltage-sensitive Ca^{2+} channels that will subsequently depress release of neurotransmitter from the terminal (see Figure 22–1).
- These joint actions often lead to powerful, receptor-mediated inhibition of neuronal excitability.

DRUG AND RECEPTOR INTERACTIONS

- Binding to the opiate receptor for most agents is competitive and reversible.
- Classically the following are the classes of agents that bind with the opiate receptor: those agents, full agonists (fentanyl, morphine) and partial agonists

(which produce a limited activation even at full occupancy [buprenorphine]), that when bound activate the downstream pathways to varying degree and those agents, antagonists, that have no effect when bound and thereby prevent the actions of other agents with affinity for the receptor (eg, naloxone) classes of agents. The property that endows these characteristics to the drug is broadly referred to as intrinsic activity.

- Currently, there is an appreciation that, additionally, it is possible to conceive the fact that opiate receptors exist in several active states and different ligands may preferentially stabilize the receptor in one active state over another, a property referred to as "ligand bias." There is not space here to discuss this additional complexity, but the point is that different opiate agonists acting at the mu opioid receptor in different tissues may display different properties.

TOLERANCE AND DESENSITIZATION

- Persistent agonist activation of families of G protein–coupled receptors often results in a progressive, time-dependent loss of effect, otherwise referred to as tolerance. For opiates, there is at the cellular level an acute desensitization and with chronic exposure a longer lasting tolerance. Dose–response curves show that with persistent exposure, the curves are typically shifted in parallel to the right. These changes are reversible with drug removal. An alternate way of expressing the issue is that it takes more drug to produce a given effect.
- The mechanisms of the acute desensitization and tolerance are uncertain. The nature of the dose–response curve shifts suggests a loss of functionally coupled receptors on the cell surface. Such an uncoupling *could* reflect changes in G protein coupling and/or loss of cell surface binding sites. Additional cellular mechanism could include counterregulatory processes such as superactivation of downstream systems such as those for adenylate cyclase.
- Receptor internalization is believed to be the initial step in receptor recovery from desensitization, leading to reinsertion of nondesensitized/reactivated receptors in the cell membrane.
- Although internalization removes the receptor from the membrane, this activity is, in fact, believed to serve as a means of rapidly uncoupling the receptor and allowing it to externalize for subsequent activation.
- While changes in receptor–ligand coupling likely account for the changes in the analgesic dose–effect curve observed in analgesic tolerance, there is an additional argument that loss of apparent analgesic

actions may be the result of a paradoxical enhancement of pain processing initiated by continued opiate exposure (eg, opioid hyperalgesia).

OPIOID SITES OF ACTION IN ANALGESIA

- Opiates given systemically produce a potent dose-dependent analgesia with a specific structure–activity relationship (eg, sufentanil > morphine > meperidine), which is reversed by naloxone.
- These observations suggest an effect mediated by an opioid receptor.
- The essential question is: Where in the organism do opiates act to alter pain transmission?
- Defining the location of opiate action in producing analgesia involves assessing the effects of drugs delivered into specific brain sites and assessing the effects of the local drug action on behavior, for example, the response to a strong stimulus, such as a thermal stimulus applied to the paw of the rat. This induces a "pain behavior," namely, withdrawal of the stimulated paw.

SUPRASPINAL OPIATE ACTION

Microinjections and Behavioral Effects

- Examining the effects of opiates microinjected into specific sites using chronically implanted microinjection guides has shown that injections into some brain regions produce a well-defined analgesia.
- Importantly, it can be shown that the effects of the injected agonist have a pharmacology that resembles that of one or more opiate receptors (see Figure 22–2).
- Each region can have a distinct opioid receptor pharmacology.

Brain Mapping for Analgesically Coupled Opioid Receptors

- Direct injection of opiates into the brain has shown that opioid receptors that modulate pain behavior are found in several restricted brain regions.
- The location of these sites as defined in the rat is summarized schematically in Figure 22–3.
- The best characterized of these sites so identified is the mesencephalic periaqueductal gray (PAG).
- Microinjections of morphine into this region block, in a naloxone-reversible fashion, nociceptive responses in the unanesthetized mouse, rat, rabbit, cat, dog, and primate.
- This local effect serves to block not only spinally mediated reflexes (such as the tail flick) but also supraspinally organized responses.

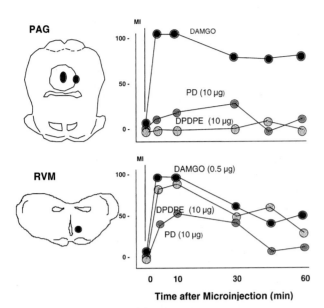

FIG. 22–2. Effects of the microinjection (0.25–0.5 μL) of receptor-selective agents DAMGO (mu), PD (kappa), and DPDPE (delta) into the mesencephalic periaqueductal gray (PAG) (top) or medulla (bottom) of an unanesthetized rat at the site indicated by the black spot and the effects on hot plate response latency. As indicated, DAMGO produces a time-dependent increase in the response latency, for example, produces analgesia in both PAG and medulla, but DPDPE and PD work only in the medulla. These effects are dose dependent and reversed by local or systemic naloxone. RVM, rostral ventral medulla.

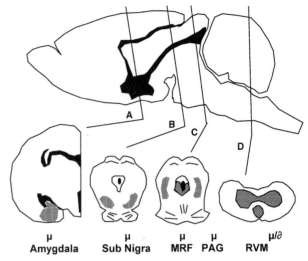

FIG. 22–3. Summary of sites within the neuraxis at which opiate injections will result in a prominent increase in the nociceptive threshold. The approximate planes of section at which the coronal sections are taken are indicated. Darkened regions indicate the cerebral aqueductal location. Light shading indicates the active regions. (A) Diencephalic: active regions within the basolateral amygdala. (B) Mesencephalic: active sites within the substantia nigra (Sub Nigra). (C) Mesencephalic: lateral regions are the mesencephalic reticular formation (MRF); the medial region is the periaqueductal gray (PAG). (D) Medulla: site indicated is the rostral ventral medulla (RVM) with the midline structure corresponding to the raphe magnus. The receptor types that result in antinociception when delivered into that region (see text for the details) are indicated.

Mesencephalic Mechanisms

- In the diversity of sites, it is unlikely that all of the mechanisms whereby opiates act within the brain to alter nociceptive transmission are identical.
- Even within a single brain region, it appears that multiple mechanisms may exist for altering pain transmission.
- Several mechanisms exist whereby opiates may act to alter nociceptive transmission. Thus, if we consider only the PAG, there are at least five mechanisms (see Figure 22–4).
  - PAG projection to the medulla serves to activate *descending* bulbospinal projections releasing serotonin and/or noradrenaline at the spinal level. Current thinking is that excitatory projections from the PAG are under the tonic inhibitory control of GABAergic interneurons. These neurons are inhibited by mu opiates, leading to a *disinhibition* and a net excitatory drive into the bulbospinal nuclei. The spinal delivery of adrenergic and serotonergic antagonists reverses the PAG morphine-induced inhibition of spinal nociceptive processing.
  - PAG outflow to the medulla, where local inhibitory interaction results in inhibition of ascending medullary projections to higher centers.
  - Opiate binding within the PAG may be preterminal on the ascending spinofugal projection. This preterminal action would inhibit input into the medullary core and mesencephalic core.
  - Outflow from the PAG can serve to act to modulate excitability of dorsal raphe and locus coeruleus, from which *ascending* serotonergic and noradrenergic projections originate to project to limbic/forebrain. Considerable evidence emphasizes the importance of these forebrain projections in modulating emotionality and may thus account for the affective actions of opiates.

SPINAL ACTION

- The local action of opiates in the spinal cord will selectively depress the discharge of spinal dorsal horn neurons activated by small (high-threshold) but not large (low-threshold) afferents (Figure 22–5).

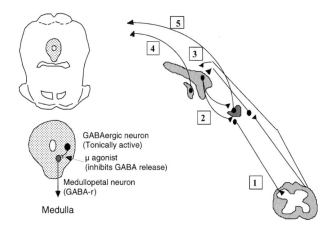

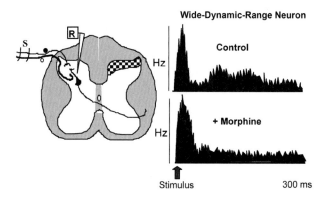

FIG. 22–4. Upper left: Mesencephalic periaqueductal gray (PAG). Lower left: Organization of opiate action within the PAG. In this schema, mu opiate actions block the release of GABA from tonically active systems that otherwise inhibit the excitatory projections to the medulla leading to activation of PAG outflow. Right: Overall organization of the mechanisms whereby a PAG mu opiate agonist can alter nociceptive processing: (1) PAG projection to the medulla that serves to activate bulbospinal projections releasing serotonin and/or noradrenaline at the spinal level. (2) PAG outflow to the medulla, where local inhibitory interaction results in an inhibition of ascending projections. (3) Opiate binding on the ascending spinofugal projection inhibits input into the medullary core and mesencephalic core. (4 and 5) Outflow from the PAG can serve to act to modulate excitability of dorsal raphe and locus coeruleus from which ascending serotonergic and noradrenergic projections originate to project to limbic/forebrain (see text for the details).

FIG. 22–5. Model for electrically activating large and small afferents while recording using single-unit microelectrodes of the activity in a single dorsal horn wide-dynamic-range neuron. As indicated on the right (showing the response over a 300-ms time trace), this brief electrical stimulus leads to an initial burst of activity reflecting the activation of the neurons by the rapidly conducting large (low-threshold) afferents followed by the activity evoked by the more slowly conducting (higher-threshold A∂ and C fibers). As indicated (bottom), the application of morphine results in a selective depression of the later discharge.

- Intrathecal administration of opioids reliably attenuates the response of the animal to a variety of unconditioned somatic and visceral stimuli that otherwise evoke an organized escape behavior in all species thus far examined.
- The mechanism of this is considered below.
  - Receptor autoradiography with opiate ligands has revealed that binding is limited for the most part to the substantia gelatinosa, the region in which small afferents show their principal termination.
  - Dorsal rhizotomies result in a significant reduction in dorsal horn opiate binding, suggesting that a significant proportion is associated with the primary afferents.
  - Confirmation of the presynaptic action is provided by the observation that opiates reduce the release of primary afferent peptide transmitters such as substance P contained in small primary afferents.
  - The presynaptic action corresponds to the ability of opiates to prevent the opening of voltage-sensitive Ca^{2+} channels, thereby preventing release.
  - A postsynaptic action was demonstrated by the ability of opiates to block the excitation of dorsal horn neurons evoked by glutamate, reflecting a direct activation of the dorsal horn.
  - The activation of potassium channels leading to a hyperpolarization is consistent with the direct postsynaptic inhibition.
- The joint ability of spinal opiates to reduce the release of excitatory neurotransmitters from C fibers as well as decrease the excitability of dorsal horn neurons is believed to account for the powerful and selective effect on spinal nociceptive processing (see Figure 22–6).

PERIPHERAL ACTION

- It has been a principal tenet of opiate action that these agents are "centrally" acting.
- However, it is evident that opiate receptor protein is synthesized in the DRG and transported to the central and the peripheral terminals.
- Direct application of opiates to the peripheral nerve can, in fact, produce a local anesthetic-like action at high concentrations, but this is most evident with agents having high lipid partition coefficients (cLogP) (eg, meperidine) and less by agents with low cLogP (morphine). Further, the effects are not naloxone-reversible. Thus, these effects on nerve conduction are not the result of an opiate receptor interaction, but are believed to reflect a "nonspecific" action, blocking sodium channels.
- In pain models examining normal animals, it can be readily demonstrated that if the agent does not readily

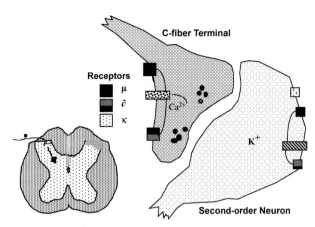

FIG. 22–6. Summary of the anticipated organization of opiate receptors in the dorsal horn regulating nociceptive processing. As indicated, mu (μ), delta (∂), and kappa (κ) bindings are high in the dorsal horn, particularly in the region associated with the termination of small unmyelinated afferents (C fibers). A significant proportion of these sites are located on the terminals of the small afferent as suggested by the loss of such binding after rhizotomy. In addition, there is a postafferent terminal localization of these sites that is apparently coupled through Gi protein to K^+ channels, leading to hyperpolarization of the neuron. Occupancy of the presynaptic mu and delta sites reduces the release of sP and/or CGRP in part by inhibition of the opening of voltage-sensitive calcium channels (see text for further discussion).

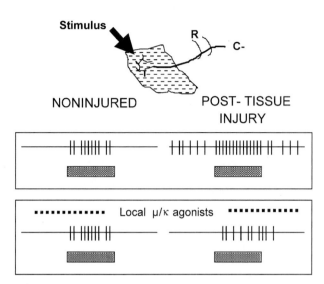

FIG. 22–7. Top: Activity arising from a single C fiber that is innervating a patch of uninjured (left) and injured (right) skin in the presence of a strong mechanical stimulus applied to the receptive field (as indicated by the horizontal bar). Note spontaneous activity and enhanced response in C fiber innervating injured skin. Similar observations are made in a variety of injury models such as in the knee joint and cornea. Bottom: The application of opioid agonists to the tissue results in suppression of the spontaneous activity otherwise noted in the C fiber. The opioids will not block activity evoked by an otherwise adequate mechanical or thermal stimulus. These effects are naloxone-reversible (see text for further discussion).

penetrate the brain, its opiate actions on acute nociception are limited.

- Alternately, studies employing the direct injection of mu opiates into peripheral sites have demonstrated that under conditions of inflammation where there is a "hyperalgesia," the local action of opiates can be demonstrated to exert a normalizing effect on the exaggerated thresholds.
- Models in which peripheral opiates appear to work are those that possess a significant degree of inflammation and are characterized by a hyperalgesic component.
- This has been demonstrated for the response to mechanical stimulation applied to inflamed paw or inflamed knee joints.
- Previous work has demonstrated that local opiates in the knee joint and in the skin can reduce the firing of spontaneously active afferents observed when these tissues are inflamed (Figure 22–7).
- It is possible, for example, that the opiates may act on inflammatory cells that are present and are releasing cytokines and products that activate or sensitize the nerve terminal.
- Application of opiates at the nerve axon will not exert opiate action locally but will have effects through systemic redistribution.
- Application of opiates at a wound site will exert opiate actions locally (and is naloxone reversible).

OPIATE MECHANISMS IN HUMANS

Supraspinal

- In humans, it is not feasible to routinely assess the site of action within the brain where opiates may act to alter nociceptive transmission.
- Intracerebroventricular opioids, however, have been employed for pain relief in cancer patients.
- An important characteristic of this action is that the time of onset is relatively rapid for even the water-soluble agent morphine.
- Gamma scans of human brain have shown that morphine, even 1 h after injection, remains close to the ventricular lumen.
- Accordingly, it seems probable that the site of opiate action in the human must lie close to the ventricular lumen.
- In this regard, preclinical studies in species such as the primate have emphasized the importance of the periaqueductal sites.

Spinal

- There is an extensive literature indicating that opiates delivered spinally can induce powerful analgesia in humans.

- The pharmacology of this action has been relatively widely studied, and it appears certain that mu, delta, and, to a lesser degree, kappa agonists are effective after intrathecal or epidural delivery.
- The effects of spinal opiates are reversed by low doses of systemic naloxone. Importantly, the activity of spinally delivered agents in modulating acute nociception in animal models, such as for the rodent hot plate, reveals an ordering of activity that closely resembles that observed in humans for controlling clinical pain states.

Peripheral

- It was shown that intra-articular morphine injections have a powerful sparing effect on subsequent analgesics.
- The appropriate controls emphasize that the effects are indeed mediated by a local action and not by a CNS redistribution.
- A wide variety of studies have been undertaken to indicate that there is a modest antihyperalgesic effect of opiates reflecting a peripheral effect.

SUMMARY

- Opiates produce a potent modulatory effect on nociceptive transmission by an action on specific receptors that reflects a modulation of afferent input at both the spinal and supraspinal levels.
- This effect reflects an action mediated by specific membrane receptors that are G protein coupled to generally depress the excitability of the cell (increased potassium conductance) and prevent transmitter release (block opening of voltage-gated calcium channels).
- In addition, these agents have strong influence over the affective component of pain by mechanisms that reflect on actions mediated at the supraspinal level though forebrain systems mediating emotionality.
- These joint effects on neuraxial function provide an important key to defining the analgesic actions exerted by these classes of receptor agonists.

BIBLIOGRAPHY

Abbadie C, Lombard MC, Besson JM, Trafton JA, Basbaum AI. Mu and delta opioid receptor-like immunoreactivity in the cervical spinal cord of the rat after dorsal rhizotomy or neonatal capsaicin: an analysis of pre- and post-synaptic receptor distributions. *Brain Res.* 2002;930:150–162.

Alvarez VA, Arttamangkul S, Dang V, et al. Mu-opioid receptors: ligand-dependent activation of potassium conductance, desensitization, and internalization. *J Neurosci.* 2002;22:5769–5776.

Andreev N, Urban L, Dray A. Opioids suppress spontaneous activity of polymodal nociceptors in rat paw skin induced by ultraviolet irradiation. *Neuroscience.* 1994;58:793–798.

Burkey TH, Ehlert FJ, Hosohata Y, et al. The efficacy of delta-opioid receptor-selective drugs. *Life Sci.* 1998;62:1531.

Chu LF, Angst MS, Clark D. Opioid-induced hyperalgesia in humans: molecular mechanisms and clinical considerations. *Clin J Pain.* 2008;24(6):479–496. doi:10.1097/AJP.0b013e31816b2f43.

Dionne RA, Lepinski AM, Gordon SM, Jaber L, Brahim JS, Hargreaves KM. Analgesic effects of peripherally administered opioids in clinical models of acute and chronic inflammation. *Clin Pharmacol Ther.* 2001;70:66–73.

Fields HL. Pain modulation: expectation, opioid analgesia and virtual pain. *Prog Brain Res.* 2000;122:245–253.

Grudt TJ, Williams JT. Opioid receptors and the regulation of ion conductances. *Rev Neurosci.* 1995;6:279–286.

Kelly E. Efficacy and ligand bias at the μ-opioid receptor. *Br J Pharmacol.* 2013;169(7):1430–1446. doi:10.1111/bph.12222.

Kent JM, Mathew SJ, Gorman JM. Molecular targets in the treatment of anxiety. *Biol Psychiatry.* 2002;52:1008–1030.

King T, Ossipov MH, Vanderah TW, Porreca F, Lai J. Is paradoxical pain induced by sustained opioid exposure an underlying mechanism of opioid antinociceptive tolerance? *Neurosignals.* 2005;14(4):194–205.

Kondo I, Marvizon JC, Song B, et al. Inhibition by spinal mu- and delta-opioid agonists of afferent-evoked substance P release. *J Neurosci.* 2005;25(14):3651–3660.

Lazorthes YR, Sallerin BA, Verdie JC. Intracerebroventricular administration of morphine for control of irreducible cancer pain. *Neurosurgery.* 1995;37:422–428.

Levac BA, O'Dowd BF, George SR. Oligomerization of opioid receptors: generation of novel signaling units. *Curr Opin Pharmacol.* 2002;2:76–81. doi:10.1016/j.neuropharm.2013.03.039.

Lord JA, Waterfield AA, Hughes J, Kosterlitz HW. Endogenous opioid peptides: multiple agonists and receptors. *Nature.* 1977;267:495–499.

Martin WR. History and development of mixed opioid agonists, partial agonists and antagonists. *Br J Clin Pharmacol.* 1979;7(suppl 3):273S–279S.

Martin WR, Eades CG, Thompson JA, Huppler RE, Gilbert PE. The effects of morphine- and nalorphine-like drugs in the nondependent and morphine-dependent chronic spinal dog. *J Pharmacol Exp Ther.* 1976;197:517–532.

Minami M, Satoh M. Molecular biology of the opioid receptors: structures, functions and distributions. *Neurosci Res.* 1995;23:121–145.

Ninkovic M, Hunt SP, Kelly JS. Effect of dorsal rhizotomy on the autoradiographic distribution of opiate and neurotensin receptors and neurotensin-like immunoreactivity within the rat spinal cord. *Brain Res.* 1981;230:111–119.

Nunes-de-Souza RL, Graeff FG, Siegfried B. Strain-dependent effects of morphine injected into the periaqueductal gray area of mice. *Braz J Med Biol Res.* 1991;24:291–299.

Pasternak GW. Studies of multiple morphine and enkephalin receptors: evidence for mu1 receptors. *Adv Exp Med Biol.* 1988;236:81–93.

Pasternak GW. The pharmacology of mu analgesics: from patients to genes. *Neuroscientist.* 2001;7:220–231.

Pasternak GW. Opioids and their receptors: are we there yet? *Neuropharmacology*. 2014;76:198–203.

Ramberg DA, Yaksh TL. Effects of cervical spinal hemi-section on dihydromorphine binding in brainstem and spinal cord in cat. *Brain Res*. 1989;483:61–67.

Stein C, Clark JD, Oh U, et al. Peripheral mechanisms of pain and analgesia. *Brain Res Rev*. 2009;60:90–113.

Stein C, Machelska H, Binder W, Schafer M. Peripheral opioid analgesia. *Curr Opin Pharmacol*. 2001;1:62–65.

Wallace M, Yaksh TL. Long-term spinal analgesic delivery: a review of the preclinical and clinical literature. *Reg Anesth Pain Med*. 2000;25:117–157.

Wang WH, Lovick TA. The inhibitory effect of the ventrolateral periaqueductal grey matter on neurones in the rostral ventrolateral medulla involves a relay in the medullary raphe nuclei. *Exp Brain Res*. 1993;94:295–300.

Wei LN, Loh HH. Regulation of opioid receptor expression. *Curr Opin Pharmacol*. 2002;2:69–75.

Williams JT, Ingram SL, Henderson G, et al. Regulation of μ-opioid receptors: desensitization, phosphorylation, internalization, and tolerance. *Pharmacol Rev*. 2013;65(1):223–254. doi:10.1124/pr.112.005942.

Yaksh TL. Inhibition by etorphine of the discharge of dorsal horn neurons: effects on the neuronal response to both high-and low-threshold sensory input in the decerebrate spinal cat. *Exp Neurol*. 1978;60:23–40.

Yaksh TL. Direct evidence that spinal serotonin and noradrenaline terminals mediate the spinal antinociceptive effects of morphine in the periaqueductal gray. *Brain Res*. 1979;160:180–185.

Yaksh TL. Spinal opiate analgesia: characteristics and principles of action. *Pain*. 1981;11:293–346.

Yaksh TL. Pharmacology and mechanisms of opioid analgesic activity. *Acta Anaesthesiol Scand*. 1997;41(1 Pt 2):94–111.

Yaksh TL, Rudy TA. Narcotic analgesics: CNS sites and mechanisms of action as revealed by intracerebral injection techniques. *Pain*. 1978;4:299–359.

23 LOCAL ANESTHETICS IN CLINICAL PRACTICE

Anand C. Thakur, MD

HISTORICAL PERSPECTIVE

- The use of local anesthetics as an analgesic and anesthetic has been known for centuries. Cocaine obtained from the leaves of the coca plant (*Erythroxylon coca*) is well known to the indigenous tribes of South America for centuries.
- In 1885, Gaedicke used cocoa leaves to isolate the alkaloid erythroxylin.
- In 1860, Albert Niemann isolated cocaine from the *Erythroxylon* extract.

- In 1884, Sigmund Freud, renowned father of psychoanalysis, shared his knowledge about the mouth-numbing properties of cocaine with fellow intern Karl Koller, an Austrian ophthalmologist, at Vienna's City Hospital.
- Koller was the first person to recognize the tissue-numbing properties of cocaine.
- In 1884, he demonstrated the use of topical cocaine for eye surgery. This led to the widespread use of cocaine as a local anesthetic in many diverse medical fields from ear, nose, and throat surgery to dentistry.
- In the 1940s, Holger Erdtman in Stockholm, Sweden, was a young researcher who was examining the alkaloid pesticide gramine and via analytic testing, which then was tasting of the chemical compound, noted that this compound numbed the lips and tongue.
- In 1943, Erdtman's assistant Nils Lofgren synthesized lidocaine from a series of aniline derivatives.
- After four relatively "simple" changes in molecular structure, lidocaine was produced. Sweden remains the birthplace and progenitor of local anesthetics such as bupivacaine and ropivacaine.

MECHANISM OF ACTION OF LOCAL ANESTHETICS

- Local anesthetics act by way of blockade/deactivation of sodium channels in a reversible fashion. The propagation of action potentials is blocked by local anesthetics at the sodium channel in peripheral central spinal or epidural nerves.
- Peripheral nerves are mixed nerves containing both afferent and efferent fibers that may be either myelinated or unmyelinated.
- The mechanism of local anesthetic blockade in the central neuraxis is the same as for peripheral nerves but also involves blockade of sodium channels of the spinal nerve roots both intradural and extradural.
- Neuraxial administration of local anesthetics allows for multiple actions at different sites within the spinal cord. Blockade of sodium and potassium channels in the dorsal horn inhibits propagation of nociceptive impulses.
- Neuraxial administration of local anesthetics in clinically significant doses inhibits release of substance P and possibly augments analgesia by presynaptic inhibition as well.

BASIC NEURAL ANATOMY

- The basic composition of the nerve fiber is as follows: an individual axon is surrounded by a sheath called the endoneurium composed of non glial cells.

- Nerve fibers are gathered into bundles and fascicles. These fascicles are surrounded by connective tissue, called the epineurium.
- All mammalian nerves greater than 1 μm in diameter are myelinated.
- Myelinated nerve fibers are further repeatedly covered by Schwann cells. This forms a bilayer lipid membrane.
- Nodes of Ranvier separate segmented myelinated regions.
- Unmyelinated nerve fibers (diameter less than 1 μm) are lightly encased by Schwann cells and do not have nodes of Ranvier.
- Increasing degrees of myelination and nerve diameters leads to increased conduction velocity.
- Myelin acts like electrical installation of wires and allows for saltatory conduction of nerve impulses.

HOW LOCAL ANESTHETICS BLOCK NERVES

- Peripheral and central nerves are made up of cells. A lipoprotein membrane separates the stable internal axoplasm from the volatile external cellular environment.
- This is the focal point of ion local anesthetic action. This lipoprotein cellular membrane is transversed by protein-lined, ion-transmitting channels (sodium, potassium, ATPase channel) that allow for the conduction and propagation of electrical signals.
- The baseline state of electrical activity of the cell is generated by the intracellular potassium ion concentration and potassium ion gradient. This is called the resting membrane potential.
- The resting membrane potential is roughly −90 mV.
- There are two main ion gradients working to maintain the resting membrane potential. There is active outward transport of the sodium ions and inward transport of potassium ions.
- An action potential is generated by an influx of sodium ions down its concentration gradient, across the sodium/potassium/ATPase channel into the intracellular matrix.
- Threshold potential is a critical potential in which a rapid self-sustaining inward current of sodium ions results in depolarization.
- After this phase is complete, the cell reverts to its resting state with the use of the sodium/potassium/ATPase pump.
- Local anesthetics cause a reversible blockade of the sodium channel. This leads to a temporary stabilization or deactivation of the sodium channel. The cell is not allowed to reach the threshold potential.

- After local anesthetic blockade, an action potential cannot be propagated down the axonal segment. Local anesthetics block the inward sodium current that allows for cellular propagation of the action potential. The resting membrane potential remains unchanged and the blocked nerve remains polarized.
- Local anesthetics cause depolarizing and stabilizing types of blockade. This is similar to neuromuscular blockade by curare, which is a depolarizing agent.
- Local anesthetics act at the intracellular binding site of the sodium channel. They induce voltage-dependent conformational changes in the sodium channel via electrostatic forces that keep the channel in a closed confirmation.
- This closed conformation does not allow for sodium ion passage into the cell. Thus, the cell is rendered deactivated. In this setting, there is no propagation of action potentials.
- It is important to note that the local anesthetics exist in dynamic equilibrium. Local anesthetics exist in dynamic equilibrium of two forms: an uncharged base and a pronated quaternary amine.
- It is most likely the pronated quaternary amine that is responsible for the predominant effects of local anesthetics. The uncharged, hydrophilic molecule cannot pass through the semipermeable nerve membrane. The neutral/uncharged face form diffuses easily through the lipophilic membrane.
- After local anesthetic diffuses through the semipermeable nerve sheath and membrane, it is pronated and forms the discharged cationic form allowing attachment to the receptor.
- Another mechanism by which local anesthetics block nerve conduction is lipid solubility. The uncharged local anesthetics in the base form pass through the lipophilic membrane. On entry into the cell via lipid solubility, the local anesthetic disassociates into the cationic form. This cation then blocks and locks the sodium channel.

THE MINIMUM BLOCKING CONCENTRATION

- The minimal blocking concentration (C_m) is the dose of local anesthetic that effectively stops nerve impulse propagation.
- For myelinated nerves, the C_m is different; three successive nodes of Ranvier must be blocked by local anesthetic for nerve conduction to be stopped.
- Nerve impulses can skip over one or two blocked nodes of Ranvier, but usually not over three successive nodes.
- CBL is critical blocking length for a nerve. This value is proportional to the diameter of the nerve and spans

three nodes that must be blocked by local anesthetic to ensure effective blockade. Thicker motor nerves have a longer distance between nodes. The internodal distance between smaller fibers, such as A-delta or C fibers (pain fibers), is much less.

USE-DEPENDENT/FREQUENCY-DEPENDENT BLOCKADE

- The sodium channel exists in dynamic flux of several conformational states. Local anesthetics can bind to these different conformational states.
- Excitation is when the sodium channel changes from a resting-closed state to an activated-open state. Postdepolarization channel is in an inactivated-closed state.
- Local anesthetics bind more easily to the activated and inactivated states than to the resting state. Consequently, repeated depolarization allows for more effective local anesthetic binding.
- This repeated depolarization obviously leads to a more effective conduction blockade with repetitive stimulation.
- This phenomenon is known as frequency-dependent or use-dependent blockade.

PHYSICAL CHEMISTRY OF LOCAL ANESTHETICS

- Local anesthetics are organic amines with either an ester or an amide linkage separating the lipophilic ringed head from the hydrophilic hydrocarbon tail.
- Local anesthetic amines are weakly basic, lipid soluble, water insoluble (hydrophobic), and unstable.
- Local anesthetics are stored as a hydrochloride salt (acidic-stable), and when combined with water they ionize to form local anesthetic cation (positively charged quaternary amine) and acid anion (uncharged amine) that exist in equilibrium.
- The Henderson–Hasselbalch equation is given as follows:

  - $pK_a = pH - \log\left[\dfrac{\text{base}}{\text{conjugate acid}}\right]$

  - Here, pK_a is the dissociation constant (the likelihood of an acid to stay in a charged or an uncharged state).
  - If the concentration of base equals the concentration (log 1 = 0) of acid, then $pK_a = pH$.
  - Lower pK_a values represent a greater percentage of local anesthetic in an unionized fraction. Benzocaine's pK_a is 3.5. It exhibits as a highly lipophilic neutral base under physiologic conditions. Benzocaine penetrates tissue membranes quite easily but requires a

high concentration because relatively few cations are present for sodium channel blockade.
  - pK_a values of commonly used local anesthetics are between 7.6 and 8.9. This implies that less than half of the molecules exist in the unionized state. The onset of blockade may be slowed in this state.
  - Sodium bicarbonate can be added to local anesthetics to decrease acidity and increase the unionized fraction to increase the speed of onset of local anesthetic blockade.
  - Infection can cause a localized tissue acidosis that hampers local anesthetic activity.
- Lipid solubility:
  - Lipid solubility of local anesthetics affects both tissue penetration and uptake in nerve membrane.
  - Lipid solubility is determined by comparing the solubility of a compound in a polar solvent, such as octanol, with solubility in water. This is the participation coefficient.
  - Lipid solubility roughly follows and predicts local anesthetic potency and duration of action (along with protein binding), and varies inversely with latency or time of onset of local anesthetic effect.
- Differential local anesthetic blockade:
  - Neurons and nerve fibers are classified by conduction velocity. They are stratified into three basic types: A, B, and C.
  - Conduction velocity is increased by greater diameter and myelination.
  - Most peripheral nerves are mixed in nature containing a combination of myelinated and nonmyelinated fibers that carry both afferent and efferent activities.
  - Group A fibers: large myelinated, somatic afferent and efferent fibers.
  - Group B fibers: smaller myelinated, preganglionic and autonomic efferent fibers.
  - Group C fibers: smallest fibers and unmyelinated afferent axons.
  - Differential nerve blockade allows blockade of the (pain-carrying) A-delta and C fibers without interfering with the motor fibers that allow for ambulation.
  - Solid blockade of even the thickest nerve fibers requires that at least three successive nodes of Ranvier are bathed in local anesthetic.
  - Blocks for pain relief are usually done with the weakest possible concentration of local anesthetic solution; thus, large volumes are usually needed to decrease the likelihood of incomplete block and allow for nerve penetration.
  - In a mixed nerve, the nerve fibers closer to the outer layer (innervating proximal regions) of the nerve fascicle are blocked first by diffusion of local anesthetic

and the inner core (innervating distal regions) is blocked subsequently.

○ This explains why local anesthetic blockade produces a proximal anesthesia with subsequent involvement of distal structures.

- Clinical potency use of local anesthetic:
  ○ Clinical potencies for local anesthetics are influenced by multiple factors including local anesthetic diffusion and nerve fiber type.
- Tachyphylaxis:
  ○ Tachyphylaxis is a clinical condition in which repeated administration of the same dose of local anesthetic leads to decreased efficacy.
  ○ The exact mechanism for tachyphylaxis has not been identified, although possible peripheral and central theories have been proposed.
  ○ The peripheral theory postulates a possible pharmacokinetic mechanism. This involves following radiolabeled lidocaine concentrations after repeated injection, which shows decreased local anesthetic content in nerves and skin after repeated injection.
  ○ There is also a potential central theory involving spinal cord sensitization and "windup." This involves smaller dosing intervals during which tachyphylaxis does not develop. If the dosing interval between repeated injections is increased, this allows for the return of pain. Tachyphylaxis results more quickly.
  ○ Tachyphylaxis occurs for peripheral nerve blocks, central neuraxial blocks, and all local anesthetic compounds (amides, esters, and both short- and long-acting local agents).

ADDITIVES TO LOCAL ANESTHETICS

- Epinephrine:
  ○ The addition of epinephrine to a local anesthetic can increase the duration of blockade and intensity of blockade, and decrease systemic absorption of local anesthetic.
  ○ Epinephrine's mechanism of action involves vasoconstriction but is not completely identified. Most local anesthetics produce a relative vasodilation.
  ○ Ropivacaine is not greatly affected by the use of epinephrine.
  ○ Epinephrine counteracts the inherent basilar debilitating properties of most local anesthetics.
  ○ Epinephrine also has an α_2-adrenergic receptor interaction in the brain and spinal cord. This may account for direct analgesic effects from the use of epinephrine with local anesthetics.
- Alkalinization:
  ○ The addition of bicarbonate for alkalinization of local anesthetics cannot increase the amount of local anesthetic existing in the neutral lipid-soluble form that can more easily cross the lipid neural bilayer membrane.
  ○ Alkalinization of local anesthetics can be achieved by adding bicarbonate, keeping the pH within the normal range. The pK_a of the lipid-soluble, neutral form of local anesthetic ranges from 7.6 to 8.9.
  ○ The clinical effect of alkalinizing plain solutions of local anesthetic varies with the type of local anesthetic and the type of regional block performed. Clinical data suggest that alkalinization works best with lidocaine for axillary block, lidocaine and bupivacaine for epidural block, and mepivacaine for sciatic and femoral blocks.
- α_2 agonist:
  ○ When added to local anesthetics, α_2 agonists such as clonidine act via both spinal and supraspinal adrenergic receptors.
  ○ Clonidine has a direct inhibitory action on peripheral A fibers and C fibers.
  ○ The exact mechanism of action is still undecided. There appears to be both a central neuraxial (possible reduction in spinal cord metabolism and vasoconstriction of blood flow) and a peripheral analgesic synergy of action.
  ○ Clonidine works effectively and synergistically in peripheral, epidural, and intrathecal administration with local anesthetics to increase local anesthetic activity.

SYSTEMIC ANALGESIA FROM LOCAL ANESTHETICS

- Intravenous lidocaine (1–5 mg/kg) has been used for the treatment of postoperative, cancer, and chronic neuropathic pain states. The mechanism of action involves impulse conduction blockade in peripheral nerves.
- Although the mechanism is again not clearly elucidated, both a peripheral and a central mechanism have been proposed.
- The peripheral mechanism involves decreased spontaneous activity in injured peripheral C fibers, A-delta fibers, and dorsal root ganglia.
- The central mechanism involves central sensitization ("windup"), in addition to nociceptive reflexes and hippocampal pyramidal cells in the spinal cord.

CLINICAL PHARMACOKINETICS

- The systemic absorption of local anesthetics can lead to both central nervous system and cardiovascular toxicity.

- Factors that influence the extent of absorption of local anesthetics are as follows:
  ○ Injection site
  ○ Dose
  ○ Physiochemical properties
  ○ Use of epinephrine
- Rate of systemic absorption varies directly with blood flow and vascularity. Increased vascularity, versus fat deposition, will have more rapid and complete uptake of local anesthetic.
- Generally rate of absorption going from highest to lowest is as follows: intercostal > caudal > epidural > brachial plexus > sciatic/femoral.
- The dose relationship between total anesthetic load and systemic absorption/peak blood levels is linear. It is not affected by anesthetic concentration and/or speed of injection.
- More potent local anesthetics with greater lipid solubility and protein binding will result in lower systemic concentrations and C_{max}.

TOXICITY OF LOCAL ANESTHETICS

- Central nervous system toxicity of local anesthetics is a dose-dependent process.
- Central nervous system toxicity presents as a circumoral numbness and facial tingling restlessness, vertigo, tinnitus, and slurred speech. Tonic–clonic seizures are an end point.
- Local anesthetic potency for systemic CNS toxicity directly parallels actual local anesthetic blocking potency.
- CNS toxicity can be increased in certain medical conditions such as acidosis and increased pco_2, arterial hypoxemia, and increased cerebral perfusion or decreased protein binding (of local anesthetics) states.
- Speculative mechanism of actions of local anesthetic neurotoxicity involves injury to Schwann cells, inhibition of fast axonal transport, and disruption of the blood–nerve barrier.
- Local anesthetics are neuronal depressants. In the central nervous system, depression of cortical inhibitory neurons causes unopposed excitatory pathway activity. This leads to a possible onset of seizure activity.
- If seizure activity occurs, airway management and cardiopulmonary resuscitation may be required. Supportive treatment can involve benzodiazepines or propofol to help reduce central nervous system seizure activity.

INTRATHECAL LIDOCAINE

- Intrathecal lidocaine (5% in 7.5% dextrose) administered via small-bore intrathecal catheter and single-shot spinal administration has resulted in a high incidence (20%–40%) of transient neurologic symptoms (TNSs).
- Multiple factors play a role in the etiology of TNSs such as ambulatory anesthesia status, lidocaine, and a lithotomy position.
- Because of the multifactorial possible etiology, TNS does not appear to be concentration dependent.
- TNS does not usually show neurologic deficits and electrophysiologic changes, and is successfully managed conservatively with NSAIDs and trigger point injections.
- TNS as a neurologic entity is under question.

CARDIOVASCULAR TOXICITY OF LOCAL ANESTHETICS

- The cardiovascular system can better tolerate the toxic effects of local anesthetics than can the central nervous system. This is a dose-dependent phenomenon. Local anesthetic potency for CVS toxicity directly reflects anesthetic potency of the agent.
- Bupivacaine, etidocaine, ropivacaine, and levobupivacaine have a different cardiovascular toxicity than does lidocaine.
- Lidocaine toxicity is manifested by hypertension, bradycardia, and hypoxia.
- Bupivacaine toxicity is manifested by sudden cardiovascular collapse and ventricular dysrhythmias, and is markedly resistant to resuscitation techniques.
- Both ropivacaine and levobupivacaine are single isomer compounds and not racemic. They offer a 30%–50% reduction in cardiotoxic profile and are still capable of cardiovascular collapse and ventricular dysrhythmias.
- Cardiac toxicity is a reflection of local anesthetic blockade of sodium channels, the impact of which is felt in impaired automaticity and conduction of cardiac impulses. This is identified on EKG as widening of the QRS complex and prolongation of the PR interval.
- Systemic cardiovascular toxicity: nucleus tractus solatarii in the medulla in part regulates autonomic control of the cardiovascular system. Bupivacaine diminishes activity in this region prior to the development of hypotension in rats. Also direct intracerebral injection of bupivacaine can elicit dysrhythmias and cardiovascular collapse.
- Bupivacaine also has a peripheral effect on the autonomic and vasomotor systems that may contribute to its cardiovascular toxicity. Bupivacaine peripherally inhibits sympathetic reflexes. There is also a direct vasodilating component to bupivacaine that may augment cardiovascular collapse.

- Local cardiovascular toxicity:
  - Although all local anesthetics block cardiac conduction through a dose-dependent blockade of sodium channels, bupivacaine has a much stronger binding affinity to both the resting and the inactivated sodium channels than does lidocaine.
  - Bupivacaine also dissociates much more slowly from sodium channels during diastole. Lidocaine fully dissociates from sodium channels during diastole and little accumulation occurs. Bupivacaine dissociates slowly during diastole and accumulates at normal physiologic heart rates between 60 and 180 bpm.
  - Bupivacaine toxicity rescue: administration of 20% intravenous lipid has been advocated for the treatment of sudden cardiac collapse following bupivacaine administration.
  - The mechanism of action of lipid rescue is not fully clear. It has been postulated that lipid is able to extract bupivacaine or other lipophilic agents from aqueous plasma or tissue targets, thus reducing the effective concentration. Solutions for lipid rescue are lipid emulsions.
  - Propofol is not administered for this purpose. High doses of propofol as needed for lipid rescue would be potentially lethal.
  - Lipidrescue.org, the American Society of Regional Anesthesia, and Task Force on Local Anesthetic Systemic Toxicity are good resources.

ALLERGIC REACTIONS

- The incidence is less than 1%. Most adverse reactions to local anesthetic are due to additives or systemic toxicity from excess plasma concentration of local anesthetic.
- Tachycardia and palpitations may come from the systemic absorption of epinephrine.
- Amino ester local anesthetics that produce metabolites such as *para*-amino benzoic acid are more likely to produce hypersensitivity-type reactions than are amino-amides.

IN SUMMATION/KEY POINTS

- Local anesthetics as a class of medication have contributed greatly to the field of medicine.
- Local anesthetics with different potency use and side effects are commonly used in regional anesthesia and pain medicine.
- A clear understanding of neuroanatomy in electrophysiology is necessary prior to the use of local anesthetics in pain medicine.

- A more detailed explanation of each specific local amide or ester local anesthetic can be found in any standard textbook of anesthesiology.
- Local anesthetics can be potentiated by epinephrine, alkalinization, opioids, and α_2 agonists.
- Toxicity profile of local anesthetics, both CNS and cardiovascular, should be recognized.

BIBLIOGRAPHY

Abram SE, Yaksh TL. Systemic lidocaine blocks nerve injury induced hyperalgesia and nociceptive driven spinal sensitization and rats. *Anesthesiology.* 1997;86:1262–1272.

Chang KSK, Yang M, Andersen MC. Clinically relevant concentrations of bupivacaine inhibited rat aortic barrier receptors. *Anesth Analg.* 1994;78:501.

Eisenach JC, De Kock M, Klimscha W. L4 to adrenergic agonist for regional anesthesia. A clinical review of clonidine (1984–1985). *Anesthesiology.* 1996;85:655.

Groban L, Deal DD, Vernon JC, et al. Cardiac resuscitation after incremental overdose with lidocaine, bupivacaine, levo bupivacaine, and ropivacaine in anesthetized dogs. *Anesth Anal.* 2001;92:37–43.

JAW Wildsmith Professor Emeritus at the University of Dundee–Lidocaine. A More Complex Story Then 'Simple' Chemistry Suggests. Vol 43, History of Anaesthesia Society.

Ladd LA, Chang DH, Wilson KA, et al. Effects of CNS site directed carotid arterial infusions of bupivacaine, levo bupivacaine and ropivacaine in sheet. *Anesthesiology.* 2002;97:418–428.

Liu SS, Hodgson PS. Local anesthetics. In: Barash PG, Cullen BF, Stoelting RF, eds. *Clinical Anesthesia.* Philadelphia: Lippincott-Raven; 2006:453–471.

Liu SS, McDonal SB. Current issues in spinal anesthesia. *Anesthesiology.* 2001;94:888–906.

Miller RD, Pardo MC. *Basics of Anesthesia.* 6th ed. Philadelphia: Elsevier/Churchill Livingstone; 2011:130–142.

Ohmura S, Kawada M, Ohta T, et al. Systemic toxicity and assist patient in bupivacaine, levo bupivacaine, or ropivacaine infused rats [comment]. *Anesth Anal.* 2001;93:743–748.

Pickering AE, Waki H, Headley PM, Paton JF. Investigation of systemic bupivacaine toxicity using in situ perfused working heart–brainstem preparation of the rat. *Anesthesiology.* 2002;97:1550–1556.

Raja SN, Fishman S, Liu S, et al. Benzon Essentials of Pain Medicine and Regional Anesthesia. 2nd ed. 2005:558–565.

Rosenberg PH, Veering BT, Urmey WF. Maximum recommended dose is of local anesthetics: a multifactorial concept. *Reg Anesth Pain Med.* 2004;29:564–575.

Sinnot CJ, Cogswell LP III, Johnson A, Strichartz GR. On the mechanism by which epinephrine potentiates lidocaine and peripheral nerve block. *Anesthesiology.* 2003;98:181–188.

Tucker GT. Safety and numbers. The role of pharmacokinetics in the local anesthetic toxicity: the 1993 ASRA lecture. *Reg Anesth.* 1994;19:155.

Ueda W, Hirakawa M, Mori K. Acceleration of epinephrine absorption by lidocaine. *Anesthesiology.* 1985;63:717.

Waldman S, Winnie A. *Interventional Pain Management*. 1st ed. 1996:151–163.

Walker SM, Goudas LC, Cousins MJ, Carr DB. Combination spinal anesthesia chemotherapy: a systematic review. *Anesth Analg*. 2002;95:674–715, 202.

24 MISCELLANEOUS DRUGS

Timothy Furnish, MD
Mark S. Wallace, MD

INTRODUCTION

- Some drugs are known to result in analgesia in certain pain syndromes.
- The coadministration of these agents with traditional analgesics such as the opioids, NSAIDs, and acetaminophen may enhance analgesic efficacy.

MONOCLONAL ANTIBODIES

- The use of monoclonal antibodies is an emerging field in pain management. There are no agents approved specifically for pain but several that are approved for rheumatoid arthritis (RA) with the effect of reducing pain. Others have been investigated specifically for pain including anti-nerve growth factor (NGF).
- Monoclonal antibodies on the market for RA include anti-TNF agents and one anti-IL6 antibody.
- Advantages include long half-life, novel approach, and lack of typical analgesic adverse effect profile.
- Disadvantages include high cost, IV or SQ route of administration, and risks of surgery.

ALPHA-2 AGONISTS

- α_2 agonists are mostly used for acute pain with the exception of tizanidine (see the section "Muscle Relaxants").
- α_2 agonists exhibit opioid-sparing effects with significant sedation but without respiratory depression. Hypotension and bradycardia are potentially limiting adverse effects.
- Clonidine: studied in a wide variety of routes including intravenous, intrathecal, epidural, oral, transcutaneous, and perineural. Systemic administration reduces opioid requirements postoperatively. Intrathecal clonidine improves the analgesic efficacy of intrathecal morphine. When combined with local anesthetics,

clonidine can increase the duration of peripheral nerve blocks.
- Dexmedetomidine: Not widely studied for pain. There is evidence for an opioid-sparing effect in postoperative pain, but limited evidence for reducing pain intensity.

BENZODIAZEPINES

- Benzodiazepines are frequently used as an adjuvant in the treatment of acute pain; however, the use in chronic pain is controversial. The exception is clonazepam, which has anticonvulsant activity and is used in the treatment of neuropathic pain. Diazepam also has anticonvulsant properties.
- The analgesic efficacy is not well established, but these agents appear to alter the unpleasantness of the pain experience.
- Benzodiazepines have muscle relaxant properties and may be used as a muscle relaxant and antispasmodic (see below).

CANNABINOIDS

- The two cannabinoid receptors are CB1 and CB2.
- CB1 is located in the brain, spinal cord, and on primary sensory nerve terminals. CB2 is found on microglia, monocytes, macrophages, and B and T lymphocytes.
- Activation of CB1 receptors reduces pain transmission.
- Activation of CB2 on peripheral cells has been shown to decrease inflammatory cell mediator release, plasma extravasation, and the sensitization of afferent terminals.
- The term cannabinoid refers to a variety of compounds that are (1) derived from cannabis plants (phytocannabinoids), (2) endogenous cannabinoids (referred to as endocannabinoids), and (3) synthetic cannabinoids.
- The main psychoactive compound in cannabis is delta-9-tetrahydrocannabinol (THC).
- Other major cannabinoids found in the cannabis plant are cannabidiol (CBD) and cannabinol (CBN). CBD is the second most abundant compound in the plant next to THC. It is less psychoactive than THC and appears to enhance the effects of THC.
- Clinical trials with inhaled cannabis have shown it to be effective in chronic pain.
- Cannabis-based extracts (CBME) are derived by extracting compounds directly from the marijuana plant. There are currently two CBME that have undergone clinical trials, Cannador and Sativex. Cannador is a CBME delivered in oral capsules with differing THC:CBD ratios. Sativex is a sublingual spray

containing both THC and CBD that is currently in phase III trials for cancer pain.

- There are two synthetic cannabinoids on the market (dronabinol and nabilone) and one in clinical trials (ajulemic acid). Dronabinol is an oral synthetic THC that has been on the market since 1985 to treat nausea associated with chemotherapy and as an appetite stimulant in HIV/AIDS. It recently went generic, which may eliminate some of the cost issues that precluded the use in the treatment of pain. Nabilone is a semi-synthetic analogue of THC that is about 10 times more potent with a longer duration. In the United States, it is FDA approved to treat chemotherapy-induced nausea. Both have had mixed results in treating chronic pain. Ajulemic acid is a synthetic analogue of THC currently in clinical trials for pain.

DISEASE-MODIFYING ANTIRHEUMATIC DRUGS

- The use of DMARDs in the treatment of RA, psoriatic arthritis (PsA), and ankylosing spondylitis (AS) has been associated with an improvement in pain from these conditions. The studies of these drugs have not used pain as a primary end point but typically do report the effects on pain.
- Nonbiologic DMARDs include sulfasalazine, methotrexate, cyclosporine, and hydroxychloroquine.
- Most studies show improvement in pain with initiation of nonbiologic DMARDs for RA and PsA. Only sulfasalazine has been shown to reduce pain in AS.

CNS STIMULANTS

AMPHETAMINES

- Amphetamines are sometimes coadministered with opioids to treat opioid-induced sedation.
- They are occasionally used to treat depression.
- The amphetamines may enhance the analgesic effect of the opioids.
- The mechanism of amphetamine potentiation of opioid analgesia is unknown. The amphetamines stimulate the release of catecholamines in the central nervous system that may result in analgesia.

CAFFEINE

- Caffeine enhances the analgesic effect of aspirin and acetaminophen.
- It is used in a variety of pain syndromes including cancer, headache, and postoperative pain.
- The mechanism of action for relieving pain is unclear.

CORTICOSTEROIDS

- The corticosteroids have been proven efficacious in advanced cancer pain including diffuse bony metastasis, tumor infiltration of neural structures, and spinal cord compression.
- The pain relief may be the result of a direct analgesic action, reduction in swelling due to anti-inflammatory activity, or modulation of pain transmission pathways.
- Corticosteroids have also been shown to reduce pain from inflammatory arthopathies, and complex regional pain syndrome, but no good evidence exists for systemic administration for radiculopathy.
- Long-term relief of pain from corticosteroids may result from cytosolic receptors that carry the steroid to the cell nucleus resulting in changes in gene expression.
- Significant adverse effects of steroid administration are immune suppression, myopathy, Cushing syndrome, osteoporosis, hypertension, hyperglycemia, increased appetite, and insomnia.

MUSCLE RELAXANTS

- The use of the muscle relaxants is usually limited to the treatment of acute muscle problems with placebo-controlled studies showing short-term efficacy in low back pain.
- Because of abuse potential, dependence, and lack of long-term efficacy data, the use of the muscle relaxants for chronic pain is controversial.
- Muscle relaxants can be classified as either antispasticity agents or antispasmodic agents. Antispasticity agents are used for upper motor neuron conditions such as cerebral palsy or multiple sclerosis. There is no clear clinical efficacy difference between the antispasticity agents.
- Antispasmodic agents are used to treat musculoskeletal conditions such as acute low back pain or muscle strain.
- Site of action:
  - The muscle relaxants act at several sites important to muscle tone:
    - Direct effect on skeletal muscle fiber (dantrolene—rarely used due to significant risk of hepatotoxicity)
    - Polysynaptic reflexes (benzodiazepines, baclofen, tizanidine, other muscle relaxants)
    - Descending facilitatory systems (benzodiazepines, other muscle relaxants)

BACLOFEN

- Antispasmodic effect is thought to be secondary to GABA-B activity at the spinal cord level that inhibits evoked release of excitatory amino acids.

- Baclofen is indicated for the treatment of spasticity secondary to spinal cord injury.
- There exists anecdotal evidence that baclofen may have intrinsic analgesic efficacy.
- Common signs of baclofen withdrawal include hallucinations, autonomic dysfunction, and altered mental status.

BENZODIAZEPINES

- Antispasmodic effect is thought to be neuronal inhibition secondary to postsynaptic GABA-A activity at the spinal cord level.
- Long-term use for chronic pain or spasticity is controversial due to disturbances in REM sleep, dependence, and difficulties in withdrawing the drug.

TIZANIDINE

- Tizanidine is a centrally acting α_2-adrenergic agonist that reduces spasticity by increasing presynaptic inhibition of motor neurons in the spinal cord.
- It is similar in structure to clonidine but has 1/10th to 1/50th of the potency of clonidine in lowering blood pressure.
- It is indicated for the treatment of spasticity secondary to spinal cord injury and multiple sclerosis.
- It may have intrinsic analgesic activity secondary to the α_2-adrenergic agonist effect.
- Adverse effects of tizanidine include somnolence and dry mouth.

OTHER SKELETAL MUSCLE RELAXANTS

- Examples of centrally acting muscle relaxants include carisoprodol, metaxalone, chlorzoxazone, cyclobenzaprine, methocarbamol, and orphenadrine citrate.
- Mechanisms of action are not well understood but may be due to inhibition of interneuronal activity in the descending reticular formation and spinal cord.
- There is no evidence that any one muscle relaxant is more efficacious than the others.
- Cyclobenzaprine is structurally similar to the tricyclic antidepressants. Most recent and largest clinical trial data support the use of cyclobenzaprine for short term.
  - Side effects include sedation and anticholinergic effects including dry mouth.
- Long-term bedtime dosing may be beneficial in the treatment of fibromyalgia.
- Carisoprodol: metabolized to meprobamate—a DEA-scheduled drug with abuse potential.

- Metaxalone: limited and old efficacy data:
  - Least sedating of the muscle relaxants with a short elimination half-life

NMDA RECEPTOR ANTAGONISTS

- The *N*-methyl-D-aspartate (NMDA) ionophore is located on postsynaptic neurons in the dorsal horn.
- The release of glutamate from the presynaptic terminal activates the NMDA ionophore channel causing an influx of calcium, which initiates a cascade of effects resulting in spinal "windup."
- Binding sites that influence the influx of calcium include:
  - A magnesium binding site within the channel that when occupied inhibits channel opening
  - A glycine binding site that must be occupied in order for the channel to open
  - A polyamine site that regulates NMDA ionophore excitability
- The use of ketamine for chronic pain has been limited due to the IV route of administration and narrow therapeutic window with significant psychomimetic effects.
- Ketamine has benefit for late-stage cancer pain, especially in the opioid-tolerant patient. In postsurgical pain, the use of ketamine has been shown to reduce pain scores, postoperative opioid requirements, and nausea. Ketamine infusions have also shown benefit in complex regional pain syndrome.

BIBLIOGRAPHY

Bell RF, Dahl JB, Moore RA, Kalso EA. Perioperative ketamine for acute postoperative pain. *Cochrane Database Syst Rev.* 2009.

Chan AKM, Cheung CW, Chong YK. Alpha-2 agonists in acute pain management. *Expert Opin Pharmacother.* 2010; 11:2849–2868.

Chessell IP, Dudley A, Billinto A. Biologics: the next generation of analgesic drugs? *Drug Discov Today.* 2012;17:875–879.

Chou R, Huffman LH. Medications for acute and chronic low back pain: a review of the evidence for an American Pain Society/American College of Physicians clinical practice guideline. *Ann Intern Med.* 2007;147:505–514.

Fields H. *Pain.* New York: McGraw Hill; 1987.

Forrest WH, Brown BW, Brown, CR, et al. Dextroamphetamine with morphine for the treatment of postoperative pain. *N Engl J Med.* 1977;296:712–715.

Graceley RH, McGrath P, Dubner R. Validity and sensitivity of ratio scales of sensory and affective verbal pain descriptors: manipulation of affect by diazepam. *Pain.* 1978;5:19–29.

Hocking G, Cousins MJ. Ketamine in chronic pain management: an evidence-based review. *Anesth Analg.* 2003;97:1730–1739.

Irving G, Wallace M. *Pain Management for the Practicing Physician.* New York: WB Saunders; 1996:37–47.

Laska EM, Sunshine A, Mueller F, et al. Caffeine as an adjuvant analgesic. *JAMA.* 1986;251:45–50.

Leppert W, Buss, T. The role of corticosteroids in the treatment of pain in cancer patients. *Curr Pain Headache Rep.* 2012;16:307–313.

Mackey S, Feinberg S. Pharmacologic therapies for complex regional pain syndrome. *Curr Pain Headache Rep.* 2007;11:38–43.

Max MB, Gilron IH. Antidepressants, muscle relaxants, and N-methyl-D-aspartate receptor antagonists. In: Loesser J, ed. *Bonica's Management of Pain.* Philadelphia: Lippincott, Williams and Wilkens; 2001:1710–1726.

Pertwee RG. The diverse CB1 and CB2 receptor pharmacology of three plant cannabinoids: delta 9-tetrahydrocannabinol, cannabidiol, and delta-9-tetrahydrocannabivarin. *Br J Pharmacol.* 2008;153(2):199–215.

Russo EB, Hohmann AG. Role of cannabinoids in pain management. In: *Comprehensive Treatment of Chronic Pain by Medical, Interventional, and Integrative Approaches: The American Academy of Pain Medicine Textbook on Patient Management.* New York, NY: Springer; 2013:181–197.

See S, Ginzburg R. Skeletal muscle relaxants. *Pharmacotherapy.* 2008;28:207–213.

Steiman AJ, Pope JE, Thiessen-Philbrook H, et al. Non-biologic disease modifying antirheumatic drugs (DMARDs) improve pain in inflammatory arthritis: a systematic literature review of randomized controlled trials. *Rheumatol Int.* 2013;33:1105–1120.

Wallace MS. Pharmacologic treatment of neuropathic pain. *Curr Pain Headache Rep.* 2001;5:138–150.

ACUTE PAIN MANAGEMENT

25 INTRAVENOUS AND SUBCUTANEOUS PATIENT-CONTROLLED ANALGESIA

Anne M. Savarese, MD

INTRODUCTION

- Patient-controlled analgesia (PCA) is a method of pain relief that allows patients to self-administer small doses of opioids on demand, accompanied by the option of a continuous infusion, using a programmable infusion device.
- Versatile routes and pharmacologic agents exist for PCA administration; this chapter focuses on intravenous and subcutaneous routes of opioid analgesia.

RATIONALE

- After initial loading doses establish effective analgesia, frequent small doses of self-administered opioid maintain a patient's plasma opioid concentration above the minimal effective analgesic concentration (MEAC), and below higher concentrations at which unwanted side effects occur.
- Analgesic administration is simplified so that patients self-select when and how much medication they receive to achieve optimal pain relief.
- Immediate access, avoidance of injections, independence from nursing requests, better pain relief, acceptable side effects, and a sense of control contribute to patient acceptance and satisfaction with this technique.
- PCA technology permits flexible titration and efficiently adjusts to the wide interindividual variability in analgesic requirements between patients and even within patients.

- Variability in patient-specific opioid requirements during PCA therapy results from differences in pharmacokinetics, pharmacodynamics, pain intensity, psychological makeup, anxiety, and previous painful experiences.
- Programmable features and PCA device engineering contribute to the excellent overall patient safety and efficacy of this technique.

ADVANTAGES

- Superior pain relief with better patient satisfaction compared with conventional parenteral "on-demand" opioid analgesia.
- Painless routes of administration (intravenous or subcutaneous/clysis).
- Avoids peaks, valleys, fluctuations, and delays in pain relief associated with conventional modes of opioid administration.
- Provides prompt and lasting comfort.
- Flexible, titratable, and individualized therapy.
- Facilitates rapid establishment of analgesia as well as equianalgesic transitions.
- Potential for fewer opioid-related side effects compared with intermittent bolus administration.
- Enhanced sense of control over the pain experience for the patient.
- Decreased nursing burden compared with conventional methods.
- Safe application in most hospital environments and clinical practice settings.

DISADVANTAGES

- Requires specialized equipment (the PCA infusion device or "pump") and secure IV access.

- Requires patient self-awareness and cognitive understanding of the principles of PCA therapy for safe and effective use.
- Potential for operator and/or mechanical errors in prescribing, programming, or delivery.

INDICATIONS

- Relief of moderate to severe acute pain.
- Postoperative pain.
- Burns/trauma.
- Sickle cell crisis/pancreatitis/painful medical conditions
- Cancer pain/painful conditions related to cancer treatment.

CONTRAINDICATIONS

- History of device tampering with prior PCA use or prior opioid diversion or substance abuse.
- Developmental disability/cognitive impairment that limits understanding of PCA therapy or limits successful interface with the pump.
- Patient or parent/family refusal.

INTRAVENOUS OPIOID PCA: "HOW TO DO IT"

THE PCA PRESCRIPTION

- The clinician selects an opioid analgesic in a standard concentration and then programs the PCA pump parameters, including the clinician loading dose, the PCA or patient demand/bolus dose, the dosing interval or "lockout," the time-based cumulative dose limit, and the optional "background" continuous/basal infusion.
- Efficacy and safety of IV PCA are probably more significantly related to these prescribed parameters than the choice of any particular opioid analgesic.
- The PCA microprocessor programs, stores, and retrieves data, so that the patient's pattern of analgesic use and cumulative consumption can be reviewed. Suggested prescriptions for IV PCA are found in Table 25-1.

CHOICE OF OPIOID

- The ideal agent for IV PCA should be rapid in onset, be intermediate in duration, be lacking in potentially toxic metabolites, have a broad safety margin, and be readily available, inexpensive, and stable in solution.
- Clinicians typically choose morphine, hydromorphone, and fentanyl for IV PCA.
- Use of meperidine is discouraged for PCA because of the risk of normeperidine accumulation and Central Nervous System (CNS) toxicity with repetitive administration.
- Initial choice of opioid is influenced by practitioner familiarity and preference, as well as patient factors such as prior drug responses, clinical status, comorbid conditions, and expected clinical course.
- As individual patient's responses vary, the clinician must be prepared to switch agents on an equianalgesic basis if the patient fails to achieve adequate relief or if dose-limiting or intolerable side effects occur.
- Opioids for IV PCA should be compounded in standard concentrations, preferably equianalgesic on a volume basis, to facilitate safe and convenient conversions during PCA therapy. "Smart" technology such as bar code labeling of PCA infusion bags or syringes may decrease the risk for programming and medication errors.

ADJUNCTS TO OPIOIDS FOR INTRAVENOUS PCA

- Adjunct nonopioid medications may be used to supplement opioid IV PCA.
- These may diminish opioid consumption (aka "opioid-sparing"), decrease the incidence and severity of side effects (especially nausea, vomiting, and sedation), and improve pain relief as well as contribute to enhanced overall patient satisfaction.
- NSAIDs (ketorolac), α-agonists (clonidine, dexmedetomidine), and NMDA antagonists (ketamine) have been shown to provide these advantages when used in combination with IV PCA opioids.
- Low-dose IV naloxone (0.25–1 mcg/kg/h) may decrease the incidence and severity of opioid-associated adverse effects.

TABLE 25-1 **Suggested Intravenous PCA Prescriptions for Opioid-naïve Adult Patients**

DRUG	STOCK SOLUTION (mg/mL)	LOADING DOSE (mg)	PCA DOSE (mg)	LOCKOUT (min)	BASAL RATE (mg/h)	1-H LIMIT (mg)
Morphine	1	2–5	0.5–2.5	5–10	0.5–1	8–15
Hydromorphone	0.2	0.4–0.8	0.1–0.4	5–10	0.1–0.4	1.2–2.4
Fentanyl	0.020	0.020–0.050	0.025–0.050	5–10	0.010–0.050	0.080–0.200

CLINICIAN LOADING DOSE

- Successful PCA therapy requires that an analgesic plasma level be established by one or more loading doses before the patient begins to maintain this level by self-administering smaller PCA demand doses.
- During ongoing PCA therapy, some patients with large or fluctuating analgesic requirements may need upward titration of their PCA prescription preceded by reloading.
- The clinician loading dose feature allows initial and subsequent loading doses to be administered via the PCA device, rather than by separate syringe boluses.
- This facilitates convenient and rapid titration to effective analgesia, and records all administered opioid doses in the PCA history software, thereby improving patient safety, limiting diversion, and simplifying opioid tracking.

PCA DEMAND OR BOLUS DOSE

- The optimal PCA dose should provide measurable and satisfactory pain relief with minimal side effects.
- The patient must "feel" the effect of an adequate dose to encourage patient interaction and prevent frustration with the PCA device.
- Too large of a dose will lead to unpleasant (nausea, pruritus, dysphoria) or even potentially dangerous (sedation, confusion, respiratory depression) side effects, which may inhibit the patient from interacting with the PCA device or necessitate interruption or discontinuation of PCA therapy. Most critical events occur within the first 24 h of postoperative use of IV opioids, so vigilant attention to dosing is warranted especially when initiating IV PCA.
- Decreased starting doses are suggested for patients with advanced age, hepatic or renal insufficiency, preexisting respiratory or neurologic impairment, congestive heart failure, morbid obesity, or sleep apnea.
- Increased starting doses are appropriate for opioid-tolerant patients and those using opioids to control preexisting pain.
- In general, if the patient consistently receives more than three to four PCA doses per hour, PCA "demands" significantly exceed delivered doses, and pain scores remain unacceptable, then an upward titration of 25%–50% in the PCA dose is indicated.

DOSING INTERVAL OR "LOCKOUT"

- The lockout is the programmed delay between the last delivered dose and the next possible dose, despite the number of demands made by the patient to the PCA device.
- The dosing interval should reflect the time to peak effect for the prescribed opioid, so that successive doses are not administered before the patient "feels" the effect of the preceding self-administered dose.
- This is a critical programming feature affecting both safety and efficacy of PCA.
- The lockout interval protects the patient from repetitive doses (despite demands) over too short a period, while permitting an adequate interval for successive doses to be successfully delivered so that an effective analgesic plasma concentration is achieved, especially during active periods with increased analgesic requirements.

TIME-BASED CUMULATIVE DOSE LIMIT

- This parameter allows the clinician to restrict the patient's cumulative opioid consumption to a time-based limit, typically 1 or 4 h.
- This feature permits the flexibility of a "generous" PCA dose and "short" lockout, while still protecting the patient from an excessive cumulative dose over the specified period.
- This is particularly useful when prescribing for patients with expected periods of increased analgesic requirements, such as physical therapy and dressing changes.

BACKGROUND CONTINUOUS/BASAL INFUSION

- For most adult patients, the routine use of a background or concurrent opioid infusion is not recommended, as it results in increased opioid consumption, increased side effects, increased risk for respiratory depression, and no real improvement in sleep, quality of pain relief, or patient satisfaction.
- Therapy must be individualized, and clinical experience suggests that some adult patients (such as those who are opioid-tolerant) may benefit from a continuous infusion.
- Children and adolescents may benefit more from background infusions than adults.
- In general, for acute pain patients the basal should provide about one third of the expected total hourly opioid requirement, while for chronic or cancer pain patients the reverse ratio is suggested, and the basal should provide about two thirds of the expected total hourly opioid requirement.

INTRAVENOUS OPIOID PCA: TIPS FOR SUCCESS

- PCA technology facilitates on-demand analgesia tailored to the individual patient's needs, but it is not to be mistaken for a "one size fits all" or "set it and forget it" therapy. The success, efficacy, and safety of PCA are enhanced by:

○ Management by a dedicated acute pain service (APS) staffed with pain management specialists (physicians and nurses) and support from clinical pharmacists.

○ Prescribing of PCA, as well as supplemental analgesics, sedatives, and transition analgesics, restricted to one team only, ideally an APS.

○ Establishment of institutional policies, standardization of opioid formulations, standardized PCA order sets, clinical decision-making support for dosing, opioid conversions, and IV to oral transitions, and side effect management, as well as management guidelines to ensure consistent clinical practice.

○ Staff education about PCA and pain management in general.

○ Patient/family education about PCA therapy (see Table 25-2).

○ Proactive side effect management, especially for common "nuisance" side effects such as pruritus and nausea (see Table 25-3).

○ Standardized and frequent assessment/monitoring of vital signs, pain scores, sedation levels, side effects, patient responses to interventions, and pump prescription/programming verification. Currently there is no consensus regarding the efficacy of costly technology-supported monitoring (eg, continuous pulse oximetry or capnography) in improving safety with IV opioid PCA.

○ "Built-in" PCA delivery system safety features, such as "smart" pump technology, locked drug reservoirs, tamper resistance, security locks and programming access codes, antisyphon valves, antireflux valves,

---

TABLE 25-2   PCA Teaching Tips for Patients and Families

1. Demonstrate how to use the pump to give pain medication, and have the patient return the demonstration
2. Instruct the patient in the use of an appropriate assessment tool (pain scale)
3. Inform the patient that the goal of PCA therapy is a resting pain score (PS) of 0–3, and a dynamic PS of ≤5 on a 0–10 pain scale, where 0 = no pain and 10 = the worst pain possible
4. Instruct the patient and family members that only the patient is to activate the PCA demand button
5. Explain that the lockout interval is set so that the patient cannot receive additional medication until the last dose has had some effect, regardless of how often the demand button is pressed
6. Instruct the patient to "premedicate" by activating the PCA demand button once or twice about 10–15 minutes before engaging in activities such as getting out of bed, ambulating, coughing, using incentive spirometry, and participating in physical therapy or dressing changes
7. Instruct the patient to notify the nurse for unrelieved pain despite using the PCA pump, nausea/vomiting, itching, dysphoria/confusion, and difficulty passing urine or stool
8. Instruct the patient to notify the nurse of any unexpected change in the site, severity, or quality of the pain being treated, as this may represent a new medical or surgical condition requiring investigation or treatment
9. Instruct the patient and family members to notify the nurse if the pump alarms. Be sure the patient can correctly identify the "normal" sound the pump makes when delivering medication
10. Refute common myths about opioid-based acute pain management; that is, inform the patient and family that the risk for addiction is negligible, that overdose is unlikely given the pump's safety features, and that inadequate analgesia or unpleasant side effects will be aggressively managed
11. Counsel the patient that concurrent use of unprescribed medications, such as street drugs and alcohol, increases the risk for serious side effects, and may disqualify the patient from receiving PCA therapy
12. Basal rates need to be used with caution due to possibility of overdose
13. These are typical starting doses that can be modified by increasing or decreasing these doses based on the clinical setting

---

TABLE 25-3   Opioid-related Side Effect Management for Adult Patients on PCA Therapy

SIDE EFFECT	INTERVENTION
Nausea/vomiting	Reduce the dose of opioid
	Ondansetron 4–8 mg IV q6h
	or
	Dolasetron 12.5–25 mg IV q12h
	or
	Prochlorperazine 10–25 mg IV q6h
	or
	Metoclopramide 10–20 mg IV q6h
	or
	Droperidol 0.625–1.25 mg IV q6h
	Switch opioid
Pruritus	Reduce the dose of opioid
	Diphenhydramine 25–50 mg IV q6h
	or
	Hydroxyzine 25–50 mg PO q6h
	Switch opioid
	Naloxone 0.25–1.0 µg/kg/h IV continuous infusion
Urinary retention	Reduce the dose of opioid
	Bladder catheterization
	Naloxone 100-µg IV push × 1
	Bethanechol 0.05 mg/kg SC × 1
Constipation	Stool softener and stimulant laxative in combination, for example, Senokot
Respiratory depression	Stop any background continuous/basal infusion
	Remove the PCA button from the patient's reach
	Stimulate the patient and call for help
	Remain with the patient and continue frequent assessments
	Provide supplemental oxygen
	Assess airway patency, respiratory effort, and Spo2
	Provide airway management (chin lift, jaw thrust, BVM ventilation) as appropriate
	Administer naloxone 100 mcg IVP q3–5 min
	Consider naloxone IV infusion 0.5–3 µg/kg/h
	Avoid coadministration of any other respiratory depressants (eg, sedatives/hypnotics)
	Depending on episode severity and patient response, consider resuming PCA at a decreased dose without basal or, alternatively, moving patient to a monitored setting

and user-friendly interfaces to diminish the risks for operator programming errors.
  ○ Ongoing institutional quality management and improvement.

DISCONTINUING PCA THERAPY

- Adult postoperative patients are usually ready to transition from IV PCA to oral analgesics when normal gastrointestinal function is restored and opioid consumption is about 50 mg parenteral morphine equivalents over the preceding 24 h.
- For patients with mild to moderate pain, conventional fixed combination agents (eg, acetaminophen/oxycodone) are usually sufficient.
- The first dose of oral analgesic is given while the patient still has access to the PCA pump; if at the time of peak effect for the oral agent the patient is comfortable, the pump is discontinued, and the transition oral analgesics are continued.
- For patients with more severe pain or documented higher opioid requirements, long-acting or sustained-release oral opioids (eg, methadone, morphine [MS Contin], oxycodone hydrochloride [OxyContin]) should be considered.
- Patients with significant ongoing opioid requirements who are otherwise ready to transition but still cannot take enteral medications are candidates for long-acting transdermal fentanyl (Duragesic).
- The long-acting agent is begun, the background continuous/basal infusion is stopped, and the patient is allowed access to PCA demand doses for about another 18–24 h.
- Ultimately an equianalgesic conversion is made so that about two thirds to three fourths of the expected 24-h requirement is achieved by the long-acting agent, with the remainder provided in immediate-release or short-acting opioids.

SUBCUTANEOUS (CLYSIS) OPIOID PCA

- Clysis administration of opioid analgesics is conceptually similar to intravenous analgesia when provided in a continuous plus demand paradigm (ie, basal plus PCA mode).
- It provides more rapid and reliable absorption, as well as essentially painless administration, when compared with intramuscular injections.
- It finds application in patients with limited intravenous access who, in all other respects, meet eligibility criteria for opioid PCA.
- Typical patients for clysis opioid PCA are pediatric, elderly, debilitated, or in hospice, with significant

acute pain superimposed on chronic pain, such as that from malignancy or end-stage medical conditions.
- The only real contraindication is localized infection at the site for placement of the indwelling subcutaneous needle, and because there are multiple suitable skin sites, this contraindication is an infrequent impediment.
- The key differences compared with intravenous PCA are:
  ○ Clysis cannot accommodate rapid titration or dose adjustments such as the intravenous route; clysis does provide adequate prolonged analgesia.
  ○ The rate-limiting step in prescribing clysis is the amount of fluid volume the subcutaneous tissue depot can absorb; in general, volumes greater than 1.0 mL/h are not recommended.
  ○ Compounding the opioid analgesic solution must account for this hourly volume restriction; in general, opioids are concentrated to about 10 times what would be used for conventional IV PCA analgesia; most often morphine and hydromorphone are used.
  ○ Many patients managed with clysis opioid analgesia are opioid tolerant, so double-check that the solution and programming will deliver appropriate individualized doses while respecting the hourly volume restriction.
- Preferred sites are the infraclavicular area, abdomen, lateral aspect of the thigh, or flexor aspect of the forearm, as these provide easy inspection for site "healthiness," minimize needle motion/dislodgement, and allow adequate patient mobility after attachment to PCA pump tubing.
- Be sure to choose sites away from scars, wounds, or ostomy sites.
- The skin is topically anesthetized with EMLA and aseptically prepared with chlorhexidine or povidone, a preflushed sterile 25- or 27-gauge steel butterfly or specialty subcutaneous needle is inserted, and then a sterile transparent dressing is applied with benzoin adhesive.
- The pump prescription should provide almost all the expected hourly requirement as the basal, with only a few PCA demand doses per day for incident pain.
- Sites may be rotated electively at about five days, or sooner if redness, irritation, or leakage occurs.
- Side effect management is similar to that for intravenous opioid PCA.

BIBLIOGRAPHY

American Society of Anesthesiologists Task Force on Pain Management. Practice guidelines for acute pain management in the perioperative setting: an updated report by the American Society of Anesthesiologists Task Force on

Pain Management, Acute Pain Section. *Anesthesiology.* 2012;116(2):248–273.

Grass JA. Patient-controlled analgesia. *Anesth Analg.* 2005;101:S44–S61.

Hong D, Flood P, Diaz G. The side effects of morphine and hydromorphone patient-controlled analgesia. *Anesth Analg.* 2008;107:1384–1389.

Hudcova J, McNicol E, Quah C, Lau J, Carr DB. Patient controlled opioid analgesia versus conventional opioid analgesia for postoperative pain. *Cochrane Database Syst Rev.* 2006;(4): CD003348.

Joint Commission. *Sentinel Event Alert Issue 49: Safe Use of Opioids in Hospitals.* August 8, 2012.

Macintyre PE. Intravenous patient-controlled analgesia: one size does not fit all. *Anesthesiol Clin North America.* 2005;23:109–123.

Werner MU, Soholm L, Rotbell-Nielsen P, Kehlet H. Does an acute pain service improve postoperative outcome? *Anesth Analg.* 2002;95:1361–1372.

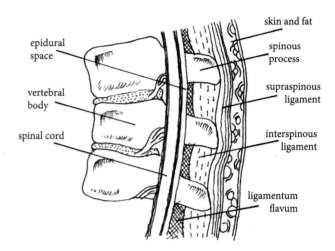

FIG. 26-1. Anatomy of the epidural space.

26   EPIDURAL ANALGESIA

Nicole Khetani, MD

Jon Y. Zhou, MD

Eugene R. Viscusi, MD

BACKGROUND AND HISTORY

- Epidural analgesia has become a cornerstone of acute pain management.
- Since 1901, when Corning described the epidural space, and the first application of the use of cocaine in the epidural space, and through the pioneering efforts of Edwards, Hingson, Pages, Dogliotti, Tuohy, and Bromage, epidurals have become a standard modality for anesthesia. In the United States, Dr. Brian Ready has been a driving force behind the establishment of epidural analgesia as the modality of choice for postoperative pain control.
- Improvements in technique, equipment, and pharmacological science have made the technique one of the most widely used in the anesthesiologist's arsenal.

ANATOMY

- The epidural space exists between the dura and the ligamentum flavum. Since the dura and ligamentum flavum adhere to one another, the epidural space is

a "potential" space that surrounds the dural sac (see Figure 26-1 and Table 26-1):
  ○ Anteriorly, it is bounded by the posterior longitudinal ligament.
  ○ Posteriorly, it is bounded by the ligamentum flavum and the periosteum of the laminae.
  ○ Laterally, the intervertebral foramina containing their neural elements abut the epidural space.
  ○ The epidural space is continuous with the paravertebral space via the intervertebral foramina.

TABLE 26-1   **Main Features of Spinal Anatomy**

Cervical region	Very thin ligamentum flavum
	C7 and T1 have almost horizontal spinous processes
	C7 is the most prominent cervical spine (vertebra prominens)
	Lamina are shaped like narrow rectangles
	Usually exhibits marked negative pressure (especially if seated)
Thoracic region	Very narrow lateral epidural space
	Ligamentum flavum is thicker than in cervical region, but thinner than midlumbar
	T5 through T9 spinous processes are the most angulated, making midline approach difficult
	Spinal cord is narrowest in the thoracic region
	Usually exhibits negative pressure (especially when seated)
Lumbar region	Widest epidural space
	Spinal cord ends at about L1–2 (in adults)
	Ligamentum flavum is the thickest
	Spinous processes have the least angulation
	Lumbar region has very prominent lateral epidural veins

- ○ Superiorly, the space is anatomically closed at the foramen magnum where the spinal dura attaches to the dura of the cranium.
- ○ Caudally, the epidural space ends at the sacral hiatus and is closed by the sacrococcygeal ligament.
- The epidural space contains areolar connective tissue, fat, lymphatics, arteries, veins, and the spinal nerve roots as they exit the dural sac and pass through the intervertebral foramina.
- Posteriorly, the epidural space is entered by passing through the skin and thin subcutaneous tissue between the vertebral spinous processes, piercing the two relatively soft supraspinous and interspinous ligaments, and entering the often leathery tough ligamentum flavum that posteriorly bounds the epidural space. Especially in the elderly, the ligamentum flavum can be calcified (making it difficult to distinguish from bone) or uncharacteristically soft.
- Lacunae in the midline (especially in the thoracic region) may result in false loss of resistance when placing an epidural.

EPIDURAL MEDICATIONS

GENERAL COMMENTS REGARDING EPIDURAL MEDICATIONS

- All medications placed in the epidural space must be free of preservatives.
- It is of utmost importance to maintain sterility when preparing epidural infusions or when drawing up bolus drugs.
- The incidence of contamination or medication error is lower when infusions are prepared centrally by the hospital pharmacy. Standard concentrations and additives should be established with the pharmacy.
- Standardization of epidural analgesic medications for the institution may reduce costs and minimize waste by allowing batch preparation.
- Epidural medications must be appropriately labeled (see Figure 26-2).
- Epidural catheters must be readily identifiable by medical and nursing staff to prevent unintended injection or infusion of inappropriate agents. Brightly colored

> **FOR EPIDURAL ADMINISTRATION ONLY**

FIG. 26-2. Typical epidural medication label.

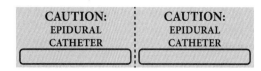

FIG. 26-3. Typical epidural catheter label.

flag-type labels near the injection port end of the catheter work well for this purpose (see Figure 26-3).
- The principles of contamination control and proper compounding procedures must meet USP <797> requirements in health care settings to ensure compound sterile preparations' sterility and accuracy. All epidural infusions must be prepared in a pharmacy (ISO class 2, under a sterile vacuum hood). The intent of USP <797> is to prevent harm to patients from incorrect ingredients and from microbial contamination (nonsterility) in compound sterile preparations. In addition, any medication delivered into the epidural space should be drawn up immediately prior to administration.

DELIVERY METHODS

- In the past, epidural medications were delivered as single-shot boluses, on an as-needed basis. This practice, however, inevitably leads to periods of inadequate analgesia and increased severity of unwanted side effects resulting from high peak medication levels.
- Newer methods employ continuous and patient-controlled epidural analgesia (PCEA) infusions to alleviate the shortcomings of periodic bolus dosing.
- The PCEA method allows for a continuous level of epidural analgesia with small boluses initiated by the patient to cover periods of increased discomfort (eg, transfers or physical therapy).
- Continuous versus intermittent bolus dosing provides superior analgesia with lower incidence and severity of side effects.
- Several types of delivery devices are available for use in delivering epidural medications.
  - ○ *Syringe pumps*: Deliver contents of the syringe during a specified period (minutes, hours, or days). Typically, however, these pumps cannot accommodate the quantities of medication in the concentrations usual for epidural analgesia. Syringe pumps are best used for intrathecal drug delivery and pediatric acute pain management.
  - ○ *Peristaltic pumps*: Deliver medications from a flexible reservoir via tubing that is squeezed between rollers that create a positive displacement of a given volume of fluid with each cycle. Peristaltic pumps

TABLE 26-2 Common Infusion Rates of Epidural Solutions

Thoracic catheter	4–10 mL/h
Lumbar catheter	10–18 mL/h

can accommodate larger volumes (50–1000 mL) than are possible with syringe pumps and are typically employed for epidural analgesia. Peristaltic pumps permit various flow rates and more PCEA options.

  o *Elastomeric reservoir pumps*: Force fluid from an elastomeric pressurized medication reservoir through a flow regulator. These devices are less well suited for in-hospital epidural drug administration because of limited available flow rates.

- Delivery rates for adult epidural analgesic solutions are usually between 4 and 20 mL/h. The lower rates are used for thoracic epidural infusions; the higher rates are used for lumbar infusions (Table 26-2).

LOCAL ANESTHETICS

- Local anesthetics play the central role in epidural analgesia but require adequate "spread" within the epidural space to produce a segmental block. Poor distribution may produce a "patchy" or one-sided block.
- The major sites of action for epidural local anesthetics are the spinal nerve roots and dural cuff regions, where there is a relatively thin dural cover. Only a small fraction of local anesthetic diffuses into the subarachnoid space.
- In epidural analgesic applications, as opposed to spinal and epidural anesthesia, selection of the local anesthetic is typically not dependent on the drug's onset time or duration of action. The particular local anesthetic is chosen primarily because of its block density and side effect profile.
- The local anesthetics used most frequently for epidural analgesic purposes are bupivacaine and ropivacaine.
- Bupivacaine, the most widely studied local anesthetic, has been associated with significant cardiotoxicity and motor (vs sensory) blockade.
- Commercially available bupivacaine is a racemic mixture of the *R* and *S* isomers. The *R* isomer is more cardiotoxic than the *S* moiety.
- Ropivacaine, the *S* isomer of the propyl analog of bupivacaine, has a safer cardiotoxic profile than the bupivacaine enantiomers.
- The most common side effects associated with epidural local anesthetics are hypotension, numbness, and motor block. These effects can be managed by decreasing the infusion rate or concentration of local anesthetic.

  o Hypotension, resulting from epidural-induced sympathectomy, can be minimized or reversed by increasing intravascular volume with crystalloid or colloid. This hypotension can be difficult to treat in thoracic surgery patients, who are often maintained on the "dry side" by the surgical service. Treatment with boluses of adrenergic agents (phenylephrine and ephedrine) may be used as a temporizing measure until fluid volume can be increased. If a continuous infusion is required, dopamine is the drug of choice. Inotropic agents are preferred over "afterload" agents that might trigger the Bezold–Jarish reflex. With thoracic epidurals, hypotension may be accompanied by bradycardia.

  o Sensory block, to some degree, is an obvious result of epidural local anesthetics.

  o Some patients may be disturbed by numbness to light touch in certain areas. Reducing the concentration of local anesthetic in the epidural infusion may reduce the level of sensory blockade at the expense of pain relief.

  o Using ropivacaine instead of bupivacaine may reduce the motor block component while maintaining adequate sensory analgesia.

  o Motor block-limiting ambulation is less likely to be a concern with an epidural placed in the thoracic region. A thoracic epidural catheter can provide adequate pain relief after most surgical procedures (except those in the lower extremity).

OPIOIDS

- Opioids have played a significant historical role in epidural analgesia. Nearly every available preservative-free opioid preparation has been used.
- The mechanism of action of epidural opioids requires penetration across the dura into the cerebrospinal fluid (CSF). Hence, spread of drug within the epidural space is less important than with local anesthetics.
- Opioids may be used alone or, more commonly, as an adjunct to local anesthetic analgesia. Because the mechanism of action differs with these two agents, opioids may be utilized to improve poor distribution within the epidural space.
- Although the various opioids differ slightly in pharmacokinetics, they share side effects to varying degrees. When adding opioids to epidural analgesia, always increase monitoring for respiratory depression and sedation and administer, as needed, medications

TABLE 26-3 Typical Concentrations for Epidural Opioids

Morphine	0.025–0.05 mg/mL
Hydromorphone	5–10 μg/mL
Fentanyl	2–5 μg/mL
Sufentanyl	1–2 μg/mL

to treat nausea, pruritus, sedation, and respiratory depression.

- o *Nausea*: Treat with ondansetron, prochlorperazine, or low-dose naloxone.
- o *Pruritus*: Treat with an antihistamine, such as diphenhydramine, low-dose naloxone, or a small dose of oral naltrexone.
- o *Respiratory depression*: Although rare at the typically low opioid concentrations used in epidural analgesia, respiratory depression can be reversed with naloxone. Naloxone should be administered in 40-μg boluses, until the desired effect is reached. Excessive naloxone administration can result in acute withdrawal syndrome consisting of tachycardia, tachypnea, hypertension, and severe pain. Naloxone-induced acute withdrawal syndrome can result in stroke, myocardial ischemia, or myocardial infarction.
- o *Sedation*: Although less problematic in the in-hospital setting, sedation may also be antagonized with naloxone.
- o *Neuraxial effects*: An agonist–antagonist may be used to treat neuraxial opioid side effects but may cause dysphoric reactions.
- Epidural morphine and hydromorphone produce a local analgesic effect, followed by redistribution to the central compartment CSF. The efficacy of epidural morphine and hydromorphone is enhanced by placement of the epidural catheter at the correct interspace (center of surgical manipulation).
- Epidural infusions with a local anesthetic (with or without opioid) reduce postoperative pain and shorten postoperative ileus after abdominal surgery. The best effects are found with the catheter tip located at the interspace at the center of surgical manipulation (Table 26-3).
- The ASA guidelines on obstructive sleep apnea recommend avoidance of opioids for at-risk patients, using local anesthetics alone.

OTHER ADDITIVES

- Agents may be added to epidural preparations to enhance efficacy. Although many preservative-free agents are used in the epidural space, few are approved for this purpose.

- Any medication used in the epidural space MUST be free of preservatives to avoid potential neurotoxicity.
- Epinephrine and clonidine may enhance epidural analgesia.
  - o Clonidine stimulates postsynaptic α_2 receptors in the dorsal horn interneurons, producing analgesia.
  - o The recommended starting dose for epidural clonidine infusion is 30 μg/h. Data for doses above 40 mg/h are lacking.
  - o Side effects of epidural clonidine include decreased heart rate and blood pressure. Patients receiving epidural clonidine should be closely monitored during the first 24 h of treatment for hypotension, bradycardia, and excess sedation.
  - o Epinephrine (in concentrations of 2–3 μg/mL) may enhance epidural analgesia, possibly by a mechanism of action similar to that of clonidine, without causing bradycardia or hypotension.

ADJUNCTS TO EPIDURAL ANALGESIA

- Acute pain management is best served using multimodal therapy.
- Intravenous patient-controlled analgesia (PCA) infusions may be safely used in conjunction with epidural local anesthetics.
- Opioids can be used in either the epidural or intravenous PCA; avoid simultaneous use in both.
- Anxiety can be an important component of postoperative pain. Some patients benefit from addition of anxiolytic medication to their analgesic therapy.
- Care must be taken when using benzodiazepines with opioids due to resulting synergy in producing respiratory depression and decreased level of consciousness.
- Muscle spasm can complicate analgesia and may not respond well to systemic opioids or epidural analgesia. Small doses of benzodiazepines (eg, diazepam 2.5–5 mg) may relieve spasms. As stated above, the additive effects of these agents on sedation and respiratory depression must be considered.

EPIDURAL ANALGESIA FOR THE CHRONIC PAIN PATIENT WITH ACUTE PAIN

- Patients who chronically take pain medications at home pose a challenge with respect to management of acute postoperative pain.
  - o Chronic pain may cause neurologic changes that sensitize the response to noxious stimuli.

○ Chronic pain patients on opioids often require higher doses of opioids because of tolerance.

○ Patients chronically taking opioids require opioid medication equivalent to their baseline dosage, as a minimum, to prevent acute withdrawal.

○ It is generally advisable to continue baseline opioids throughout the perioperative period (oral opioids, transdermal opioids) when possible.

○ Parenteral opioids administered using intravenous PCA only (without a basal rate) may be insufficient to control pain. A basal opioid infusion (equivalent to a portion of the baseline opioid requirements) may be necessary if a patient is unable to continue routine oral opioids. The risk of respiratory depression may be higher with continuous intravenous infusions compared to patient-controlled administration.

○ Chronic pain patients who use a fentanyl transdermal patch should continue using the patch throughout the perioperative period (it is neither necessary nor desirable to discontinue the patch preoperatively).

○ Chronic pain patients who use extended-release pain medications at home should be continued or restarted on their at-home medication as soon as possible postoperatively.

• Nonsteroidal anti-inflammatory drugs (NSAIDs) or COX-2 inhibitors and acetaminophen may be used as around-the-clock adjuncts to epidural analgesia.

• Oral or transdermal clonidine may be a helpful adjunct for the chronic pain patient with acute pain.

• Chronic opioid exposure may increase the risk of respiratory depression in the perioperative period.

EQUIPMENT

• Epidurals must be performed in an area designed with cardiovascular monitoring and airway and cardiopulmonary support, such as a dedicated block room or the operating room. The procedure may also be performed in a separate area of the patient holding room as long as monitoring and emergency equipment and drugs are available.

• Sterile epidural kits are prepackaged with all the necessary equipment and medications for performing the procedure. Most kits are disposable.

• Most epidural catheters have a "dead space" equal to approximately 0.3 mL.

• Epidural catheters are manufactured in 16–21 gauge and are approximately 100 cm in length. Most are made of polyamide nylon. Modern catheters have centimeter markers and a radiopaque distal tip. Ideally, 3–5 cm of catheter should reside in the epidural space for maximum efficacy.

• On removing an epidural catheter, visually inspect and record that the tip is intact.

• In studies of obstetric patients, lateral-hole epidural catheters have demonstrated the best block spread.

• Common epidural catheters include the single-terminal-opening and the three-lateral-opening types. The three-holed design may have arisen from a desire to produce lateral full-bore equivalent flow with the minimum number of holes while at the same time maintaining catheter tensile strength. As manufacturing techniques improved, the holes were moved closer to the end, thereby minimizing the probability of a multicompartment block.

• "Successful" test dosing of a multiport epidural catheter may not rule out intrathecal or intravascular placement. One port can be intrathecal, while others are epidural. Fluid pressure exerted during test dosing is greater than that during continuous pump infusion. This difference may result in unequal flow distribution between the ports such that all or most of the test dose exits an epidural port.

PLACING THE EPIDURAL

• Because the epidural is a "potential" space between the ligamentum flavum and the dura, take care to stop advancing the needle as soon as the tip exits the ligamentum flavum, or the dura may be punctured.

• Select an interspace for needle insertion that will allow the physician to thread a catheter in to the spine, such that the tip of the catheter lies at the segment of the spinal cord that modulates pain transmission for the relevant part of the body.

• The epidural may be placed using the midline or paramedian approach.

○ The midline approach is favored in the lumbar region, where the spinous processes are nearly horizontal in the seated patient.

○ A paramedian approach may be advisable when placing a thoracic epidural, especially between T5 and T9, where the spinous processes almost overlap. When placing a thoracic epidural using the midline approach, angle the needle 50°–60° (up from the back plane) to pass between the two adjacent spines (see Figure 26-4).

• Once the tip of the epidural needle is situated in the epidural space, thread the epidural catheter 3–5 cm.

○ Never withdraw the catheter from the needle once it has passed the epidural needle tip. Doing so may

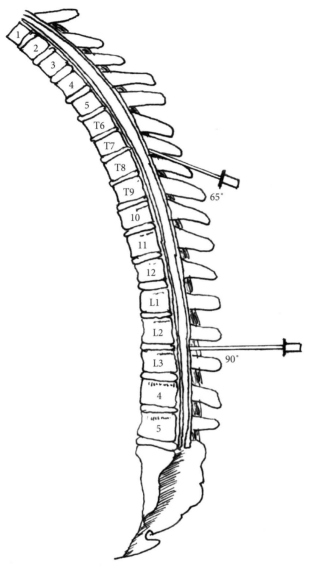

FIG. 26-4. Epidural "angle of attack."

shear the catheter tip, leaving it in the epidural space. Withdraw the entire assembly (needle and catheter) and reinsert after inspection of the catheter and replacement of the needle stylet.

○ The catheter should advance easily into the epidural space. Ease in advancing the catheter into the epidural space provides another confirmation of correct placement.

○ Without fluoroscopic guidance, the epidural catheter cannot reliably be directed one way or the other once it leaves the tip of the epidural needle.

○ Advancing the catheter more than 5 cm increases the potential for knotting or could place the catheter tip too far from the intended center of epidural action to allow for adequate analgesia.

○ Catheters placed 3 cm or less into the epidural space have a tendency to come out.

ACTIVATING THE EPIDURAL

• Before the epidural catheter can be used for infusion of analgesic medication, confirm that the tip lies within the epidural space and not within an epidural vein or the intrathecal space.

• A small dose of lidocaine containing epinephrine is used as a "test dose":

○ About 3 cm³ of 1.5 or 2% lidocaine (45–60 mg) with epinephrine (5–10 μg) is used for this purpose.

○ If the catheter tip rests intravascularly, the 5 or 10 μg of epinephrine should cause an increase in heart rate (15–20 bpm) easily seen on the monitor.

○ If the catheter tip rests intrathecally, the test dose will result in a wide dense block (sensory and motor). The dose is small enough not to result in a high spinal.

• A "negative" test dose does not eliminate the possibility of intrathecal or intravascular catheter placement. Constant vigilance is required whenever epidural analgesia is used.

○ Elderly patients and those taking β-blocking medication may not display a significant heart rate increase from intravascular injection of the few micrograms of epinephrine in the test dose.

○ It may take 10 min or more for the full manifestations of an intrathecal test dose to be seen particularly in the thoracic region. Profound hypotension and bradycardia may be early signs.

○ As stated previously, multiport catheters may allow one or more ports to be intrathecal, while others are within the epidural space. Test dosing may inject medication preferentially through some (but not other) ports.

• Treat every epidural catheter bolus dose as potentially intrathecal or intravascular. Bolus epidural medications incrementally rather than all at once.

• Although it has become standard practice, negative aspiration of the epidural catheter does not rule out intravascular or intrathecal placement.

• If the test dose is positive for intravascular or intrathecal placement, the catheter can be withdrawn 1 cm and retested. This can be repeated several times as long as a sufficient length of catheter remains in the epidural space (at least 1 cm). Often it is easier simply to remove the epidural catheter and reinsert it one interspace above or below.

EPIDURAL COMPLICATIONS

- Complications of epidural analgesia include inadequate analgesia, excessive blockade, unintentional intrathecal or intravascular injection and its sequelae, and the potentially more serious infections or hematomas that can lead to neurologic damage (Table 26-4).
- A study of more than 1000 patients who had postoperative epidural analgesia showed a 20% incidence of inadequate analgesia resulting from catheter dislodgement. There was 1 subarachnoid catheter migration, 3 intravascular migrations, 40 catheter leaks, 57 catheter site inflammations, and 5 catheter infections requiring antibiotic treatment.
- Early recognition and management are the keys to minimizing poor outcome.
- Epidural infection is a rare complication of epidural anesthesia. Usually the source of infection arises from blood-borne spread secondary to infection elsewhere in the body. A review of 50,000 epidural anesthetics did not show a single epidural or intrathecal infection. However, smaller studies cite the incidence of epidural abscess closer to 1:10,000. Relative

TABLE 26-4 Epidural Complications

COMPLICATION	COMMENTS	TREATMENT
Headache	May be result of dural puncture (incidence 1–2%)	Analgesia Bed rest Hydration
	Usually self-limiting	Blood patch if prolonged
Backache	At insertion site	Analgesics and reassurance
	Usually transient	With fever or neurologic deficit—requires careful attention
Sympathetic blockade	May cause significant hypotension	Hydration Vasopressors
High blockade	Respiratory distress (intercostal block)	Resuscitation Cease epidural infusion
	Bradycardia (high thoracic block)	
	Unconsciousness (total spinal block)	
	Dermatome block higher than T4	
	Numbness or tingling in fingers or arms	
	Horner's syndrome	
Nerve damage	Rare and usually transient	Investigation Neurology consult

TABLE 26-5 Epidural Abscess Versus Hematoma

	ABSCESS	HEMATOMA
Time course	Insidious and slow Hours to days	Acute and abrupt Minutes to hours
Typical symptoms	Starts with local back pain and tenderness percussion	Starts with local back pain and tenderness to percussion
	Weakness progresses over hours or days, often abruptly ending in a cauda equine syndrome, paraplegic or quadriplegic pattern	Weakness progresses very rapidly to cauda equine syndrome or paresis
	Fever and leukocytosis are usual	Bowel and bladder dysfunction often occurs with lumbar lesions
	Bowel and bladder dysfunction often occurs with lumbar lesions	
	Sepsis	
	Mental status changes	
Diagnosis	MRI with gadolinium is the study of choice	MRI with gadolinium is the study of choice
Treatment	Surgical decompression, with medical treatment reserved for early/mild cases or those not fit for surgery	Surgical decompression

contraindications to epidural placement include local infection at the intended insertion site and sepsis (Table 26-5).

EPIDURALS IN PATIENTS WITH ANTICOAGULATION

- The actual incidence of neurologic dysfunction as a consequence of hemorrhagic complications after neuraxial blockade is unknown.
- The complication rate for serious neurologic injury resulting from epidural placement has been quoted as anywhere from 1:3000 in some patient populations to less than 1:150,000 epidural and less than 1:220,000 spinal anesthetics. Most of these complications were attributed to detergent contamination or toxic drug injection through the needle, causing ascending arachnoiditis.
- The risks of bleeding concerns are increased in patient populations that have an underlying coagulopathy and an indwelling neuraxial catheter during sustained pharmacological anticoagulation (ie, heparin or low-molecular-weight heparin).

- The American Society of Regional Anesthesia and Pain Medicine (ASRA) has guidelines for patients receiving neuraxial and peripheral anesthesia in combination with antithrombotic therapy that are based on expert consensus statements and adverse events.
- Each type of anticoagulant used for thrombolytic therapy has specific recommendations in relation to receiving a neuraxial block or removal of neuraxial catheters. In particular, newer agents have prolonged half-lives and may be difficult to reverse without the administration of blood products. For example, fondaparinux (Arixtra) has a plasma half-life of 21 h, and in a recent study of 3600 patients who had a neuraxial block in combination with Arixtra thromboprophylaxis, 1 patient developed a spinal hematoma. The majority of the patients screened had strict controls and were included only if the epidural was obtained in a single attempt (less than 40% of neuraxial blocks were successful in one attempt). Thus, use of neuraxial blockade in patients on fondaparinux may not be clinically practical. The current ASRA guidelines do not recommend neuraxial catheters for patients on fondaparinux, and single-shot injections are recommended only under conditions used in clinical trials (single needle pass, atraumatic needle placement).
- In one study of 5704 orthopedic patients on chronic fondaparinux, neuraxial catheters were removed 36 h after the last fondaparinux dose with the next dose of fondaparinux to be administered 12 h after catheter removal. No neuraxial hematomas were observed.
- Newer anticoagulants such as rivaroxaban (Xarelto) and dabigatran (Pradaxa) are being used increasingly. ASRA guidelines mention using extra caution when using neuraxial anesthesia techniques concurrently but do not provide firm recommendations. It is not advisable to start these agents with epidural catheters concurrently until further information is provided. The European Society of Anesthesiology (ESA) recommends holding rivaroxaban 22–26 h prior to neuraxial block. If a catheter is placed, the epidural catheter should be removed at least 18 h after the last dose of rivaroxaban, with the next dose to not be administered until at least 6 h after removal.
- The ESA also recommends stopping dabigatran for seven days prior to neuraxial blockade. The epidural catheter should be removed at least 6 h before initiation of therapy.
- Generally, with the newer anticoagulants agents mentioned above, central neuraxial blocks should not be performed and epidural catheters should be removed only after at least two half-lives have elapsed, the half-life depending on renal function, for the specific anticoagulant involved.

EPIDURAL ANALGESIA MANAGEMENT

- The primary goals of an acute pain management service are to offer a wide variety of services in addition to epidural postoperative pain management. These services must be seamlessly integrated into the hospital infrastructure to be effective.
- Establishing a well-coordinated and effective acute pain management service requires strong institutional support and collaboration among anesthesiologists, surgeons, nurses, pharmacists, and administrators. In our experience, once established, an effective acute pain management service becomes an expected part of perioperative patient care.
- Optimal analgesia requires therapeutic fine-tuning to maximize benefits with minimal side effects. This can be accomplished only with close patient surveillance. A nurse-based acute pain management service is the most effective way to provide this level of service.
  - With appropriate training and well-designed protocols, nurses and nurse clinicians can be empowered to assess pain and side effects and to adjust therapy at "the point of care."
  - Physicians maintain the role of deciding in what circumstances epidural analgesia is appropriate and perform the procedure.
  - Nurses manage the epidural when patients are returned to "the floor," using physician-determined protocols.
- Carefully designed plans or protocols may include epidural analgesia, traditional NSAIDs, COX-2 inhibitors, acetaminophen, and opioids.
- Standard physician orders facilitate a uniform approach to epidural and adjunct analgesia management. Although standard orders should allow for some degree of customization to accommodate individual patient needs, the vast majority of situations can be managed using standardized orders. An example of such standardized epidural orders is provided in Figure 26-5.
- The appropriate level of epidural analgesia surveillance "on the floor" requires cooperation from floor nurses, who must be trained to recognize and record the most common problems of epidural analgesia (eg, pain, pruritus, respiratory depression, sedation, and excessive motor blockade). A standardized flow sheet for recording epidural (and other analgesic) parameters can be used.

Thomas Jefferson University Hospital
J *Jefferson Health System*

MR# _____

LW Acct# _____

Name _____

||||| *0 1 9 4 0 0   0 1 0 2* |||||

Department of Anesthesia
Epidural / Intrathecal Analgesia Order Form

Complete or Imprint with Address-O-Plate

No administration (po, subq, IM or IV) of any narcotics, sedatives, hypnotics, tranquilizers, antiemetics or antihistamines unless part of this protocol or ordered by anesthesiology.

IMPORTANT: DO NOT WRITE IN MARGINS

Allergies _____

1. This patient has   ☐ Epidural catheter   ☐ Intrathecal catheter   ☐ Neither

2. This patient's primary mode of therapy is either *(choose a or b)*:
   a. Continuous infusion of
   ☐ **Bupivacaine** _____ % (final concentration)   ☐ **Ropivacaine** _____ % (final concentration)
   ☐ **Fentanyl** _____ mcg / ml (final concentration)   ☐ **Morphine** _____ mg / ml (final concentration)
   ☐ **Hydromorphone** _____ mcg/ml (final concentration) ☐ **Epinephrine** _____

   Total volume _____ mls (qs using preservative free normal saline)
   to infuse at _____ **ml / hr** (Basal Rate).

   ☐ **Patient controlled epidural**   PCA Dose _____ ml.
   Lockout interval _____ min.
   Hourly Limit _____ ml.

   b. Single shot   ☐ **EPIDURAL**   ☐ **INTRATHECAL**   injection
   Medication _____ Dose _____ Time _____

3. Have naloxone 0.4mg available at bedside. Prior to administration, qs naloxone 0.4mg to 10ml with 0.9% NaCl and notify APMS service

4. Heparin lock or IV at all times.

5. Please label patient's door and medication cardex **"Intraspinal Analgesia."**

6. For solutions containing narcotics, monitor resp. rate and sedation level as follows:
   Infusions   q _____ hr x _____, then q _____ hr for duration of therapy.
   Following Bolus   Resp. rate q 15 min. x 2.

7. For infusions containing local anestetic, monitor motor score, B.P., and HR as follows:
   Infusions   q 4 hr. for duration of therapy.
   Following Bolus   q 5 min. x 4.

8. Monitor pain score q 4 hr.

9. **Treatment of side effects**
   Itching   Diphenhydramine Hydrochloride (Benadryl) 25–50 mg IVPB / IM q 4 hr. prn.
   Nausea/Vomiting   _____
   Urinary Retention   Straight cath. q 8hr. prn; may place foley cath if patient requires second straight cath.

10. For sleep *(if resp. rate > 12 / min. and patient is easily arousable)*: Benadryl (diphenhydramine) 25–50 mg IVPB / IM / PO, qHS pm.

11. Call _____ pain service at beeper _____ for following:

    a. Resp. rate < 10. In the event of **severe** respiratory depression (RR<5), house officer or nurse may administer naloxone diluted to 10ml with 0.9% NaCl for final concentration of 0.04mg/ml. Administer 1ml (0.04mg) slowly over 1 minute, repeating 1ml doses as needed, up to 3ml over 3 minutes.

    b. Altered mental status or patient becomes difficult to arouse.

    c. Inadequate analgesia.

    d. Pruritus or Nausea and Vomiting not controlled by above measures.

    e. Problems with Intraspinal catheter.

    f. Increasing motor block.

12. Other _____

APMS RNs Only

☐ Follow thoracic epidural protocol

☐ Follow lumbar epidural protocol

☐ Alternate plans

  ☐ Epidural local and IV
    PCA opioid

  ☐ Other _____

  _____
  _____
  _____
  _____
  _____
  _____

Signature	Date Ordered	Time Ordered

Form 0194-00 (Rev. 1/02)   White: Chart Copy • Yellow: Pharmacy Copy   MJUG 01.4265

FIG. 26-5. Example of standardized epidural orders.

BIBLIOGRAPHY

Acute Pain Management Guideline Panel. Acute pain management in adults: operative procedures, quick reference guide for clinicians. *J Pharm Care Pain Symptom Control.* 1993;1(1):63–84.

American Society of Anesthesiologists Task Force on Perioperative Management of patients With Obstructive Sleep Apnea. Practice guidelines for the perioperative management of patients with obstructive sleep apnea. *Anesthesiology.* 2008;104:1081–1093.

Block BM, Liu SS, Rowlingson AJ, Cowan AR, Cowan JA Jr, Wu CL. Efficacy of postoperative epidural analgesia: a metaanalysis. *JAMA.* 2003;290:2455–2463.

Brown BL, Fink BR. The history of neural blockade and pain management. *Neural Blockade Clin Anesth Manage Pain.* 1998;3(1):3–34.

Brull R, McCartney CJ, Chan VW, El-Beheiry H. Neurological complications after regional anesthesia: contemporary estimates of risk. *Anesth Analg.* 2007;104(4):965–974.

Correll DJ, Viscusi ER, Grunwald Z, et al. Epidural analgesia with intravenous morphine patient-controlled analgesia: postoperative outcomes measures after mastectomy with immediate TRAM flap breast reconstruction. *Reg Anesth Pain Med.* 2001;26:444–449.

Hermanides J, Hollmann MW, Stevens MF, Lirk P. Failed epidural: causes and management. *Br J Anaesth.* 2012;109(2):144–154.

Horlocker TT, Wedel DJ, Rowlingson JC, et al. Regional anesthesia in the patient receiving antithrombotic or thrombolytic therapy: American Society of Regional Anesthesia and Pain Medicine evidence-based guidelines (third edition). *Reg Anesth Pain Med.* 2010;35:64.

Jørgensen H, Wetterslev J, Møiniche S, Dahl JB. Epidural local anaesthetics versus opioid-based analgesic regimens on postoperative gastrointestinal paralysis, PONV and pain after abdominal surgery. *Cochrane Database Syst Rev.* 2000;(4):CD001893.

Kastango ES. *The ASHP Discussion Guide for Compounding Sterile Preparations.* American Society of Health-System Pharmacists. 2009:1–13. Accessed 7/06.

Manion SC, Brennan TJ. Thoracic epidural analgesia and acute pain management. *Anesthesiology.* 2011;115:181–188.

Marret E, Remy C, Bonnet F; Postoperative Pain Forum Group. Meta-analysis of epidural analgesia versus parenteral opioid analgesia after colorectal surgery. *Br J Surg.* 2007;94:665–673.

Miaskowski C, Crews J, Ready LB, Paul SM, Ginsberg B. Anesthesia-based pain services improve the quality of postoperative pain management. *Pain.* 1999;80(1):23–29.

Peyton PJ, Myles PS, Silbert BS, Rigg JA, Jamrozik K, Parsons R. Perioperative epidural analgesia and outcome after major abdominal surgery in high-risk patients. *Anesth Analg.* 2003;96(2):548–554.

Rawal N. 10 years of acute pain services—achievements and challenges. *Reg Anesth Pain Med.* 1999;24(1):68–73.

Rigg JR, Jamrozik K, Myles PS, et al. Epidural anaesthesia and analgesia and outcome of major surgery: a randomised trial. *Lancet.* 2002;359(9314):1276–1282.

Singelyn FJ, Verheyen CC, Piovella F, Van Aken HK, Rosencher N; EXPERT Study Investigators. The safety and efficacy of extended thromboprophylaxis with fondaparinux after major orthopedic surgery of the lower limb with or without a neuraxial or deep peripheral nerve catheter: the EXPERT Study. *Anesth Analg.* 2007;105(6):1540–1547.

Tuman KJ, McCarthy RJ, March RJ. Effects of epidural anesthesia and analgesia on coagulation and outcome after major vascular surgery. *Anesth Analg.* 1991;73:696–704.

Viscusi ER, Jan R, Warshawsky D. An acute pain management service with regional anesthesia: how to make it work. *Tech Reg Anesth Pain Manage.* 2002;6(2):40–49.

Wheatley RG, Schug SA, Watson D. Safety and efficacy of postoperative epidural analgesia. *Br J Anaesth.* 2001;87(1):47–61.

27 PERIPHERAL NERVE BLOCKS AND CONTINUOUS CATHETERS

Juan Egas, MD
Einar Ottestad, MD
Sean Mackey, MD, PhD

GENERAL PRINCIPLES

- Peripheral nerve blocks and/or continuous perineural catheters can be used in the management of both acute and chronic pain. They are especially effective in the perioperative period when a balanced, multimodal therapeutic approach is used. Preoperative neural blockade techniques can be used with monitored anesthesia care as the sole anesthetic or in conjunction with general anesthesia.

- Because of technologic and pharmacologic advances in recent years, the use of nerve blocks for both inpatient and outpatient pain management has dramatically increased. Although anatomic and nerve stimulator approaches to peripheral nerve blocks have a long history of safety and efficacy, a current trend is using ultrasound guidance for these techniques.

BENEFITS AND RISKS

- Peripheral nerve blockade for acute pain management is associated with significantly improved postoperative pain control with less opioid use, decreased incidence of postoperative nausea and vomiting, improved hemodynamic stability, and a reduced time to discharge.

- Contraindications to peripheral nerve blockade include patient refusal and localized infection.

- Relative contraindications include preexisting neurologic deficit, coagulopathy, and bacteremia. For certain procedures surgeons may prefer to confirm intact nerve function after surgery prior to analgesic neural blockade in the recovery room, and the use of local anesthetic blocks can make it difficult to validate normal neural function.

• Risks associated with peripheral nerve blockade include local anesthetic toxicity, nerve damage, bleeding, infection, and failed/inadequate block. Specific nerve blocks also carry site-specific risks depending on surrounding anatomy.

• Local anesthetic toxicity initially manifests neurologically with perioral numbness and tinnitus. As plasma levels of local anesthetics increase, the patient may have altered mental status that can progress to seizures. The final consequence to intravascular injection is cardiovascular collapse.

• At high systemic doses, local anesthetics can be cardiotoxic and result in arrhythmias. Evidence suggests that bupivacaine is significantly more arrhythmogenic than other local anesthetics. Newer agents such as ropivacaine and levobupivacaine have a duration of action similar to that of bupivacaine with less arrhythmogenic potential.

• Persistent paresthesias are rare and, if they do occur, normally resolve within six weeks.

METHODS

• Peripheral nerve blocks should be performed only by practitioners who have a thorough understanding of the relevant functional neuroanatomy, surrounding anatomic landmarks including vascular supply, and the resources and skills to handle potential complications. Blocks should be performed in a monitored setting with resuscitation equipment readily available. Lipid emulsion bolus and infusion has been shown to reverse local anesthetic systemic toxicity and guidelines are available.

• Most practitioners use mild to moderate sedation during block placement with a combination of anxiolytic and analgesic medications. If a paresthesia technique is being used, mild sedation is preferred. Except in pediatric or unusual cases, nerve blockade should not be performed under general anesthesia.

• Local anesthetic selection is dependent on the practitioner's desired onset time and duration of action:
  ○ Two percent lidocaine and 1.5% mepivacaine have a rapid onset coupled with a short duration of action.
  ○ 0.5% bupivacaine, 0.5% ropivacaine, and 0.5% levobupivacaine have an extended duration of action but a slower onset time.

• Administration of local anesthetic solutions should always begin with a 1-cm^3 test dose (to rule out intraneural injection) followed by incremental dosing with close monitoring of the patient. Frequent aspiration should be performed to minimize intravascular injection.

• Patients should be advised as to the expected duration of sensory and motor blockade. If a short-acting local anesthetic is given for a case expected to result in significant postoperative pain, then a plan should be devised to address the patient's pain control when the block wears off. Patients are sometimes advised to take an oral pain medicine as the block is abating to prevent a sudden onset of acute pain.

• Additional agents can be added to the solution to achieve desired effects (Table 27-1).

• Nerve localization can be performed based on anatomic location in combination with ultrasound guidance with or without a nerve stimulator. When a nerve stimulator is used, continued motor twitches at a current of <0.5 mA indicate appropriate needle placement. A current of <0.2 mA may suggest intraneural needle tip placement and the needle should be adjusted. The use of ultrasound guidance does not guarantee avoidance of intraneural injection.

• When using ultrasound guidance, ideally the hypoechoic local anesthetic fluid should be seen surrounding the target nerve in what is called the "donut" sign.

• A stimulating needle with appropriate current, ultrasound guidance, and the use of a blunt-tipped needle can help minimize intraneural injections. These can be recognized by pain and increased resistance during injection, or visualization of nerve expansion or swelling on ultrasound imaging during injection.

• Although ultrasound guidance may offer several advantages compared to stimulator technique, such as faster onset, higher success rate, and lower doses of local anesthetic, this is not well established in the literature. In addition, there may be less risk of iatrogenic puncture of surrounding structures (such as lungs and major blood vessels).

TABLE 27-1   Effects of Additives on Neural Blockade

MEDICATION	DOSE	EFFECT	COMMENT
Epinephrine	1/200,000–400,000	Marker of intravascular injection. Increases block duration	Increased duration of action with lidocaine or mepivacaine
Sodium bicarbonate	1 cm^3 in 10 cm^3	Decreased onset time	Precipitates with bupivacaine, ropivacaine, levobupivacaine
Clonidine	0.5 mcg/kg	Improves block quality and increases duration	High doses have increased side effects
Opioids	Numerous	Improves block quality and increases duration	Evidence lacking

UPPER EXTREMITY

- The brachial plexus is composed of the nerve roots C5 to T1, which combine to form the superior, middle, and inferior trunks. These trunks further divide to form the lateral, medial, and posterior cords, which then give off the peripheral nerves of the upper extremity (Table 27-2).
- Brachial plexus blocks are mainly performed in four anatomic regions: interscalene groove, supraclavicular, infraclavicular, and axillary.
- Rescue blocks can be performed at the level of the midhumerus, elbow, and wrist for inadequate blocks. Although rescue blocks more distal in the limb may improve surgical anesthesia, tourniquet pain may be an issue with an upper arm tourniquet.

INTERSCALENE BLOCK

- The interscalene block is performed predominantly for shoulder surgery. Although the interscalene block includes the axillary and supraclavicular nerves that provide the majority of shoulder joint innervation, the coverage of the inferior trunk of the brachial plexus is poor. As such, this block is not indicated for forearm or hand surgery. The supraclavicular nerves that provide cutaneous innervation to the shoulder might require separate cutaneous infiltration.
- In this location, the brachial plexus is lateral to the carotid artery, posterior to the sternocleidomastoid, and between the anterior and middle scalene muscles. The interscalene groove is palpated at the level of C6 or the cricoid cartilage and the plexus is usually at a depth of 1–3 cm. For a paresthesia or nerve stimulator approach, the needle is inserted in the groove and directed medial and caudally until an appropriate response is obtained. If a nerve stimulator is used, deltoid or biceps motor response correlates with adequate blockade. Diaphragmatic movement indicates stimulation of the phrenic nerve that passes over

the anterior scalene and the needle should be directed posteriorly.
- For an ultrasound-guided block, the brachial plexus is identified vertically aligned between the two scalene muscles. A needle is directed using an in-plane technique with a needle entry lateral to the transducer. The goal is to place the needle in the interscalene groove and confirm the spread of local anesthetic around the brachial plexus. With care, deeper infiltration in the tissues can increase the chance of covering the lower trunk.
- Typical doses for landmark or stimulation techniques of local anesthetic range from 30 to 40 cm³. With ultrasound guidance, appropriate anesthesia can be obtained with lower volumes ranging from 10 to 20 mL. Lower volumes provide an advantage of a lesser likelihood of blocking the phrenic nerve without a significant difference in pain scores and opioid consumption 24 h after surgery.
- Site-specific consequences of this block include a high percentage of temporary ipsilateral diaphragmatic paralysis, Horner syndrome, and less frequently a recurrent laryngeal nerve block with temporary vocal cord paralysis. These are expected with an interscalene block and may precipitate respiratory distress in patients with underlying pulmonary disease. Rarely, this block is associated with complications such as pneumothorax, seizures (due to intra-arterial injection), and epidural/intrathecal injection resulting in a high spinal.

SUPRACLAVICULAR AND INFRACLAVICULAR BLOCKS

- Performed at the level of the cords of the brachial plexus, these blocks are excellent for surgeries distal to the midhumeral level. Although both blocks can be performed using nerve stimulation, the presence of the dome of the lung may favor ultrasound guidance, especially for the supraclavicular block. In fact, the incidence of pneumothorax has decreased since the implementation of ultrasound guidance.
- The preferred technique for supraclavicular brachial plexus block utilizes ultrasound guidance. Initial scanning localizes the subclavian artery. Several structures surrounding the artery can be visualized: underneath, there are two linear hyperechoic structures corresponding to the first rib and apical pleura. Lateral and superficial to the artery, a series of hypoechoic nodules resembling a bundle of grapes correspond to the brachial plexus. The needle is then inserted using an in-plane technique in a lateral to medial direction toward the brachial plexus (Figure 27-1).
- The infraclavicular brachial plexus uses the coracoid process as the main anatomic landmark. For the

TABLE 27-2 **Upper Extremity Nerve Distribution**

NERVE	MOTOR	SENSORY
Musculocutaneous	Arm flexion	Lateral forearm
Median	Lateral deviation of wrist and grip of thumb, index, and middle finger	Medial aspect of palm including thumb, index and middle finger
Ulnar	Medial deviation of wrist and grip of fourth and fifth fingers	Lateral aspect of hand including fourth and fifth fingers
Radial	Arm, wrist, and finger extension	Extensor surfaces of arm and hand

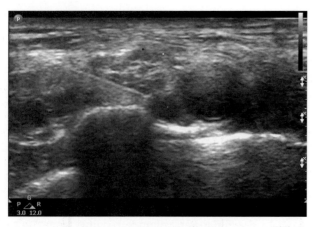

FIG. 27-1. Supraclavicular block. Needle directed at a "bundle of grapes" lateral to the round subclavian artery. The lines of the pleura and first rib are seen deep to the needle.

anatomic or nerve stimulator approach, the needle entry site is 2 cm medial and 2 cm caudal from the coracoid process with the needle directed perpendicular to all planes. A nerve stimulator is used to achieve motor response distal to the wrist.

- When using ultrasound to perform an infraclavicular block, the median, lateral, and posterior cords are identified medial, lateral, and posterior to the axillary artery caudal to the clavicle. The axillary artery is 3–5 cm deep and lies underneath the fascia of the pectoralis minor muscle. Visualization of the cords is not necessarily required since a successful block can be achieved by injecting local anesthetic around the artery aiming to achieve a U-shaped spread around the artery.
- Local anesthetic solution of 20–40 cm³ is the typical dose for stimulation technique in contrast to 20–30 mL for the supraclavicular and infraclavicular ultrasound-guided blocks.
- These techniques may prove to be superior to the axillary block because of better patient tolerance, decreased tourniquet pain, lower incidence of incomplete block, and they can be performed with the patient's arm at the side.

AXILLARY BLOCK

- The major arm nerves surround the axillary artery: the median nerve is superficial and lateral to the artery, ulnar nerve is medial, and the radial nerve is posterior. The musculocutaneous nerve is found in the fascial layers between the biceps and coracobrachialis muscles.
- The axillary block is frequently performed for surgeries distal to the elbow. Once the axillary artery is identified in the proximal arm using palpation, a transarterial technique can be used in which half of the local anesthetic is injected deep to the artery and

the other half superficial to the artery. Nerve stimulation can be used to identify each of the four peripheral nerves based on specific motor response and each can be blocked. Finally, ultrasound can identify the artery for a periarterial injection followed a separate injection to the musculocutaneous nerve.

- Local anesthetic doses of 20–40 cm³ are deposited depending on the technique used. With ultrasound guidance, each of the four nerves can also be visualized and independently blocked with much lower volumes of local anesthetic.
- Tourniquet pain is better tolerated if a medial upper arm superficial ring block is performed to anesthetize the intercostobrachial and medial brachial cutaneous nerves.

LOWER EXTREMITY

- The neuroanatomy to the lower extremity is composed of the lumbar and lumbosacral plexuses. The lumbar plexus is derived from the ventral rami of L1 through L3 with part of L4 and occasionally contributions from T12. The lumbosacral plexus is derived from L4 through S3. Although it is common to provide complete upper extremity anesthesia with a single injection at the brachial plexus, regional anesthesia approaches in the lower extremity often require two separate injections—one for each component of the lumbar and sacral plexuses (Table 27-3).
- All blocks use 20–30 cm³ of local anesthetic and may be performed with an ultrasound machine, a nerve stimulator, or both.

SCIATIC NERVE BLOCK

- The sciatic nerve derives from the ventral rami of L4–S3 of the lumbosacral plexus. The sciatic nerve leaves the pelvis and enters the gluteal compartment through the greater sciatic foramen and then travels between the greater trochanter and ischial tuberosity,

TABLE 27-3 Lower Extremity Nerve Distribution

NERVE	MOTOR	SENSATION
Femoral	Leg extension	Anterior thigh and knee, medial aspect of lower leg by saphenous nerve
Lateral femoral cutaneous	None	Lateral thigh
Obturator	Hip adductors	Medial distal thigh
Tibial	Plantar flexion and inversion of foot	Heel and plantar foot
Common peroneal	Dorsiflexion and eversion of foot	Dorsal foot
Sural	None	Lateral foot

deep to the gluteus maximus and superficial to the quadratus femoris. At the level of the popliteal fossa, it is accompanied by the popliteal artery and vein, both running 1–2 cm medially and deep to the nerve. At this level, it divides into the tibial nerve medially and the common peroneal nerve laterally.

- The sciatic nerve is most commonly blocked in three different areas: the gluteal, subgluteal, and popliteal regions. The sciatic nerve may be visualized better with a low-frequency curvilinear ultrasound probe in the gluteal and subgluteal regions, and with a high-frequency linear probe at the popliteal fossa. Blocks of the sciatic nerve have the slowest onset times and the longest durations of the peripheral nerve blocks.

- The tibial nerve provides sensation to the heel and plantar aspect of the foot and performs plantar flexion and inversion. The common peroneal nerve provides sensation to the lateral lower leg and dorsal aspect of the foot and performs dorsiflexion and eversion.

- The classic anatomic gluteal approach has the patient in Sim's position (lateral decubitus with operative leg up and bent at the knee with nonoperative leg straight), the anterior approach and the lateral popliteal approach have the patient supine, and the posterior popliteal approach has the patient prone.

- For the classic posterior approach, a line is drawn from the greater trochanter to the posterior superior iliac spine. A second line is drawn from the greater trochanter to the sacral hiatus. From the midpoint of the first line, a third line is drawn perpendicular and where this line intersects the second line is the location of needle placement. With a nerve stimulator, ankle dorsiflexion or plantar flexion is the goal.

- One can use the same landmarks and the aid of a curvilinear low-frequency probe for identification of the sciatic nerve deep to the gluteus maximus, superficial to the quadratus femoris, and between the greater trochanter and ischial tuberosity. Then the needle is inserted using an in-plane technique and advanced in a lateral to medial direction toward the nerve.

- The posterior popliteal approach is often performed for ankle and foot surgery. With the patient prone and the leg supported at the ankle, the needle is inserted at a 30°–45° angle 8 cm above the popliteal skin crease and 1 cm lateral to the midline. Since the sciatic nerve may have split into its two components at this level, some practitioners search for both the common peroneal and tibial nerves and anesthetize them individually.

- For the ultrasound-guided popliteal fossa block, the sciatic nerve can be identified with the use of a linear high-frequency probe between the biceps femoris and semitendinosus muscles, superficial to the popliteal blood vessels. A needle is inserted using an in-plane technique and in a horizontal orientation toward the sciatic nerve. The goal is to inject the local anesthetic

outside the epineurium that encases both the common peroneal and tibial nerves. Proximal and distal scanning of the sciatic nerve will identify the location of the sciatic bifurcation into the tibial and common peroneal nerves to ensure both are blocked (Figure 27-2).

- In patients who are unable to move from the supine position, the sciatic nerve can be reached by both the anterior approach and the lateral popliteal approach.

- Both Beck and Chelly have described anatomic bony landmarks for the anterior approach. An additional technique helpful in obese patients is to place the needle 2.5 cm distal to the inguinal crease and 2.5 cm medial to the femoral artery. The needle is then directed 10°–15° from the vertical plane with the leg externally rotated.

- Using ultrasound at the level of the lesser trochanter with a curvilinear probe placed in the anteromedial aspect of the thigh, the sciatic nerve is 6–8 cm deep, medial to the femur and immediately deep to the adductor magnus muscle.

- The lateral popliteal nerve block is performed with needle insertion perpendicular to the vertical plane 7 cm above the lateral femoral epicondyle between biceps femoris and vastus lateralis. Once femur contact is made, the needle is grasped 2 cm above the skin. The needle is redirected 30°–45° posteriorly and advanced approximately 2 cm beyond the depth required to make

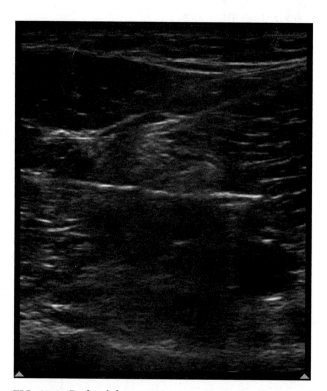

FIG. 27-2. Popliteal fossa sciatic nerve block. Needle directed immediately deep to sciatic nerve and superficial to popliteal artery and vein.

femur contact. The degree of approach is adjusted until appropriate stimulation is achieved.
- The ultrasound-guided lateral popliteal block is identical to the prone popliteal block except for positioning and a lateral thigh needle entry point.

LUMBAR PLEXUS BLOCK

- The lumbar plexus includes the obturator, lateral femoral cutaneous, and femoral nerves. There are two main anatomic approaches used to block the lumbar plexus: the posterior or psoas compartment block and the anterior or fascia iliaca block. These blocks are performed for both hip and knee surgery. Fascia iliaca blocks have been proposed for the treatment of pain after a hip fracture.
- A psoas compartment block can be performed and will reliably block all three nerves of the lumbar plexus. A line is drawn between the iliac crests with the patient in prone or in Sim's position. Along this line, 5 cm from midline, a needle is directed perpendicular to the skin until quadriceps stimulation occurs, confirming correct placement.
- Ultrasound guidance is used to identify the L4 transverse process with the psoas muscle deep to the transverse process. The needle is advanced in plane immediately deep to the transverse process. Since the lumbar plexus is not visible on ultrasound, stimulation is still useful to confirm quadriceps contraction prior to injection.
- The fascia iliaca block can be performed under ultrasound guidance or anatomic landmarks technique. This block is usually performed 1 cm below the junction of the lateral and medial third of the inguinal ligament and 3 cm lateral to the femoral artery. For an anatomic approach, the needle is inserted perpendicular to the skin with the target end point being through the second "pop." The first perceived fascial layer is the fascia lata and the second is the targeted fascia iliaca. Ultrasound guidance has a higher success rate of blocking all three branches of the lumbar plexus. In the same location, the needle is advanced using an in-plane technique along the fascia iliaca plane and this is followed by an injection of local anesthetic with confirmation of the spread along this fascial plane.
- The femoral nerve block is frequently performed and well tolerated for knee surgery. The nerve is located at the level of the inguinal crease lateral to the femoral artery. If a nerve stimulator is used, one is looking for quadriceps contraction. Ultrasound is easily able to visualize the femoral artery and adjacent nerve for the block. With either technique, using increased volumes and distal pressure a "3–1" block (lateral femoral cutaneous, femoral, and obturator nerves) may be achieved; however, the obturator nerve is often not anesthetized.

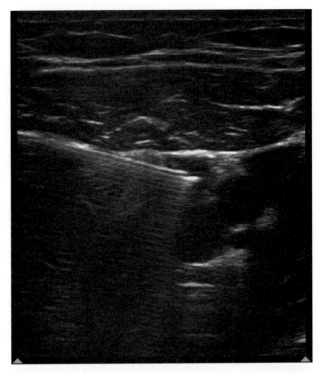

FIG. 27-3. Adductor canal block. Needle directed deep to sartorius muscle adjacent to femoral artery and superficial to femoral vein.

- The terminal sensory branch of the femoral nerve is the saphenous nerve that innervates the knee through its infrapatellar branches and continues to provide sensation to the anteromedial leg and ankle. The nerve runs in the adductor canal deep to the sartorius muscle and adjacent to the femoral artery in conjunction with the motor branch of the vastus medialis. A saphenous nerve block can provide additional analgesia to foot and ankle surgery using a sciatic nerve block and can also be used as a single shot or catheter technique for knee surgery. This block provides an equivalent degree of analgesia to femoral nerve blocks for total knee replacement surgery with the advantage of minimal muscle weakness due to preservation of the majority of quadriceps muscle strength (Figure 27-3).

CONTINUOUS CATHETERS

- All of the previously described blocks can be performed as either "one-shot" or continuous catheter placements.
- No evidence supports one type of catheter placement system over another. They can be divided into the plastic introducer catheter with stimulating guide and the insulated Tuohy needle introducer. There are also catheters with a metallic stylet that allow stimulation. Use of ultrasound guidance allows direct visualization

of the catheter tip when fluid is injected to ensure coverage of the target nerve.

- Common postoperative regimens include 0.2% ropivacaine (6–10 cm³/h), 0.125–0.25% bupivacaine (6–12 cm³/h), and 0.125–0.25% levobupivacaine (6–12 cm³/h).
- Drug delivery systems have been developed that are now allowing patients to go home with continuous catheters in place.
- There are several advantages of using continuous infusions in the outpatient setting such as significant decreases in postoperative opioid requirements and decreased side effects and early home discharge. This technique is indicated for patients who are expected to have moderate to severe postsurgical pain >24h. Appropriate sterile technique, patient education, and patient selection are crucial for a safe outpatient infusion. Patients are often required to have a "caretaker" during infusion. Conservative application of this technique is recommended since complications may take longer to be identified in medically unsupervised patients.
- The future of continuous catheters will be significantly affected if extended-duration long-acting local anesthetics become available. A single injection technique is faster and less cumbersome than placement of a perineural catheter.

BIBLIOGRAPHY

Brown DL. *Atlas of Regional Anesthesia*. 2nd ed. Philadelphia: WB Saunders; 1999.

Bruce BG, Green A, Blaine T, Wesner L. Brachial plexus blocks for upper extremity orthopaedic surgery. *J Am Acad Orthop Surg*. 2012;20:38–47.

Chelly JE. *Peripheral Nerve Blocks—A Color Atlas*. Philadelphia: Lippincott; 1999.

Chelly JE, Casati A, Fanelli G. *Continuous Peripheral Nerve Block Techniques*. London: Mosby; 2001.

Choquet O, Morau D, Biboulet P, Capdevila X. Where should the tip of the needle be located in ultrasound-guided peripheral nerve blocks? *Curr Opin Anesthesiol*. 2012;25(5):596–602.

Dolan J, Williams A, Murney E, Smith M, Kenny GN. Ultrasound guided fascia iliaca block: a comparison with loss of resistance technique. *Reg Anesth Pain Med*. 2008;33(6):526–531.

Groban L. Central nervous system and cardiac effects from long-acting amide local anesthetic toxicity in the intact animal model. *Reg Anesth Pain Med*. 2003;28:3–11.

Hadzic A. *Hadzic's Peripheral Nerve Blocks and Anatomy for Ultrasound-guided Regional Anesthesia*. 2nd ed. McGraw-Hill 2012.

Haslam L, Landown A, Lee J, van der Vyver M. Survey of current practices: peripheral nerve block utilization by ED physicians for treatment of pain in the hip fracture patient population. *Can Geriatr J*. 2013;16(1):16–21.

Liu SS, Salinas FV. Continuous plexus and peripheral nerve blocks for postoperative analgesia. *Anesth Analg*. 2003;96:263–272.

Moayer N, van Geffen G, Bruhn J, Chan V, Groen G. Correlation among ultrasound, cross-sectional anatomy, and histology of the sciatic nerve; a review. *Reg Anesth Pain Med*. 2010;35:442–449.

Murphy DB, Chan VWS. Upper extremity blocks for day surgery. *Tech Reg Anesth Pain Med*. 2000;4:19–29.

Stai P, Karnwal A, Kakazu C, Tokhner V, Julka S. Efficacy of ultrasound-guided subsartorial approach to saphenous nerve: a case series. *Can J Anesth*. 2010;57:683–688.

Van Elstrate AC, Poey C, Lebrum T, Pastureau F. New landmarks for the anterior approach to the sciatic nerve block: imaging and clinical study. *Anesth Analg*. 2002;95:214–218.

Warman P, Nichols B. Ultrasound-guided nerve blocks: efficacy and safety. *Best Pract Res Clin Anaesthesiol*. 2009;23:313–326.

Weinberg G. Lipid emulsion infusion: resuscitation for local anesthetic and other drug overdose. *Anesthesiology*. 2012;117(1):180–187.

28   ABDOMINAL PAIN

Elliot S. Krames, MD

INTRODUCTION

- The abdomen is one of the most common sites of regional pain. According to a 2000 survey, 21.8% of respondents stated that they experienced either abdominal pain or discomfiture one month before answering the survey. The prevalence of recurrent abdominal pain in children in Western societies ranged from 0.3% to 19% (median 8.4).
- Pain in the abdomen is usually caused by disorders of viscera in the abdominal cavity or pelvic cavity. The next most common cause of abdominal pain is referred pain from diseases of the thorax.
- The somatic and visceral nerve supplies of both regions have a common segmental distribution within the spinal cord, the so-called viscero–somatic convergence.
- The physiologic mechanisms of visceral pain share similarities and differences with somatic pain mechanisms.

CLASSIFICATION

- Abdominal pain can be classified into pain caused by abdominal visceral disease, musculoskeletal pain, neuropathic pain, and other pain etiologies.

ABDOMINAL VISCERAL DISEASE

- Visceral pain is:
  ○ Not evoked from all viscera (liver, kidney, lung, and most solid viscera are not sensitive to pain)
  ○ Not always linked to visceral injury (cutting the intestines causes no pain, while bladder stretching is painful without any discernible injury)
  ○ Diffuse and poorly localized (with few "sensory" visceral afferents and extensive divergence in the central nervous system [CNS])
  ○ Referred to other locations (viscerosomatic convergence in the CNS)
  ○ Accompanied by motor and autonomic reflexes (nausea, vomiting, diaphoresis, pallor, lower back muscle tension with renal colic, etc)
  ○ *Unreferred parietal pain* is acute, intense, sharp, localized, and aggravated by movement, and may be localized to the abdominal/thoracic wall directly over the site of inflammation/injury (eg, right lower quadrant pain in acute appendicitis).
  ○ *Referred parietal pain* is remote from the pain generator site (eg, shoulder pain from diaphragmatic irritation).

MUSCULOSKELETAL PAIN

- Musculoskeletal pain, pain that affects muscles, tendons, ligaments, and bone, is most usually focal; however, some diseases such as fibromyalgia can cause generalized musculoskeletal pain. Examples of focal abdominal musculoskeletal pain include, but are not limited to, rib fracture/dislocation, slipping rib syndrome, intercostal cartilage fracture/subluxation, trauma with secondary abdominal wall hemorrhage, and postoperative pain. Thoracic spine disorders can refer anteriorly.

NEUROPATHIC PAIN

- Neuropathic pain has recently been redefined by the neuropathic pain special interest group of the International Association for the Study of Pain (IASP) as pain arising as direct consequence of a lesion or disease affecting the somatosensory system.

- Spinal cord lesions or compression of the spinal cord involving lower thoracic levels cause dull, aching, poorly localized abdominal neuropathic pain.
- Thoracic root inflammation/lesions cause sharp, burning neuropathic pain in a segmental distribution (examples include herpes zoster, herniated disks, and vertebral tumors).
- Intercostal neuropathy can cause anterior abdominal pain.

OTHER PAIN ETIOLOGIES

- Systemic, hematologic, and endocrine disorders can cause various types of abdominal pain (examples include porphyria causing severe, episodic, deep abdominal pain and diabetes mellitus, a known cause of abdominal pain).
- Inflammatory bowel disorders include Crohn disease, colitis and proctitis, and inflammatory bowel disease.
- Vascular diseases, such as rupture of an abdominal aortic aneurysm (AAA) and occlusion of the superior mesenteric artery, cause abdominal pain and/or back pain.

ANATOMY OF THE ABDOMEN

BOUNDARIES

- For descriptive purposes, the abdomen can be divided into nine regions:
  - Right and left hypochondriac
  - Epigastric
  - Right and left lumbar
  - Umbilical
  - Right and left inguinal (iliac)
  - Hypogastric
- The abdomen is bounded:
  - Anteriorly by the rectus abdominis muscles, the aponeuroses of the external oblique, and the internal oblique
  - Laterally by the external and internal oblique muscles, the rectus abdominis, the iliac muscles, and the bones
  - Posteriorly by the lumbar vertebral column, the psoas and quadratus lumborum muscles, the diaphragmatic crura, and the posterior iliac bones
  - Superiorly by the diaphragm
  - Inferiorly by the superior aperture of the pelvis

COMPONENTS

Muscles

- Anterolateral: flat muscular sheets (the external and internal obliques, the rectus abdominis).

- Posterior: psoas major/minor muscles, quadratus lumborum, and iliacus muscles.
- Diaphragm: superior boundary.

Peritoneum

- Parietal: serous membrane lining the abdominal wall.
- Visceral: serous membrane reflected over the viscera.
- The parietal and visceral peritoneal layers are derived from the somatopleural and splanchnopleural layers of the lateral mesoderm plate.

Omenta

- Greater omentum: a two-layer peritoneal fold that descends downward from the stomach and duodenum in front of the small intestine, and then reflects upward to the level of the transverse colon.
- Lesser omentum: the peritoneal fold extending from the stomach and first portion of the duodenum to the liver.

Mesenteries

- The mesenteries are the collective of peritoneal folds that contain blood vessels, nerves, and lymph vessels. When stretched, the mesenteries provoke painful stimuli.

Nerves/Plexuses

- The parietal peritoneum derives its nerve supply from the spinal nerves, which also supply the corresponding muscles and skin.
- The visceral peritoneum derives its nerve supply from the autonomic nervous system that supplies the viscera.
- In conscious patients, pain can be elicited by chemical and thermal noxious stimuli to the parietal peritoneum but not to the viscera, which respond to mechanical noxious stimuli such as stretch and tension.
- See Figure 28-1.

Vagus Nerves

- Vagus nerves supply parasympathetic, preganglionic fibers, and sensory fibers to the abdominal viscera except the left half of the transverse colon and descending colon, which are supplied by the sacral parasympathetic nerves.
- Vagal efferents have parasympathetic preganglionic cell bodies located in the medulla.
- Vagal afferents have pseudounipolar sensory cells in the inferior vagal ganglion (nodose), located just caudad to the jugular foramen.

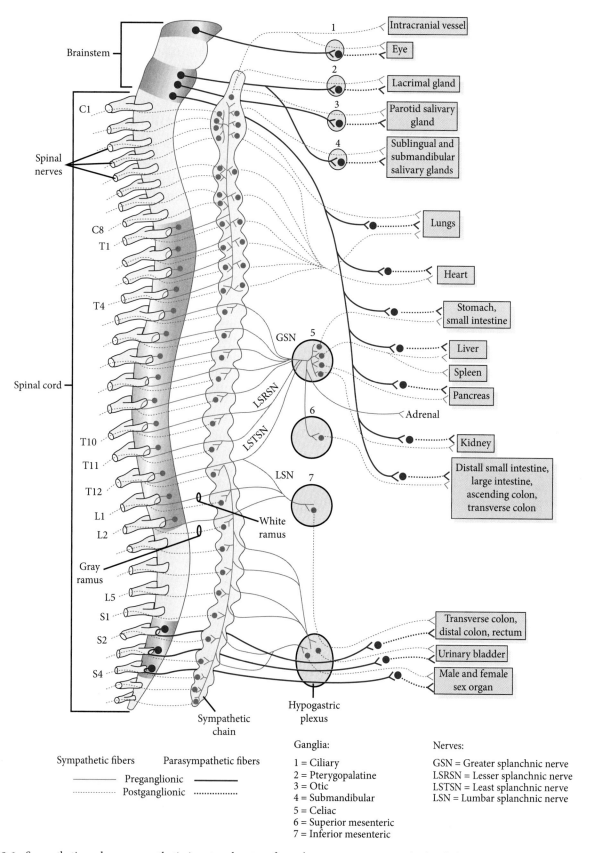

FIG. 28-1. Sympathetic and parasympathetic input and output from the nervous system to the head, thoracic, abdominal, and pelvic structures.

Sympathetic Nerves

- Sympathetic efferents supply the abdominal viscera with cell bodies in the T5 to L2 spinal segments.
- Axons pass through the sympathetic chains without synapsing via splanchnic nerves to end in three prevertebral ganglia: the celiac, the aorticorenal, and the inferior mesenteric ganglia. Here they synapse with postganglionic neurons.

Celiac Plexus

- The celiac plexus is the largest prevertebral plexus, with parasympathetic and sympathetic efferent and afferent fibers within the ganglia.
- The celiac plexus is located inferior to the diaphragm, posterior to the stomach, just anterior to the aorta at the L1/L2 vertebral body levels, and surrounding the celiac artery.

Superior and Inferior Hypogastric Plexuses

- These plexuses are the continuation of the abdominal aortic plexus portion of the celiac plexus.
- They contribute sympathetic, parasympathetic, and afferent nerves to the pelvic viscera.
- The superior hypogastric plexus is located anterior to the S1 vertebral body, and the inferior hypogastric plexus lies on either side of the rectum within the sacral pelvis.

Intrinsic (Enteric) Nervous System

- This consists of cell bodies and short axons within the gastrointestinal tract.
- *The interstitial cells of Cajal* (ICC) is a type of interstitial cell found in the gastrointestinal tract that serves as a pacemaker that creates the bioelectrical slow wave potential that leads to contraction of the smooth muscle. See Figure 28-2.

- *Auerbach plexus* lies between the longitudinal and circular muscle layers within the intestinal viscera.
- *Meissner plexus* is in various muscle and submucosal layers within the intestinal viscera.

EVALUATION OF THE PATIENT

- Evaluation of the patient should include a detailed patient-derived history, review of pertinent medical records, review of pertinent laboratory and/or imaging studies, and a complete physical examination.

PATIENT-DERIVED HISTORY SHOULD INCLUDE THE FOLLOWING QUESTIONS

- What are the characteristics of the abdominal pain: its rapidity of onset, quality, intensity, location, duration, and aggravating and/or alleviating factors?
- What are the effects of: eating, swallowing, belching, deep breathing, flatus, defecation, urination, trunk movements, and supine/prone positions?
- What are any associated symptoms: nausea, vomiting, dyspnea, hematemesis, hemoptysis, melena, weakness, and/or numbness?

Are there generalized associated nonabdominal signs and symptoms?

- Noted in detail are previous medical history, drugs taken (licit and illicit), family history, social history, toxic exposures, and patient age.

Any previous workup or surgical intervention from other specialists is also noted.

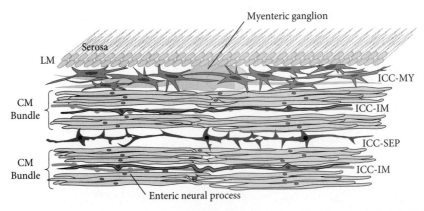

FIG. 28-2. The interstitial cells of Cajal pace slow waves of the gastrointestinal tract. (Reproduced, with permission, from Magrina JF, Pawlina W, Kho RM, Magtibay PB. Robotic nerve-sparing radical hysterectomy: feasibility and technique. *Gynecol Oncol.* 2011;121(3): 605–609.)

PHYSICAL EXAMINATION

Vital Signs

- Tachycardia and hypotension or orthostatic hypotension indicating hypovolemia/shock, bradycardia from acute gastric dilation, unilateral blood pressure gradient from acute aortic dissection, tachypnea with metabolic acidosis, fever indicating infection, and so on.

Inspection

- General appearance:
  ○ Patients with renal or biliary colic may writhe in bed constantly.
  ○ Patients with peritonitis lie still, avoid the slightest motion, and may draw up their legs to reduce intra-abdominal pressure.
- Respiratory rate is increased in patients with peritonitis, obstruction, or hemorrhage.
- Skin: Patients with abdominal visceral disease may have jaundice, scleral icterus, or spider angiomas.
- Hands: Patients may present with muscle atrophy. Nailbed lunula (the white half-moon at the proximal edge of the *nail bed*) is increased in patients with cirrhosis.
- Face: There may be temporal wasting with visceral disease, lip/tongue telangiectasias from Osler–Weber–Rendu syndrome, or Cushingoid facies.
- Abdomen: Increased intra-abdominal pressure may cause an everted umbilicus. Cachexia may be the result of severe malnutrition or cancer. Protuberance of the abdomen may result from obesity, gaseous distension, ascites, or organomegaly. Ecchymoses of abdomen or flanks might be due to hemorrhagic pancreatitis, strangulated bowel, or hemoperitoneum.
- Hernias: Valsalva maneuver may cause inguinal, umbilical, or femoral area hernias.
- Superficial veins: caput medusae from portal hypertension, cephalad draining veins from vena caval obstruction.

Auscultation

- Supine: absence of bowel sounds in ileus secondary to peritonitis; borborygmi—high-pitched "tinkles"; hyperperistalsis in early obstruction.
- Succussion splash: The physician applies the stethoscope, shakes the patient side-to-side, and listens for sloshing from stomach or colon distension.
- Bruits: abdominal aorta or renal artery stenosis.
- Peritoneal friction rubs: during inspiration with hepatic or splenic pathology.

Percussion

- Abdomen: tympany from gas in stomach or bowels; suprapubic dullness in bladder distention or uterine enlargement.
- Liver: 10-cm width is normal at midclavicular line.
- Spleen: The physician percusses at the lowest intercostal space at the left midaxillary line. Splenic enlargement can cause percussion changes from resonance to dullness on full inspiration.
- Ascites: shifting dullness sensitive; fluid wave specific.

Palpation

- Palpation begins in an area away from the pain.
- For light palpation, the flat of the hand, not the fingertips, is used.
- For deep palpation to ascertain organ size, the left hand is placed over the right and steady pressure is gently applied with the left hand.
- "Guarding" refers to muscle spasm. "Involuntary guarding" occurs when the patient cannot eliminate the response. "Rigidity of the muscle" describes a tense and boardlike abdominal wall. Rigidity implies peritonitis.
- *Fothergill sign* differentiates between an intra-abdominal and an intramuscular cause of spasm. First, after the patient relaxes the abdominal muscles, the physician palpates the abdomen. The physician then asks the patient to contract the abdominal muscle by placing his or her head on the chest; the physician palpates the abdomen again. If tenderness is less during abdominal contraction, then the process is intra-abdominal.
- Rebound: The physician performs deep, slow palpation away from the suspected area of inflammation. The palpating hand is then quickly removed. If pain is felt after release of pressure, this "rebound" suggests peritoneal inflammation on that side.
- Palpation for the liver: The physician places his or her left hand posteriorly between the 12th rib and the iliac crest; the right hand is placed in the right upper quadrant below the area of liver dullness. Enlargement of edge of the liver most likely indicates cirrhosis, hepatitis, vascular congestion, or neoplasm.
- Murphy sign: If the patient suddenly stops inspiratory efforts during liver palpation because of pain on inspiration, the cause may be acute cholecystitis.
- Spleen: The physician palpates during deep inspiration with the patient lying on the right side. A palpable spleen suggests congestion, tumor, or infection.
- Kidneys: Palpable kidneys with costovertebral angle tenderness suggest kidney disease.

Rectal Exam

- Irregularities, undue tenderness, or masses are noted.
- The physician palpates for prostate nodules or asymmetries.
- An occult blood test on residual fecal matter is performed.

Testicular Exam

- Evidence of torsion or inflammation is sought.
- Epididymitis or orchitis may present with hypogastric discomfort.

Pelvic Exam

- A bimanual and speculum exam should be performed on all women with abdominal pain, especially on women of reproductive age.
- The patient is checked for adnexal masses (ectopic pregnancy, ovarian tumor, abscess, cyst, or torsion); cervical motion tenderness (pelvic inflammatory disease); discharge, bleeding, or tissue in vault (possible spontaneous abortion); and uterine tenderness (endometritis, fibroids, or carcinoma). Cultures for *Chlamydia trachomatis* and *Neisseria gonorrhoeae* should be taken.

Special Maneuvers

- Iliopsoas test: The patient lies on his or her unaffected side and extends at the hip against resistance. The test is positive if the maneuver produces abdominal pain. Appendicitis will cause pain on the right side with this maneuver.
- Obturator test: The patient is placed supine with the hip flexed and knee joint bent. The hip is then rotated internally and externally. Pain occurs if there is inflammation adjacent to the obturator muscle.

DIFFERENTIAL DIAGNOSIS

INTRA-ABDOMINAL DISEASE

- Parietal peritoneal inflammation may be due to generalized bacterial or chemical peritonitis, localized peritonitis from either pancreatitis or appendicitis, or mesenteric traction/distension from a tumor.
- Obstruction of a hollow viscus includes obstruction of the small or large intestine, obstruction of the biliary system, ureteral obstruction, or obstruction of the uterus.
- Examples of rapid capsular distension of a solid viscus include liver capsule stretching from hepatitis or common bile duct obstruction, stretching of the splenic capsule from hemorrhage or acute splenomegaly, and renal capsule stretching from pyelonephritis.
- Examples of acute ischemia include mesenteric thrombosis/embolism; splenic thrombosis/embolism; hepatic infarction/toxemia; torsion of the ovary, testicle, gallbladder, spleen, or appendix; vascular rupture; and sickle cell anemia.

EXTRA-ABDOMINAL DISEASE

- Thoracic viscera: pulmonary (pneumonia, pulmonary embolism), cardiac (myocardial infarction/ischemia), esophageal (rupture, spasm), and so on.
- Neuropathic disorders: spinal cord (compression, tumor), mechanical radiculopathy (herniated disk), infectious radiculopathy (herpes zoster), and so on.
- Musculoskeletal disorders: rib fracture, costal cartilage fracture, costochondritis, myofascial pain syndromes, trauma, rectus sheath hematoma, slipping rib syndrome, and so on.

METABOLIC DISORDERS AND TOXINS

- Exogenous: iron, lead, mercury, aspirin, arsenic, alcohols, acidic/alkali caustic compounds, black widow venom, and so on.
- Endogenous: acute intermittent porphyria, uremia, diabetes/diabetic ketoacidosis, and so on.

PSYCHOLOGICAL DISORDERS

- Anxiety, depression, hypochondriasis, somatoform disorder, and conversion disorder.

DIAGNOSTIC STRATEGIES

ACUTE ABDOMINAL PAIN

- This pain is a great challenge to the primary care physician, gastroenterologist, emergency room physician, surgeon, and pain physician. The history and physical examination are the foundation of the evaluation.
- Figure 28-3 shows the initial algorithm for the evaluation of a patient who is hemodynamically unstable or has a rigid abdomen. These patients may need rapid fluid resuscitation and immediate transfer to the operating room.
- Patients who are stable without a rigid abdomen are best evaluated by localizing the signs and symptoms. First, whether the pain is well or poorly localized is determined, as shown in Figure 28-4.
- A differential diagnosis might be established if the pain is well localized to the epigastrium or one of the four quadrants of the abdomen, as shown in Figure 28-5.
- It is important to realize that women of childbearing age have many possible causes of abdominal pain. Pregnancy testing and speculum and bimanual examinations should be part of the workup in this population, and pelvic ultrasound is often helpful.

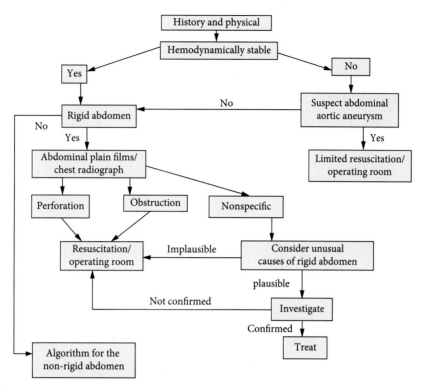

FIG. 28-3. Acute abdominal pain: algorithm for the nonrigid abdomen. (Reproduced, with permission, from Martin RF, Rossi RL. The acute abdomen, an overview and algorithms. *Surg Clin North Am.* 1997;77:1227.)

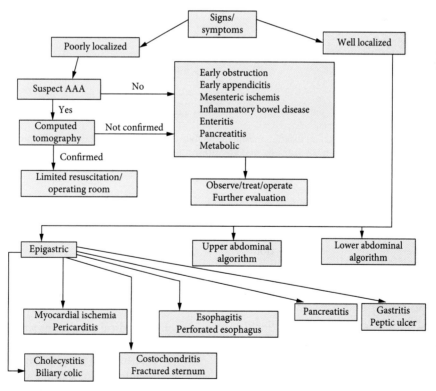

FIG. 28-4. Determines whether the acute abdominal pain is well or poorly localized, creating an algorithm from this observation. (Reproduced, with permission, from Martin RF, Rossi RL. The acute abdomen, an overview and algorithms. *Surg Clin North Am.* 1997;77:1227.)

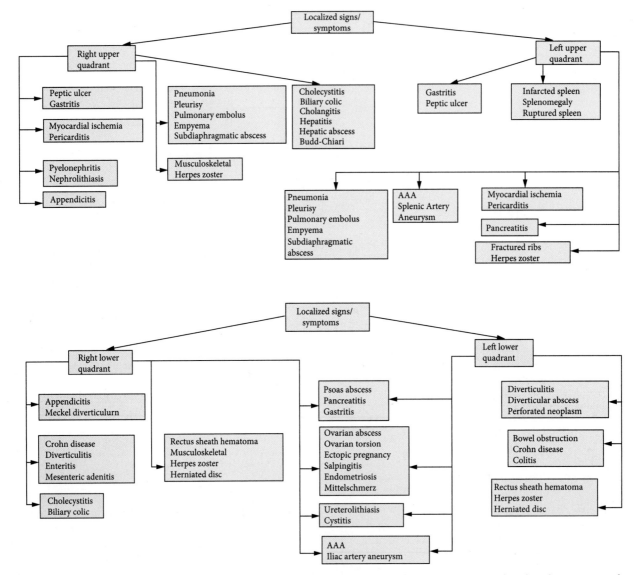

FIG. 28-5. A differential diagnosis based on location in one of the four quadrants of the abdomen. (Reproduced, with permission, from Martin RF, Rossi RL. The acute abdomen, an overview and algorithms. *Surg Clin North Am.* 1997;77:1227.)

Pediatric Population

- Causes of acute abdominal pain in children are best divided on the basis of age (see Figure 28-6).
- In infants, intussusception is the most common cause of pain.
- In children, appendicitis, gastroenteritis, adenitis, pneumonia, and constipation are common.
- In adolescents, appendicitis, pelvic inflammatory disease, ovarian cysts, gastroenteritis, and urinary tract infections should be considered.

Geriatric Population

- The prevalence and frequency of AAA, a manifestation of atherosclerosis, increases with age. Most

(75%) AAAs are asymptomatic when diagnosed but can be palpated on routine exam. All older patients with backache should have an abdominal exam to rule out AAA. Abdominal, flank, or back pain may indicate imminent rupture. Syncope, hypotension, or a pulsatile tender mass may be present. Mesenteric ischemia or infarction causes abdominal distension and pain.

- Five medical conditions should always be ruled out in the elderly patient with acute abdominal pain:
  - Inferior wall myocardial infarction
  - Pneumonia or pulmonary infarct
  - Diabetic ketoacidosis
  - Pyelonephritis
  - Inflammatory bowel disease

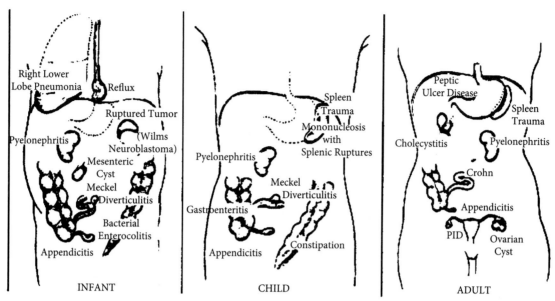

FIG. 28-6. Differential diagnosis based on age. (Reproduced, with permission, from Hatch EI. The acute abdomen in children. *Pediatr Clin North Am.* 1985;32:1151.)

- Other possible causes of abdominal pain in the elderly include constipation, drug-induced pain from polypharmacy (eg, nonsteroidal anti-inflammatory drug [NSAID]-caused gastritis, erythromycin, immunosuppressants, antibiotics causing colitis), trauma (elder abuse), bowel obstruction, and peritonitis.

- Table 28-1 shows acute causes of abdominal pain.

CHRONIC ABDOMINAL PAIN

- History and physical examination form the foundation for evaluating chronic abdominal pain.
- Table 28-2 notes various pertinent historical considerations, and Table 28-3 lists various physical findings.
- It is important to determine the *pattern of pain*. Chronic abdominal pain can be classified into chronic intermittent pain, chronic unrelenting pain with an identifiable cause, and chronic intractable pain. Table 28-4 is a useful guide for making a differential diagnosis.
  - Chronic intermittent abdominal pain is usually explained by a discrete physiologic disorder, and often the underlying condition can be treated.
  - Chronic unrelenting abdominal pain is usually caused by a clear pathophysiologic abnormality, such as chronic pancreatitis or metastatic cancer.
  - Chronic intractable abdominal pain is present most of the time for at least six months. Typically, these patients have had extensive diagnostic testing and surgical procedures without definitive results. More

than 50% have suffered childhood physical or sexual abuse. Pain at other locations and other somatic symptoms are common.

Special Considerations

Acute Intermittent Porphyria

- Patients with AIP suffer from recurrent bouts of severe abdominal pain, constipation, and peripheral neuropathy; have "port wine" urine; and may have associated neuropsychiatric disorders.
- AIP is autosomal dominant with incomplete penetrance.
- The pain is usually characterized as crampy, poorly localized, and commonly precipitated by prescription and recreational drugs. Smoking may trigger an attack.
- Urinary porphobilinogens are increased and account for the "port wine" color.
- Therapy with heme albumin, hematin, or heme arginate administered intravenously may lead to rapid recovery. Opiate analgesics for pain and phenothiazines for nausea are useful.

Abdominal Migraine

- This migraine variant is associated with recurrent abdominal symptoms, usually vomiting and epigastric pain.
- Headache may or may not be present.
- Pathophysiology of this disorder remains unclear.

TABLE 28-1   Causes of Abdominal Pain

I. Intra-abdominal disease
   A. Parietal peritoneal inflammation
      1. Generalized peritonitis
         a. Primary bacterial infection (eg, pneumococcal, streptococcal, enteric bacillus)
         b. Bacterial contamination (eg, perforated appendix, pelvic inflammatory disease, ruptured hepatic abscess)
         c. Chemical peritonitis (eg, perforated ulcer, pancreatitis, ruptured ovarian cyst, rupture of follicle)
      2. Localized peritonitis (eg, acute appendicitis, cholecystitis, peptic ulcer, colitis, regional enteritis, abdominal abscess, Meckel diverticulitis, pancreatitis, gastroenteritis, hepatitis)
      3. Distension or traction of mesentery (eg, tumor)
   B. Mechanical obstruction of hollow viscus that leads to increased tension, stretching
      1. Obstruction of small or large intestine (eg, tumor, adhesions, hernia, volvulus, intussusception)
      2. Obstruction of biliary system (eg, gallstones, strictures, tumors)
      3. Obstruction of ureter (eg, calculi, external tumors, kinking)
      4. Obstruction of uterus (eg, tumor, childbirth)
   C. Rapid distension of capsule of solid viscus that leads to increased tension or stretching
      1. Capsule of liver (eg, toxic or viral hepatitis, rapidly growing tumor, common duct obstruction)
      2. Capsule of spleen (eg, acute splenomegaly, hemorrhage, abscess, cyst, tumor)
      3. Capsule of kidney (eg, pyelonephritis, hemorrhage, abscess, ureteral obstruction)
   D. Acute ischemia
      1. Mesenteric embolism or thrombosis
      2. Splenic embolism or thrombosis
      3. Hepatic infarction or toxemia
      4. Rapid torsion of gallbladder, spleen, ovarian cyst, testicle, appendix
      5. Vascular rupture
      6. Sickle cell anemia

II. Extra-abdominal disease
   A. Thoracic visceral disease
      1. Pneumonia, pulmonary embolism, pneumothorax
      2. Acute myocardial infarction, myocarditis, angina pectoris
      3. Esophageal rupture, esophageal spasm
   B. Neuropathic and musculoskeletal disorders
      1. Diseases of the spinal cord (eg, tumor, tabes dorsalis, spinal cord compression)
      2. Infectious or mechanical radiculopathy (eg, herpes zoster, postherpetic neuralgia, compression by disorders of the spine)
      3. Fracture of lower ribs leading to neuropathy and neuralgia
      4. Fracture or dislocation of the lower costal cartilages
      5. Myofascial pain syndromes, trauma to abdominal muscles, polymyositis

III. Metabolic disorders and toxins or poisons
   A. Exogenous causes
      1. Spider bite (eg, black widow)
      2. Lead and other heavy metal poisoning
   B. Endogenous causes
      1. Uremia
      2. Porphyria
      3. Diabetes mellitus
      4. Allergic diseases

IV. Abdominal pain primarily of psychological origin
   A. Irritable bowel syndrome
   B. Anxiety states
   C. Depression
   D. Hypochondriasis
   E. Operant abdominal pain

Source: Reproduced, with permission, from Bonica J, Graney D. General considerations of abdominal pain. In: Loeser J, Butler S, Chapman C, Turk D, eds. *Bonica's Management of Pain.* 3rd ed. Philadelphia: Lippincott Williams & Wilkins; 2001:1235.

TABLE 28-2   Pertinent Elements in History When Evaluating Abdominal Pain

PERTINENT HISTORICAL ELEMENT	RELATED CONDITION
Follows ingestion of drugs or medications	Acute intermittent porphyria
Related to medications	Pancreatitis
Related to menstrual cycle	Endometriosis
	Mittelschmerz
Related to eating	Mesenteric ischemia
	Pancreatitis
	Biliary disease
Related to neurologic abnormalities	Abdominal migraine
	Abdominal epilepsy
	Acute intermittent porphyria
Related to body position	Nerve entrapment syndrome
	Nerve root compression
	Vertebral body fracture
	Rib tip syndrome
Fever and arthralgias	Familial Mediterranean fever

Source: Reproduced, with permission, from Zackowski SW. Chronic recurrent abdominal pain. *Emerg Med Clin North Am.* 1998;16:877.

TABLE 28-3   Possible Physical Findings Associated With Abdominal Pain

PHYSICAL FINDING	RELATED CONDITION
Jaundice	Choledocholithiasis
	Gallstone pancreatitis
Purpura or retinal cytoid bodies	Autoimmune process
Distended abdomen	Intermittent bowel obstruction
Spasm and rigidity of abdominal wall	Lead poisoning
Palpable mass	Hernia
	Neoplasm
Focal neurologic finding	Nerve root compression
	Vertebral body fracture
Anal fissure	Crohn disease
Dark red "port wine" urine	Acute intermittent porphyria
Occult blood in stool	Colonic or gastric malignancy
	Crohn disease
	Peptic ulcer disease
	Ulcerative colitis
Carnett test positive	Abdominal wall hernia
	Cutaneous nerve entrapment
	Myofascial pain syndromes
	Rectus sheath hematoma
	Rib tip syndrome

Source: Reproduced, with permission, from Zackowski SW. Chronic recurrent abdominal pain. *Emerg Med Clin North Am.* 1998;16:877.

TABLE 28-4   Differential Diagnosis of Abdominal Pain

Chronic intermittent abdominal pain
  Abdominal epilepsy
  Abdominal migraine
  Abdominal wall
    Cutaneous nerve entrapment syndromes
    Abdominal wall hernia
    Myofascial pain syndromes
    Rectus sheath hematoma
    Rib tip syndrome
  Acute intermittent porphyria
  Ampullary stenosis
  Autoimmune disorders
  Cholelithiasis
  Crohn disease
  Diabetic radiculopathy
  Endometriosis
  Familial Mediterranean fever
  Familial pancreatitis
  Heavy metal poisoning
  Intermittent intestinal obstruction
    Intussusception
    Internal hernia
    Abdominal wall hernia
  Mesenteric ischemia
  Nerve entrapment syndromes
  Ovulation (ie, mittelschmerz)
  Ulcerative colitis
  Vertebral nerve root compression
Chronic unrelenting abdominal pain with an identifiable cause
  Autoimmune processes
  Chronic pancreatitis
  Intra-abdominal malignancies
    Gastric or hepatic metastases
    Lymphoma
    Metastatic malignancy
    Pancreatic or biliary tree cancer
  Nerve entrapment syndrome
  Occult intraperitoneal abscess
  Osteoporosis
Chronic intractable abdominal pain
  Chronic pancreatitis
  Functional dyspepsia
  Intra-abdominal malignancies
  Irritable bowel syndrome
  Psychiatric disorders
    Somatization
    Psychogenic (conversion) pain
    Hypochondriasis
    Munchausen syndrome
    Malingering

Source: Reproduced, with permission, from Zackowski SW. Chronic recurrent abdominal pain. *Emerg Med Clin North Am.* 1998;16:877.

Abdominal Epilepsy

- This disorder is associated with paroxysmal abdominal symptoms including periumbilical and right upper quadrant pain, bloating, and diarrhea.
- All patients have neurologic symptoms including headache, blurred vision, confusion, blindness, or fatigue. Temporal lobe seizure activity is found on EEG.

- Anticonvulsants have efficacy with both abdominal and neurologic symptoms.

Familial Mediterranean Fever

- Episodic abdominal pain, fever, peritoneal signs, arthritis, and leukocytosis in patients of Mediterranean descent might be associated with this disorder.
- Autosomal recessive, it usually begins at 5–15 years of age.
- There are no diagnostic tests for this disorder.
- Chronic colchicine therapy reduces the number of attacks and may help during acute attacks.

Functional Dyspepsia

- This may cause persistent or recurrent pain or discomfort in the epigastric or upper abdomen area. It is associated with bloating and early satiety.
- Other conditions, under the rubric of organic dyspepsia, are associated with these symptoms.
- Functional dyspepsia has no identifiable structural or biochemical abnormality.
- Antisecretory and promotility (eg, cisapride, metoclopramide) agents are useful therapies.

PATHOPHYSIOLOGY OF VISCERAL PAIN

OVERVIEW

- The neurologic mechanisms of visceral pain differ from those involved with somatic pain.
- The perception and psychological processing of visceral pain differ from those of somatic pain. Most visceral sensations, whether from vagal or spinal afferents, do not reach consciousness.
- Gastrointestinal innervation has been categorized as parasympathetic or sympathetic, but it is more appropriate to designate the pattern by the name of the nerves involved (vagus, pelvic, hypogastric nerves) (see Figure 28-7).
- Afferent fibers convey mechanical, thermal, chemical, and osmotic changes to modulating neurons in the spinal cord. Further information is sent to the brainstem, hypothalamus, limbic system, thalamus, and cerebral cortex.
- More than 90% of vagal afferents are unmyelinated C fibers; the rest are myelinated Aδ and Aβ fibers.
- Intrinsic afferents control and coordinate local gastrointestinal function. They contribute indirectly to visceral sensations by changes in secretomotor activity (see Figure 28-8).

NEUROPHYSIOLOGY

- The cell bodies of vagal afferents are in the nodose ganglia, and those of spinal afferents are in the dorsal

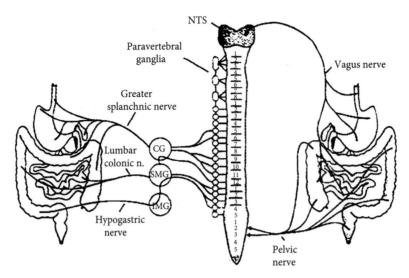

FIG. 28-7. Representation of visceral sensory innervation of the gastrointestinal tract. The nerves that are associated with the sympathetic nervous system are on the left. These spinal visceral afferent fibers traverse both prevertebral (CG, celiac ganglion; IMG, inferior mesenteric ganglion; SMG, superior mesenteric ganglion) and paravertebral ganglia en route to the spinal cord. On the right, the pelvic and vagus nerve innervation to the sacral cord and brainstem. (Reproduced, with permission, from Gebhart GF. Visceral pain: peripheral sensitisation. *Gut.* 2000;47:iv56.)

root ganglia. These afferents then project to the brainstem and spinal cord (see Figure 28-8).

- Visceral and somatic information converge in the spinothalamic, spinoreticular, and dorsal column pathways. This "viscerosomatic convergence" can result in referred pain (see Figure 28-9).
- Nerve terminals within the gastrointestinal wall convey mechanosensory information. Vagal afferents have low thresholds of activation and reach maximum

responses within physiologic levels of distension. Spinal afferents can respond beyond the physiologic level and encode both physiologic and noxious levels of stimulation. Vagal afferents are involved with physiologic regulation and modulate sensory experience. Spinal afferents mediate pain.

- Afferents are thought to have collateral branches to blood vessels and enteric ganglia to modify local blood flow and reflex pathways.

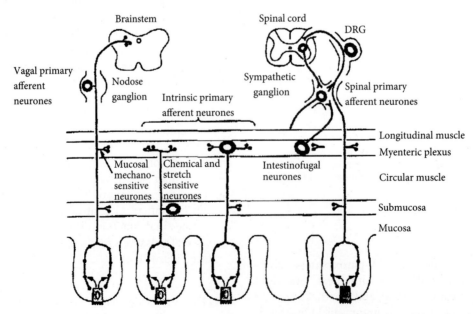

FIG. 28-8. Arrangement of the primary afferent neurons within the intestine, and central connections. (Reproduced, with permission, from Grundy D. Neuroanatomy of visceral nociception: vagal and splanchnic afferent. *Gut.* 2002;51:i2.)

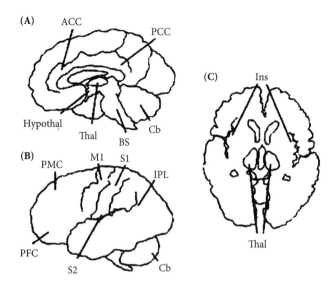

FIG. 28-9. Principal cerebral structures activated in functional imaging studies of somatic and visceral stimulation. (A) Medial view of right hemisphere. ACC, anterior cingulated cortex; PCC, posterior cingulated cortex; Hypothal, hypothalamus; Thal, thalamus; BS, brainstem; Cb, cerebellum. (B) Lateral view of left cerebral hemisphere. PFC, prefrontal cortex; PMC, premotor cortex; M1, primary motor cortex; S1, primary somatosensory cortex; S2, secondary somatosensory cortex; IPL, inferior parietal lobule. (C) Cerebral cross-sectional view at the level of the insulae and thalami. Ins, insula. (Reproduced, with permission, from Ladabaum U, Minoshima S, Owyang C. Pathobiology of visceral pain: molecular mechanisms and therapeutic implications, V. Central nervous system processing of somatic and visceral sensory signals. *Am J Physiol Gastrointest Liver Physiol.* 2000;279:G1.)

- Spinal afferents use calcitonin gene-related protein (CGRP) and substance P transmitters that may contribute to inflammation.
- Visceral afferents may play a cytoprotective role by increasing mucosal blood flow.
- Mechanosensitivity: Vagal afferents branch in circular and longitudinal muscle layers that respond to tension generated from passive stretch or active contraction. However, other vagal sensory endings called IGLE surround myenteric ganglia. These fibers may respond to muscle stretch/contraction. Spinal afferents can be influenced by many chemical mediators from injury and/or inflammation. Bradykinin and prostaglandins may potentiate each other and lead to hypersensitivity. Previously insensitive fibers may become sensitive during inflammation.

TRANSMISSION

- Traditional theory held that the viscera were innervated by separate classes of sensory receptors, some concerned with autonomic regulation and some with

sensation and pain, or that a single type of receptor sent normal signals in response to low frequencies of activation (nonnoxious) but signaled pain at high frequencies.
- Research, however, shows that high- and low-threshold receptors are present in viscera.
- For high-threshold receptors, the relationship between stimulus intensity and nerve activity (encoding) is evoked by stimuli entirely within the noxious range.
- Low-threshold receptors are intensity-encoding receptors with a low threshold to natural stimuli and encoding that spans the range of stimulation intensity from innocuous to noxious.
- Another theory is that silent nociceptors (unresponsive afferent fibers) exist and become activated only in the presence of inflammation.
- These fibers are concerned only with tissue injury and inflammation (not with mechanical stimuli).
- The importance of these *silent nociceptors* has not been established.
- The strongest evidence is that both high-threshold and intensity-encoding receptors contribute to peripheral encoding of noxious stimuli.
- Brief, acute, visceral pain initially triggers high-threshold afferents. Extended visceral stimulation (ie, hypoxia and inflammation) sensitizes high-threshold receptors and activates silent nociceptors. The CNS receives a barrage of afferent stimuli, initially from the acute injury; then central mechanisms amplify and sustain the peripheral input.
- Also, damage and inflammation of the viscus alter its normal pattern of motility and secretion. This changes the environment around the nociceptor endings, which increases excitation of sensitized nociceptors and excites distant fibers. The resultant discharges may be greater in magnitude and duration than the initial injury. Therefore, visceral pain may persist after the initial injury has begun resolving.

BIOCHEMISTRY

- Two classes of unmyelinated primary afferents innervate somatic and visceral tissues. One expresses peptide neurotransmitters, such as substance P and CGRP, and the other does not. They also terminate in different lamina of the spinal dorsal horn.
- Somatic fibers contain both classes, but visceral belong only to the peptide class. Therefore, peptides are particularly important to future therapy for visceral pain. Some preliminary data suggest that substance P may have a specific role in visceral hyperalgesia. Several receptor antagonists for substance P are being tested and may lead to new therapies for visceral pain.

CENTRAL SENSITIZATION

- In somatic nociceptive systems, the frequency-dependent increase in neuronal excitability is known as "windup." Visceral nociceptor neurons do not "wind up" as somatic neurons do. Prolonged noxious stimuli evoke increased excitability of viscerosomatic neurons in the spinal cord. These highly selective changes occur only on cells driven by the conditioning visceral stimulus. This increase in excitability may be due to the properties of the activated neuronal network and/or to the release of certain transmitters. Positive feedback loops between spinal and supraspinal structures may be prominent and could be responsible for the enhanced autonomic and motor reflexes seen with visceral pain.
- Transmission of pain was once thought to occur via crossed spinothalamic and spinoreticular pathways (ascending the contralateral side of the spinal cord after crossing the gray matter). Investigators have found three new pathways, however, that carry visceral nociception: the dorsal columns (the dorsal column pathway), the trigeminoparabrachio-amygdaloid, and spinohypothalamic pathways.
- *N*-Methyl-D-aspartate (NMDA) receptors in the spinal cord may play an important regulatory role. NMDA receptor antagonists blocked visceral pain perception in rats but did not affect painful stimuli of somatic tissues.
- Substance P and the neurokinin 1 receptor may play a role in persistent visceral pain at the spinal cord level.
- Many cerebral areas are involved in signal processing as well.
- PET and functional MRI scans show several cerebral structures activated during somatic pain, including the anterior cingulate cortex, insula, thalamus, somatosensory areas, prefrontal cortex, inferior parietal cortex, lentiform nucleus, hypothalamus, periaqueductal gray, and cerebellum. Studies of gastrointestinal distension showed a similar pattern of activity (illustrated in Figure 28-9).

PERIPHERAL SENSITIZATION

- Low-threshold or intensity-encoding receptors respond within the physiologic range. They also respond to distending stimuli in the noxious range of >30 mm Hg. The response magnitude in the noxious range is greater than that of the high-threshold fibers, which do not respond until the stimulus is at or exceeds noxious levels.
- In patients with irritable bowel syndrome (IBS), the response shifts leftward, suggesting visceral hyperalgesia. Visceral afferent neurons should exhibit sensitization (primary hyperalgesia), therefore, and the spinal neurons on which they terminate should change their excitability (secondary hyperalgesia).
- Experimental inflammation of viscera awakens silent afferent fibers that become sensitive to mechanical stimuli.

INFLAMMATORY AND NONINFLAMMATORY MEDIATORS

- Local tissue injury releases chemical mediators (potassium, hydrogen ions, ATP, bradykinin, etc) and inflammatory mediators (eg, prostaglandin E_2 [PGE_2]). These substances activate nerve endings and trigger release of algesic mediators (eg, histamine, serotonin, nerve growth factor) from other cells and afferent nerves. This sensitizes afferent nerve terminals causing an increased response to painful stimuli.
- Activation of immunocytes (ex-mast cells) and local adrenergic nerve fibers results in a state of prolonged or permanent sensitization.
- Stress alters perception of visceral pain, possibly because of increased mast cell degranulation.

LABORATORY STUDIES

ACUTE ABDOMINAL PAIN

- Laboratory tests are helpful to aid in diagnosis and to assist in preparation for an operation, if needed.
  - Complete blood count (CBC) and differential
  - Liver function tests
  - Serum electrolytes
  - Serum creatinine
  - Blood urea nitrogen
  - Amylase or lipase
  - Urinalysis
  - Urine or serum pregnancy test

CHRONIC ABDOMINAL PAIN

- In chronic recurrent abdominal pain, tests may identify a discrete cause. Laboratory studies should be ordered only if their results may alter diagnosis or therapy. CBC, erythrocyte sedimentation rate (ESR), and liver function tests may lead to a diagnosis. A pregnancy test should be performed in women.

IMAGING

IMAGING FOR ACUTE ABDOMEN

- X-rays: upright, kidneys, ureter, bladder (KUB), and upright chest films.

- CT scanning is the standard for detecting most causes of acute abdominal pain. It is highly sensitive for appendicitis, diverticulitis, intestinal ischemia, pancreatitis, intestinal obstruction, and perforated viscus. Helical CT reduces artifact from respiration and reduces scanning times. CT scans are enhanced greatly by the use of gastrointestinal and intravenous contrast administration. Helical CT angiography can also allow accurate assessment of thoracoabdominal vessels.
- Ultrasound is most useful in pelvic imaging. A full bladder acts as an acoustic window for pelvic images. Vaginal ultrasound provides images of the uterus and adnexa. For suspected cholelithiasis and cholecystitis, ultrasound is the initial imaging method of choice (the liver acts as an acoustic window).
- MRI is not the modality of choice for acute abdomen due to high cost, artifact from bowel motion, patient limits of tolerance, and lack of ready availability.

IMAGING FOR CHRONIC ABDOMINAL PAIN

- X-rays: Upright, KUB, and upright chest films should be performed in the patient without an obvious diagnosis. Upright x-rays during an attack may show dilated loops of bowel caused by intermittent obstructing hernia or intussusception, for example.
- Sigmoidoscopy or barium enema may show ischemic colitis or endometriosis.
- CT scan may reveal various pancreatic or biliary tract lesions, masses, or dilated bowel loops.
- Ultrasound may reveal biliary tract abnormalities.

TREATMENT

THE TREATMENT OF CHRONIC PAIN SYNDROMES: INTRODUCTION

- The goals of pain therapies are to:
  - Reduce intensity of pain
  - Improve physical and emotional functioning
  - Reduce drains on health care resources
- The pain-treating physician should know and understand all of the appropriate "tools of the trade" for the treatment of chronic pain of both terminal illness and nonmalignant origin.
- These tools include all of the modalities and therapies, conservative or invasive, used for treating chronic, nonmalignant, AIDS-related, and cancer-related pain syndromes. These therapies can be broadly categorized as noninvasive and invasive (see Table 28-5).

TABLE 28-5   Invasive and Noninvasive Therapies for Chronic Pain Syndromes

NONINVASIVE THERAPIES	INVASIVE THERAPIES
Exercise	Pharmacologic pain medicine
Cognitive behavioral therapy	Anesthetic blocking techniques
Physical and occupational therapy	Neuromodulatory techniques
Chiropractic manipulation	Surgery
Nutritional therapy	Neuroablation
Massage therapy	
Psychotherapy	
Alternative therapies	

Noninvasive Therapies

- Cognitive and behavioral therapies to improve locus of self-control, increase awareness and understanding of the painful experience, promote activity that is not harmful or activating of the painful experience, increase relaxation time, promote behavior that is healing, and reduce behavior that perpetuates the chronic painful experience.
- Rehabilitational pain medicine.
- Alternative pain-relieving therapies, such as acupuncture, acupressure, meditation and relaxation, nutrition, Qigong, and so on.

Invasive Therapies

- Pharmacologic interventions:
  - Nonopioid analgesics, including centrally acting nonopioids (such as methotrimeprazine, tramadol, and acetaminophen) and peripherally and centrally active NSAIDs
  - Opioid analgesics
  - Adjuvant medications: agents that are labeled for other medical purpose but have analgesic or coanalgesic properties, including the heterocyclic antidepressants; serotonin-specific reuptake inhibitor (SSRI) antidepressants; membrane-stabilizing drugs, such as anticonvulsants; local anesthetic oral analogs and local anesthetics; α_1 blocking agents; β blockers; calcium channel blockers; and so on
- Peripheral nerve blocks.
- Sympathetic nerve blocks.
- Neurodestructive procedures (for malignant pain only).
- Neuromodulatory procedures: These would include spinal cord stimulation, sacral nerve root stimulation, or a combination of both.
  - Deep brain and motor cortex stimulation
  - Intrathecal and epidural delivery of opioid and nonopioid analgesics
  - Surgical interventions

THINKING ALGORITHMICALLY: USING A PAIN TREATMENT CONTINUUM

Algorithm for Cancer-Related Pain

- The 1980s saw the introduction of the World Health Organization guidelines for pain management for the dying patient. This attempt to simplify pain management for cancer patients underscores simple interventions that can be used by technologically advanced as well as technologically deprived societies.
- These guidelines group cancer-related pain syndromes by severity and intensity into mild, moderate, and severe pain and recommend "tailoring" the strength and potency of pain medications to the severity of the pain syndrome.
  - Nonopioid analgesics are suggested for mild to moderate cancer pain.
  - Weak to moderate-strength opioids, such as codeine and hydrocodone in combination with nonopioid and adjunctive medications, are suggested for moderately severe cancer pain.
  - Potent opioids, such as morphine, hydromorphone, and methadone, together with nonopioids and adjuvant medications, are suggested for strong and severe cancer-related pain.

- By following these guidelines, physicians should be able to control the pain of 50–80% of patients dying of cancer.
  - For the cancer patient who does not respond to this approach, consideration should be given for sympatholysis with alcohol or phenol for the appropriate patient.

Algorithm for Chronic Nonmalignant Pain

- In 1999, Krames introduced an algorithm for the management of chronic pain including abdominal pain based on the KISS principle, "Keep it sweet and simple." This algorithm biased interventions based on low cost and low invasiveness and relegated more costly and more invasive therapies to "last-resort" therapies. See Figure 28-10.
- Because the original Krames Pain Treatment Continuum was based on only cost and levels of invasiveness and not comparative efficacy, many patients underwent continuous trials of therapies that failed before finding a therapy that worked.
- Not all patients responded to trials of "less costly, less invasive" treatments.
- Based on a new set of evaluative tools, the SAFE principles (*s*afety, *a*ppropriateness, time to *f*iscal

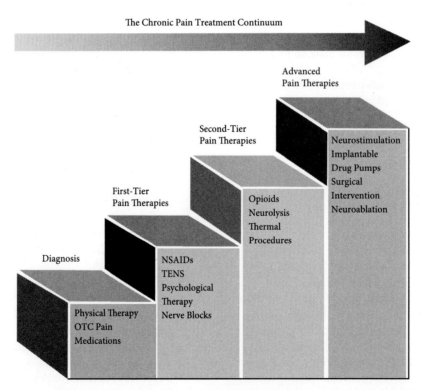

FIG. 28-10. A Pain Treatment Continuum based on the KISS principle, keep it sweet and simple. This algorithm relegates more costly and more invasive therapies to last-resort therapies. (Reproduced, with permission, from Krames ES. Interventional pain management: appropriate when less invasive therapies fail to provide adequate analgesia. *Med Clin North Am.* 1999;83(3):7870–7808.)

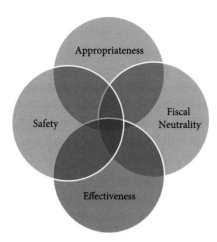

FIG. 28-11. The SAFE principles, a set of evaluative tools to compare therapies in a Venn diagram. (Reproduced, with permission, from Poree L, Krames ES, Pope J, et al. Spinal cord stimulation as treatment for complex regional pain syndrome should be considered earlier than last-resort therapy. *Neuromodulation.* 2013;16(2):125–141.)

neutrality, and efficacy), Krames et al have introduced comparative analysis to therapies in a Pain Treatment Continuum based on review of the literature and up-to-date information. See Figure 28-11.

ACUTE ABDOMINAL PAIN

- Depending on the diagnosis, treatment may include acute fluid resuscitation measures, surgery, opioid analgesics, antibiotics, and other modalities.

CHRONIC ABDOMINAL PAIN

- Depending on the diagnosis, treatment of patients with chronic recurrent abdominal pain may include surgical interventions (eg, incarcerated hernias, neoplasms with hemorrhage or causing acute obstruction).
- Treatment of patients with chronic, unrelenting, abdominal pain, either cancer-related or nonmalignant, should follow a pain treatment algorithm based on up-to-date analysis of appropriate issues/principles, the SAFE principles.
- Treatments should be performed within a multidisciplinary pain treatment center.
- Learning coping mechanisms, accepting that there may not be a diagnosis for their pain, and learning relaxation strategies are useful treatment goals for these patients.
- Appropriate interventions include:
  - Sympathetic blocks with local anesthetics of the celiac plexus or superior hypogastric plexus. Such

blocks have limited therapeutic value but may be used for diagnosis of visceral pain.
  - Although sympatholysis with neurolytics has historically been used, the general consensus is that the risk/benefit is unfavorable for chronic nonmalignant pain.
  - Continuous epidural blockade.
  - Spinal cord stimulation.
  - Intrathecal analgesia.

BIBLIOGRAPHY

Al-Chaer ED, Lawand NB, Westlund KN, Willis WD. Visceral nociceptive input into the ventral posterolateral nucleus of the thalamus: a new function for the dorsal column pathway. *J Neurophys.* 1996;76(4):2661–2674.

Berkley KJ. On the significance of viscerosomatic convergence. *APS J.* 1993;2(4):239–247.

Bonica J, Graney D. General considerations of abdominal pain. In: Loeser J, Butler S, Chapman C, Turk D, eds. *Bonica's Management of Pain.* 3rd ed. Philadelphia: Lippincott Williams & Wilkins; 2001:1235.

Bueno L, Fioramonti J. Visceral perception: inflammatory and non-inflammatory mediators. *Gut.* 2002;51:i19.

Cervero F. Visceral pain: central sensitization. *Gut.* 2000;47:iv59.

Cervero F, Laird JMA. Visceral pain. *Lancet.* 1999; 353:2145.

Chitkara DK, Rawat DJ, Talley NJ. The epidemiology of childhood recurrent abdominal pain in Western countries: a systematic review. *Am J Gastroenterol.* 2005;100(8):1868–1875.

Dang C, Aguilera P, Dang A, et al. Acute abdominal pain: four classifications can guide assessment and management. *Geriatrics.* 2002;57:30.

Geber C, Baumgärtner U, Schwab R, et al. Revised definition of neuropathic pain and its grading system: an open case series illustrating its use in clinical practice. *Am J Med.* 2009;122(10 suppl):S3–S12.

Gupta H, Dupuy DE. Advances in imaging of the acute abdomen. *Surg Clin North Am.* 1997;77:1245.

Kapural L, Narouze SN, Janicki TI, Mckhail N. Spinal cord stimulation is an effective treatment for the chronic intractable visceral pelvic pain. *Pain Med.* 2006;7(5):440–443.

Krames E, Monis S, Poree L, Deer T, Levy R. Using the SAFE principles when evaluating electrical stimulation therapies for the pain of failed back surgery syndrome. *Neuromodulation.* 2011;14(4):299–311.

Krames E, Poree LR, Deer T, Levy R. Implementing the SAFE principles for the development of pain medicine therapeutic algorithms that include neuromodulation techniques. *Neuromodulation.* 2009;12(2):104–113.

Krames E, Poree LR, Deer T, Levy R. Rethinking algorithms of pain care: the use of the S.A.F.E. principles. *Pain Med.* 2009;10(1):1–5.

Krames ES. Interventional pain management: appropriate when less invasive therapies fail to provide adequate analgesia. *Med Clin North Am.* 1999;83(3):7870–7808.

Krames ES, Foreman R. Spinal cord stimulation modulates visceral nociception and hyperalgesia via the spinothalamic tracts and the postsynaptic dorsal column pathways: a literature review and hypothesis. *Neuromodulation.* 2007;10(3):224–237.

Krames ES, Mousad DG. Spinal cord stimulation reverses pain and diarrheal episodes of irritable bowel syndrome: a case report. *Neuromodulation.* 2004;7(2):82–88.

Ladabaum U, Minoshima S, Owyang C. Pathobiology of visceral pain: molecular mechanisms and therapeutic implications, V. Central nervous system processing of somatic and visceral sensory signals. *Am J Physiol Gastrointest Liver Physiol.* 2000;279:G1.

MedlinePlus. Osler–Weber–Rendu syndrome [NIH Web site]. Available at: www.nlm.nih.gov/medlineplus/ency/article/000837.htm. Accessed June 18, 2014.

Poree L, Krames ES, Pope J, et al. Spinal cord stimulation as treatment for complex regional pain syndrome should be considered earlier than last resort therapy. *Neuromodulation.* 2013;16(2):125–141.

Sanders K, Koh S, Ward S. Interstitial cells of Cajal as pacemakers in the gastrointestinal tract. *Annu Rev Physiol.* 2006;68:307–343.

Sandler RS, Stewart WF, Liberman JN, Ricci JA, Zorich NL. Abdominal pain, bloating, and diarrhea in the United States: prevalence and impact. *Dig Dis Sci.* 2000;45(6):1166–1171.

Spaeth M. Fibromyalgia syndrome review. *J Musculoskelet Pain.* 2009;17(2):195–201.

29   UPPER EXTREMITY PAIN

Matthew Meunier, MD

INTRODUCTION

- Upper extremity pain can be related to acute trauma, the delayed effects of trauma, degenerative changes, local and remote neurologic compromise, and vascular compromise, as well as local or systemic inflammatory disease.

NEED TO RULE OUT ACUTE TREATABLE CAUSES

- A history of recent trauma should be evaluated with plain x-rays, with a minimum of two 90° orthogonal views of the affected part.
- Special attention to fracture or subluxation should be given.
- Referral to an appropriate specialist should occur to treat the underlying injury.

- A sensation of painful "sliding in and out of joint" can be a sign of chronic instability and again should be evaluated by an appropriate specialist prior to starting any pain control regimen.
- Patients with instability may well have normal-appearing radiographs.
- Degenerative conditions in the hand, wrist, elbow, or shoulder need to be ruled out.
- Typical subjective clues include a feeling of pain at the end of range of motion, pain worsening following activity, a feeling of stiffness, and localization of discomfort to a specific location.
- Radiographs with osteoarthritis will show a characteristic narrowing of the joint space with osteophytes typically present at the margins of the joint.
- Finally, all radiographs should be evaluated for the possibility of neoplastic activity, either primary or metastatic.

COMPRESSIVE NEUROPATHY

- Chronic compression of a nerve can be a cause of regional pain.
- The most commonly involved are the median nerve at the carpal tunnel and the ulnar nerve at the cubital tunnel.

CARPAL TUNNEL SYNDROME

- Carpal tunnel syndrome (CTS) is compression of the median nerve under the transverse carpal ligament. (The *carpal tunnel* is defined as the space bordered by the hook of the hamate, the triquetrum and pisiform at the ulnar side, and the scaphoid, trapezium, and flexor carpi radialis sheath on the radial side. The transverse carpal ligament is the roof, and the concave arch of carpal bones is the floor. The narrowest portion is at the level of the capitate.)
- Normal pressure in the carpal tunnel is 0–5 mm Hg, can rise to 30 mm Hg at rest in CTS, and is >90 mm Hg with wrist flexion or extension in patients with CTS.
- It is a collection of symptoms rather than a diagnostic finding. Classic symptoms include night pain that wakes the patient from sleep, pain with maximal wrist flexion or extension, decreased grip strength, and decreased dexterity.
- The exam should include Phalen test (maximal wrist flexion for 30 s with distal subjective changes), Durkan test (direct compression over carpal tunnel with distal subjective changes), and Tinel test (percussion along the path of the median nerve with radiation to fingertips).

- Electrodiagnostic testing is used to confirm nerve conduction compromise rather than a diagnosis of CTS.
- In addition, thenar atrophy and thenar motor strength, as well as subjective sensation and two-point discrimination, should be evaluated (normally <5 mm).

CUBITAL TUNNEL SYNDROME

- The ulnar nerve can be compressed in the cubital tunnel at the elbow causing pain and numbness in the ulnar border of the forearm and hand, with, classically, numbness of the small finger.
- In addition, atrophy of the first dorsal interosseous muscle (radial border of index finger metacarpal), clawing of the small finger (Duchenne sign), weakness of small finger adduction (Wartenberg sign), flattening of the palmar arch (Masse sign), and weakness of grip and pinch are later findings of chronic ulnar nerve compromise.
- The cubital tunnel is a fibrous sheath at the level of the elbow, terminating in the proximal portion of the flexor carpi ulnaris.
- Prolonged elbow flexion, direct pressure over the medial forearm or elbow, and idiopathic causes can all result in ulnar nerve compression.
- In the exam, increased numbness and tingling in the small finger with elbow flexion (elbow flexion test) and pain and distal radiation of tingling when ulnar nerve percussion at the elbow is performed (Tinel sign) are observed. Decreased subjective sensation in the small finger is often present. Decreased grip strength, decreased pinch strength, ulnar-sided digital clawing, and first dorsal interosseous atrophy are all later findings.
- Electrodiagnostic testing will classically show slowing of the conduction velocity at the elbow to less than 45 m/s.

OTHER SITES OF COMPRESSION

- Other sites of compression include the median nerve in the forearm (most commonly under the pronator teres), the radial nerve in the axilla (quadrangular space syndrome) or forearm (most commonly under the supinator), and the ulnar nerve in Guyon's canal (ulnar border of carpal tunnel).
- These are all far less frequent than carpal tunnel or cubital tunnel syndrome and often present with a deep aching sensation.
- Finally, in any patient with suspected idiopathic nerve compression, cervical spine pathology needs to be ruled out.

ELECTROPHYSIOLOGIC TESTING

- Prolonged distal latency, decreased amplitude, increased area, and decreased conduction velocity can all indicate compromise of the nerve.

TREATMENT

- The mainstay of treatment remains splinting in a position to decrease pressure on the affected nerve (wrist straight for the median nerve, elbow at approximately 45° for the ulnar nerve).
- Splints should be worn at the minimum at night and, preferably, as much as tolerated during the day.
- For CTS, a local anesthetic and steroid (1 cm³ of lidocaine or marcaine combined with 1 cm³ of Kenalog or similar steroid) are injected into the carpal tunnel combined with splinting or surgical release. The injection point is 1 cm proximal to the wrist flexion crease and 1 cm ulnar to the palmaris longus tendon (or approximately 1 cm radial to flexor carpi ulnaris). The needle should be oriented 45° to the long axis of the arm in both the radial–ulnar and palmar–dorsal planes, aiming distally. Injection directly into the median nerve should be avoided. If resistance is felt, repositioning should occur. Injection around the ulnar nerve at the cubital tunnel is not recommended.

POSTTRAUMA: CRUSH, NEUROMA, DYSVASCULAR CONDITIONS

- Chronic pain can be a complication following upper extremity trauma.
- The effects of residual articular incongruity can often lead to degenerative arthrosis.
- The mainstay of treatment is nonsteroidal anti-inflammatory medication; however, some patients find this is inadequate for pain control requirements.
- Surgical options include arthrodesis, allograft replacement, and total joint prosthetic replacement and should be explored prior to commencement of a complex medication regimen.

NERVE TRAUMA CAN LEAD TO CHRONIC PAIN

- An area of intense sensitivity with distal radiation of an "electric shock," particularly in the area of previous trauma, should raise suspicion for a neuroma.
- Occasionally surgical treatment can be effective, typically burying the neuroma under a muscular or fat flap.
- Traumatized nerves in continuity (ie, with brachial plexus or upper extremity traction injuries) can be quite painful.

- If compression from scar or local tissues, intraneural fibrosis, and neuroma in continuity has been ruled out, then medical treatment may well be needed for control of symptoms.
- Historically the primary treatment has been Neurontin (mechanism unknown); however, recent evidence suggests that antidepressants such as amitriptyline have been at least equally effective in controlling chronic nerve pain symptoms.

TRAUMA CAN LEAD TO CHRONIC ARTERIAL INSUFFICIENCY OR TO CHRONIC VENOUS CONGESTION

- Arterial insufficiency often causes a claudication-type pain, most common with increasing levels of activity, or in more severe cases, ischemic pain occurs.
- In addition, patients often complain of stress- or cold-induced symptoms.
- The most severe group may even present with vascular insufficiency ulceration distal to the level of compromise.
- Although it may sound obvious, the first line of treatment is smoking cessation, cold avoidance, and stress reduction.
- In addition, surgical evaluation for possible reconstruction should be considered.
- For persistent symptoms, beta blockade and calcium channel blockade can also be effective treatment.
- Sympathetic blockade with local injections can be useful in establishing the diagnosis, but is unlikely to offer long-term relief.
- Venous stasis can also be a cause of pain, most likely related to pooling of blood, increased local pressures, and deoxygenation of pooled blood.
- Treatment is directed at improving venous return and typically includes compressive garments and avoiding dependent positioning.

VASCULOPATHY: SCLERODERMA, BUERGER DISEASE

- Chronic vaso-occlusive and vasospastic conditions can often lead to ischemic pain.
- The most commonly encountered include systemic sclerosis (scleroderma and CREST), thromboangiitis obliterans (TAO, or Buerger disease), and Raynaud phenomenon and syndrome.
- Raynaud phenomenon is common in the early stages of almost all of the vasculopathic conditions and classically has three phases: blanching (white), cyanosis (blue), and rubor (red).

- These phases correlate with the initial vasospasm and vascular insufficiency (white), vascular pooling and deoxygenation (blue), and subsequent reactive hyperemia (red).
- The hyperemic phase is accompanied by a classic burning pain sensation. Later, cases often present with digital contracture and ulceration. Frank gangrene is unfortunately not all that uncommon.
- In all vaso-occlusive conditions the primary goal of treatment is to limit vascular spasm. Unfortunately, success is unpredictable and often of limited long-term effectiveness.
- As with posttraumatic vasculopathy, calcium channel blockade, stellate ganglion, or brachial plexus blocks, although not providing a cure, may allow modification of symptoms and allow digital ulcerations to heal.

COMPLEX REGIONAL PAIN SYNDROME

- Following occasionally even incidental trauma, hypersensitivity to stimuli can occur in an injured limb.
- The diagnosis is suspected in patients who show allodynia (pain in a specific dermatomal distribution to normal stimuli) and hyperesthesia (increased sensitivity to stimulation) to a normal stimulus.
- Classic findings include pain out of proportion to normal stimuli, loss of motion in the affected extremity, hyperhidrosis, shiny red skin, and increased hair growth on the affected limb.
- Diagnosis is based on the presence of certain signs and symptoms.
- Prior to undergoing treatment, it is paramount that underlying causes of chronic pain, particularly compressive neuropathy, be ruled out.
- Type I CRPS, or classic reflex sympathetic dystrophy, is not related to a defined nerve injury. In type II, a neural injury is present.
- Treatment centers on controlling pain and improving function.
- Treatment of CRPS incorporates a multidisciplinary approach; however, current diagnostic criteria do not predict the success of specific treatment regimens.
- Aggressive, but careful, hand therapy is essential in the recovery of function.
- In addition, treatment of the underlying causes, the allodynia and hyperesthesia, and any psychologic factors is part of a potentially successful program.
- Approximately 80% of patients diagnosed and treated within one year of onset have an improvement or full recovery from CRPS.
- In patients with symptoms lasting longer than one year approximately 50% have significant impairment despite adequate treatment.

BIBLIOGRAPHY

Cooney WP. Somatic versus sympathetic mediated chronic limb pain: experience and treatment options. *Hand Clin.* 1997;13:355–361.

Gelberman RH, Eaton RG, Urbaniak JR. Peripheral nerve compression. *Instr Course Lect.* 1994;43:31–53.

Koman LA, Poehling GG, Smith TL. Complex regional pain syndrome: reflex sympathetic dystrophy and causalgia. In: Green DP, Hotchkiss RN, Pederson WC, eds. *Green's Operative Hand Surgery.* 4th ed. New York: Churchill Livingstone; 1999.

Mackinnon SE. Pathophysiology of nerve compression. *Hand Clin.* 2002;18:231–241.

Troum SJ, Smith TL, Koman LA, Ruch DS. Management of vasospastic disorders of the hand. *Clin Plast Surg.* 1997; 24:121–132.

Wilson PR. Post-traumatic upper extremity reflex sympathetic dystrophy. *Hand Clin.* 1997;13:367–372.

30 LOWER EXTREMITY PAIN

Andrew Albert Indresano, MD
Robert Scott Meyer, MD

INTRODUCTION

- Evaluation of pain in the lower extremity can be a diagnostic challenge.
- A thorough assessment requires a precise understanding of both primary pain generators and referred pain in specific areas of the extremity.
- Questions regarding the characteristics of the pain, including its location, onset, duration, quality, radiation, severity, and aggravating and alleviating factors, are important, and frequently a preliminary diagnosis can be made on history alone.
- A detailed physical examination is critical, and with this added information the correct diagnosis can usually be reached with confidence.
- This chapter provides a detailed differential diagnosis of lower extremity pain by region, with tips on history, physical exam findings, and diagnostic tests that will help determine the correct diagnosis.

SACROILIAC JOINT PAIN

- The diagnosis of sacroiliac joint pain can be difficult due to its anatomic location, and disorders of this joint are frequently underdiagnosed.
- The sacroiliac joint is commonly affected by osteoarthritis and is also a characteristic feature of patients with spondyloarthropathies such as ankylosing spondylitis (often the initial pain generator in this disease entity) and psoriatic arthritis. Patients with a history of intravenous drug use may present with a septic arthritis of the sacroiliac joint.
- A typical pain pattern of sacroiliac disease is the involved buttock area with referral to the low back, the posterior thigh, and, occasionally, the groin. It is very important to rule out sacroiliac joint pain and dysfunction in patients with low back pain as it may be the primary cause of the back pain in up to 30% of these patients.
- The physical examination of the sacroiliac joint includes palpation of the posterior joint and several provocative maneuvers. The joint can be stressed by distraction, compression, and rotation of the pelvis. Patrick test or *fabere* sign (flexion, abduction, external rotation, and extension of the hip) typically reproduces the pain in the buttock area. If this test causes groin pain, the hip joint is the more likely pain generator.
- Plain radiographs, including AP and oblique views of the pelvis, may be helpful in documenting sacroiliac joint arthritis and are less expensive than a CT scan. The latter, however, is the preferred study to qualify the degree of osteoarthritis. In cases of septic arthritis, inflammatory arthritis, or other disorders where soft tissue imaging of the joint is important, MRI is the modality of choice.
- An injection of anesthetic and steroid into the sacroiliac joint, along with an arthrogram for confirmation of appropriate location, is extremely useful in confirming the diagnosis of sacroiliac joint pain and dysfunction.

HIP PAIN

- Intra-articular causes of hip pain include osteoarthritis, inflammatory arthritis, septic arthritis, osteonecrosis, femoroacetabular impingement (FAI) and labral pathology, and femoral neck stress fractures. Common extra-articular causes of pain include greater trochanteric bursitis, snapping hip, iliopsoas bursitis/tendonitis, muscle strains about the hip, and referred pain such as facet joint arthritis of the low back, lumbar radiculitis, and sacroiliac joint pathology see Table 30-1.
- It is important for the patient to relate where the hip pain is located. Lateral hip pain implies greater trochanteric bursitis, whereas groin pain is typically seen with iliopsoas bursitis/tendonitis or intra-articular causes, particularly arthritis. Buttock pain can also occur with intra-articular conditions, but referred pain from the back or sacroiliac joint should be considered. It is not uncommon for groin pain from

TABLE 30-1   Differential Diagnosis of Hip Pain

Extra-articular causes
  Referred pain from the lumbar spine or sacroiliac joint
  Greater trochanteric bursitis
  Iliopsoas tendonitis
  Coxa saltans (snapping hip)
  Muscle strains and contusions
Intra-articular causes
  Labral pathology
  Loose bodies
  Osteonecrosis of the femoral head
  Osteoarthritis, inflammatory arthritis, septic arthritis
  Femoral neck stress fractures

intra-articular causes, particularly arthritis, to radiate down into the thigh and medial knee.

- A focused history should include exposure to risk factors for osteonecrosis such as alcohol use, corticosteroid use, clotting disorders, and previous hip trauma. A history regarding overuse syndromes or amenorrhea in a young woman may lead to the diagnosis of a femoral neck stress fracture or musculotendinous strain. A history of audible snapping or clicking implies the presence of etiologies such as coxa saltans (snapping hip), iliopsoas bursitis, and labral pathology. Patients with hip arthritis usually give a history of mechanical symptoms such as locking, clicking, and catching.

- Typical physical examination findings in patients with arthritis include limited hip range of motion—particularly internal rotation, hip joint contractures (positive Thomas test), limb shortening, and a positive Trendelenburg sign or gait. A Patrick test should be performed to help rule out sacroiliac pain and a strait leg raise and neurologic examination performed to rule out lumbar radiculitis. A good screening test for intra-articular hip pathology, particularly arthritis, is the Stinchfield test. The patient is asked to actively elevate a straight leg off the exam table, which increases the intra-articular hip pressure. The examiner then adds some gentle manual resistance. The test is positive if it causes typical groin, thigh, or buttock pain, sometimes associated with yielding weakness.

- A hip apprehension test may be useful in the diagnosis of hip anterior labral pathology and FAI. In this test, also known as the impingement test, the patient has pain with flexion, adduction, and internal rotation of the hip joint while supine. A click may also be reproduced with this maneuver.

- Plain radiographs to look for arthritis should include an AP pelvis and AP and lateral views of the symptomatic hip. A hip stress fracture or osteonecrosis of the femoral head may not be apparent on plain films, and further advanced imaging such as MRI should be obtained if clinical suspicion is high. An MRI arthrogram may be useful in the diagnosis of hip labral pathology; however, physicians should strongly consider whether the findings on MRI arthrogram will alter treatment strategy for an individual patient with a clinical suspicion of labral pathology given the low negative predictive value for this test.

- Iliopsoas bursography for suspected iliopsoas bursitis with audible snapping may be useful.

- Diagnostic and/or therapeutic extra- and intra-articular injections about the hip are often very useful. Common examples include a greater trochanteric bursa injection, an intra-articular hip joint injection, an iliopsoas bursa injection, a sacroiliac joint injection, and lumbar spine injections such as facet joint and epidural injections (Table 30-1).

KNEE PAIN

- Intra-articular causes of knee pain include arthritis, articular cartilage injuries, meniscus tears, ligament tears, tendon tears, subchondral insufficiency fracture of the femoral condyle (entity more commonly known as spontaneous osteonecrosis of the knee [SONK]), an inflamed plica, and patellofemoral pain syndrome. Extra-articular etiologies include iliotibial band syndrome, patellar or quadriceps tendonitis, pes anserine tendonitis or bursitis, and referred pain from the hip and lumbar spine. Also in the differential diagnosis, particularly in a patient with a recent injury or surgical procedure to the knee, is complex regional pain syndrome see Table 30-2.

- It is useful to ask the patient to describe the exact location of the pain and even to point to where the pain is located. Anterior knee pain is suggestive of patellar or quadriceps tendonitis or patellofemoral pathology. Lateral knee pain may represent iliotibial band tendonitis, a lateral meniscus tear, or lateral compartment arthritis. Medial knee pain may represent pes anserine tendonitis or bursitis, a medial meniscus tear, and medial compartment arthritis. Low back pain may radiate to the medial or lateral knee depending on its dermatomal distribution, and hip pain classically refers to the medial knee via the obturator nerve.

- A focused history should include questions regarding mechanical problems, such as clicking, catching, locking, and giving way. These symptoms usually point to an internal derangement such as a meniscus tear or arthritis. Questions with respect to associated injuries or surgery, along with a history of temperature and skin color changes, may lead to a diagnosis of complex regional pain syndrome.

TABLE 30-2 Differential Diagnosis of Knee Pain

Extra-articular causes
   Referred pain from the lumbar spine or hip joint
   Iliotibial band syndrome
   Patellar or quadriceps tendonitis
   Pes anserine tendonitis
Intra-articular causes
   Meniscal tear
   Chondral injuries
   Insufficiency fracture/osteonecrosis
   Ligament injury
   Tendon injury
   Symptomatic plica
   Patellofemoral pain syndrome
   Osteoarthritis, inflammatory arthritis, septic arthritis

- A screening examination of the lumbar spine, along with a neurologic examination of the lower extremities, as well as a good examination of the hip, is very useful in ruling out causes of referred pain to the knee, particularly when the clinical suspicion is high.
- Useful physical examination findings for the diagnosis of meniscus tears include focal joint line tenderness and positive provocative maneuvers such as McMurray test. A thorough exam should also include range of motion of the knee, a ligament stability exam, and competency of the patellar and quadriceps tendon. Tenderness in the medial parapatellar region may represent plica syndrome, and a knee joint effusion may represent chondral injuries or osteoarthritis. Other typical exam findings in cases of arthritis include deformity of the knee, limited range of motion, and crepitus in the knee. Typical findings of complex regional pain syndrome include temperature changes, skin color changes, and pain out of proportion to exam findings, and are discussed in more detail in other chapters.
- Physical examination findings for extra-articular causes of knee pain typically involve tenderness to palpation of the involved structure, such as the patellar or quadriceps tendon, pes anserine insertion, and insertion of the iliotibial band at Gerdy's tubercle.
- AP and lateral plain radiographs are useful in the workup of knee pain and should always be weight bearing. A Rosenberg view is useful for detecting early evidence of tibiofemoral osteoarthritis and should also be a weight-bearing film. A merchant view should also be taken to evaluate the patellofemoral compartment. Advanced imaging such as MRI can be extremely helpful for suspected meniscal, chondral, and ligament injuries and for subchondral insufficiency fractures or osteonecrosis.
- As in other areas of the lower extremity, differential diagnostic injections may be quite useful. An injection of anesthetic and steroid into the pes anserine bursa, for example, may help differentiate between a medial meniscus tear and pes tendonitis/bursitis.
- Treatment is effective if the differential diagnosis is narrowed to a short list. Physical therapy and nonsteroidal anti-inflammatory drugs are used for the majority of extrinsic causes. Corticosteroid injections are also commonly useful. Treatment of proximal pathology such as herniated nucleus pulposus in the spine or hip pathology to diminish the referred pain in the knee can also be provided when necessary.
- On failure of nonoperative therapy, treatment of intrinsic causes include arthroscopy for meniscal or chondral pathology, osteotomy for limb malalignment, and arthroplasty for symptomatic and significant osteoarthritis (Table 30-2).

LEG (CALF) PAIN

- Common extrinsic causes of leg pain include referred pain from the lumbar spine, such as radiculitis and neurogenic claudication, and referred pain from the hip or knee.
- Common intrinsic causes of leg pain include periostitis (shin splints), tendonitis/muscle strain, gastrocnemius muscle tear (tennis leg), tibial or fibular stress fracture, acute or chronic compartment syndrome (CCS), vascular claudication, deep venous thrombosis, varicose veins, and ruptured popliteal cyst see Table 30-3.
- Both history and physical examination are important in distinguishing neurogenic from vascular claudication. Vascular claudication is typically a cramping pain that is brought on by walking a certain time or distance and is relieved by stopping walking. Neurogenic claudication is also brought on by walking but may occur with standing as well. This pain is typically relieved by assuming a specific posture such as sitting or bending forward. A detailed neurovascular examination is critical and will help confirm the diagnosis. Having a patient ride a stationary bike is a classic test to help determine if the symptoms are related to vascular claudication (pain with stationary bike riding) or neurogenic claudication (typically will not cause associated pain).
- Periostitis is a typical overuse injury seen in running and jumping, and individuals who overpronate at the foot and ankle may be more susceptible to this injury. Exam findings include tenderness to palpation either over the medial tibia or posteromedial tibial border and overlying skin changes such as swelling or redness. Similar history and exam findings are present in a tibial stress fracture, although the exam findings may be more focal. A bone scan or MRI is often very useful in the diagnosis of a stress fracture.
- Exertional or CCS of the calf may occur in any of the four compartments of the leg; however, anterior

TABLE 30-3   Differential Diagnosis of Leg (Calf) Pain

Extrinsic causes
  Lumbar radiculitis
  Neurogenic claudication
  Referred pain from hip or knee
Intrinsic causes
  Periostitis (shin splints)
  Tendonitis/muscle strain
  Gastrocnemius muscle tear (tennis leg)
  Stress fracture
  Acute or chronic compartment syndrome
  Vascular claudication
  Deep venous thrombosis
  Varicose veins
  Ruptured popliteal cyst

compartment syndrome is the most common. Unlike shin splints or tibial stress fracture, pain from CCS may occur after a typical period of time or distance during activity. Associated symptoms include weakness and numbness. Physical examination findings may be completely absent in the resting patient, but fascial defects may be noted. In the exercising patient weakness, numbness, and pain on passive stretch of the muscles in the involved compartment are common. Confirming the diagnosis of CCS can be difficult, but elevation of intramuscular pressures is the hallmark.

- Deep venous thrombosis and ruptured popliteal cyst may present with similar findings of calf pain. In both cases the calf is usually swollen; in fact, there are reported cases of compartment syndrome due to ruptured popliteal cysts. The calf may be tender to palpation, and Homans sign (calf pain with passive dorsiflexion of the ankle) may be positive in both conditions. Calf ultrasonography is usually helpful in making the correct diagnosis.
- A tear of the medial gastrocnemius (tennis leg) also presents as a painful, swollen calf. As with ruptures of the Achilles tendon, the patient frequently reports a history of feeling like the calf was struck with an object and a "pop" is felt. On examination there is focal tenderness and swelling at the medial head of the gastrocnemius and Thompson test for a ruptured Achilles tendon is negative (Table 30-3).

FOOT AND ANKLE PAIN

- Extrinsic causes of foot and ankle pain include referred pain from the lumbar spine, hip, knee, or leg.
- Intrinsic causes of foot and ankle pain include tendonitis (Achilles tendon, posterior tibial tendon, peroneal tendons), ligament sprains, stress fractures, metatarsalgia, Morton's neuroma, plantar fasciitis, tarsal tunnel

syndrome, vascular claudication, osteochondral lesions of the talus, and arthritis of the ankle, hindfoot, midfoot, or forefoot see Table 30-4.
- Plantar fasciitis is very common and usually presents as medial heel pain that is worse on first rising in the morning or after rest. This pain may be relieved by stretching, night splinting, or local steroid injections.
- Ankle pain with mechanical symptoms of catching, clicking, or locking, and occasional or persistent swelling is suggestive of an osteochondral lesion of the talus or tibiotalar arthritis.
- Pain along a particular course of a tendon with focal swelling is suggestive of tendonitis and may be exacerbated by passive stretching of the tendon. An acute or subacute loss of the foot's medial arch (flatfoot deformity) is commonly associated with posterior tibial tendon insufficiency. In such cases the deformity will be associated with the "too many toes sign" where the foot viewed from behind will be abducted and "too many" toes will appear on the outside of the forefoot.
- Metatarsal stress fractures and stress fractures of the tarsal navicular or distal fibula are usually associated with an increase in specific activities such as running.
- Ankle sprains are usually associated with a history of an inversion injury to the ankle, and the pain is typically at the anterolateral ankle joint. Deltoid ligament sprains are less common and are associated with pain in the medial ankle. High ankle sprains (syndesmosis sprains) may be distinguished from typical lateral ankle sprains by a positive "squeeze test" (compression of the tibia and fibula at the mid or distal calf). Prolonged pain in the ankle following an ankle sprain may be caused by a syndesmosis sprain, tendon tear, or osteochondral injury to the talus, and in such cases an MRI is often useful.
- Pain during weight bearing in an interspace between the toes, particularly the third interspace, is suggestive of a Morton's neuroma. Associated symptoms include numbness, burning pain, and cramping in the forefoot or toes.
- Tarsal tunnel syndrome is similar to its counterpart in the hand, carpal tunnel syndrome. Entrapment of the posterior tibial nerve in its tunnel is frequently associated with pain, numbness, and tingling in the plantar aspect of the foot. The pain is usually activity related and reduced by rest. A positive Tinel sign may be present over the tarsal tunnel, and electrodiagnostic testing may be helpful in making the diagnosis as well.
- Arthritis is common in the foot and ankle and is typically associated with stiffness and activity related pain. Common sites of osteoarthritis include the tibiotalar joint, subtalar joint, talonavicular and calcaneocuboid

TABLE 30-4 Differential Diagnosis of Foot and Ankle Pain

Extrinsic causes
  Referred pain from the lumbar spine, hip, knee, or leg
Intrinsic causes
  Tendonitis
  Ligament sprains
  Stress fractures
  Metatarsalgia
  Morton's neuroma
  Plantar fasciitis
  Tarsal tunnel syndrome
  Vascular claudication
  Osteochondritis dissecans of the talus
  Arthritis of the ankle, hindfoot, midfoot, or forefoot
  Subtalar or tibiotalar arthritis

joints, tarsometatarsal (Lisfranc) joints, and the metatarsophalangeal joint of the hallux. Differential injections of a local anesthetic and steroid are sometimes useful for both diagnostic and therapeutic purposes, particularly in cases of concomitant ankle and hindfoot arthritis (Table 30-4).

Bibliography

Ahmad M, Tsang K, Mackenney PJ, Adedapo AO. Tarsal tunnel syndrome: a literature review. *Foot Ankle Surg.* 2012;18(3):149–152.

Allen WC, Cope R. Coxa saltans: the snapping hip revisited. *J Am Acad Orthop Surg.* 1995;3:303–308.

Anderson K, Strickland SM, Warren R. Hip and groin injuries in athletes. *Am J Sports Med.* 2001;29:521–533.

Braun J, Sieper J, Bollow M. Imaging of sacroiliitis. *Clin Rheumatol.* 2000;19:51–57.

Byrd JW. Labral lesions: an elusive source of hip pain case reports and literature review. *Arthroscopy.* 1996;12:603–612.

Curl W. Popliteal cysts: historical background and current knowledge. *J Am Acad Orthop Surg.* 1996;4:129–133.

Deland JT. Adult-acquired flatfoot deformity. *J Am Acad Orthop Surg.* 2008;16(7):399–406.

Dowd GS, Hussein R, Khanduja V, Ordman AJ. Complex regional pain syndrome with special emphasis on the knee. *J Bone Joint Surg Br.* 2007;89(3):285–290.

Easley ME, Latt LD, Santangelo JR, Merian-Genast M, Nunley JA 2nd. Osteochondral lesions of the talus. *J Am Acad Orthop Surg.* 2010;18(10):616–630.

Edwards DJ, Lomas D, Villar RN. Diagnosis of the painful hip by magnetic resonance imaging and arthroscopy. *J Bone Joint Surg Br.* 1995;77:374–376.

Frymoyer J. Degenerative spondylolisthesis: diagnosis and treatment. *J Am Acad Orthop Surg.* 1994;2:9–15.

Fulkerson JP. Patellofemoral pain disorders: evaluation and management. *J Am Acad Orthop Surg.* 1994;2:124–132.

Gill L. Plantar fasciitis: diagnosis and conservative management. *J Am Acad Orthop Surg.* 1997;5:109–117.

Hungerford DS. Pathogenesis of ischemic necrosis of the femoral head. *Instr Course Lect.* 1983;32:252–260.

James SL. Running injuries to the knee. *J Am Acad Orthop Surg.* 1995;3:309–318.

Lavernia CJ, Sierra RJ, Grieco FR. Osteonecrosis of the femoral head. *J Am Acad Orthop Surg.* 1999;7:250–261.

Lyons JC, Peterson LF. The snapping iliopsoas tendon. *Mayo Clin Proc.* 1984;59:327–329.

Mankin HJ. Nontraumatic necrosis of bone (osteonecrosis). *N Engl J Med.* 1992;326:1473–1479.

Mont MA, Hungerford DS. Non-traumatic avascular necrosis of the femoral head. *J Bone Joint Surg Am.* 1995;77:459–474.

Mont MA, Marker DR, Zywiel MG, Carrino JA. Osteonecrosis of the knee and related conditions. *J Am Acad Orthop Surg.* 2011;19(8):482–494.

Parvizi J, Leunig M, Ganz R. Femoroacetabular impingement. *J Am Acad Orthop Surg.* 2007;15(9):561–570.

Pedowitz RA, Hargens AR, Mubarak SJ, Gershuni DH. Modified criteria for the objective diagnosis of chronic compartment syndrome of the leg. *Am J Sports Med.* 1990;18:35–40.

Reurink G, Jansen SP, Bisselink JM, et al. Reliability and validity of diagnosis acetabular labral lesions with magnetic resonance arthrography. *J Bone Joint Surg Am.* 2012;94(18):1643–1648.

Schwarzer AC, Aprill CN, Bogduk N. The sacroiliac joint in chronic low back pain. *Spine (Phila Pa 1976).* 1995;20(1):31–37.

Teitz CC, Hu SS, Arendt EA. The female athlete: evaluation and treatment of sports-related problems. *J Am Acad Orthop Surg.* 1997;5:87–96.

Weinfeld S, Myerson MS. Interdigital neuritis: diagnosis and treatment. *J Am Acad Orthop Surg.* 1996;4:328–335.

Wuest T. Injuries to the distal lower extremity syndesmosis. *J Am Acad Orthop Surg.* 1997;5:172–181.

31 HEADACHES

Joel R. Saper, MD
Arnaldo Neves Da Silva, MD

EPIDEMIOLOGY

- Primary headache disorders are highly prevalent conditions affecting tens of millions of US citizens and hundreds of millions of individuals worldwide.
- The lifetime prevalence of common headache disorders can be more than 78%, with migraine prevalence greater than 20% in adult women.
- The economic and quality-of-life burden of migraine alone is substantial, with the most disabled half of migraine sufferers accounting for more than 90% of migraine-related work loss.
- Barriers to successful care include failure to properly diagnose, underestimation by both the professional and public of the morbidity of these conditions, and denied access to appropriate treatment.

PRIMARY AND SECONDARY HEADACHES

- *Primary headaches* include those in which intrinsic dysfunction of the nervous system, often, but not always, genetic in origin, predisposes to increased vulnerability to headache attacks. Examples include cluster headache (CH) and migraine.
- *Secondary headaches* are those in which the headache is secondary to an organic or physiologic process, intracranially or extracranially.
- According to the International Classification of Headache Disorders, the primary headache entities include migraine, tension-type headache, trigeminal autonomic cephalgia, and other primary headache disorders. In this chapter, we will focus on the headache diagnoses most frequently seen in clinical practice:
  1. Migraine:
     a. With aura
     b. Without aura
     c. Chronic
  2. Tension-type headache:
     a. Episodic
     b. Chronic
  3. Trigeminal autonomic cephalgia:
     a. CH
     b. Paroxysmal hemicrania (PH)
     c. Hemicrania continua (HC)
     d. Short-lasting, unilateral neuralgiform headache with conjunctival injection and tearing (SUNCT)
  4. Other primary headache disorders:
     a. Primary thunderclap headache
     b. New daily persistent headache (NDPH)
- Secondary headaches can arise from more than 300 conditions, among which are ischemic, metabolic, intracranial, cerebrospinal fluid (CSF) hypotension/hypertension, infectious, endocrine, and cervicogenic disorders.

MIGRAINE

- *Migraine* is a complex neurophysiologic disorder characterized by episodic and progressive forms of head pain, in association with numerous neurologic and nonneurologic (autonomic, psychophysiologic) accompaniments. These can precede, accompany, or follow the headache itself (see Table 31-1).
- Migraine is classified into three major subtypes:
  ○ *Migraine with aura*: Heralding neurologic events lasting 30 min to 1 h occur before the head pain attacks (only 20% of migraine attacks).

TABLE 31-1   Migraine Without Aura

Diagnostic criteria:

A. At least five attacks fulfilling criteria B–D
B. Headache attacks lasting 4–72 hours (untreated or unsuccessfully treated)
C. Headache has at least two of the following four characteristics:
  1. Unilateral location
  2. Pulsating quality
  3. Moderate or severe pain intensity
  4. Aggravation by or causing avoidance of routine physical activity (eg, walking or climbing stairs)
D. During headache at least one of the following:
  1. Nausea and/or vomiting
  2. Photophobia and phonophobia
E. Not better accounted for by another ICHD-3 diagnosis

  ○ *Migraine without aura*: Attacks of migraine and accompaniments occur without clear-cut preheadache neurologic symptomatology.
  ○ *Chronic migraine*: In this often progressive form of migraine intermittent attacks occur at increasing frequency, eventually reaching 15 or more days per month. Of these 15 days, 8 days must fulfill episodic migraine criteria. By definition, *chronic migraine* occurs on a backdrop of episodic *migraine without aura*, often accompanied by comorbid neuropsychiatric phenomena. *Chronic migraine* is frequently associated with medication overuse and "rebound" (now referred to as *medication overuse headache*) (see later). Comorbid conditions associated with migraine, particularly *chronic migraine*, include depression, anxiety and panic disorders, bipolar disorder, obsessive-compulsive disorder, character disorders, and perhaps fibromyalgia.

CLINICAL SYMPTOMATOLOGY OF MIGRAINE

- 80% to 90% of cases have a family history.
- The 3:1 female:male gender ratio is thought to be related primarily to the adverse influence of estrogen on migraine mechanisms.
- Attacks generally last 4–72 h *for episodic migraine*.
- Attacks are often accompanied by a wide range of autonomic and cognitive symptoms.
- In complex cases, particularly *chronic migraine*, an association with several neuropsychiatric comorbid disorders, including depression, panic/anxiety syndromes, sleep disturbance, and obsessive-compulsive disorder, is likely.
- Predisposed individuals are particularly vulnerable to attack provocation (triggering) by certain extrinsic and intrinsic events, including hormonal fluctuation

(ie, menstrual periods, use of oral contraceptives), weather changes, certain foods, skipped meals and fasting, extra sleeping time, and stress.

PATHOPHYSIOLOGY OF MIGRAINE

- Migraine is a brain disorder that generally renders the brain overly sensitive and overly responsive to a variety of internal and external stimuli. Trigeminal/cervical connections and cervical activation may be important phenomena in the clinical manifestations, pathogenesis, and treatment. Key features of current pathophysiologic concepts include:
  - Trigeminal-mediated perivascular (neurogenic) inflammation resulting in painful vascular and meningeal tissue
  - The perivascular and systemic release of vasoactive neuropeptides, particularly calcitonin gene-related peptide (CGRP)
  - The development of allodynia and central sensitization as attacks progress
  - The presence of an active "modulator zone" in the dorsal raphe nucleus of the midbrain during migraine attacks
  - Activation and threshold reduction of neurons in the descending trigeminal system following C2–3 cervical stimulation
  - The deposition of nonheme iron in the brainstem, roughly correlated to increasingly frequent attacks
  - A yet-to-be-defined relationship to nitrous oxide, and numerous other neurohormonal peptide and receptor dynamics, including those involving glial cells and release of proinflammatory cytokines

TENSION-TYPE HEADACHE

- This controversial disorder is classified into both episodic and chronic forms. Episodic forms have certain features that overlap with *migraine without aura*, although there is a general absence of throbbing pain and autonomic accompaniments. *Chronic tension-type headache* overlaps in clinical features with *chronic migraine*. Both forms of *tension-type headache* may be present in patients who have otherwise typical migraine headaches. Tension-type headaches are usually bilateral and pressing/tightness in quality. Typically, as noted earlier, tension-type headaches are not associated with nausea but phonophobia and photophobia can be present. Some authorities believe that tension-type headaches are variant form of migraine, but they are listed as a distinct entity in the classification systems.

MEDICATION OVERUSE HEADACHE (FORMERLY REBOUND HEADACHE)

- Rebound headache (or medication overuse headache) is a self-sustaining headache condition characterized by persisting and recurring headache (usually migraine forms) against a background of chronic, regular use of centrally acting analgesics, ergotamine tartrate, or triptans. The key features of this condition include:
  - Weeks to months of excessive use of the above agents, with usage exceeding two to three days per week
  - Insidious increase in headache frequency
  - Dependable and predictable headache, corresponding to an irresistible escalating use of offending agents at regular, predictable intervals
  - Evidence of psychologic and/or physiologic dependency
  - Failure of alternate acute or preventive medications to control headache attacks
  - Reliable onset of headache within hours to days of the last dose of symptomatic treatment
- See Table 31-2 for current ICHD summary definition of MOH.

TRIGEMINAL AUTONOMIC CEPHALGIAS

These disorders are characterized primarily by the presence of short-lasting, variable-duration (seconds [SUNCT] to 3 h [CH]) headache attacks associated with autonomic features. HC, which is now listed as a trigeminal autonomic cephalgia, does not have short-lasting attacks.

Trigeminal autonomic cephalgia attacks may be mimicked by intracranial pathological disturbances. These usually involve the pituitary or parapituitary region. The pituitary gland and region must be carefully imaged in atypical cases and perhaps even in typical cases of TACs.

CLUSTER HEADACHE

- *CH* is a relatively rare disorder that affects more men than women in a ratio of 3:1. Current concepts on pathophysiology suggest disturbances within the hypothalamus with relevant involvement of autonomic systems and alterations in melatonin function.

TABLE 31-2 Medication Overuse Headache (MOH)

Diagnostic criteria:

A. Headache occurring on ≥15 days per month in a patient with a preexisting headache disorder
B. Regular overuse for >3 months of one or more drugs that can be taken for acute and/or symptomatic treatment of headache
C. Not better accounted for by another ICHD-3 diagnosis

Melatonin "fine-tunes" endogenous cerebral rhythms and homeostasis.

- Clinical features of CHs include:
  - Presence of headache cycles or bouts (clusters) lasting weeks to months, occurring one or more times per year or less, during which repetitive headache attacks occur.
  - Individual attacks lasting 1–3 h.
  - Attacks associated with focal (orbital, temporal, or unilateral) facial pain, accompanied by lacrimation, nasal drainage, pupillary changes, and conjunctival injection.
  - Attacks commonly occur during sleeping times or napping.
  - High likelihood of blue or hazel-colored eyes; ruddy, rugged, lionized facial features; and long history of smoking and excessive alcohol intake.
- Table 31-3 lists the clinical distinctions between CH and migraine.
- *CH* may occur in its episodic form (bouts or cycles of recurring headaches followed by a period of no headache [interim], lasting weeks to years) or in a chronic form without an interim period, with headache attacks daily for years without interruption. Treatment differences may exist.

TABLE 31-3 Clinical Features Distinguishing Between Cluster and Migraine Headaches

FEATURE	CLUSTER	MIGRAINE
Location of pain	Always unilateral, periorbital; sometimes occipital referral	Unilateral, bilateral
Age at onset (typical)	Onset 20 years or older	10–50 years (can be younger or older)
Gender difference	Majority male	Majority female in adulthood
Time of day	Frequently at night, often same time each day	Any time
Frequency of attacks	1–6 per day	1–10 per month in episodic form
Duration of pain	30–120 min	4–72 h
Prodrome	None	Often present
Nausea and vomiting	2%–5%	85%
Blurring of vision	Infrequent	Frequent
Lacrimation	Frequent	Infrequent
Nasal congestion/ drainage	70%	Uncommon
Ptosis	30%	1%–2%
Polyuria	2%	40%
Family history of similar headaches	7%	90%
Miosis	50%	Absent
Behavior during attack	Pacing, manic, and histrionic	Resting in quiet, dark room

Reproduced, with permission, from Saper JR, Silberstein SD, Godeon CD, Hamel RL. *Handbook of Headache Management*. 2nd ed. Baltimore: Lippincott Williams & Wilkins; 1999.

- In addition to *CH*, several short-lasting headache entities are recognized and currently classified along with CH in the category referred to as the *trigeminal autonomic cephalgias*.

These include:

- CH
- Chronic paroxysmal hemicrania (CPH) and episodic paroxysmal hemicrania (EPH)
- SUNCT syndrome
- PH: short-lasting attacks (2–30 min) of strictly unilateral orbital, supraorbital, or temporal pain occurring several times per day. Attacks are associated with ipsilateral conjunctival injection, lacrimation, nasal stuffiness/rhinorrhea, miosis, ptosis, and/or eyelid edema, and forehead and facial sweating. Absolute response to indomethacin is a diagnostic criterion.
- SUNCT syndrome: attacks of short-lasting, strictly unilateral headaches (seconds to minutes), occurring at least once a day and often up to multiple attacks and usually associated with prominent lacrimation and redness of the ipsilateral eye. SUNCT is not responsive to indomethacin.
- HC: persistent unilateral headaches (although unilaterally may alternate sides) with ipsilateral conjunctival injection, lacrimation, nasal drainage, eye "grittiness," meiosis, ptosis, eyelid edema, and occasional facial and forehead sweating. Migraine features such as photophobia are frequently seen. Cervical and cervicogenic features overlap with HC. A diagnostically reliable response to indomethacin is characteristic of HC.

THUNDERCLAP HEADACHE

Primary thunderclap is a severe headache of sudden abrupt onset that resembles that of a ruptured aneurysm often in the absence of intracranial pathology. Thunderclap-type presentations may occur as a result of many headache conditions including some of the following:

- Subarachnoid hemorrhage
- Intracerebral hemorrhage
- Cerebral vein thrombosis
- Arterial dissection
- Pituitary apoplexy
- Reversible cerebral vasoconstrictive syndrome (RCVS) (see later)
- "Crash migraine"
- Sudden CSF hypotension/leak
- Acute cervical disk herniation
- Acute occipital/cervical junction events

OTHER HEADACHES

- Among the other headaches is NDPH that is a distinct subtype of a primary headache, the onset of which is characterized by the patient's ability to recall specifically the onset of the pain. The pain is continuous (or at least within 24h becomes continuous) and lasts at least three months. It typically occurs in patients without a previous history of headache. NDPH may have features similar to that of migraine or tension-type headache and is characteristically difficult to treat.

TREATMENT OF PRIMARY HEADACHES AND RELATED PHENOMENA

KEY TREATMENT PRINCIPLES

- Diagnosing the specific primary headache entity; ruling out secondary headaches
- Determining attack frequency and severity
- Establishing the presence or absence of comorbid illnesses (psychiatric, neurologic, medical, etc)
- Identifying confounding factors and other barriers to improvement, including external or internal phenomena, such as:
  - MOH
  - Psychologic, comorbid illnesses and medication factors
  - Hormonal disturbances (estrogenic disorders, etc)
  - Use of or exposure to toxic substances
- Identifying previous treatment successes and failures
- Many others

TREATMENT MODALITIES

- Nonpharmacologic (self-help, behavioral modification, biofeedback, physical therapy, etc)
- Pharmacologic
- Interventional treatment including:
  - Neuroblockade (nerve, facet, epidural space)
  - Radio-frequency and cryolysis procedures
  - Implantations and stimulation
- Hospital/rehabilitation programs

NONPHARMACOLOGIC TREATMENTS FOR PRIMARY HEADACHES

- A variety of factors related to health, habits, and education can assist patients with headache:
  - Education on provocation and relief measures
  - Reduction of medication overuse; treatment of MOH (rebound) headache (see later)
  - Discontinuation of smoking
  - Regular eating and sleeping patterns (maintaining sameness)
  - Exercise
  - Biofeedback and behavioral treatment (cognitive behavioral therapy)
  - Physical therapy treatment for neck disorders
  - Other psychotherapeutic interventions

TREATMENT OF MOH

MOH (formerly rebound) requires treatment because continued use renders patients refractory to effective treatment and is also potentially toxic. The available evidence demonstrates progressive worsening of the pathophysiology of headache making the primary process worse in exchange for short-term relief. Outpatient and inpatient strategies are available, depending on the quantity and frequency of medication overusage, the type of medication used, and the specific characteristics of each case, including the neurobehavioral features of that individual. Evidence suggests that chronic receptor/brain changes occur secondary to overuse, particularly the opioids but even with simple analgesics. Generally, these changes require weeks, if not months, of chronic use and do not occur after a single week or so of excessive usage to treat an acute exacerbation of headache, although psychologic dependency may develop. Evidence suggests that these receptor changes are similar to those seen in addiction.

The following principles of treatment apply:

- Gradual or rapid discontinuation of offending agent (taper if opioid- or barbiturate-containing).
- Aggressive treatment of resulting severe headache.
- Hydration, including intravenous fluids and support in severe cases (treat nausea, etc).
- The development of pharmacologic prophylaxis.
- Implementation of behavioral therapies.
- Use of infusion or hospitalization venues for advanced and severe conditions, including those accompanied by opioid and/or barbiturate dependency or significant behavioral factors.
- Medication overuse headaches, which most likely result from chronic changes to receptors, must be distinguished from headaches resulting from exposure to toxic substances or other agents or drugs. These have a direct provocative influence.

PHARMACOLOGIC TREATMENT OF MIGRAINE

- Table 31-4 lists pharmacologic agents used in headache management and clinical information regarding their use.

TABLE 31-4   **Selected Drugs Used in the Pharmacotherapy of Head, Neck, and Face Pain**[a,b]

DRUG NAME	mg/DOSE	STANDARD DAILY ADMINISTRATION	NOTES
Symptomatic drugs			
Analgesics			
Excedrin[c]	—	Varies	Avoid more than 2 d/wk of use
NSAIDs			
Naproxen sodium (PO)[c]	275–550	bid–tid	Avoid extended, daily use
Indomethacin (PO)	25–50	bid–tid	Avoid extended, daily use
Indocin SR (PO)	75	1 qd or bid	Avoid extended, daily use
Indomethacin (PR)	50	bid–tid	Avoid extended, daily use
Meclofenamate (PO)	50–200	bid	Avoid extended, daily use
Ibuprofen (PO)[c]	600–800	bid–tid	Avoid extended, daily use
Ketorolac (PO)	10	qid	Avoid extended, daily use
Ketorolac (IM)	30	tid	Avoid extended, daily use; appears particularly valuable when ergot derivatives and narcotics must be avoided and parenteral therapy is necessary; no more than occasional, short-term use is advisable because of renal toxicity, most likely in predisposed patients
Diclofenac oral powder		Single 50 mg dose at headache onset	Avoid extended, daily use
Diclofenac nasal spray			
Special migraine drugs			
Isometheptene combinations[c] (Midrin, etc)	—	2 caps at onset, 1–2q30–60 min	Max 5–6 caps/d; 2 d/wk
Dihydroergotamine (DHE)[c] (IM/IV)	0.25–1	0.25–1 mg SC, IM, IV tid	Can be used 2 or 3 times/d in conjunction with antinauseant, analgesic, etc; IM more effective than SC
Antimigraine			
DHE	1	1 spray each nostril (2 mg/spray); repeat in 15 min (4 sprays = 2 mg)	Use no more than 2 or 3 times/wk, on separate days
Nasal spray		An inhalant form is not yet approved at the time of this publication	
Inhalant—not approved at the time of this publication but expected[c]			
Triptans			
Sumatriptan (parenteral)[c]	6 SC	May repeat in several hours	
Sumatriptan (oral)	25–50	Take at HA onset; may repeat at 2 hours; max 100 mg/d	
Sumatriptan (nasal spray)[c]	5 or 20	1 spray in 1 nostril only; may repeat in 2 hours; max 40 mg/24 hours	
Sumatriptan[c] iontophoretic patch		1 at onset; may repeat in 2 hours; max 10 mg/24 hours	
Zolmitriptan (oral)[c]	2.5–5	1 at onset; may repeat in 2 hours; max 10 mg/24 hours	Triptans cannot be used within 24 hours of ergotamine-related meds or other triptans; should not be used in presence of cardiovascular and/or cerebrovascular, severe hypertension, Prinzmetal angina, or peripheral vascular disorders; no more than 2 doses in 24 hours; limit 2 d/wk usage
Zolmitriptan (ZMT)[c]	2.5–5	1 at onset; may repeat in 4 hours; max 5 mg/24 hours	
Naratriptan (oral)[c]	2.5	1 at onset; may repeat in 4 hours; max 20 mg/24 hours	
Rizatriptan (oral)[c]	5–10	1 at onset; may repeat in 4 hours; max 20 mg/24 hours	
Rizatriptan (MLT)[c]	5–10	1 at onset; may repeat; max 25 mg/24 hours	
Almotriptan[c]	12.5	1 at onset; may repeat after 6–8 hours; max 5 mg/24 hours	
Frovatriptan[c]	2.5		
Eletriptan	20, 40		
Antinauseants/neuroleptics/antihistamines			
Chlorpromazine			
PO	25–100	bid–tid	Limit 3 d/wk, except for persistent nausea; avoid extended use; monitor for hypotension and cardiac rhythm effects (QT interval)
Supp	25–100	bid–tid	
IM	25–100	bid–tid	
IV	2.5–10	bid–tid	
Metoclopramide (PO—tablet and syrup)	10–20	tid	
(Parenteral)	10	tid	

(Continued)

TABLE 31-4 Selected Drugs Used in the Pharmacotherapy of Head, Neck, and Face Pain[a,b] (*Continued*)

DRUG NAME	mg/DOSE	STANDARD DAILY ADMINISTRATION	NOTES
Promethazine			Limit 3 d/wk, except for persistent nausea; avoid extended use; monitor for hypotension and cardiac rhythm effects (QT interval)
PO	25–75	tid	
IM	25–75	tid	
Perphenazine		bid–tid	
PO	4–8	bid	
IM	5	tid	
Diphenhydramine (IV, IM)	25–50	tid	Anticholinergic effects
Hydroxyzine (PO, IM)	25–75	bid–tid or at hs tid–qid	Can be used as a symptomatic or preventive treatment
Cyproheptadine (PO)	2–4		Can be an effective preventive in childhood migraine
Steroids			
Prednisone (PO)	40–60	In 1 or divided doses	4- to 10-d program; avoid repeated use
Preventive drugs[d]			
Tricyclic antidepressants			
Amitriptyline	10–150	Divided doses or hs	
Nortriptyline	10–100		Bedtime dose aids sleep disturbance
Doxepin	10–150		
Other antidepressants			
Fluoxetine	20	20–80 mg/d in divided dose	
MAO inhibitors			
Phenelzine	15–60	15–90 mg/d in divided dose	Dietary and medication restrictions mandatory; hypotension can be severe
β-Adrenergic blockers			
Propranolol[c]	20–50	tid–qid (standard dose)	
Atenolol	50–100	bid	
Timolol[c]	10–20	bid	Monitor cardiac function, BP, pulse, lipids
Metoprolol	50–100	bid	
Nadolol	20–120	bid	
Calcium channel antagonists			
Verapamil	80–160	tid–qid	
Nimodipine	30–60	tid	Monitor cardiac function, BP, pulse, lipids; eliminated by kidneys
Diltiazem	30–90	tid	
Ergotamine derivatives			After 6 mo therapy, review cardiac, pulmonary, and retroperitoneal regions for fibrotic changes; carefully observe contraindications
Methysergide[c]	1–2	tid, 5 times/d	
Methylergonovine	0.2–0.4	tid–qid	
Anticonvulsants			
Valproic acid[c]	125–500	1–2 g/d in divided doses	Monitor hepatic and metabolic (platelets) parameters carefully; consider dose reduction when used with antidepressants, lithium, verapamil, phenothiazines, benzodiazepines, other anticonvulsants; observe warnings carefully; avoid using with barbiturates and perhaps benzodiazepines
Valproic acid (ER)[c]	250–1000	500 mg to 1 g/d, once per day dosing	
Valproic acid (IV)	250–750	1000–3000 mg/d	
Gabapentin	100–400	1800–3600 mg/d	May cause sedation and other CNS adverse effects
Topiramate	25–50	25 mg bid, tapered slowly to 200–400 mg/d	Sedation, cognitive impairment, abdominal cramps, and risk for renal stones are limiting features; liver function disturbances, acute myopia, and closed-angle glaucoma (in first month) require careful monitoring and immediate discontinuation; weight loss may occur
OnabotulinumtoxinA[c]			In recent years, several studies have demonstrated the efficacy of onabotulinumtoxinA for chronic migraine. It is increasingly used in the prophylaxis of chronic migraine headaches. It is not effective in episodic migraine
Others			
Baclofen	10–20	tid–qid	Increase and decrease dose slowly and allow tolerance to develop; taper when discontinuing
Tizanidine	2–8	2–8 mg tid or prn; max dose 32–36 mg/d	May be used as abortive or preventive agent; sedation, hypotension, liver function disturbances must be considered and monitored; careful use with other α-adrenergic agonist agents such as clonidine and hepatotoxic agents is recommended; max dose is 36 mg/d
Lithium	150–300	bid–tid	Reduce dose in conjunction with verapamil, other calcium channel antagonists, and NSAIDs; monitor metabolic parameters

(*Continued*)

TABLE 31-4   Selected Drugs Used in the Pharmacotherapy of Head, Neck, and Face Pain[a,b] (Continued)

DRUG NAME	mg/DOSE	STANDARD DAILY ADMINISTRATION	NOTES
Oxygen inhalation	100% O_2 with mask	7–15 L/min for 10–15 min	Must be used at onset of attack of cluster headache; avoid around extreme heat or flame, such as cigarettes
Melatonin	3–15	Usually hs	Its value in cluster headache is currently tentative but promising; risks in asthma and vasoconstrictive diseases remain to be defined

[a]Modified with permission from Saper JR, Silberstein SD, Godeon CD, Hamel RL. *Handbook of Headache Management.* 2nd ed. Baltimore: Lippincott Williams & Wilkins; 1999.

[b]Few of the medications listed in this table either are approved specifically for headache or have been shown by controlled studies to be effective for headache. Their inclusion reflects that they have been recommended from various sources as possibly useful for the treatment of some cases of headache.

[c]Drugs that have been approved by the Food and Drug Administration (FDA) for the treatment of migraine, cluster headache, or tension-type headache.

[d]Avoid sustained use for more than six months without trial reduction.

- The pharmacologic treatment of headache involves the use of *abortive (acute)* and *preventive* medications. *Abortive (acute) treatments* are used to terminate evolving or existing attacks. *Preventive treatment* is implemented to reduce the frequency of attacks and prevent overuse of acute medications. Most patients with frequent headache require combination treatment. *Preemptive treatment* is a short-term preventive course of therapy used in anticipation of a predictable event, such as a menstrual period or vacation-related headache.

Acute Treatment of Migraine

- Simple and combined analgesics (acetaminophen, aspirin, nonsteroidal anti-inflammatory drugs [NSAIDs], and others).
- Mixed barbiturate- and opioid-containing analgesics (barbiturate and simple analgesics: aspirin ± acetaminophen, ± caffeine), often avoided because of the likelihood of dependency and misuse.
- Ergot derivatives, including dihydroergotamine (DHE).
- Use of one or several triptan medications, including sumatriptan, naratriptan, almotriptan, rizatriptan, zolmitriptan, frovatriptan, and eletriptan.
- The triptans represent narrow-spectrum, receptor-specific (serotonin [5-HT_1]) agonists that stimulate the 5-HT_1b and 5-HT_1d receptors to reduce neurogenic inflammation. The ergot derivatives are broader-spectrum agents, affecting serotoninergic receptors and also α-adrenergic and dopamine receptors (and others). While many patients respond well to the triptans, others appear to require the broader influence of ergot derivatives. Experienced clinicians are adept at administering several of the triptans as well as the ergots. Short-acting, rapidly effective triptans include almotriptan, sumatriptan, rizatriptan, zolmitriptan, and eletriptan, while naratriptan and frovatriptan

have the longest half-lives. Several delivery formats are available in addition to tablets: injection (sumatriptan), nasal spray (sumatriptan and zolmitriptan), and rapidly dissolving forms (zolmitriptan and rizatriptan). Recently a sumatriptan iontophoretic patch has been introduced and an inhalant form of DHE is currently before the FDA. Approval is expected.
- Patients who have not responded to less potent medications require triptans or ergots for maximum benefit.
- Acute medications are used in conjunction with antinauseants and in combination with each other for maximum efficiency (do not combine ergots and triptans). Clinicians must be familiar with important contraindications and safety warnings of each of these medication groups as well as adverse effects and influence on hepatic metabolism, particularly when these drugs are used in combination with others.
- Finally, for reasons that are not fully understood but perhaps related to the cervical/trigeminal connections, occipital nerve blocks may relieve acute migraine attacks in some individuals. This method has been historically used by anesthesiologists but is increasingly employed by neurologists and others treating headache. Long-term relief is unknown, but short-term relief is frequently seen, and can be useful in overall treatment programs.

Preventive Treatment of Migraine

- The following medications are useful in the prevention of migraine:
  - Tricyclic antidepressants (particularly amitriptyline, nortriptyline, and doxepin).
  - β-Adrenergic blockers (particularly propranolol and nadolol).
  - Calcium channel blockers (verapamil, etc) are only occasionally helpful in migraine, but sometimes offer a value in selected cases.

- Anticonvulsants (valproic acid, gabapentin, topiramate).
- Ergot derivatives (methylergonovine and methysergide).
- Monoamine oxidase inhibitors (MAOIs) (for refractory cases).
- Others: selective serotonin reuptake inhibitors (SSRIs), neuroleptics, tizanidine, and onabotulinumtoxinA for chronic migraine.

- Tricyclic antidepressants and β-blockers are well-established, first-line medications for preventive treatment of migraine in those patients who do not have contraindications or restrictions to either medication. Calcium channel blockers are generally not as effective for migraine, but better for CH (see below). The anticonvulsants have considerable value and are particularly useful in the presence of neuropsychiatric comorbidity or other conditions, such as seizures and bipolar disorders, that might accompany migraine. During the last few years, topiramate has gained popularity for episodic and chronic migraine. Risks include nephrolithiasis and metabolic acidosis as well as cognitive impairment at the higher dosages. However, topiramate is an effective drug for many patients at a dose range of 100 to 200 mg per day in divided doses. It does not contribute to weight gain as many other antimigraine preventive drugs do.
- The SSRIs are helpful for neuropsychiatric comorbid conditions, such as depression and panic and anxiety disorders, but generally do not have a strong antimigraine influence. Some patients with migraine-related headaches benefit from the antidopaminergic influence of the new neuroleptics, although the potential for adverse effects limits their widespread use. Tizanidine, an α-adrenergic agonist, has been shown effective in an adjunctive, preventive role. OnabotulinumtoxinA is increasingly administered for the prevention of chronic migraine. It is likely to work through a central mechanism and perhaps both central and peripheral mechanisms, but that is not clearly delineated at this time.
- The treatment of *chronic migraine* is generally similar to that of episodic migraine. Recently onabotulinumtoxinA and topiramate have been shown effective for chronic migraine. Treatment is directed at both the daily or almost daily pain and periodic attacks. Because of the likely presence of a progressive course, medication overuse, and neuropsychiatric comorbidity in this population, a more comprehensive approach beyond medications alone is required. This includes cognitive behavioral therapy and other forms of psychotherapy and family therapy. Organic illness must be ruled out with appropriate testing in patients with frequent or daily headache and in those with neurologic findings (see Table 31-5).

TABLE 31-5 Recommended Seven-Day Prednisone Program[a]

DAY	BREAKFAST (mg)	LUNCH (mg)	DINNER (mg)
1	20 (4 pills)	20	20
2	20	20	20
3	20	15 (3 pills)	15
4	15	15	10 (2 pills)
5	10	10	10
6	10	5 (1 pill)	5
7	5	5	

[a]Five-milligram tablets; dispense 60 tablets.

- Occipital nerve stimulation is of interest. Several studies have been published on the treatment of chronic migraine with suboccipital stimulators. These studies demonstrate modest to moderate benefit in patients with chronic migraine. These data are not yet compelling, but interest exists in potential value of neurostimulation of the occipital and vagus nerves for headaches and it is expected that there will be further well-designed studies.

TREATMENT OF CLUSTER HEADACHE

- CH responds and is treated differently than migraine. Because CH attacks generally occur numerous times daily (one to eight times), the use of abortive medications is limited to only a few agents that are safe for such frequent use.

Acute Treatment of Cluster Headache

- Oxygen inhalation (7–15 L/min, 100% oxygen via mask)
- Triptans/ergot (avoid more than two usage days per week)
- Indomethacin, which is occasionally useful for CH but more effective for CPH and EPH (see Table 31-4)

Preventive Treatment of Cluster Headache and Other TACs

- *CPH* and *EPH*, as well as HC, are characteristically sensitive to treatment with indomethacin at a dose of 25–50 mg three times daily. SUNCT syndrome may respond to lamotrigine or gabapentin.
- Verapamil (short acting) at a dose of 120–160 mg three to four times daily (Table 31-4). Care must be taken to monitor ECG for rhythm disturbances.
- Lithium.
- Divalproex/topiramate.
- Melatonin 6–15 mg at night.
- Seven-day prednisone burst (steroids are generally effective for CH prevention, and short-term trials can be dramatically effective, but risks limit utility) (Table 31-6).

TABLE 31-6 Selective Diagnostic Tests

Physical examination
Metabolic evaluation
    Hematologic
    ESR/CRP
    Endocrinologic
    Chemistry
    Toxicology (drug screens, etc)
Standard x-rays
Neuroimaging
    CT/CTA/CTV
    MRI/MRA/MRV
Dental and otologic exam
Lumbar puncture
Radioisotope/CT myelogram
Diagnostic blockades
Arteriography

ESR, erythrocyte sedimentation rate; CRP, C-reactive protein; MRA, magnetic resonance angiography; MRV, magnetic resonance venography.

- Ergot derivatives (methylergonovine/methysergide).
- Occipital nerve blockade.
- For intractable cases, hospitalization or infusion treatments are recommended (see below). In some cases surgical intervention is required, but surgical treatment is limited due to the likelihood of postsurgical painful sequelae. Occipital nerve injection is effective in treating some attacks, and subcutaneous occipital stimulation has recently been reported.

TREATMENT OF OTHER PRIMARY HEADACHE DISORDERS

For NDPH, no predictably reliable treatment exists. Hospitalization with aggressive infusion and multimodal treatments can be successful.

- Recently much interest has focused on the concept of reversible vasospasm (*reversible cerebral vasoconstriction syndrome*). This disorder manifests as acute severe headache that may include recurrent thunderclap attacks due to the spasm of cerebral arteries rather than due to the standard mechanism of migraine. It can occur in patients with migraine. Characteristically, the vasospasm is provoked by vasoconstrictive or vasoactive agents and recreational drugs such as marijuana. SSRIs, triptans, and ergots are frequently involved. The treatment includes removal of the provocative agent and treatment with intravenous or high-dose oral calcium channel blockers. Careful preventive action against ischemic events as a consequence of the vasoconstriction is necessary. Stroke is a complication of severe vasospasm.

DIAGNOSTIC TESTING AND SECONDARY HEADACHE DISORDERS

- More than 300 entities may produce symptoms of headache, many of which mimic the primary headache disorders. The clinician has the burden of ruling in and ruling out potentially relevant conditions in patients with recurring or persistent headache. Diagnostic testing includes a wide range of studies, including metabolic, endocrinologic, toxic, dental, traumatic, cervical, infectious, and space-occupying. Disturbances of CSF pressure, ischemic disease, and allergic conditions must be considered. Table 31-6 lists diagnostic tests that should be considered in intractable or variant cases.
- Important specific conditions to consider are many but include those of the jaw or dental structures, sphenoid sinuses (must specifically image and evaluate for sphenoid sinusitis), carotid and vertebral dissection syndromes, cerebral venous occlusion, and CSF pressure disturbances. Acute sphenoid sinusitis can be a fatal disorder with acute cranial nerve disturbances and present with vertex or other headaches.
- Increasing interest has also been focused on disorders of CSF pressure. Low-pressure and high-pressure syndromes can be occult and not clearly evident. Papilledema is not a reliable finding in all cases of intracranial hypertension, and low-pressure syndromes may be very subtle with opening pressures in the normal range. When performing an LP, opening and closing pressures, as well as volume removed, must be recorded and the patient must be in the lateral decubitus position. Pressures obtained when patients are prone are unreliable and often misleading. Standard ranges for normal and abnormal pressures are quite variable, and individual patients may experience abnormal phenomena even when the pressures are in normal range during the LP.
- Because of the relevance of cervical spine to the descending trigeminal system and headache physiology (trigeminal cervical connection), disturbances at the level of the upper cervical spine and its nerves and joints have become important targets for the treatment of otherwise pharmacologically resistant headaches. Premature or excessive use of interventional procedures is unwarranted, but when selective and expertly administered, they clearly have a role in the overall spectrum of diagnosis and treatment for headache conditions. Even more advanced treatments, such as implantable and noninvasive neurostimulators, are on the horizon. The influence of cervical dorsal horn connections to descending trigeminal circuits appears to be a "window" of therapeutic opportunity at the cervical level, even in the absence of pathophysiology

(C1, C2, and C3 levels are intimately related to referral of pain anteriorly including the frontal and orbital regions).

REFERRAL AND HOSPITALIZATION

- It is advisable to refer intractable and other difficult-to-treat patients to headache specialists, specialized clinics, and tertiary centers. Hospitalization is required for many complex patients whose medication misuse or the presence of intractable pain and behavioral/neuropsychiatric symptomatology has reached an intensity and complexity that make outpatient therapy no longer appropriate (see below). Aggressive and thorough diagnostic assessment is mandatory to either rule out organic, toxic, or physiologic illness or define unrecognized provocative factors.

HOSPITALIZATION/INFUSION PROGRAMS

- Intractable headache patients can respond to the more aggressive therapeutic environment and milieu in specialty inpatient programs when outpatient therapy has failed to establish efficacy. Hospitalization and infusion program should be considered when:
  - Symptoms are severe and refractory to standard outpatient treatment.
  - Headaches are accompanied by drug overuse or toxicity not treatable as an outpatient.
  - The intensity of neuropsychiatric and behavioral comorbidity renders outpatient treatment ineffective.
  - Confounding medical illness is present.
  - The presence of treatment urgency in a desperate patient exists.
- The principles of hospitalization include:
  - Interrupt daily headache pain with parenteral protocols (see below).
  - Discontinue offending analgesics if rebound is present.
  - Implement preventive pharmacotherapy.
  - Identify effective abortive therapy.
  - Treat behavioral and neuropsychiatric comorbid conditions.
  - Employ interventional modalities when indicated.
  - Provide education.
  - Provide discharge and outpatient planning.
- A variety of parenteral agents can be used during hospitalization and in infusion programs to control attacks, particularly during rebound withdrawal:
  - DHE (0.25–1 mg IV or IM, three times daily)
  - Diphenhydramine (25–50 mg IV or IM, three times daily)
  - Various neuroleptics (ie, chlorpromazine 2.5–10 mg IV, three times daily)
  - Ketorolac (10 mg IV or 30 mg IM, three times daily)
  - Valproic acid (250–750 mg IV, three times daily)
  - Magnesium sulfate (250–1000 mg IV, two to three times daily)
  - Steroid infusions (methylprednisolone, etc)
- These protocols can also be used for emergency department treatment of acute episodic migraine.

WHEN TO USE OPIOIDS

- Experience and data support the *avoidance* of sustained opioid administration in the chronic headache population, except in the rarest of circumstances. Use in acute situations when other treatments are contraindicated remains appropriate if use is infrequent and patient is reliable and compliant, but dose and amounts of prescriptions should be limited and monitored carefully. Sustained opioid administration can be administered in the following very limited circumstances:
  - When all else fails following a full range of advanced services, including detoxification
  - When contraindications to other agents exist
  - In the elderly or during pregnancy
- Except in the elderly or during pregnancy, patients must be refractory to aggressive therapies before opioids are administered regularly. Approximately one half of those maintained on opioids demonstrated noncompliant drug-related behavior. Despite reports of pain reduction, a major improvement in function was not noted in a significant percentage of patients. Subsequent observation has suggested less than 15% of patients benefit. Risks from chronic opioid use for headache overcome advantages in most cases. Only a small, select group of patients who are elderly with comorbid contraindications to standard drugs or others who cannot tolerate standard drugs would be eligible, but even in these cases individual selection is necessary and widespread use is strongly discouraged.

BIBLIOGRAPHY

Argoff CE. A focused review of the use of botulinum toxins for neuropathic pain. *Clin J Pain.* 2002;18:S177–S181.

Aurora SK, Dodick DW, Turkel CC, et al; PREMPT 1 Chronic Migraine Study Group. OnabotulinumtoxinA for treatment of chronic migraine: results from the double-blind, randomized, placebo-controlled phase of the PREEMPT 1 trial. *Cephalalgia.* 2010;30(7):793–803.

Bartsch T, Goadsby PJ. Stimulation of the greater occipital nerve (GON) enhances responses of dural responsive convergent neurons in the trigeminal cervical complex in the rat. *Cephalalgia.* 2001;21:401–402.

Boes CJ, Dodick DW. Refining the clinical spectrum of chronic paroxysmal hemicrania: a review of 74 patients. *Headache.* 2002;42:699–708.

Burns B, Watkins L, Goadsby PJ. Treatment of medically intractable cluster headache by occipital nerve stimulation: long-term follow-up of eight patients. *Lancet.* 2007;369:1099–1106.

Burstein RH, Cutrer FM, Yarnitsky D. The development of cutaneous allodynia during a migraine attack. *Brain.* 2000;123:1703–1709.

Charles A. The evolution of a migraine attack—a review of recent evidence. *Headache.* 2013;53(2):413–419.

Cohen AS, Burns B, Goadsby PJ. High-flow oxygen for treatment of cluster headache: a randomized trial. *JAMA.* 2009;302(22):2451–2557.

Diener HC, Dodick DW, Aurora SK, et al; PREEMPT 2 Chronic Migraine Study Group. OnabotulinumtoxinA for treatment of chronic migraine: results from the double-blind, randomized, placebo-controlled phase of the PREEMPT 2 trial. *Cephalgia.* 2010;30(7):804–814.

Diener HC, Dodick DW, Goadsby PJ, Lipton RB, Olesen J, Silberstein SD. Chronic migraine—classification, characteristics and treatment. *Nat Rev Neurol.* 2012;8(3):162–171.

Evans RW. New daily persistent headache. *Headache.* 2012;52(suppl 1):40–44.

Ferrari MD, Roon KL, Lipton RB, et al. Oral triptans (serotonin 5-HT$^{1b/1d}$ agonist) in acute migraine treatment: a meta-analysis of 53 trials. *Lancet.* 2001;358:1668–1675.

Ferraro S, Grazzi L, Muffatti R, et al. In medication-overuse headache, fMRI shows long-lasting dysfunction in midbrain areas. *Headache.* 2012;52:1520–1534.

Front CJ, Dodick DW, Bosch EP. SUNCT responsive to gabapentin. *Headache.* 2002;42:525–526.

Goadsby PJ. Short-lasting primary headaches: focus on trigeminal autonomic cephalgias. *Curr Opin Neurol.* 1999:12(3): 273–277.

Goadsby PJ, Lipton RB, Ferrari MD. Migraine: current understanding and treatment. *N Engl J Med.* 2002;246:257–270.

Johnston, MM, Jordan SE, Charles AC. Pain referral patterns of the C1 to C3 nerves: implications for headache disorders. *Ann Neurol.* 2013;74:145–148 [Epub ahead of print].

Lake AE 3rd, Saper JR, Hamel RL. Comprehensive inpatient treatment of refractory chronic daily headache. *Headache.* 2009;49(4):555–562.

Leone M, D'Amico D, Moschiano F, et al. Melatonin vs. placebo in the prophylaxis of cluster headache: a double-blind pilot study with parallel groups. *Cephalalgia.* 1996;16:494–496.

Limmroth V, Katsarav AZ, Fritsche G, et al. Features in medication overuse headache following overuse of different acute headache drugs. *Neurology.* 2002;59:1011–1014.

Linde M, Mulleners WM, Chronicle EP, McCrory DC. Topiramate for the prophylaxis of episodic migraine in adults. *Cochrane Database Syst Rev.* 2013;6:CD010610.

May A, Bahra A, Buchel C, et al. PET and MRA findings in cluster headache and MRA in experimental pain. *Neurology.* 2000;55:1328–1535.

Mokri B. Spontaneous low pressure, low CSF volume headaches: spontaneous CSF leaks. *Headache.* 2013;53(7):1034–1053.

Nixdorf DR, Heo G, Major PW. Randomized control trial of botulism toxin A for chronic myogenous orofacial pain. *Pain.* 2002;99:465–473.

Noseda R, Burstein R. Migraine pathophysiology: anatomy of the trigeminovascular pathway and associated neurological symptoms, cortical spreading depression, sensitization, and modulation of pain. *Pain.* 2013;(13):389–388.

Headache Classification Committee of the International Headache Society (IHS). The International Classification of Headache Disorders, 3rd edition (beta version). *Cephalalgia.* 2013;33(9):629–808.

Palmisani S, Al-Kaisy A, Arcioni R, et al. A six year retrospective review of occipital nerve stimulation practice—controversies and challenges of an emerging technique for treating refractory headache syndromes. *Headache Pain.* 2013;14(1):67.

Peres MF, Rozen TD. Melatonin in the preventive treatment of chronic cluster headache. *Cephalalgia.* 2001;21:993–995.

Saper JR. What matters is not the differences between triptans, but the differences between patients. *Arch Neurol.* 2001;58:1481–1482.

Saper JR, Da Silva AN. Medication overuse headache: history, features, prevention and management strategies. *CNS Drugs.* 2013;27:867–877 [Epub ahead of print].

Saper JR, Dodick DW, Silberstein SD, et al. Occipital nerve stimulation for the treatment of intractable chronic migraine headache: ONSTIM feasibility study. *Cephalalgia.* 2011;31(3):271–285.

Saper JR, Evans RW. Oral methylergonovine maleate for refractory migraine and cluster headache prevention. *Headache.* 2013;53(2):378–381.

Saper JR, Jones JM. Ergotamine tartrate dependency: features and possible mechanisms. *Clin Neurophrmacol.* 1986;9(3):244–256.

Saper JR, Lake AE III. Borderline personality disorder and the chronic headache patient: review and management recommendations. *Headache.* 2002;42:663–674.

Saper JR, Lake AE 3rd, Bain PA, et al. *Headache.* 2010;40(7):1175–1193.

Saper JR, Lake AE III, Cantrell DT, Winner PK, White JR. Chronic daily headache prophylaxis with tizanidine: a double-blind, placebo-controlled, multicenter outcome study. *Headache.* 2002;42:570–582.

Saper JR, Silberstein SD, Godeon CD, Hamel RL. *Handbook of Headache Management.* 2nd ed. Baltimore: Lippincott Williams & Wilkins; 1999.

Silberstein SD, Freitag F, Dodick DW, Argoff C. Asthma E; Quality Standards Subcommittee of the American Academy of Neurology and American Headache Society. Evidence-based guideline update: pharmacologic treatment for episodic migraine prevention in adults: report of the Quality Standards Subcommittee of the American Academy of Neurology and the American Headache Society. *Neurology.* 2012;78(17):1337–1347.

Silberstein SD, Lipton RB, Dodick DW. *Wolff's Headache and Other Head Pain.* 8th ed. New York: Oxford University Press; 2007 [ISBN-13: 9780195326567].

Silberstein SD, Peres MF, Hopkins MM, et al. Olanzapine in the treatment of refractory migraine and chronic daily headache. *Headache.* 2002;42:515–518.

Srikiatkhachorn A, Puanguiyom MS, Govitrapon P. Plasticity of 5-HT^{2a} serotonin receptor in patients with analgesic-induced transformed migraine. *Headache.* 1998;38:534–539.

Watkins LR, Milligan ED, Maier SF. Glial activation: a driving force for pathological pain. *Trends Neurosci.* 2001;24(8):450–455.

Weiller CA, May A, Limmroth V, et al. Brainstem activation and spontaneous human migraine attacks. *Nat Med.* 1995;1:658–660.

Welch KM, Nagesh V, Aurora SK, Gelman N. Periaqueductal gray matter dysfunction in migraine: cause or the burden of illness. *Headache.* 2001;41:629–637.

Yancy H, Lee-Iannotti JK, Schwedt TJ, Dodick DW. Reversible cerebral vasoconstriction syndrome. *Headache.* 2013;53(3):570–576.

32 LOW BACK PAIN

Michael J. Dorsi, MD
Allan J. Belzberg, MD, FRCSC

EPIDEMIOLOGY AND RISK FACTORS

- Low back pain (LBP) is pain arising from the spinal or paraspinal structures in the lumbosacral region. It extends approximately from the iliac crests to the coccyx.
- Radicular leg pain, or sciatica, may accompany LBP but should be regarded as a separate entity with a distinct pathophysiology.
- LBP is the fifth most common reason for all physician visits and the second most common symptomatic reason (upper respiratory symptoms are first).
- 50% to 80% of adults experience LBP.
- LBP is the leading cause of disability and lost production in the United States, with associated direct and indirect costs estimated to exceed $50 billion per year.
- Despite the widespread opinion that 75%–90% of patients with acute LBP recover within about six weeks, irrespective of their treatment, pain may persist in up to 72% and disability in up to 12% of patients one year after their first episode of LBP.
- The predictors for LBP include:
  1. Poor physical fitness and comorbidity
  2. Social class, occupation, and employment status
  3. Increasing age up to 55 years
  4. Obesity
  5. Dimensions of spinal canal
  6. Smoking
  7. Substance abuse history
  8. Hard physical labor
- Predictors of chronicity and disability include:
  1. Radicular leg pain
  2. Poor self-rated health status
  3. A positive straight leg test
  4. Reduced elasticity/flexibility of the lumbar spine
  5. Poor coping strategies
  6. High levels of distress, depression, and somatization
  7. Lower activity level
  8. Anxiety

ETIOLOGY AND PATHOPHYSIOLOGY

- LBP can be arbitrarily classified based on symptom duration.
- The biological basis, natural history, and response to therapy differ for each category.
- *Transient pain* is short-lived (a few hours) and is usually activity-related. Patients rarely seek medical attention for transient pain unless the frequency of painful episodes becomes intolerable.
- *Acute pain*, by definition, resolves within three months. The onset of symptoms is spontaneous in approximately half of cases, with trauma accounting for the rest.
- *Chronic LBP* persists without change for months to years and may develop into a chronic pain syndrome marked by personality dysfunction and psychosocial and medical comorbidities.
- The differential diagnosis for LBP includes mechanical and nonmechanical causes (Table 32-1).
- Most patients have mechanical LBP.

TABLE 32-1 Differential Diagnosis of LBP

MECHANICAL LBP	NONMECHANICAL LBP	VISCERAL DISEASE
Lumbar strain or sprain	Neoplasia	Pelvic organs
Degenerative disease	Metastatic carcinoma	Prostatitis
Disks (spondylosis)	Multiple myeloma	Endometriosis
Facet joints	Lymphoma and leukemia	Chronic pelvic inflammatory disease
Diffuse idiopathic skeletal	Spinal cord tumors	Renal disease
Hyperplasia	Retroperitoneal tumors	Nephrolithiasis
Spondylolysis	Infection	Pyelonephritis
Spondylolisthesis	Osteomyelitis	Vascular disease
Herniated disk	Septic discitis	Abdominal aortic aneurysm
Spinal stenosis	Paraspinal or epidural	Aortoiliac disease
Osteoporosis with compression fracture	Abscess	Gastrointestinal disease
Fractures	Endocarditis	Pancreatitis
Congenital disease	Inflammatory arthritis	Cholecystitis
Severe kyphosis	Ankylosing spondylitis	Perforated bowel
Severe scoliosis	Reiter syndrome	
Paget disease	Psoriatic spondylitis	
	Inflammatory bowel disease	
	Polymyalgia rheumatica	

Reproduced, with permission, from Atlas SJ, Deyo RA. Evaluating and managing acute low back pain in the primary care setting. *J Gen Intern Med.* 2001;16:120.

- The specific pathology or exact anatomic source of pain cannot be determined by physical examination or diagnostic testing in 50%–80% of patients with mechanical LBP.
- A pathologic diagnosis is attainable in most patients with LBP of nonmechanical origin.
- Pain can arise from anterior structures:
  1. Discs
  2. Vertebral bodies
  3. Ligaments
  4. Muscles (ie, psoas)
- Pain can arise from midline structures:
  1. Spinal cord
  2. Nerve roots
- Pain can arise from posterior structures:
  1. Facet joints
  2. Ligaments
  3. Sacroiliac joints
  4. Paraspinal muscles

HISTORY

- Adequate history taking is essential to determine if mechanical back pain is present and to exclude "red flag" conditions, such as tumors, fractures, infections, cauda equina syndrome, and spinal osteomyelitis, that could be life-threatening or result in permanent neurological dysfunction if not treated (Table 32-2).

SEVERITY

- Although LBP may be severe, it is rarely described as excruciating; excruciating pain might indicate a new fracture, infection, or metastatic disease.

LOCATION

- Nonspecific LBP often radiates to the buttocks, hips, groin, and thighs. Radicular pain below the knee suggests nerve root compression, especially if it follows a dermatomal pattern.

TABLE 32-2 Red Flags Requiring Immediate Attention

Recent trauma
Mild trauma or strain with a history of osteoporosis
Unexplained weight loss
History of cancer
Fever
Pain worse at night
Bowel/bladder dysfunction
Intravenous drug use
Pain not relieved in the supine position/awakes patient from sleep

TIMING

- Pain severity commonly waxes and wanes over the course of a day. Pain that is constantly severe or that peaks at night when recumbent should heighten suspicions that it has a neoplastic etiology.

ALLEVIATING/AGGRAVATING FACTORS

- Back and leg pain associated with stocking-glove sensory loss or a feeling of leg heaviness during walking that is relieved by sitting or leaning forward is suggestive of neurogenic claudication due to spinal stenosis.
- Mechanical LBP due to spondylosis is typically exacerbated by increased activity and relieved by rest. Lying supine typically offers some relief.
- Postures that maximize axial loading (erect, sitting) typically exacerbate LBP.

ASSOCIATED SYMPTOMS

- Stiffness and fatigue commonly accompany LBP.
- Muscle weakness, sensory loss, and changes in bowel and bladder function suggest nerve root compression and may warrant further investigation.
- Weight loss, low-grade fever, failure to improve, age greater than 50 years, and elevated sedimentation rate should increase concerns about neoplastic disease.
- Alerting features of spinal infection include fever, new-onset neurologic deficits, diabetes, immunocompromise, previous surgical procedure, intravenous drug use, and an elevated sedimentation rate.

PHYSICAL EXAMINATION

INSPECTION

- With the patient erect, assess posture, symmetry, and spinal curvature.
- Asymmetric muscle spasm may produce asymmetry at the hip level or may cause new-onset scoliosis.
- Careful inspection involves evaluating muscle bulk and checking for atrophy.

PALPATION

- Assess spinous processes, paraspinal muscles, ribs, sacroiliac joints, sciatic notches, and hips for tenderness.
- Examine the abdomen to determine if an aneurysm is present.
- Palpate for lymphadenopathy if the history is suggestive of neoplastic or infectious etiology.
- Palpate pulses in lower extremities.

RANGE OF MOTION

- Ask the patient to flex, extend, and rotate laterally to determine range limitations.
- Assess range of motion about the hip in patients with buttock or groin symptoms.

GAIT

- Normal gait, toe walking, and/or heel walking provide a gross assessment of functional strength.
- Flexed posture when walking is commonly seen with spinal stenosis or hip joint pathology.

MOTOR STRENGTH

- Examine strength in all muscle groups.
- Motor weakness, especially when it is asymmetric, can help identify an involved nerve root (Table 32-3).
- Subtle weakness of plantar flexion may be uncovered by repetitive motion testing.

DEEP TENDON REFLEXES

- Diminished reflexes are consistent with nerve root compression (Table 32-3).
- Hyperreflexia may suggest upper motor neuron injury in the spinal cord or centrally.

SENSATION

- Light touch and pinprick sensation should be assessed in a dermatomal pattern (Table 32-3).

TABLE 32-3 Physical Examination Findings Associated With Specific Nerve Root Impingement

NERVE ROOT	MUSCLE (MOTION)	SENSORY	DEEP TENDON REFLEX
L2	Iliopsoas (hip flexion)	Anterior thigh, groin	None
L3	Quadriceps (leg extension)	Anterior/lateral thigh	Patellar
L4	Quadriceps, ankle dorsiflexors (heel walking)	Medial ankle/foot	Patellar
L5	Ankle dorsiflexors, extensor hallucis longus (first toe dorsiflexion)	Dorsum of foot	None
S1	Gastrocnemius (toe walking)	Lateral plantar foot	Achilles

DIAGNOSTIC SIGNS

- Straight leg raise that reproduces back pain is nonspecific but may predict a poor prognosis.
- A positive straight leg raise is highly suggestive of nerve root compression of the L5 or S1 roots.
- Extension of the hip stretches the femoral nerve and may reproduce symptoms stemming from pathology at the L3 or L4 segment.
- A contralateral "straight leg raise" that results in ipsilateral pain suggests a free fragment disc herniation.
- Internal/external rotation of the hip may detect hip or sacroiliac joint pathology.

IMAGING

- Many imaging modalities are available for imaging the lumbar spine. Each has its own advantages, disadvantages, and indications (Table 32-4).
- In most cases of acute LBP, imaging studies are unnecessary.
- Imaging provides valuable anatomic information but may not be helpful in identifying the cause of a patient's pain or in guiding management.
- In general, for patients under the age of 50 with acute LBP without a history of trauma, systemic disease, or neurologic deficit, the use of imaging should be delayed at least one month.
- Imaging is indicated in patients with clinical history and exam findings suggestive of "red flag" conditions, history of recent trauma, or persistent pain refractory to conservative treatment.
- Imaging studies are appropriate in patients older than 50 who are more likely to have compression fractures, degenerative changes, and spinal stenosis.
- Plain radiographs in two views, anteroposterior and lateral, should be the initial modality of choice in most patients.
- Lateral oblique, flexion, and extension views should be reserved for confirmation of findings on initial films or for use when there is prior fusion or suspicion of instability.
- Many plain film findings, such as degenerative disc disease, vertebral osteophytes, facet joint arthropathy, transitional vertebrae, Schmorl nodes, and spina bifida occulta, are present in close to one half of the population and asymptomatic in most.
- The best study for evaluation of the lumbar spine is MRI.
- For patients with previous back surgery, gadolinium enhancement helps differentiate scar tissue from recurrent disc herniation.
- CT scanning is superior for imaging bony anatomy, metastases to the spine, and trauma.

TABLE 32-4   Imaging Modalities for Low Back Pain

MODALITY	DEMONSTRATES	RECOMMENDED FOR	DISADVANTAGES
Plain x-rays	Lumbar alignment Size of vertebral bodies, discs, neural foramina	Possible fractures Arthropathy Spondylolisthesis	Do not detect disc bulges, focal herniations, intraspinal masses, or small paraspinous lesions
	Bone density Fractures Osteophytes	Tumors Infections Stenosis Congenital deformities	Radiation exposure

CT	Cross-sectional images of spine	Bony/joint pathology
		   Arthropathy
		   Fractures
		   Tumors
		Lateral disc herniation
		Stenosis
		   Spinal canal
		   Neuroforaminal
		   Lateral recess
		Contraindication to MRI
			Cost
			Contrast required to image intrathecal anatomy
			Radiation exposure

MRI	Details of spinal cord
	Cauda equina
	Discs
	Paraspinal soft tissue
		Disk herniation
		Spinal stenosis
		Osteomyelitis
		Tumors
		   Spinal cord
		   Nerve roots
		   Nerve sheath
		   Paraspinal soft tissue
		Cauda equina syndrome
			Cost
			Poor for bony anatomy

- CT myelography is indicated for patients with a contraindication to MRI (Table 32-5) or those with spinal instrumentation. This is the most sensitive test for spinal nerve compression but carries significantly greater risk than does MRI.

MANAGEMENT

- Since 1994, 11 countries have published guidelines for diagnosis and management of LBP, which are generally followed with individual modification.
- Appropriate management involves formulating an accurate diagnosis.

TABLE 32-5   Contraindications to MRI

Cardiac pacemaker
Implanted cardiac defibrillator
Aneurysm clips
Carotid artery vascular clamp
Neurostimulator (noncompatible; please note MRI-compatible leads have recently been developed and may be available at the time of this publication)
Insulin or infusion pump (read package insert as compatibility is possible with some equipment)
Implanted drug infusion device (relative and is device specific)
Bone growth/fusion stimulator
Cochlear, otologic, or ear implant
Significant claustrophobia

- For patients with acute, nonspecific LBP, the primary treatment emphasis should be nonoperative care, time, reassurance, and education.

NONOPERATIVE CARE

Patient Education

- Reassure the patient that full recovery is expected.
- Maintain an active and educational relationship with the patient.
- Future plans, diagnostic studies, and therapies should be discussed with the patient if symptoms persist.

Patient Comfort

- Pain relief and return of function are primary goals.
- Work with the patient to find an effective therapeutic regimen.

Physical Activity

- Bed rest is not effective for LBP or radiculopathy and may be harmful.
- Maintaining a normal activity level may result in a faster return to work, less chronic disability, and fewer recurrent problems but may have little or no beneficial effect for acute LBP or radiculopathy.

- Exercise may initially cause a slight increase in symptoms but overall may prove beneficial for preventing debility and improving weight control.
- Light aerobic exercises, such as swimming, walking, and using a stationary bicycle, may begin when the patient can sit comfortably and may be increased as tolerated.
- Strenuous activities, such as heavy lifting, twisting, and sitting/standing for prolonged periods, should be avoided until symptoms have resolved.
- Specific back exercises during the acute phase are not beneficial and may worsen symptoms.

Oral Medications

- NSAIDs and acetaminophen are first-line medications for acute LBP. No intraclass differences in efficacy have been demonstrated for NSAIDs. The favorable side effect profile of acetaminophen supports its use before undergoing trials with NSAIDs.
- Addition of a muscle relaxant may benefit patients with muscle spasms or trouble sleeping.
- During the acute phase, adding opiates to NSAIDs has no demonstrated clear benefit and may add troubling side effects.
- Opioid use should be limited to patients with pain refractory to NSAIDs. Long-term use of opioids to treat chronic LBP, although controversial, has become commonplace. However, this treatment has recently been challenged with trends to reduce use of opioids to treat chronic LBP.
- Oral corticosteroid use is controversial; some studies demonstrate lasting benefit and others show short-lived or no benefits.

Other Conventional Therapies

- There are no long-term studies demonstrating efficacy of epidural steroid injections for chronic nonradicular LBP, but these injections may be effective in patients with acute lumbosacral radicular pain or patients with known disc herniations.
- Injecting other sites with local anesthetics and steroids to treat chronic LBP, including facet joints, trigger points, ligaments, and sacroiliac joint injections, may provide transient relief during acute LBP episodes and provide diagnostic information for chronic back pain as well.
- Although studies deny efficacy for bracing, traction, physical modalities, behavioral therapy, transcutaneous electrical nerve stimulation, acupuncture, or "back school," many of these therapies can provide pain relief during the approximately six weeks it takes to heal the underlying cause of acute LBP.

SURGICAL INTERVENTION

- Only 1% of LBP sufferers have a medical condition requiring surgical intervention.
- Surgical intervention should be reserved for patients with an identifiable pathology on imaging studies that is consistent with history and physical examination findings.
- Immediate surgery is reserved for patients with identifiable and correctable pathology causing incapacitating pain, progressive neurologic deficits, impaired bowel or bladder function, cauda equina syndrome, or extremely hazardous conditions (eg, infection or neoplasm).
- In cases of new-onset mechanical LBP, delaying surgery until the patient has had at least one month of nonoperative treatment is appropriate in most cases.
- In the absence of a new neurologic deficit, if the patient is improving slowly, it is reasonable to delay surgery until symptoms plateau at an unacceptable level.
- Surgery on the lumbar spine corrects two abnormalities: compression of nerve roots and spinal instability.
- The procedures most frequently performed include discectomy, laminectomy, spinal fusion, and vertebroplasty/kyphoplasty.
- Satisfactory relief of pain is achieved in 16%–95% of lumbar spinal fusions, with better results achieved with laminectomy and discectomy.

MANAGEMENT PLAN

- Overall, the prognosis remains favorable for patients presenting with acute LBP.
- The detailed history and physical examination identify those few patients with underlying conditions who require immediate attention.
- For most patients, imaging and aggressive interventions should be delayed until the patient has undergone four to six weeks of nonoperative care.
- Patients should be reassured that LBP only rarely leads to disability.
- Patients should be encouraged to return to normal activity and begin light aerobic exercises immediately while avoiding strenuous activities until symptoms resolve.
- Over-the-counter analgesics, NSAIDs, and acetaminophen are the first-line medications for pain relief.
- If pain is refractory to NSAIDs, opiates may be prescribed.
- If symptoms have resolved or are improving by four to six weeks, there is no need for further investigation.
- If symptoms progress or stabilize at an unacceptable level, clinical reassessment and imaging are mandated.
- Plain radiographs serve as the initial imaging study. MRI follows and is considered the diagnostic imaging study of choice.

- If there is bony pathology on plain radiographs or a history of trauma, a CT scan is indicated.
- Surgical intervention is an option only for patients with identifiable pathology on imaging studies that is consistent with their clinical presentation.
- Early surgical consideration is given to patients with a neurologic deficit due to nerve root compression, incapacitating pain, or a progressive neurologic deficit.
- Evidence of a cauda equina syndrome with loss of bowel or bladder control is an indication for emergent imaging and surgical decompression.

BIBLIOGRAPHY

Atlas SJ, Deyo RA. Evaluating and managing acute low back pain in the primary care setting. *J Gen Intern Med.* 2001;16:120.

Battie MC, Bigos SJ, Fisher LD, et al. Anthropometric and clinical measures as predictors of back pain complaints in industry: a prospective study. *J Spinal Disord.* 1990;3:195.

Biering-Sorensen F. A prospective study of low back pain in a general population. II. Location, character, aggravating and relieving factors. *Scand J Rehabil Med.* 1983;15:81.

Deyo RA, Phillips WR. Low back pain: a primary care challenge. *Spine.* 1996;21:2826.

Frymoyer JW, Cats-Baril WL. An overview of the incidences and costs of low back pain. *Orthop Clin North Am.* 1991;22:263.

Green LN. Dexamethasone in the management of symptoms due to herniated lumbar disc. *J Neurol Neurosurg Psychiatry.* 1975;38:1211.

Hagen KB, Hilde G, Jamtvedt G, et al. Bed rest for acute low back pain and sciatica. *Cochrane Database Syst Rev.* 2000:CD001254.

Hart LG, Deyo RA, Cherkin DC. Physician office visits for low back pain: frequency, clinical evaluation, and treatment patterns from a U.S. national survey. *Spine.* 1995;20:11.

Hoffman RM, Wheeler KJ, Deyo RA. Surgery for herniated lumbar discs: a literature synthesis. *J Gen Intern Med.* 1993;8:487.

Koes BW, Scholten RJ, Mens JM, et al. Efficacy of epidural steroid injections for low-back pain and sciatica: a systematic review of randomized clinical trials. *Pain.* 1995;63:279.

Modic MT, Masaryk TJ, Ross JS, et al. Imaging of degenerative disk disease. *Radiology.* 1988;168:177.

Pincus T, Burton AK, Vogel S, et al. A systematic review of psychological factors as predictors of chronicity/disability in prospective cohorts of low back pain. *Spine.* 2002;27:E109.

Rozenberg S, Delval C, Rezvani Y, et al. Bed rest or normal activity for patients with acute low back pain: a randomized controlled trial. *Spine.* 2002;27:1487.

Taylor VM, Deyo RA, Cherkin DC, et al. Low back pain hospitalization: recent United States trends and regional variations. *Spine.* 1994;19:1207.

Torgerson WR, Dotter WE. Comparative roentgenographic study of the asymptomatic and symptomatic lumbar spine. *J Bone Joint Surg Am.* 1976;58:850.

Turner JA, Ersek M, Herron L, et al. Patient outcomes after lumbar spinal fusions. *JAMA.* 1992;268:907.

van Tulder MW, Cherkin DC, Berman B, et al. The effectiveness of acupuncture in the management of acute and chronic low back pain: a systematic review within the framework of the Cochrane Collaboration Back Review Group. *Spine.* 1999;24:1113.

van Tulder MW, Koes BW, Bouter LM. Conservative treatment of acute and chronic nonspecific low back pain: a systematic review of randomized controlled trials of the most common interventions. *Spine.* 1997;22:2128.

van Tulder MW, Scholten RJ, Koes BW, et al. Nonsteroidal anti-inflammatory drugs for low back pain: a systematic review within the framework of the Cochrane Collaboration Back Review Group. *Spine.* 2000;25:2501.

White K, Williams F, Greenberg B. The ecology of medical care. *N Engl J Med.* 1961;265:885.

33 NECK PAIN

Mikiko Murakami, DO
Sudhir Diwan, MD, DABIPP

DEFINITION

- Neck pain: Pain in the region we call the neck is defined by four anatomical borders—superiorly by the superior nuchal line, bilaterally by the lateral margins of the neck, and inferiorly by a transverse line through the T1 spinous process.
- Extensive variation exists in the way that neck pain is defined in the literature. Axial neck pain is separate from cervical radicular pain, but many surveys do not distinguish between the two.
- Cervical radiculopathy is a neurologic condition characterized by neurologic function: some combination of sensory loss, motor loss, and impaired reflexes in a segmental distribution. Axonal pain can be elicited secondary to nerve ischemia or compression of the dorsal root ganglion. Cervical radicular pain may be caused by the inflammation of the cervical nerve roots, caused by disc protrusions leaking inflammatory exudates. Radicular pain can also be caused by noninflammatory lesions such as tumors, cysts, and osteophytes by direct compression of neural structures.
- Segmental innervation of muscles is a better guide to the distribution of radicular pain than the dermatomes. Segmental innervation of deep tissues is

not the same as that of the skin. For example, muscles (myotomes) of the shoulder are innervated by C5 and C6, while skin over the shoulder (dermatomes) is innervated by C4 and C5. Nonetheless, the exact diagnosis can be confusing with referred pains and overlap dermatomes.

EPIDEMIOLOGY AND FACTS

- Prevalence of neck pain in the United States: Because of the discrepancies in the definition of neck pain, the data regarding the prevalence have been varied. Chronic persistent neck pain with or without upper extremity pain in the adult population has a prevalence of 48% for women and 38% for men, and is persistent in 22% of women and 16% of men. A total of 50%–70% patients experience re-occurring neck pain within five years.
- Prevalence of neck pain in the world: The Global Burden of Disease 2010 Study estimated that the global point prevalence of neck pain (axial with or without radicular pain) was 4.9% and disability-adjusted life years increased from 23.9 million in 1990 to 33.6 million in 2010, and concluded that out of all 291 conditions studied in the Global Burden of Disease 2010 Study, neck pain ranked 21st in terms of overall burden and 4th highest in terms of disability.
- Neck pain-contributing factors: Neck pain prevalence is generally higher in women, office and computer workers, high-income countries, and urban areas. Many environmental, personal, and past medical history factors influence the onset and course of neck pain, including a history of low back pain and psychological factors.
- Etiologies of pain in the private office setting: Bogduk and Yin attempted to determine causes of neck pain in the private office setting, and found among the 46% of patients who completed investigations the following: prevalence of zygapophyseal joint pain, 55%; prevalence of discogenic pain, 16%; and prevalence of lateral atlantoaxial (AA) joint pain, 9%.
- Whiplash, neck pain, and headache: Lord et al (1994) showed that after whiplash, 55% have chronic neck pain and 71% of patients also have a headache. The third occipital nerve headache is a common condition in patients with chronic neck pain and headache after whiplash. Diagnostic third occipital nerve blocks can help make this diagnosis. The patients with a positive diagnosis are significantly more likely to be tender over the C2–C3 zygapophyseal joint. The prevalence of third occipital nerve headache is 27%, and among

those with dominant headache the prevalence was as high as 53%.

ANATOMY

- The largest interlaminar space: C6/7 or C7/T1. The orientation of the facet joint in the cervical spine is relatively coronal compared with that of the thoracic or lumbar regions. This coronal orientation protects from shear injury, compared with the obliquely sagittal orientation in lumbar spine, which protect the discs from axial rotation.
- C1 vertebra (atlas): has no body and no intervertebral foramen for nerve roots.
- C2 vertebra (axis): has an odontoid process, a vertebral foramen with a short transverse process, a bifid spinous process, and a lamina, but no body.
- C3–C6: have a body, lamina, transverse process, and a spinous process. The vertebral foramen are in the transverse process. The vertebral body diameter is larger transverse, >AP.
- C7 vertebra: has a vertebral foramen but without a vertebral artery.
- Atlantooccipital (AO) joints: synovial joint, deep posterior arch, long and perforated transverse process, and concave articular surfaces articulate with occipital condyles. Allow for flexion and extension.
- AA joints: two lateral and one median joint. Dens (odontoid process) forms pivot for rotation. Stability is due to ligaments only.
- Epidural space: mostly loose areolar tissue and fat. Has an epidural venous plexus. In the cervical region, there is less tissue and fat, and larger-diameter veins. The epidural space has an AP diameter of 2 mm (at C3–C6) and 3–4 mm (at C6–T1), compared with 5–6 mm in the lumbar region.
- Vertebral artery: tortuous with a variable course, lateral to the AA joints, and medial and superior to AO joints (Figures 33-1 and 33-2). The vertebral arteries branch off the subclavian artery. The right and left branches come together at the base of the skull to form the basilar artery. Branches from the vertebral artery form one anterior and two posterior spinal arteries. Note its course around C7 (Figure 33-3).
- The front of the cervical spine and neck has sympathetic chains and ganglia, cervical and brachial plexuses, an arterial system, and venous system.
- Fifty percent AP flexion in neck is centered on the AO joint; the rest is divided evenly among other cervical vertebral articulations.
- In 1980, the MB was correctly defined by Bogduk. The medial branch travels around the articular pillar. C5

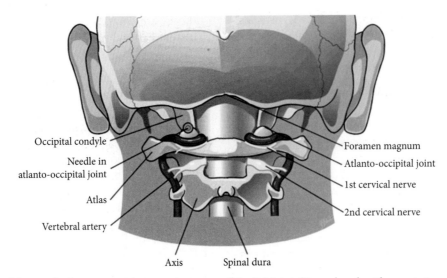

FIG. 33-1. Course of the vertebral artery over the posterior aspect of the OA joint. (Reproduced, with permission, from Waldman SD: *Atlas of Interventional Pain Management.* 3rd ed. Philadelphia, PA: Saunders Elsevier; 2009.).

runs across the centroid of the pillar and at all other levels, the medial branch path varies slightly.

- Innervation of neck:

ANATOMY	INNERVATION
Posterior neck muscles and cervical z-joints	Cervical dorsal rami
Lateral atlantoaxial joint	C2 ventral ramus

Atlantooccipital joint	C1 ventral ramus
Median atlantoaxial joint and ligaments	Sinuvertebral nerves of C1, C2, C3
Cervical spinal cord	Sinuvertebral nerves of C1, C2, C3
Prevertebral and lateral muscles of neck	Cervical ventral rami
Cervical discs	Posteriorly: by posterior vertebral plexus that lies on the floor of the vertebral canal, formed by the cervical sinuvertebal nerves
	Anteriorly: by anterior vertebral plexus that is formed by the cervical sympathetic trunks
	Laterally: by the vertebral nerve (formed by branches of cervical gray rami communicantes)

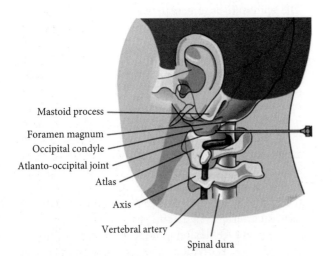

FIG. 33-2. Lateral view showing the course of the vertebral artery over the C1-2 facet joint. (Reproduced, with permission, from Waldman SD: *Atlas of Interventional Pain Management.* 3rd ed. Philadelphia, PA: Saunders Elsevier; 2009.)

The following are the differentials for neck pain that one should be aware of:

- There is no objective test that confirms the presence of neck pain.
- Serious conditions not to overlook: neoplasms, infections, and vascular disorders.
- Less serious: inflammatory arthropathy, which can be detected with appropriate imaging. Note that it is rarely a cause of neck pain alone.
- Questionable causes of neck pain: diffuse idiopathic skeletal hyperostosis and ossification of the posterior longitudinal ligament.
- Fractures, spondylosis, and osteoarthritis can be asymptomatic or symptomatic.

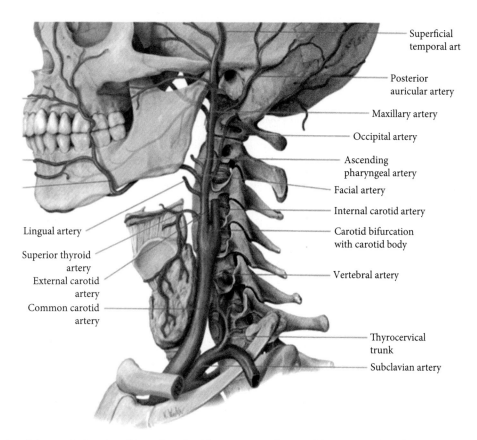

FIG. 33-3. Arteries of the cervical region. (Reproduced, with permission, from Waldman SD: *Atlas of Interventional Pain Management.* 3rd ed. Philadelphia, PA: Saunders Elsevier; 2009.)

- Systemic diseases such as fibromyalgia and polymyalgia rheumatica should not be listed as the cause of isolated neck pain.
- Psychogenic pain is outdated, not part of the DSM-IV, often a euphemism for malingering or unclear etiology.

CONSERVATIVE TREATMENTS FOR NECK PAIN

- With most mild to moderate axial neck pain, improvement will be noted in two to three weeks.
- Medications used for treatment include Tylenol, NSAID, neuropathic pain medications (gabapentin, Lyrica, amitriptyline, nortriptyline), and antidepressants (TCAs, duloxetine, venlafaxine).
- Physical therapy, manual therapy, postural modification, cervical pillows, and TENS units for home exercise have also been shown to aid in healing.
- Acupuncture: A meta-analysis published in 2012 showed that acupuncture is superior to placebo for back and neck pain, osteoarthritis, chronic headache, and shoulder pain.

INTERVENTIONAL PROCEDURES

- Common spinal procedures:
  - Cervical facet injections
  - Cervical epidural injections (interlaminar, transforaminal)
  - Cervical medial branch blocks (MBB)
  - Percutaneous radio-frequency (RF) ablation
  - Neuroaugmentation procedures
  - Stellate ganglion block procedures
  - AA and AO procedures
  - Annuloplasty
  - Nucleoplasty
  - Discography
- Less common procedures:
  - Glossopharyngeal nerve block for glossopharyngeal neuralgia
  - Styloid process injection for stylohyoid syndrome
  - Omohyoid injection for omohyoid syndrome (rupture of the inferior belly)
  - Trigger point injections for trapezius syndrome and splenius cervicis syndrome

COMPREHENSIVE EVIDENCE-BASED GUIDELINES FOR INTERVENTIONAL TECHNIQUES IN THE MANAGEMENT OF CHRONIC SPINAL PAIN (*PAIN PHYSICIAN*, 2009)—SUMMARY OF PROCEDURES

PROCEDURE	TOP INDICATIONS	COMPLICATIONS	RECOMMENDATIONS	EVIDENCE
Cervical facet or zygapophyseal joint blocks	To diagnose facet-mediated pain	Dural puncture	For pain >6/10 for >3 months	I or II-1
		Facet capsule rupture	Lack of discogenic pain, disc herniation, radiculitis	
		Paralysis		
Cervical provocation discography	Identify painful discs and depict internal derangements	Discitis	Positive if stimulation of target disc reproduces >7/10 pain	II-2
		Subdural abscess Spinal cord injury		
Medial branch block (MBB)	For facet-mediated pain	Intravascular injection	For long-term relief for chronic facet joint pain	IB or IC for cervical, thoracic, lumbar MBB
		Spinal anesthesia Dural puncture		
Medial branch neurotomy	If >80% relief with anesthetic block		Strong recommendation	II-1 or II-2
			For long-term relief for chronic facet joint pain	
Cervical interlaminar injection	Disc herniation	Spinal cord trauma	For short- and long-term relief	II-1
	Radiculopathy Spinal stenosis	Intravascular injection		

US PREVENTATIVE TASK FORCE RATINGS

The USPSTF is an independent panel of non-Federal experts in prevention and evidence-based medicine composed of primary care providers, and conducts scientific evidence reviews of a broad range of clinical preventive health care services (http://www.uspreventiveservicestaskforce.org/uspstf08/methods/procmanual4.htm). They develop recommendations for primary care clinicians and health systems. USPSTF ratings:

I: Properly powered and conducted randomized controlled trial (RCT); well-conducted systematic review or meta-analysis of homogeneous RCTs

  II-1: Well-designed controlled trial without randomization

  II-2: Well-designed cohort or case-control analytic study

  II-3: Multiple time series with or without the intervention; dramatic results from uncontrolled experiments

II: Opinions of respected authorities, based on clinical experience; descriptive studies or case reports; reports of expert committees

Algorithmic approach to diagnosis of neck pain is given in Figure 33-4.

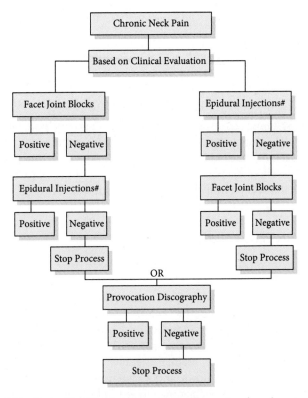

FIG. 33-4. Algorithmic approach to diagnosis of neck pain. (Reproduced from Manchikanti L, Helm S, Singh V, Benyamin RM, Datta S, Hayek SM, Fellows B, Boswell MV; ASIPP. An algorithmic approach for clinical management of chronic spinal pain. *Pain Physician.* 2009 Jul-Aug;12(4):E225-64. Originally published by BioMed Central.)

FLUOROSCOPIC GUIDANCE

- Fluoroscopic guidance: improves accuracy of needle placements.
- Always saves representative films.
- Views: lateral, anteroposterior, oblique, gun-barrel, tunnel, coaxial, and swimmer's view.

CONTRAST STUDY

- Maximizes the use of fluoroscopy and predicts the medication spread.
- Most commonly used: nonionic, hydrophilic monomer with low osmolality. Radiopacity is related to the concentration of iodine.

DIGITAL SUBTRACTION

- Identifies contrast spread in epidural, subdural, intrathecal, and intra-articular regions (Figure 33-5)
- Electronically enhanced image

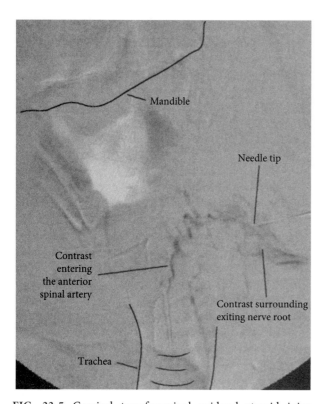

FIG. 33-5. Cervical transforaminal epidural steroid injection using digital subtraction that shows contrast entering the spinal radicular artery with flow into the anterior spinal artery. (Reproduced, with permission, from Rathmell, James: *Atlas of Image-Guided Intervention in Regional Anesthesia and Pain Medicine.* 2nd edition. Philadelphia, PA: Lipincott and Williams; 2012.)

- Reduced amount of contrast
- Live or real-time fluoroscopy with digital subtraction
- Detects intra-arterial contrast spread

CERVICAL ZYGAPOPHYSIAL JOINT (Z-JOINT) INTRA-ARTICULAR ACCESS

- Cervical z-joints are paired, planar, synovial joints formed between the inferior articular process of one vertebra and the superior articular process of the one below.
- Joint spaces are not evident in AP views, but locations can be plotted. A lateral view confirms final points of intra-articular access.
- Lateral, posterior, and oblique approaches can be used to inject.

CERVICAL TRANSFORAMINAL INJECTIONS

- Cervical transforaminal should not be performed in the absence of extensive experience. The ability to deal with rapid onset of life-threatening complications is necessary.
- The evidence for cervical transforaminal injections is poor, and there do appear to be substantive risks. The decision to proceed with transforaminal injections needs to be carefully considered.
- Insertion of the needle transversely, only utilizing the lateral view, is unsafe.
- The relationship between the superior articular process, spinal nerve, ventral ramus, vertebral artery, and radicular artery, and a needle inserted obliquely should be very well understood (Figure 33-6).
- Only nonparticulate steroid should be used.

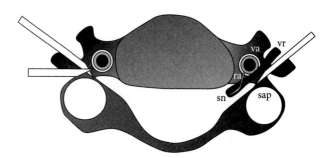

FIG. 33-6. Cross sectional illustration of the cervical spine showing the relationship of the spinal nerve (sn), vertebral artery (va), radicular artery (ra), ventral root (vr), and superior articular process (sap). (Reproduced, with permission, from Bogduk N. The anatomy and pathophysiology of neck pain. *Phys Med Rehabil Clin N Am.* 2011 Aug;22(3):367–82, vii.)

CERVICAL INTERLAMINAR EPIDURAL STEROID INJECTION

- Epidural steroid injections are one of the most commonly performed interventions in the United States for the management of chronic neck pain. Evidence for cervical interlaminar injections has been debated; at best they have had only moderate success in managing cervical radiculopathy, while there is no evidence available in the management of axial neck pain, postsurgery syndrome, or discogenic pain. Three RCTs were evaluated for cervical interlaminar injections; all three showed short-term relief, and two showed long-term relief.
- The best technique is: 1) use an AP flouroscopic view to identify the upper edge of the T1 vertebral lamina; 2) touch the lamina with the needle; 3) switch to a contralateral oblique view; 4) advance the needle over superior edge of lamina and 5) Use loss of resistance technique as you observe needle depth.

CERVICAL MEDIAL BRANCH BLOCKS

- Cervical MBB are used as a diagnostic procedure to see if a patient's pain is mediated by one or more of the medial branches of the cervical dorsal rami.
- The medial branches innervate the cervical zygapophyseal joints, the posterior arches of the typical cervical vertebrae, and certain muscles of the posterior neck. Of these, only the zygapophyseal joints may cause a focal source of chronic neck pain. This is why

this procedure can also be referred to as a zygapophyseal block.
- In patients with primary upper cervical pain and headache, the third occipital nerve (for the C2–C3 joint) should be an early target.
- In 2007, Cooper and Bogduk mapped out the distribution of pain in normal volunteers after stimulation of the zygapophyseal joints (Figure 33-7).
- In 2007, Cooper and Bogduk mapped out the distribution of pain relieved in patients with neck pain, after anesthetization of synovial joints indicated, using controlled diagnostic blocks. The density of shading is proportional to the number of patients whose pain extended into the area indicated (Figure 33-8).

CERVICAL MEDIAL BRANCH THERMAL RADIO-FREQUENCY NEUROTOMY

- RF neurotomy is a therapeutic procedure in which a Teflon-coated electrode with an exposed tip is placed onto a peripheral nerve. Alternating high-frequency electrical current concentrates around the tip, immediately heating surrounding tissues, including the target nerve.
- In 1982, Bogduk advocated a more selective targeting of cervical medial branches based on correct anatomy. In 1996, Lord et al performed an RCT placebo-controlled study and long-term follow-up sufficiently proved the efficacy of RF.
- The long-term efficacy of RF neurotomy of the medial branch was researched in 1999, showing that 71% patients had complete relief of chronic neck pain after an initial procedure. No patient who failed to respond to a first procedure responded to a repeat procedure, but if pain returned after a successful initial procedure, relief could be reinstated by a repeat procedure. Median duration of relief after a first procedure was 219 days when failures are included but 422 days when only successful cases are considered. The median duration of relief after repeat procedures was at least 219 days.
- RF ablation side effects:
  - RF C3–C7: vasovagal syncope (2%), dermoid cyst (1%), Koebner phenomenon (1%), neuritis (2%), numbness in cutaneous territory (29%), and dysesthesias (19%)
  - RF to TON: numbness (97%), ataxia (95%), dysesthesia (55%), hypersensitivity (15%), and itch (10%)
- RF for chronic neck pain from whiplash: 25 patients with chronic neck pain s/p whiplash were studied.

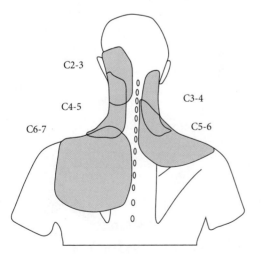

FIG. 33-7. Referred pain pattern from stimulation of the cervical facet joints. (Reproduced, with permission, from Bogduk N. The anatomy and pathophysiology of neck pain. *Phys Med Rehabil Clin N Am.* 2011 Aug;22(3):367–82, vii.)

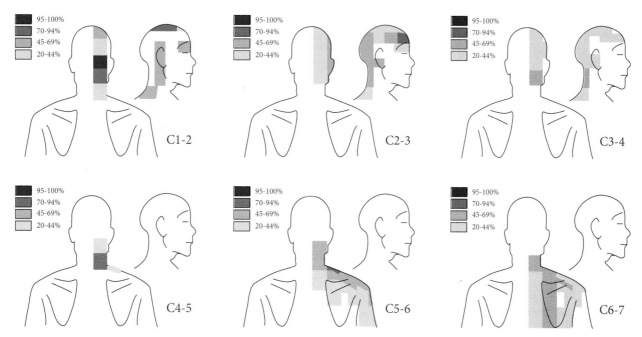

FIG. 33-8. Distribution of pain relief after anesthetizing various cervical facet levels. (Reproduced, with permission, from Bogduk N. The anatomy and pathophysiology of neck pain. *Phys Med Rehabil Clin N Am.* 2011 Aug;22(3):367–82, vii.)

An RCT showed a median of 8 days pain for recurrence of pain in control group (RF needle inserted but not turned on as sham) and the median time that elapsed before the pain returned to at least 50% of the preoperative level was 263 days in the treatment group. At 27 weeks, seven patients in the active treatment group and one patient in the control group were free of pain. Five patients in the active treatment group had numbness in the territory of the treated nerves, but none considered it troubling. It was concluded that in patients with chronic cervical zygapophyseal joint pain confirmed with double-blind, placebo-controlled local anesthesia, percutaneous RF neurotomy with multiple lesions of target nerves can provide lasting relief.

CERVICAL DISC STIMULATION (PROVOCATION DISCOGRAPHY)

- Cervical disc stimulation is designed to identify a painful intervertebral disc, which involves identifying a needle into the nucleus pulposus and injecting contrast medium in order to reproduce the pain.
- With provocation discography, a disc is stimulated while an image is obtained.
- In both cadaver studies and MRI studies, fissures on discs have been established to be age related and demonstrating them on discography is of no use. Reproduction of the patient's accustomed pain is the most important component of disc stimulation.

SURGICAL PROCEDURES

- Surgery for axial neck pain alone is not recommended. Axial neck pain with radicular symptoms can be helpful for those who fail conservative measures.
- In a 2013 systematic review, surgery was compared with conservative care for neck pain and it was found that the benefits of survey over conservative care were not clearly demonstrated.

BIBLIOGRAPHY

Benyamin RM, Singh V, Parr AT, Conn A, Diwan S, Abdi S. Systematic review of the effectiveness of cervical epidurals in the management of chronic neck pain. *Pain Physician.* 2009;12(1):137–157.

Bogduk N. The anatomy and pathophysiology of neck pain. *Phys Med Rehabil Clin N Am.* 2011;22(3):367–382, vii.

Bogduk N; International Spine Intervention Society. *Standards Committee. Practice Guidelines for Spinal Diagnostic and Treatment Procedures.* 1st ed. San Francisco: International Spine Intervention Society; 2004.

Cooper G, Bailey B, Bogduk N. Cervical zygapophyseal joint pain maps. *Pain Med.* 2007;8(4):344–353.

Diwan S, Manchikanti L, Benyamin RM, et al. Effectiveness of cervical epidural injections in the management of chronic neck and upper extremity pain. *Pain Physician.* 2012;15(4):E405–E434.

Hoy D, March L, Woolf A, et al. The global burden of neck pain: estimates from the Global Burden of Disease 2010 study. *Ann Rheum Dis.* 2014;73:1309–1315.

Lord SM, Barnsley L, Wallis BJ, Bogduk N. Third occipital nerve headache: a prevalence study. *J Neurol Neurosurg Psychiatry.* 1994;57(10):1187–1190.

Lord SM, Barnsley L, Wallis BJ, McDonald GJ, Bogduk N. Percutaneous radio-frequency neurotomy for chronic cervical zygapophyseal-joint pain. *N Engl J Med.* 1996;335(23):1721–1726.

Manchikanti L, Abdi S, Atluri S, et al. An update of comprehensive evidence-based guidelines for interventional techniques in chronic spinal pain. Part II: guidance and recommendations. *Pain Physician.* 2013;16(2 suppl):S49–S283.

Manchikanti L, Boswell MV, Singh V, et al. Comprehensive evidence-based guidelines for interventional techniques in the management of chronic spinal pain. *Pain Physician.* 2009;12(4):699–802.

Manchikanti L, Falco FJ, Diwan S, Hirsch JA, Smith HS: Cervical radicular pain: the role of interlaminar and transforaminal epidural injections. *Curr Pain Headache Rep.* 2014; 18(1):389.

McDonald GJ, Lord SM, Bogduk N. Long-term follow-up of patients treated with cervical radiofrequency neurotomy for chronic neck pain. *Neurosurgery.* 1999;45(1):61–67 [discussion 67–68].

Merskey H, Bogduk N; International Association for the Study of Pain. Task Force on Taxonomy. *Classification of Chronic Pain: Descriptions of Chronic Pain Syndromes and Definitions of Pain Terms.* 2nd ed. Seattle: IASP Press; 1994.

Oda J, Tanaka H, Tsuzuki N. Intervertebral disc changes with aging of human cervical vertebra. From the neonate to the eighties. *Spine.* 1988;13(11):1205–1211.

Parfenchuck TA, Janssen ME. A correlation of cervical magnetic resonance imaging and discography/computed tomographic discograms. *Spine.* 1994;19(24):2819–2825.

Rathmell J. *Atlas of Image-guided Intervention in Regional Anesthesia and Pain Medicine.* 2nd ed. Philadelphia, PA: Lippincott and Williams; 2012.

Schellhas KP, Smith MD, Gundry CR, Pollei SR. Cervical discogenic pain. Prospective correlation of magnetic resonance imaging and discography in asymptomatic subjects and pain sufferers. *Spine.* 1996;21(3):300–311 [discussion 311–312].

Schünke M, Ross LM, Lamperti ED, Schulte E, Schumacher U. *Head and Neuroanatomy.* Stuttgart, NY: Thieme; 2007.

van Middelkoop M, Rubinstein SM, Ostelo R, et al. Surgery versus conservative care for neck pain: a systematic review. *Eur Spine J.* 2013;22(1):87–95.

Vickers AJ, Linde K. Acupuncture for chronic pain. *JAMA.* 2014;311(9):955–956.

Waldman SD. *Atlas of Interventional Pain Management.* 3rd ed. Philadelphia, PA: Saunders/Elsevier; 2009.

Yin W, Bogduk N. The nature of neck pain in a private pain clinic in the United States. *Pain Med.* 2008;9(2):196–203.

34 SHOULDER PAIN

Frank Falco, MD
Niteesh Bharara, MD
Anjuli Desai, MD

INTRODUCTION

- The shoulder joint is the body's most mobile joint.
- Shoulder pain accounts for 12 out of every 1000 primary care office visits.
- Shoulder pain is a very prevalent musculoskeletal disorder, with a one-year prevalence rate of 5%–47%.
- When presenting to a primary care physician, approximately 50% of all patients with new complaints of shoulder pain show complete recovery within six months. After one year, this percentage increases to 60%.
- Shoulder and neck pain account for 18% of all insurance disability payments made for musculoskeletal pain.
- Since conservative care of shoulder pain is an enormous expenditure within health care systems of most developed countries, the evaluation and rational treatment of shoulder pain are extremely important.
- Thus, it is essential to understand the causes, natural history, and potential treatments of shoulder pain syndromes.

CAUSES AND NATURAL HISTORY

- Patients with transient syndromes who receive no treatment are ubiquitous but have little medical impact.
- Shoulder pain usually relents spontaneously with symptomatic care within a month, and nearly all patients improve within three months; however, pain persists more than six months in a small percentage of patients.
- Some factors that predispose the patient to shoulder pain include unstable glenohumeral joints, weakness of scapular stabilizers, abnormal posture, and hypomobility of the cervical and thoracic spine.
- When an acute pain syndrome is associated with a significant neurologic deficit, the treatment goal may be to eliminate or control the deficit.
- Chronic pain syndromes are those that persist longer than six months and have little chance of spontaneous improvement. Because symptoms usually do not worsen, treatment is dictated by severity and the degree of interference with lifestyle.

- Transient and acute syndromes without neurologic deficits are often thought to arise from inflammation of ligaments and muscles, but symptoms such as muscle spasm, tenderness, and focal areas of myositis (also known as trigger points) may be epiphenomena, and we should not pursue ineffective therapies based on imaginary pathologic explanations.
- The common causes of shoulder pain are:
  ○ Rotator cuff impingement
  ○ Rotator cuff tendonitis/tear
  ○ Traumatic ligament, capsular injury
  ○ Adhesive capsulitis
  ○ Bicipital tendonitis
  ○ Instability of the glenohumeral joint
  ○ Subacromial bursitis
  ○ Acromioclavicular joint injury
  ○ Suprascapular nerve entrapment
  ○ Inflammatory and noninflammatory arthritis
  ○ Tumor
  ○ Infection

DIAGNOSIS

- As with all shoulder problems, diagnosis begins with a careful history.
- The origins of the pain need to be explored because management differs if the problem resulted from trauma.
- The character, timing, and nature of pain radiation provide important information.
- Pain severity is the key to treatment choice.

PHYSICAL EXAMINATION

- Physical examination is important, not to make a definitive diagnosis, but to ascertain the neurologic status of the patient. Neurologic status is a key decision-making variable in management.
- Physical examination begins with inspection for asymmetry and palpation for areas of focal tenderness in the shoulder girdle muscles and surrounding joints, followed by assessment of passive and active range of motion.
- The routine neurologic examination includes assessment of stretch reflexes in upper and lower extremities, assessment of strength, and evaluation of sensation.
- Abnormal pathologic signs such as hyperreflexia and increased tone are suggestive of an underlying neurologic process.

- If certain pathology is suspected, specific shoulder examination maneuvers could be performed to help establish a diagnosis.

IMAGING THE SHOULDER

- In the acute phase with no neurologic deficit, imaging is not required unless symptomatic management fails.
- Imaging can be considered if the history suggests trauma, infection, or tumor.
- When imaging is required, plain films with AP, lateral, and oblique views are obtained first.
- Shoulder MRI allows the best evaluation of soft tissue, and CT best reveals bony changes. Both are often required, particularly to guide surgical therapy.

Imaging Findings

- Imaging studies might show only the mild age-related changes that might be expected in asymptomatic patients.
- Imaging provides a good demonstration of bony diseases, fractures, infections, tumors, and arthritic conditions, such as inflammatory and noninflammatory arthritis.
- Correlation of the imaging studies with the clinical syndrome facilitates diagnosis and management decisions.
- If needed, electrophysiologic studies of nerve and muscle may differentiate peripheral neuropathy, primary muscle disease, and radicular syndromes.
- Electromyography is not required in most patients but helps in confirming radicular abnormality and assessing polyneuropathy syndromes.
- Most patients have nonspecific shoulder pain but no neurologic complaints or findings. Range of motion is restricted, and local areas of spasm and myositis are common.
- Shoulder pain is often complicated by neck radiation and nonspecific arm radiation.
- Diagnostic blockade within the joints and tendons encompassing the shoulder girdle might reveal repairable abnormalities.

TREATMENT

- In the absence of trauma or concurrent disease, most patients recover fully within three months when treated symptomatically with an appropriate combination of:

- Adequate analgesia
- Moderate restriction of activities for no more than a week
- Avoidance of stressors that increase the pain and of local measures, such as heat, massage, ultrasound, electrical stimulation, and restoration of range of motion
- Passive physical therapy measures for short-term pain relief

- Occasionally, patients without added symptoms experience such severe pain that symptomatic measures are inadequate; these patients should be treated as if they had a neurologic deficit.
- If the deficit is relatively minor, the patient should be treated as if the deficit did not exist.
- If the deficit is significant (it should not be allowed to become permanent) or the pain severe, imaging should be performed immediately and treatment based on the findings.

MANAGEMENT OF SPECIFIC CLINICAL PROBLEMS

Rotator Cuff Tendonitis/Shoulder Impingement

- Rotator cuff impingement refers to mechanical compression of the rotator cuff tendons, most commonly occurring between the acromion and humeral head.
- Rotator cuff impingement commonly presents with shoulder pain that is worse at night and aggravated by overhead activity.
- Unless the deficit is severe, the painful shoulder should be initially rested with avoidance of overhead activities until the pain and swelling subside.
- Additional conservative treatment includes ice, nonsteroidal anti-inflammatory medications, physical therapy with gentle stretching to maintain range of motion, and steroid injections.
- If there is a significant neurologic deficit or instability, surgery is unlikely to be prevented by conservative measures.
- Surgical treatment most commonly includes an acromioplasty, which involves acromion shaving to increase the space around the inflamed tendon.
- Outcomes are approximately equivalent, and the choice depends on the surgeon's preference and anatomic issues.

Adhesive Capsulitis

- Adhesive capsulitis is a progressive, painful loss of passive and active glenohumeral range of motion.

- The initial presentation on physical examination is often a loss of shoulder abduction and external rotation.
- Treatment includes aggressive range of motion, nonsteroidal anti-inflammatory medications, heat modalities, and steroid injections.
- If refractory to conservative treatment, manipulation under anesthesia may be considered.

Bicipital Tendonitis

- Bicipital tendonitis is an overuse injury that is often associated with overhead activities or sports.
- This commonly presents with a tender bicipital groove, and pain with resisted forward flexion of the arm with full extension at the elbow.
- Unless the deficit is severe, the painful shoulder should be initially rested with avoidance of overhead activities until the pain and swelling subside.
- Additional conservative treatment includes ice, nonsteroidal anti-inflammatory medications, and physical therapy with a progressive exercise program.
- If refractory to conservative treatment, local corticosteroid injections may be beneficial.

Acromioclavicular Joint Injury

- Acromioclavicular joint injury may be seen with falls on the adducted shoulder, which may result in fracture, dislocation, or sprain of the surrounding ligaments.
- This commonly presents with local tenderness over the acromioclavicular joint.
- Acromioclavicular joint injuries have been classified from type I to VI depending on the severity of the injury.
- For type I and II injuries, conservative treatment can be initiated with rest, ice, nonsteroidal anti-inflammatory medications, arm sling, and progressive range of motion exercises.
- For type III to VI injuries, orthopedic consultation should be obtained to determine if open reduction and internal fixation is necessary.

Shoulder Dislocation

- Shoulder dislocations account for approximately half of all the major joint dislocations seen in the emergency department.
- The most common type of shoulder dislocation is anterior dislocation, which is most commonly due to direct trauma on an outstretched arm. Additional causes of shoulder dislocations are sport injuries and falls.
- The shoulder may be partially dislocated, with the head of the humerus partially out of the glenoid, or

the shoulder may be completely dislocated, with the head of the humerus completely out of the glenoid.

- The patient may present with a visible deformity in the shoulder, swelling, pain, bruising, weakness, numbness or decreased range of motion.
- A shoulder dislocation can be readily identified by physical examination and confirmed with imaging.
- Treatment of a dislocation depends on the severity of injury. The patient may require surgery, medication, immobilization, and rehabilitation.

Shoulder Pain From Infection or Tumor

- These problems are readily identified by imaging.
- Infections may require only antibiotic therapy after verification of the organism.
- Tumors causing pain usually must be removed.

Shoulder Pain Secondary to Systemic Arthritic Conditions

- Shoulder pain is common in patients with arthritic conditions.
- Most patients are managed symptomatically.
- Some patients require operative procedures such as shoulder replacement.

CONCLUSION

- Acute shoulder pain can usually be managed symptomatically, and most occurrences spontaneously resolve within one month.
- There is no need for imaging or other diagnostic studies in such patients, and symptomatic measures are adequate during the first month.
- Symptoms or history suggestive of significant intercurrent disease, significant neurologic deficit, or intractable pain are indications for early imaging and therapy.
- Trauma is a reasonable indication for imaging.
- Symptomatic measures include adequate analgesia, local treatments to reduce spasm and inflammation, and time.
- When patients do not improve with symptomatic treatment, imaging should include plain films, MRI, frequently CT and possibly ultrasound or arthrography.
- When a specific focal diagnosis cannot be made, electrophysiologic studies and diagnostic blockade of suspect structures may be helpful when correlated with the clinical situation.
- Surgical treatment is required for instability and intractable pain.

- A spectrum of surgical procedures can be employed, and the surgery should be tailored to the patient's individual needs and the abnormalities demonstrated.

BIBLIOGRAPHY

Croft P, Pope D, Silman A. The clinical course of shoulder pain: prospective cohort study in primary care. Primary Care Rheumatology Society Shoulder Study Group. *Br Med J.* 1996;313:601–602.

Kuijpers T, van der Windt DA, van der Heijden GJ, Bouter LM. Systematic review of prognostic cohort studies on shoulder disorders. *Pain.* 2004;109:420–431.

Nygern A, Berglund A, von Koch M. Neck-and-shoulder pain, an increasing problem. Strategies for using insurance material to follow trends. *Scand J Rehabil Med Suppl.* 1995; 32:107–112.

van der Windt DA, Koes BW, De Jong BA, Bouter LM. Shoulder disorders in general practice: incidence, patient characteristics, and management. *Ann Rheum Dis.* 1995;54:959–964.

35 OROFACIAL PAIN

Bradley A. Eli, DMD, MS

INTRODUCTION

- It is estimated that more than 90% of all facial pain is the result of dental pathology. Dentists are often the first clinicians involved in diagnosis and treatment of these conditions. Within the dental field the most useful pain consultants for pain physicians will be: (1) orofacial pain trained dentist, (2) endodontist, and (3) oral maxillofacial surgeon.
- Patients whose facial pain is ultimately unrelated to dental pathology often initially exhibit multiple symptoms that result in dental overtreatment and pain mismanagement. For many patients, this results in years of misdiagnosis and mismanagement, and can lead to chronic pain pathology. To further complicate this issue, patients will often jump from provider to provider as treatment failures continue to mount. This multiple previous provider history should be examined closely and alert the pain provider that this patient likely has pain of nonodontogenic origin.

- As with all disorders a strong understanding of "what" you are treating is necessary for diagnostic success and appropriate treatment. Pain is defined as an unpleasant sensory and emotional experience associated with actual or potential tissue damage or described in terms of such damage.

TERMINOLOGY

The following terms are basic to an understanding and diagnosis of pain:

- Algesia—any pain experience following a stimulus
- Allodynia—painful response to a nonpainful stimulus
- Hyperalgesia—an increased pain response to a noxious stimulus
- Hypoalgesia—a diminished pain response to a noxious stimulus
- Hypoesthesia—a decreased sensitivity to stimulation similar to anesthesia
- Neuroma—a mass of peripheral neurons formed by a healing damaged nerve
- Neuropathic pain—aberrant sensation produced by a malfunctioning nerve
- Nociception—the reception and transmission of nociceptive messages
- Pain threshold—the lowest level of stimulation perceived as painful by the subject
- Pain tolerance—the highest level of pain a subject is prepared (able) to tolerate
- Dysesthesia—an abnormal sensation that is unpleasant
- Sensitization—the increased excitability of nerve terminals or neurons produced by trauma or inflammation of peripheral tissues

DIAGNOSTIC GROUPING

- Because of the complexity associated with regional pain of the orofacial structures, many authors have suggested classification or grouping of tissue systems as the most direct method to evaluate a problem. In both the diagnosis and treatment of orofacial pain the clinician must have a working knowledge of functional neuroanatomy, PNS and CNS pathways, descending pain modulating systems, and their related structures. CNS changes may underlie persistent pain, and the affective or emotional aspects of continuing pain often become involved. The clinician must have a solid understanding of the various categories of persistent orofacial pain in order to be an effective care coordinator or provider.

- It is important to remember that directing the most appropriate care and providing the most appropriate care may be distinct parts of an overall care plan and may involve multiple clinicians. A critically important skill provided by the pain specialist is assuring the patient's pain is appropriately managed. By taking a thorough medical history and carefully processing and diagnosing the clinical characteristics, the clinician can identify the relationships between extracranial, intracranial, musculoskeletal, vascular, neurologic, and psychological pain and provide the most direct path to an appropriate diagnosis and treatment.

EXTRACRANIAL PAIN

- Head and neck structures involved with disease and pain include eyes, ears, nose, throat, sinuses, tongue, teeth, and glands. The quality of pain within a region involving such a broad range of structures can range from mild aching to excruciating. As previously mentioned, the most common cause of pain in the orofacial region is dental pathology. One should always consider dental pathology early in the differential and continue to search diligently throughout care.
- Disease most commonly affects the region of the maxillary sinus and teeth. The typical descriptors of sinus disease are "constant," "aching," "pressure," and "fullness." Pain will often include the teeth or ear. Fever, congestion, and/or discharge may also be present. Head position or movement can often exacerbate this symptomatology.
- Some of the most difficult headache diagnoses involve this region. Headache disorders *can and do* occur anywhere within the trigeminal distribution and can be difficult to differentiate from disease. For example, midface migraine and sinus disease can look and act very similar in many ways. Careful history taking is critical to an accurate diagnosis and treatment. Recurrence and duration can often be helpful in differentiation of these specific disorders. Also, with the introduction of the specific drug class triptans, medication trial as an abortive agent can assist with the diagnosis.
- Pain of the pulpal tissues or periodontium is often of high intensity and is often easily localized on examination or by patient report. Affected teeth are often painful to palpation or percussion, and use of percussion testing is extremely helpful in the diagnostic process. In addition, pain of dental origin will often awaken a patient from sleep or keep them from sleeping. This sleep disturbance is significant in this author's experience. A thorough medical history with careful questioning is often needed to get this

subtle information from most patients, who may be unaccustomed to sharing noncritical medical information. Any tooth-related pain should be evaluated radiographically to exclude dental disease. Most CT imaging and radiology reporting do not provide an adequate evaluation of the dental structures, and if imaging is completed, this author suggests a dental provider be involved in diagnosis.

INTRACRANIAL PAIN

- Although uncommon, neoplasm, hematoma, hemorrhage, edema, aneurysm, and infection of the central nervous system can result in facial pain. Space-occupying lesions are often associated with progressive pain complaints and associated neurologic deficit or signs. Patient descriptors, including the "worst or first," have been identified as specifically pathognomonic of more serious conditions.

MUSCULOSKELETAL PAIN

- Musculoskeletal conditions are the major cause of nonodontogenic pain in the orofacial region. Included in this group are cervical spine and temporomandibular joint disturbance (TMD). Oral and facial pain may be the result of temporomandibular joint disorder, myofascial disorders, or systemic rheumatologic, collagen, or cervical spine disease.
- TMD refers to pain and dysfunction specific to the temporomandibular joint. This is often associated with dysfunctional mandibular movements or function. Palpation of the region is often associated with exacerbations of pain. Trauma is thought to be the main cause of dysfunction within the region. Microtrauma resulting from tooth grinding or jaw clinching or macrotrauma resulting from external forces such as a MVA or facial impact has been discussed in much of the literature as the etiology of such disorders.
- The temporomandibular joint is made up of three bony structures, which include the condyle, disc, and skull. Coordinated movements within this structure require maintenance of the disc between the condyle and skull. This position is further complicated by the complex movements within the temporomandibular joint, which include both rotational and translational movements. Rapid displacement can result in pressures that often disrupt the disc–condyle relationship, resulting in incoordination identified on examination as clicking or popping. Less subtle noises such as crepitation can occur with degenerative disease such as osteoarthritis (noninflammatory

arthritis) or rheumatoid arthritis. Mechanical disturbance of this joint is often associated with inflammatory events that often respond to anti-inflammatory treatment. Noise within the temporomandibular joint without pain, catching, locking, or sudden and notable change in bite position is often simply a finding requiring no more than identification. Because of the temporomandibular joint's location in relation to the ear, patients' concerns about joint noise should be addressed and explained to avoid unnecessary treatment of the TMJ.

FACIAL MUSCLE PAIN

- The most common muscle pain disorder of the orofacial region is myofascial pain. Muscle splinting, muscle spasm, and myositis are the most common acute conditions and, based on duration, may precede myofascial pain in etiology.
- Factors associated with aggravation of muscle pain include prolonged muscle tension, poor posture, parafunction, trauma, sleep disturbance, viral infection, metabolic disturbance, and specific joint pathology.
- The most common examination finding associated with muscle problems involves pain with palpation, movement anomalies, and referred pain. Pain providers who are familiar with the most common referral patterns for the head and neck muscles will save hours of confounding findings and failed treatments. Known as the myofascial pain bible, the text by Travell and Simons is your best resource for this disorder.

CERVICAL SPINE PAIN

- Disruption in spine position, structure, and movement can often refer pain into the orofacial region. Careful assessment, history, and clinical examination, including the cervical spine, are paramount to correct identification of etiology and exclusion of referred pain phenomena.

VASCULAR PAIN

- Discussion regarding vascular etiology of pain refers specifically to the discussion of headache syndromes.
- Because headache is reviewed in Chapter 31, it should be noted that migraine, as well as tension-type and cluster headaches, may occur anywhere within the trigeminal nerve supply.
- Carotidynia and temporal arteritis are localized to their specific anatomic locations.

NEUROLOGIC PAIN

- Neurologic or neuropathic pain is the result of abnormality within nociceptors. Both peripheral and central locations and mechanisms may be involved.
- Decreased inhibition and/or increased peripheral activity result in two basic types of pain: paroxysmal and continuous neuralgias.

Paroxysmal Neuralgias

- Paroxysmal neuralgias are described as intense, sharp, stabbing, electric-like pains, usually of unilateral presentation involving the specific nerve.
- The intensity of the pain is described as "the worst pain known to man." This can occur in short- or extended-duration volleys of pain. Although intensity of these types of pain is extreme, they generally do not often awaken the sleeping patient, which helps differentiate this pain from pulpal or periodontal pain.

Trigeminal Neuralgia

- Trigeminal neuralgia affects the fifth cranial nerve. It is usually unilateral and is more common in women over the age of 50. Etiology includes idiopathic, demyelination, or vascular malformations. Additional etiology theory includes pathologic (bone) cavities at the site of previous tooth extraction, periodontal lesions, and previous endodontic therapy.
- Because of the difficulty separating trigeminal neuralgia from dental etiology, it is prudent to request a workup by an endodontist. Most endodontic specialists are very familiar with this distinction and will evaluate "to eliminate" toothache as the etiology. Failure to ask for this consult can result in significant unnecessary and irreversible neurosurgical procedures.
- The majority of patients describe the classic high-intensity, triggerable pain in association with such activities as eating and talking. Even minor stimuli, such as a cold breeze, can trigger a pain episode.
- In addition to the paroxysmal nature of classic trigeminal neuralgia, a pretrigeminal neuralgia has also been described by Fromm. This is of note due to its more constant, dull aching characteristics and is often described by patients as "like a toothache." To further confound the pain provider, most neuralgias are disabled for four to eight weeks by dental procedures such as endodontic treatment (root canal) and oral surgery (tooth extraction). On return the pain is then "transferred" to the next tooth in the same arch, which is then incorrectly treated.

Glossopharyngeal Neuralgia

- Glossopharyngeal neuralgia is more rare than trigeminal neuralgia and involves branches of the glossopharyngeal and vagus nerves.
- Symptoms of pain often include the ear, throat, tonsillar pillar, and submandibular regions.
- Triggering mechanisms, including chewing, talking, and swallowing, are often the hallmark.
- Aggressive imaging of the region is recommended because of the high suspicion of regional lesion or pathology associated with this disorder.

NERVOUS INTERMEDIUS NEURALGIA

Symptoms of pain are almost always described as a "hot poker in the ear canal." It is much like trigeminal neuralgia in most other ways. It responds to a similar care plan as most of the other paroxysmal neuralgias.

DEAFFERENTATION SYNDROMES

- Partial or total loss of nerve supply to a region can result in a painful condition. This can be a direct result of traumatic injury, surgery, or a breakdown of the neural structures.
- Deafferentation-type pain is thought to involve the sympathetic nervous system, as blockade of this system may often eliminate or reduce the complaints of the patient. Characteristic descriptors used with this type of pain seem most commonly to include the words "burning," "stinging," "itching," and "crawling." It is not always present immediately at the time of injury or trauma, and may be the result of a breakdown of the central inhibition.
- A significant amount of work has been done in the area of deafferentation syndromes since the time of the first edition of this book. The author suggests clinicians who choose to evaluate or treat complex pain involving the sympathetic nervous system familiarize themselves with this continually expanding and unique field within pain medicine.

ATYPICAL ODONTALGIA

- This condition has been proposed to describe a painful condition within the oral cavity.
- Additional terms synonymous with atypical odontalgia include phantom tooth pain, atypical facial neuralgia, and idiopathic toothache.
- Four common characteristics have been identified in association with this disturbance:

○ Duration longer than four months
○ Normal radiographic examination
○ No clinical observable cause
○ Description as a toothache or tooth site pain
- Dental procedures, testing, and diagnostic block of the somatic system are rarely conclusive. Confirmation is associated with positive sympathetic nerve block.

NEUROMAS AND NEURITIS

- Neuromas and neuritis involve constant regional or localized pain.
- Neuromas are often associated with trauma or direct section of nerve tissue. Stimulation of the region is consistent for diagnostic purposes; however, treatment can be elusive due to recurrence.
- Neuritis as a systemic inflammatory response is often associated with herpes zoster viral infection. Aggressive and early identification and treatment can often decrease or eliminate the constant sequelae of a zoster episode.

PSYCHOLOGICAL PAIN

- Psychological illness with reported pain complaints is common. It requires the inclusionary criteria present for any other disease and should not be assumed.
- Once identified, treatment plans should be developed and presented as clearly and succinctly as those of the other pain etiologies discussed.
- It is important to remember that many of the currently described pain disorders were, as recently as the 1990s, considered to be psychological illnesses. Therefore, care should be exercised when allowing this diagnosis to be made by exclusion.
- It is also important to remember that with extended time, multiple treatment failures, and constant pain, patients who present with depression, fear, and feelings of hopelessness and helplessness are actually showing signs of a "normal" human.

TREATMENT

- Over the past three decades, significant progress has been made in understanding the pathophysiology of painful conditions.
- Treatment of painful conditions of the orofacial region comprises identification of the specific illness and correction of the disorder present. For disorders for which no current curative understanding exists, a management strategy is employed with the focus being on improving quality of life and decreasing unnecessary treatment.

- Management of painful conditions attempts to join the most efficient medications and treatment with little or no negative experience, side effect, or misuse potential. This goal can be quite elusive and is the subject of another chapter in this book.

BIBLIOGRAPHY

American Pain Society Quality Assurance Standards for Relief of Acute Pain and Cancer Pain. *Proceedings of the 6th World Congress on Pain.* New York: Elsevier; 1991.

Bell WE. *Orofacial Pains: Classification, Diagnosis, Management.* 4th ed. Chicago: Year Book; 1989.

Chapman CR, Syrjala KL. Measurement of pain. In: Bonica JJ, ed. *The Management of Pain.* Vol 1. 2nd ed. Philadelphia: Lea & Febiger; 1990:580–594.

de Leeuw R, Klasser G. *Orofacial Pain Guidelines for Assessment, Diagnosis and Management.* 5th ed. Quintessence; 2013.

Long D. *Contemporary Diagnosis and Management of Pain.* 2nd ed. Newtown, PA: Handbooks in Health Care; 2001.

Merskey H, Bogduk N, eds. *Classification of Chronic Pain: Descriptions of Chronic Pain Syndrome and Definitions of Pain Terms.* Seattle: IASP Press, 1994:59–76.

Okeson JP, ed. *Orofacial Pain: Guidelines for Assessment, Classification, and Management.* Carol Stream, IL: Quintessence; 1996.

Pertes RA, Gross SG, eds. *Clinical Management of Temporomandibular Disorders and Orofacial Pain.* Carol Stream, IL: Quintessence; 1995.

Pertes RA, Heir GM. Temporomandibular disorders and orofacial pain. *Dent Clin North Am.* 1991;35:123–140.

Travell JG, Simon DG. *Myofascial Pain and Dysfunction: The Trigger Point Manual.* Baltimore: Williams & Wilkins; 1999.

36 CHRONIC PELVIC PAIN

Ricardo Plancarte, MD
Faride Chejne-Gomez, MD
Jorge Guajardo-Rosas, MD
Ignacio Reyes-Torres, MD

DEFINITION

Chronic pelvic pain is defined as nonmalignant continuous or recurrent pain in structures related to the pelvis, lasting at least six months, and often associated with negative cognitive, behavioral, sexual, and emotional consequences. If nonacute and central sensitization pain mechanisms are present, then the condition is considered chronic, regardless of the time frame. The multifactorial etiology of CPP contributes to the challenges of its medical and rehabilitative management and has been described as a medical "nightmare" for clinicians. Chronic pelvic pain is not a disease; rather, it is a condition associated with dysfunction in one or usually more of the following body systems: gynecologic, urologic, gastrointestinal, musculoskeletal, and neurologic. In addition to specific organs, the following supportive structures may contribute to CPP: abdominal and pelvic floor muscles (PFMs), ligaments, tendons, fascia, blood vessels, and peripheral and central nervous systems. Surgical procedures or any organic inflammatory process, such as endometriosis or irritable bowel syndrome (IBS), may result in scarring and adhesions, leading to pain in the affected viscera, pain in the PFMs, or both. PFMs affected by adhesions or inflammation caused by an organic (pathologic) process or surgery may spasm, become shortened, and have trigger points, all of which are believed to result in pain.

EPIDEMIOLOGY

Pelvic pain is a common disorder in women, especially in the reproductive age group, with an estimated prevalence of 3.8% in women aged 15–73, resulting in about 10% of all referrals to gynecologists. This prevalence rate parallels those rates reported for asthma, low back pain (LBP), and migraine headaches. Approximately 15%–20% of women aged 18–50 years have CPP of greater than 1 year's duration. In fact, the lifetime occurrence rate of CPP may be as high as 33%. Patients with CPP may exhibit pathology that fails to correlate with the pain, and one third to one half of cases may exist with no identifiable pathology. Signs and symptoms of CPP may be evident in at least 50% of patients with preexisting sexual or physical abuse. The psychological literature suggests that women with CPP report greater psychological distress. For instance, women with CPP have elevated rates of depression, anxiety, hostility, and somatic complaints. The direct health care costs owing to CPP are estimated to be $880 million per year. Both direct and indirect costs potentially amount to greater than $2 billion per year. The individual burden of CPP ranges from years of personal suffering to missed or lost work, marital or relationship disruption, and multiple medical and/or surgical interventions.

NEUROANATOMY OF THE PELVIC AREA

- The pelvic viscera receive neurons from the sympathetic (thoracolumbar) and parasympathetic (craniosacral) systems.

- Most of the input to the pelvic, digestive, and urogenital structures (descending and sigmoid colon, rectum, vaginal fundus, bladder, prostate, prostatic urethra, testes, seminal vesicles, uterus, and ovaries) comes through the superior hypogastric plexus (SHP) (Figure 36-1).

- In females, the corpus, cervix, and proximal fallopian tubes transmit pain through sympathetic fibers that arise from T10 to L1. These fibers include neurons that are part of the uterosacral ligaments and eventually coalesce into the SHP (presacral nerve). The presacral nerve does not receive fibers from the ovaries and lateral pelvic structures, which is why a presacral neurectomy is applicable only to midline pain.

- The lateral pelvis transmits pain via parasympathetic neurons (nervi erigentes) arising from S2 to S4. The presacral nerve divides into the hypogastric nerves that eventually form the inferior hypogastric plexus (IHP), and this plexus subdivides into vesical, middle rectal, and uterovaginal (Frankenhauser) plexuses. Frankenhauser plexus lies just lateral to the uterosacral ligaments and medial to the uterine arteries and receives pain sensations only from the corpus and vagina. Unlike presacral neurectomy, which can affect bladder and rectal function, transection of Frankenhauser plexus during a laparoscopic uterosacral nerve division should not result in constipation or bladder dysfunction.

- Thoracolumbar preganglionic nerves also synapse on postganglionic nerves in sympathetic chain ganglia that mingle with autonomic sacral parasympathetic projections as well as with the pelvic somatic neuronal pathways.

- The IHP is the major neuronal coordinating center that supplies visceral structures of the pelvis and the pelvic floor. It has a posterolateral retroperitoneal component adjacent to each lateral aspect of the rectum, with interconnections between the right and the left side, and an anterior component associated with the distal extent of the hypogastric plexus, which is referred to as the "hypogastric ganglia" in males and the "paracervical ganglia" in females.

- Efferents from the IHP spread out to innervate the prostate, seminal vesicles, vas deferens, epididymis, penis, and penile corpus cavernosum in the male and the corpora of the clitoris, vagina, and urethra in the female.

- Sensations arising from the pelvic floor are conveyed mainly via the pelvic splanchnic nerve (PSN) to the sacral afferents (S2–4) of the parasympathetic system. Sensations from the testis and epididymis, however, may involve predominantly thoracolumbar (T10–L1) afferents.

- The following pathways may be interrupted by nerve blockade:
  ○ Spermatic cord (afferents from the testis)

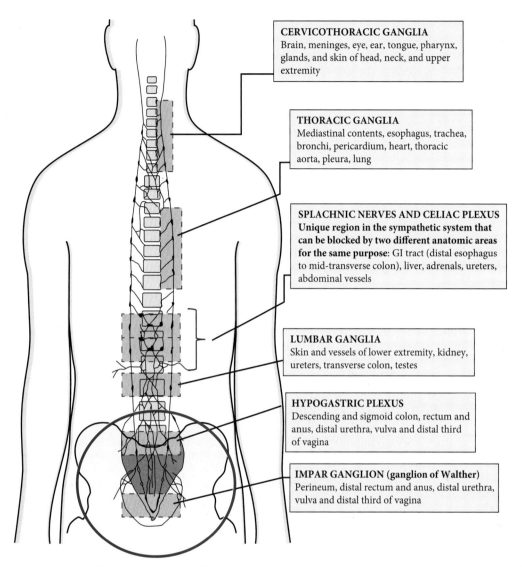

CERVICOTHORACIC GANGLIA
Brain, meninges, eye, ear, tongue, pharynx, glands, and skin of head, neck, and upper extremity

THORACIC GANGLIA
Mediastinal contents, esophagus, trachea, bronchi, pericardium, heart, thoracic aorta, pleura, lung

SPLACHNIC NERVES AND CELIAC PLEXUS
Unique region in the sympathetic system that can be blocked by two different anatomic areas for the same purpose: GI tract (distal esophagus to mid-transverse colon), liver, adrenals, ureters, abdominal vessels

LUMBAR GANGLIA
Skin and vessels of lower extremity, kidney, ureters, transverse colon, testes

HYPOGASTRIC PLEXUS
Descending and sigmoid colon, rectum and anus, distal urethra, vulva and distal third of vagina

IMPAR GANGLION (ganglion of Walther)
Perineum, distal rectum and anus, distal urethra, vulva and distal third of vagina

FIG. 36-1. Schematic outline of the sites for analgesic blockade of the sympathetic nervous system and related structures. The system is contiguous, and there is considerable overlap and variation of innervation. (Modified from Plancarte R, Amescua C, Patt RB. Sympathetic neurolytic blockade. In: Patt RF, ed. *Cancer Pain.* Philadelphia: JB Lippincott; 1993:377–425.)

- SHP
- Dorsal root ganglia
- Sympathetic ganglia (in particular, the ganglion of Walter)
- Peripheral nerves
- Pudendal nerve (PN; external anal sphincter, perineal cutaneous, and muscle branches, posterior part of the scrotum and penis [the anterior part is innervated by branches of the ilioinguinal and genitofemoral nerves that arise from L1–2 roots], clitoris, and labia majora)
- Genitofemoral nerve (cremasteric muscles, spermatic cord, and parietal and visceral structures of the tunica vaginalis)

PAIN MECHANISMS

Chronic pelvic pain mechanisms may involve:

- Ongoing acute pain mechanisms (such as those associated with inflammation or infection), which may involve somatic or visceral tissue
- Chronic pain mechanisms, which especially involve the CNS
- Emotional, cognitive, behavioral, and sexual responses and mechanism

When acute pain mechanisms are activated by a nociceptive event, as well as in the case of direct activation of the peripheral nociceptor transducers, sensitization of those transducers may also occur, thus magnifying the afferent signaling. Afferents that are not normally active may also become activated by the change, that is, there may be activation of the so-called silent afferents. Although these are mechanisms of acute pain, the increased afferent signaling is often a trigger for the chronic pain mechanisms that maintain the perception of pain in the absence of ongoing peripheral pathology.

There are a number of mechanisms by which the peripheral transducers may exhibit an increase in sensibility:

1. Modification of the peripheral tissue, which may result in the transducers being more exposed to peripheral stimulation.
2. There may be an increase in the chemicals that stimulates the receptors of the transducers.
3. There are many modifications in the receptors that result in them being more sensitive.

Central sensitization is responsible for a decrease in threshold and increase in response duration and magnitude of dorsal horn neurons. It is associated with an expansion of the receptive field. As a result, sensitization increases signaling to the CNS and amplifies what we perceive from a peripheral stimulus.

As an example, for cutaneous stimuli, light touch would not normally produce pain; however, when central sensitization is present, light touch may be perceived as painful (allodynia). In visceral hyperalgesia (so called because the afferents are primarily small fibers), visceral stimuli that are normally subthreshold and not usually perceived may be perceived. For instance, with central sensitization, stimuli that are normally subthreshold may result in a sensation of fullness and a need to void the bladder or to defecate. Stimuli normally perceived may be interpreted as pain and stimuli that are normally noxious may be magnified (true hyperalgesia) with an increased perception of pain. As a consequence, one can see that many of the symptoms of the bladder pain syndrome (BPS) (formerly known as interstitial cystitis [IC] and IBS) may be explained by central sensitization.

CAUSES OF PELVIC PAIN

NONMALIGNANT CAUSES

- Pelvic pain has many causes, some clear and some obscure. (Table 36-1 summarizes the causes of nonmalignant pelvic pain.)
- When the causes are obscure, the temptation to diagnose psychosomatic pain should be overcome, and screening should be conducted in an attempt to uncover organic causes.
- The history and physical examination must include an in-depth assessment of movement arches, sexual activity and performance, parturition, postural habits, and the minor changes that could help reveal the etiology of the pain.
- When a comprehensive evaluation excludes any underlying pathology or when the cause of pain is known but other treatments have failed, a trial of neural blockade may be undertaken to assess the pain's central sympathetic or somatic origin. The institution

TABLE 36-1   Systems Associated With Potential Sources of Pelvic Pain

GYNECOLOGIC	UROLOGIC	GASTROINTESTINAL	MUSCULOSKELETAL	NEUROLOGIC
Endometriosis	Interstitial cystitis	Irritable bowel syndrome	Pelvic floor dysfunction	Postherpetic neuralgia
Adenomyosis	Malignancy	Inflammatory bowel disease	Myofascial pain syndromes	Incisional neuroma
Pelvic congestion syndrome	Radiation cystitis	Chronic constipation	Adhesions	Visceral hyperalgesia
Adhesions	Acute recurrent cystitis	Colon malignancy	Fibromyalgia	Pudendal neuralgia
Ovarian remnant syndrome	Chronic urinary tract infection	Colitis	Muscular sprains (rectus muscle)	Entrapment neuropathy
Pelvic inflammatory disease	Urolithiasis	Hernia	Piriformis syndrome	
Malignancy	Uninhibited bladder contractions	Diverticular disease	Spondylosis	
Leiomyomata	Urethral syndrome	Diarrhea	Chronic coccygeal pain or back pain	
Symptomatic pelvic relaxation	Urethral caruncle			
Cervical stenosis	Urethral diverticulum			
Adnexal cyst				
Postoperative peritoneal cyst				
Tuberculous salpingitis				
Gärtner cyst				
Benign cystic mesothelioma				

of a differential spinal or epidural block and/or the sequential administration of more specific procedures aimed at the discrete and specific interruption of sympathetic versus somatic nerve impulses could be most helpful.

- CPP, especially urogenital pain, poses the greatest diagnostic challenge.
- CPP may be caused by:
  ○ Dysfunctional, high-pressure voiding
  ○ Intraprostatic ductal reflux
  ○ Microorganisms, such as gram-positive uropathogens (*Enterococcus* and *Staphylococcus aureus*) and gram-positive organisms (coagulase-negative *Staphylococcus*, *Chlamydia*, and *Ureaplasma*)
  ○ Cryptic, nonculturable organisms, such as biofilm bacteria, viruses, and cell wall–deficient bacteria
  ○ Autoimmune disorder
  ○ Chemical-urinary metabolites of pyrimidines and purines
  ○ Neuromuscular disorder
  ○ IC
- The diagnostic protocol consists of assessing symptoms and physical findings and conducting laboratory studies when the patient is not taking antibiotics, α blockers, nonsteroidal anti-inflammatory agents, narcotics, or analgesics.

NONMALIGNANT CAUSES SPECIFIC TO MALES

- CPP syndrome is a common urologic diagnosis in men younger than 50 years, accounts for 173 visits per urologist per year, and poses diagnostic and treatment dilemmas.
- In the United States, "chronic prostatitis," with a prevalence rate of 5%–8.8%, leads to an estimated 2 million office visits per year and causes a negative impact on quality of life similar to that in patients with unstable angina, recent myocardial infarct, or active Crohn disease.
- "Chronic prostatitis" is a misnomer; there is no proven prostate disease, and it is unlikely that the syndrome has association with the gland. The anatomic distribution of "chronic prostatitis" includes the prostate, bladder, penis, urethra, testis, epididymis, rectum, and pelvic floor.
- The medical histories of these patients tend to be remarkably similar and include a symptomatic genitourinary constellation of complaints, often coincident with a meaningful psychosocial event. In most cases, the disorder has been diagnosed as prostatitis and treated empirically with potent oral antibiotics despite a lack of microbiologic culture. A urinalysis

is generally normal. Because patients often respond dramatically to antibiotic treatment, most urologists prescribe such agents.

- Myofascial trigger points on the pelvic floor and/or abdominal wall are a common cause of "chronic prostatitis."
- Pelvic floor tension myalgia is characterized by continuous habitual contraction of the muscles of the pelvic floor (levator ani and short external rotators of the hip) and may be secondary to a local, painful inflammation. The pain is exacerbated by sitting in cars and is accompanied by suprapubic pressure, genital pain, and variable urinary symptoms. As the pain increases, the tension and contraction of the pelvic muscles also increase, creating a vicious cycle. The prostate is not usually tender, but movement of parapsoriatic fascia by palpation elicits pain.
- Treatment of trigger points and associated referred pain seeks to interrupt these reflexes with such interventions as:
  ○ Pelvic massage therapy, which involves rubbing the muscle fibers along their lengths from origin to insertion with a stripping motion. The urologist should apply as much pressure as the patient can tolerate with moderate pain. The prostate gland and surrounding endopelvic fascia should remain the primary focus of therapy.
  ○ Ischemic compression, in which specific trigger points are pressed continuously for 60–90 s.
  ○ Stretching, anesthetic injections, electrical neuromodulation, and mind–body interactions, such as progressive relaxation exercises and anorectal biofeedback.
- Well-trained physiotherapists who understand myofascial trigger points and soft tissue mobilization are needed for this labor-intensive therapy.
- It is not unusual for a patient to require several months of weekly therapy.

NONMALIGNANT CAUSES SPECIFIC TO FEMALES

- Non-oncologic CPP accounts for 10%–19% of hysterectomies (a controversial procedure for this indication) and 40% of laparoscopies.
- Pain may arise from the uterus, cervix, or ovaries and be caused by a variety of conditions, including pelvic adhesions, endometriosis, and pelvic congestion. Many of these conditions can be distinguished from levator ani syndrome and coccygodynia by history, physical examination, and, occasionally, laparoscopy. The annual prevalence of chronic pelvic pain in the primary care setting among women aged 15–73 (38/1000)

is comparable to the prevalence of asthma (37/1000) and of back pain (41/1000).

- In the premenstrual period, adnexal tenderness is often reported during a bimanual examination, and the uterus is often retroverted, boggy, and symmetrically enlarged. The patient's level of psychological distress is often high. Dysmenorrhea is a frequent complaint. Uterine pain is felt most characteristically in the hypogastrium and suprapubic regions.
- Endometriosis, when symptomatic, is often only associated with dysmenorrhea, but chronic pain may develop and become severe and constant. The identification of nonpigmented endometriosis in 1986 has increased laparoscopic recognition of this disorder. The severity of pain correlates poorly with the extent of observed disease. Hysterectomy and bilateral salpingo-oophorectomy may relieve pain in more than 90% of cases; preservation of one or both ovaries results in a small but significant recurrence rate.
- Pelvic congestion (overfilling of the pelvic venous system) may be a cause of unexplained, chronic, dull, aching pain secondary to venous stasis or ovarian varices and may be relieved by hormonal treatment. Typically, this pain increases at the end of the day, after prolonged standing, in the premenstrual period, or after nonorgasmic coitus and often is unilateral.
- Dense and vascularized pelvic adhesions may cause CPP, which may be relieved by adhesiolysis.
- Myofascial trigger points with attendant sustained muscular tension and/or painful spasms may be related to stress and autonomic hyperactivity, prolonged sitting, and/or trauma from parturition, sexual activity, or surgery.
- Women with significant central dysmenorrhea may be candidates for laparoscopic uterosacral nerve ablation (UNA). UNA should be performed only if the uterosacral ligaments are clearly visualized. It can be achieved using laser or bipolar electrodesiccation and transection/resection with scissors.
- Women with central dysmenorrhea, especially those who have failed LUNA, may benefit from laparoscopic presacral neurectomy (LPSN). Complete familiarization with retroperitoneal anatomy is essential for any surgeon performing LPSN. The superior portion of the presacral nerve runs from the bifurcation of the aorta to the junction of L5–S1 vertebral bodies. The boundaries for LPSN are superiorly, the bifurcation of the aorta; on the right, the right internal iliac artery and right ureter; on the left, the inferior mesenteric and superior hemorrhoidal arteries; inferiorly, just below the division of the right and left IHP; and deep, the periosteum of the vertebral bodies.

ANORECTAL PAIN

- Anorectal pain occurs in association with a variety of organic conditions, but the most common functional disorders are levator ani syndrome and proctalgia fugax.

Levator Ani Syndrome

- This syndrome, also known as puborectalis syndrome, chronic proctalgia, and pelvic tension myalgia, is characterized by a dull, aching, or pressurelike discomfort in the rectum that lasts several hours. Prolonged sitting and defecation precipitate the pain, and some patients experience difficult defecation or a sense of incomplete evacuation. An important clinical finding is palpable tenderness of overly contracted levator ani muscles as the examining finger moves from the coccyx posteriorly to the pubis anteriorly. Often the tenderness is asymmetric and occurs on the left side more frequently than on the right.
- The diagnostic criteria are chronic or recurrent episodes of rectal pain or aching that last 20 min or longer and have occurred for at least three months in the absence of other causes such as ischemia, inflammatory bowel disease, cryptitis, intersphincteric abscess, anal fissure, hemorrhoids, or coccygodynia.
- The role of anorectal manometry in the evaluation of such patients is not established, but increased anal channel pressures and increased electromyographic activities are often present.
- Treatment includes digital massage to tolerance three or four times per week, the use of muscle relaxants, such as diazepam and methocarbamol, and sitz baths.

Proctalgia Fugax

- Proctalgia fugax is characterized by sudden, severe, aching, gnawing, cramping, or stabbing rectal pain lasting several seconds or minutes before disappearing completely, leaving the patient asymptomatic until the next episode.
- Women are more likely than men to experience proctalgia fugax; however, no relationship exists between proctalgia fugax and IBS.
- The diagnosis depends on the absence of anorectal disease that could produce rectal pain. Although the pain occasionally may last 30 min, only 10% of patients report pain lasting longer than 5 min; occasionally, pain may awaken the patient from sleep. Reports of associated anal sphincter spasm or contractions of the puborectalis and external anal sphincter muscles have not been substantiated.
- Proctalgia fugax has been treated with clonidine, inhaled salbutamol, nitrates, diltiazem, and caudal epidural blocks.

PELVIC JOINT DYSFUNCTIONS

- A variety of dysfunctions exist within the pelvic joints, including the symphysis pubis joint. Often, symphysis pubis dysfunctions are accompanied by dysfunctions within the sacroiliac (SI) joints. These combined dysfunctions usually manifest as a rotation (anterior or posterior) or a shear (superior or inferior) of the entire bony hemipelvis (innominate).

Dysfunctional Symphysis Pubis

- With dysfunctional symphysis pubis, pain may be referred to the testicle or the vagina, or down the medial thigh toward the knee on the affected side. If the symphysis alone is dysfunctional, testicle pain occurs after heavy lifting. When the SI joints are involved, LBP occurs with somatic characteristics.
- The diagnosis is made primarily by history and physical examination but may be confirmed with plain radiographs using special stress views and with bone scans. A pelvic MRI may detect an edema within the symphysis pubis.
- Patients presenting with pelvic joint dysfunctions do not fit the standard medical paradigms for LBP or groin pain and, thus, present a diagnostic dilemma to physicians not trained in manual medicine techniques. Misdiagnosis is common. The pain does not follow a radicular pattern, and radiculopathy can be excluded with a thorough neurologic evaluation. Further complicating the presentation, secondary trigger points within the gluteus medius, piriformis, and other pelvic muscles may exist as a consequence of the joint imbalances. These trigger points refer symptoms down the leg in the nonradicular patterns of classic myofascial pain.
- Treatment: try to relocate the bone into place with external manipulation. If unsuccessful, surgery is indicated.

Sacroiliac Syndrome

- SI joint pain may result from spondyloarthropathy, pyogenic or crystal arthropathy, fracture of the sacrum and pelvis, or diastasis.
- The phenomenon of pain emanating from the SI joint in the absence of a demonstrable lesion is termed "SI syndrome" or "SI joint dysfunction" and is presumed to be a mechanical disorder.
- While definitive epidemiologic studies are lacking, SI syndrome appears to occur predominantly in women.
- Diagnostic criteria for SI syndrome include (1) pain in the region of the SI joint with possible radiation to the groin, medial buttocks, and posterior thigh; (2) reproduction of pain by physical examination techniques that stress the joint; (3) elimination of pain with intra-articular injection of local anesthetic; and (4) an ostensibly morphologically normal joint without demonstrable pathognomonic radiographic abnormalities.
- Treatment has included mild oral analgesics and anti-inflammatory agents, diagnostic/therapeutic SI joint injections with an anesthetic and corticosteroid in conjunction with or after a course of physical therapy, muscle balancing and pelvic stabilization exercises, and orthoses.

ISCHIAL SPINE AND PUDENDAL NERVE ENTRAPMENT

- Pudendal nerve entrapment (PNE) causes neuropathic pain.
- In men with PNE, aberrant development and subsequent malpositioning of the ischial spine appear to be associated with athletic activities during their youth. The changes occur during the period of development and ossification of the spinous process of the ischium.
- PNE can cause chronic perineal pain. Patients with PNE typically present with pain in the penis, scrotum, labia, perineum, or anorectal region that is exacerbated by sitting, relieved by standing, and absent when recumbent or when sitting on a toilet seat.
- In PNE, the PN is trapped between the sacrotuberous (ST) and sacrospinous (SSp) ligaments and may engage the falciform process of the ST ligament.
- Stretching of the PN from chronic constipation causes neuropathy.
- Normal vaginal delivery causes measurable neuropathy that lasts approximately three months.
- The striking common feature in all patients is that flexion activities of the hip (sitting, climbing, squatting, cycling, and exercising) induce or exacerbate urogenital pain, CPP, or prostatitis-like pain.
- Attention must be paid to (1) the transverse diameter of the ST and SP ligaments that compress the PN; (2) the dimensions of the greater sciatic notch (diameter and depth) correlated with age, weight, and body habitus; (3) the cross-sectional area of the greater sciatic notch and the piriformis muscle; and (4) sequential pelvic x-rays in youthful and maturing athletes to measure changes in position and appearance of the ischial spine.
- The primary hypothesis about the etiology is that hypertrophy of the muscles of the pelvic floor during years of youthful athleticism causes elongation and posterior remodeling of the ischial spine. The SSp ligament then rotates, causing the ST and SSp ligaments to overlap. The ligaments act like a lobster claw,

crushing the PN as it traverses the interligamentous space. In addition, in this position the PN travels a longer course because it is posterior or dorsal to the SSp ligament. In this course it may stretch over the SSp ligament or the ischial spine during squatting, sitting, or rising from a seated position. We surmise that the gluteus muscle, which is intimately attached to the ST ligament, exerts a shearing effect as it extends the hip while the pelvic floor is forced inferiorly during the Valsalva maneuver.

- Pudendal canal decompression leads to pain relief in 70%–86% of patients and to improved associated urinary and fecal incontinence in 65%–82%.

DIFFERENTIAL DIAGNOSES

- Gynecologic disease, including endometriosis, adhesions (chronic pelvic inflammatory disease), leiomyoma, pelvic congestion syndrome, and adenomyosis
- Gastrointestinal disease, including constipation, IBS, diverticulitis, diverticulosis, chronic appendicitis, and Meckel diverticulum
- Genitourinary disease, including IC, abnormal bladder function (bladder dyssynergia), and chronic urethritis
- Myofascial disease, including fasciitis, nerve entrapment syndrome, and hernias (inguinal, femoral, spigelian, umbilical, and incisional)
- Skeletal disease, including scoliosis, L1 through L2 disc disorders, spondylolisthesis, and osteitis pubis
- Psychological disorders, including somatization, psychosexual dysfunction, and depression

MALIGNANT CAUSES

- Pain is not usually an early sign of pelvic neoplasm but is associated with advanced pelvic cancer in about 75% of cases.
- Pelvic pain from malignant causes is usually visceral and occurs when an expanding tumor invades adjacent neural structures, giving rise to a neuropathic component or to somatic pain when the pelvic wall is involved. Visceral or neuropathic pain is commonly referred to the rectum, may be experienced in the lower back, hypogastrium, and perineum, and can be especially troublesome when associated with destruction of the sacrum.
- Visceral pain is the result of smooth muscle spasms of the hollow viscus, distortion of the capsule of solid organs, inflammation, traction or twisting of the mesentery, ischemia, or necrosis.
- Neuropathic pain is encountered in 60% of patients with malignant disease of soft tissues invading the nerve trunk and with sacral invasion from carcinoma of the cervix, uterus, vagina, colon, and rectum in women and from penile, prostate, and colorectal carcinoma and sarcoma in men. The infiltration of the perineal nerves results in lumbosacral plexopathies producing symptoms of sensory loss, causalgia, and deafferentation. Lumbosacral plexopathy frequently accompanies genitourinary tumors in the pelvis and occasionally develops after radiation to the area. Pain is likely to be neuropathic and is felt in the buttocks, radiating down the leg in the dermatomal distribution of the lumbar nerve roots and, perhaps, extending into the feet.

- Tumor involvement in the epidural space may resemble this pain syndrome but is more likely to be bilateral. Pain may be the initial symptom, but as the disease progresses, sensory and motor deficits may develop.
- Coccygeal plexopathy caused by tumors low in the pelvis may also mimic lumbosacral plexopathy but is more likely to be accompanied by sphincter dysfunction and perineal sensory loss.
- Somatic pain in these patients is due to stimulation of nociceptors in the integument and supporting structures (striated muscles, joints, periosteum, bones, and nerve trunks) by direct extension through fascial planes and lymphatic supplies.
- Primary treatment involves surgery, chemotherapy, and/or radiation therapy to debulk the tumor. When further antitumor therapy is not feasible, pharmacotherapy with nonsteroidal anti-inflammatory drugs (NSAIDs), opioids, and adjuvant analgesics is instituted. Invasive approaches are considered if dose-limiting side effects cannot be reversed. Early neurolytic blockade can be appropriate in the context of poor compliance with oral medication for economical or cognitive reasons. Also, infiltrating the plexus before it is rendered inaccessible by invasion of the tumor and/or the surrounding ganglions may increase the success rate.

INTERVENTIONAL TECHNIQUES

GENERAL GUIDELINES

- Lytic or local anesthetic blocks of the autonomic system need to be assessed clinically and with appropriate tests to allow proper evaluation and follow-up.
- Whether done with lytic or local anesthetic solutions, these blocks should be thoroughly explained to the patient and carried on with total consent.
- Routine coagulation tests should be conducted and inquiries made about any previous transfusion or hemorrhagic problems.

- Use of lactate Ringer's preblock infusion is mandatory to prevent hypotension.
- The help of an assistant for regular vital sign checking and proper sedation is necessary.
- Radiologic guidance (fluoroscopy or CT scan) should be used to avoid major neurologic complications.
- One must proceed gently, controlling each step with an aspiration test in each quadrant, and/or test doses, and/or dye injection before injecting a lytic solution.
- Injecting variable quantities (12–20 mL) of air may facilitate the double-contrast image visualization of the space available for the lytic or local anesthetic solution to spread, without diluting it.
- During injection, all of the patient's complaints must be respected and assessed.
- Patients should be carefully observed for 24 h postprocedure, with an emphasis on neurologic examinations.
- A proper neurosurgical environment must be available in case of a progressive neurologic complication.

NONSURGICAL INTERVENTIONS

Neurolysis

Neurolysis refers to the intentional injury of a nerve or nerves with the intent of reducing pain. Pain physicians may offer nonsurgical neurolytic treatments with chemicals (alcohol or phenol), cryoablation, or thermocoagulation. Many practitioners reserve these treatments for cancer-related pain because of the associated risks such as excessive neurologic injury, damage to nonnervous tissue, and spotty relief owing to tumor or scar tissue. For example, SHP ablation has demonstrated a 69% success rate for six months in cancer patients with intractable pelvic pain. In patients with nonmalignant pain, sequential SHP blockade with local anesthetics may attenuate central sensitization and sympathetically maintained pain, resulting in prolonged relief. Unlike alcohol, phenol exhibits local anesthetic properties that render the injection painless.

Superior Hypogastric Plexus Block

- The SHP, or presacral plexus, lies immediately anterior to the sacral promontory at the level of the L5–S1 interspace, in proximity to the bifurcation of the common iliac vessels. The SHP carries nerve fibers from the pelvic viscera (see above). It is retroperitoneal and bilateral, and contains parasympathetic nerve fibers (S2–4).
- Injection of the SHP requires radiologic guidance, with fluoroscopy or, more efficiently, CT scanning.
- The SHP block is efficacious and safe in patients with advanced cancer. Poor results should be expected in patients with extensive retroperitoneal disease overlying the plexus because of inadequate spread of the neurolytic agent.
- SHP block can serve as a less invasive diagnostic, prognostic, and therapeutic tool than such techniques as presacral neurectomy for painful pelvic conditions of nononcologic origin (ie, dysmenorrhea).
- SHP block can be used as a diagnostic tool for referred LBP (viscerosomatic convergence) from the abdomen or pelvis. One of the differential diagnoses of LBP is pain of visceral origin in the pelvis, which is sensed by the patient as LBP. In women who present with CPP and LBP, when the pelvic pain resolves with SHP block, we have observed that the LBP does also, indicating that the LBP was a secondary phenomenon referred from the pelvis and did not require primary treatment.
- When the SHP blockade is used for diagnostic/prognostic purposes, we inject 6–8 mL of 0.25% bupivacaine through each needle.
- For therapeutic (neurolytic) blocks, we use a total of 6–8 mL of 10% aqueous phenol through each needle. During manufacture, a small amount of glycerin is added to keep the phenol in solution.
- Hysterectomy is one of the most common gynecologic procedures performed to relieve CPP, but the result is not always positive. It is possible that an SHP block may predict the success of hysterectomy for CPP and, if so, prevent unnecessary hysterectomy. In a prospective clinical trial of 15 women scheduled for hysterectomy who received an SHP block, 11 had 100% relief with the SHP blockade and complete relief after hysterectomy, 2 experienced 90% pain relief with both procedures, 1 patient had 70% improvement and refused surgery, and 1 patient did not improve after SHP blockade and did not have surgery.

Technique

- The SHP can be accessed via a posterior paravertebral, transdiscal, transvascular, or transvaginal approach. We have performed more than 800 SHP blocks using the posterior paravertebral approach, with no complications and minimal side effects.
- An SHP block may be preceded by a single-shot, L4–5 epidural injection of 5–10 mL 1% lidocaine to enhance patient cooperation by reducing reflex muscle spasm, ameliorating the discomfort associated with contact of needles with periosteum, and reducing movement. Alternatively, these goals can be achieved with local infiltration of the intervening muscle planes.
- The patient assumes the prone position with padding placed beneath the pelvis to flatten the lumbar lordosis.

- The lumbosacral region is cleansed aseptically.
- The location of the L4–5 interspace is approximated by palpation of the iliac crests and spinous processes, and then is verified by fluoroscopy.
- Skin wheals are raised 5–7 cm bilateral to the midline at the level of the L4–5 interspace.
- A 7-in, 22-gauge, short-beveled needle with a depth marker placed 5–7 cm along the shaft is inserted through one of the skin wheals, with the needle bevel directed toward the midline.
- From a position perpendicular in all planes to the skin, the needle is oriented about 30° caudad and 45° medial so that its tip is directed toward the anterolateral aspect of the bottom of the L5 vertebral body.
- The iliac crest and the transverse process of L5, which sometimes is enlarged, are potential barriers to needle passage and necessitate the use of the cephalolateral entrance site and oblique trajectory described.
- If the transverse process of L5 is encountered during advancement of the needle, the needle is withdrawn to the subcutaneous tissue and redirected slightly caudad or cephalad. The needle is again advanced until the body of the L5 vertebra is encountered or until its tip is observed fluoroscopically to lie at its anterolateral aspect.
- If the vertebral body is encountered, gentle effort may be made to advance the needle further. If this is unsuccessful, the needle is withdrawn and, without altering its cephalocaudal orientation, is redirected in a slightly less mesiad plane so that its tip is "walked off" the vertebral body. The needle tip is advanced approximately 1 cm past the depth at which contact with the vertebral body occurred, at which point a loss of resistance or "pop" may be felt, indicating that the needle tip has traversed the anterior fascial boundary of the ipsilateral psoas muscle and lies in the retroperitoneal space. At this point the depth marker should, depending on the patient's body habitus, lie close to the level of the skin.
- The contralateral needle is inserted in a similar manner, using the trajectory and the depth of the first needle as a rough guide.
- Biplanar fluoroscopy is used during needle passage to verify needle placement. Anteroposterior views should demonstrate the needle tip's locations at the level of the junction of the L5 and S1 vertebral bodies, and lateral views should confirm placement of the needle tip just beyond the vertebral body's anterolateral margin.
- Injection of 3–4 mL of water-soluble contrast medium through each needle is recommended to further verify accuracy of placement.
- In the anteroposterior view, the spread of the contrast medium should be confined to the paramedian region. In the lateral view, a smooth posterior contour corresponding to the anterior psoas fascia indicates that needle depth is appropriate.
- Alternatively, computerized axial tomography may be used, permitting visualization of the vascular structures.
- Additional precautions include careful aspiration before injection and the use of "test" doses of local anesthetic. Vascular puncture with a risk of subsequent hemorrhage and hematoma formation is possible due to the close proximity of the bifurcation of the common iliac vessels. Intramuscular or intraperitoneal injection may result from an improper estimate of needle depth. These and less likely complications (subarachnoid and epidural injection, somatic nerve injury, renal or ureteral puncture) usually can be avoided by careful observation of technique (Table 36-2).

Ganglion Impar Blockade (Ganglion of Walther)

- The ganglion impar is a solitary retroperitoneal structure located at the level of the sacrococcygeal junction that marks the termination of the paired paravertebral sympathetic chains.
- Ganglion impar denervation has been performed in cancer patients with persistent perineal or rectal pain, but randomized controlled trials to support this therapy have not yet been performed. Pain physicians treating CPP due to cancer should consider pretreatment with local anesthetics prior to injection of alcohol for neurolysis owing to significant pain on injection and burning or shooting sensations after injection.
- Although the anatomic interconnections of the ganglion impar are poorly understood, its sympathetic component likely predominates.
- Blocking the ganglion impar (ganglion of Walther) can relieve intractable neoplastic perineal pain of sympathetic origin.
- The first report of interruption of the ganglion impar for relief of cancer perineal pain appeared in 1990. All 16 patients (13 women, 3 men, ranging in age from 24 to 87 years, median 48 years) had advanced cancer (9 cervix, 2 colon, 2 bladder, 2 rectum, 2 endometrium), and pain had persisted in all cases despite surgery and/or chemotherapy and radiation, analgesics, and psychological support. Each patient had localized perineal pain characterized as burning and urgent (in eight) or of a mixed character (in eight). Pain was referred to the rectum (seven), perineum (six), or vagina (three). After preliminary local anesthetic blockade and subsequent neurolytic block, eight patients experienced complete (100%) relief of pain, and the remainder experienced significant reductions in pain (90% for one, 80% for two, 70% for one, and 60% for four) as determined with a visual analog

TABLE 36-2 Efficacy of Hypogastric Plexus Block

AUTHOR	YEAR	TYPE OF STUDY	FOLLOW	PATIENTS	EFFICIENCY	COMPLICATION	RECOMMENDATION
Plancarte and colleagues	1990	Series of cases	Until the death	28	Pain reduction in basal 70%	(-)	1C
Ina and colleagues	1992	Series of cases	Unspecified	8	Total pain relief	(-)	1C
De León and colleagues	1992	Series of cases	1 year	26	Baseline pain relief in 67%, while monitoring a 67% reduction of oral morphine consumption	(-)	1C
Amaral and colleagues	1993	Series of cases	Unspecified	5	Total pain relief	(-)	1C
Plancarte and colleagues	1995	Series of cases	3 weeks	14	Baseline pain relief in 70% and reduced opioid consumption by 50%	(-)	1C
Wechsler and colleagues	1995	Comparative clinical trial		5	The bilateral posterior technique showed better pain relief compared with the unilateral approach and the anterior approach	Intraperitoneal injection of local anesthetic	1B
Chan and colleagues	1997	Case report	2 weeks	1	Baseline pain relief in 80%	Right leg hypoesthesia	1C
Plancarte and colleagues	1997	Series of cases	6 months	227	Pain relief in 72% and reduction in opioid consumption by 40%	No long-term complications	1C
Ghassan and colleagues	1997	Series of cases	Unspecified	3	Total pain relief	(-)	1C
Rosenberg and colleagues	1998	Case report	8 months	1	Visceral pain relief in 90%	(-)	1C
Ghassan and colleagues	1999	Series of cases	2 weeks	3	Total pain relief	(-)	1C
Agüero and colleagues	1999	Series of cases	6 months	16	Baseline pain relief in 87% and decreased opioid consumption by 88.9%	(-)	1C
Stevens and colleagues	2000	Case report	Unspecified	1	Total pain relief	(-)	1C
Cariati and colleagues	2002	Series of cases	160 days	10	Baseline pain relief in 70% and decreased drug consumption by 90%	(-)	1C
Erdine and colleagues	2003	Series of cases	3 months	20	Baseline pain relief in 75%, decrease in opioid consumption by 75%	(-)	1C
De Oliveira and colleagues	2005	Randomized clinical trial	8 weeks	60	Total pain relief, improved quality of life, decreased nausea and vomiting, and reduced analgesic consumption after a week in the early intervention group, compared with the group that made this management later		1B
Turker and colleagues	2005	Series of cases	12 months	3	Baseline pain relief in 80% till death; one patient required a second procedure after 12 months	(-)	1C
Kitoh and colleagues	2005	Series of cases	3 months	35	Baseline pain relief in 90%, combining celiac plexus block + superior mesenteric plexus and superior hypogastric	Diarrhea, hypotension	1C
Michalek and colleagues	2005	Series of cases	3 days and 7 months	2	Baseline pain relief in 85%	(-)	1C
Gamal and colleagues	2006	Randomized clinical trial	3 months	30	There were no differences in pain relief between the groups transdiscal approach and classic approach to pain relief in 70%	Vascular puncture, puncture of the urinary system, longer duration of the procedure in the classical approach group	1B
Mishra and colleagues	2008	Series of cases	2 months	2	Baseline pain relief in 80%	(-)	1C
Dooley and colleagues		Case report	Unspecified	1	Baseline pain relief in 80%	(-)	1C
Possover and colleagues	2009	Series of cases	21 months	4	Total pain relief and recovery urinary function after placement of a neurostimulation electrode in the superior hypogastric plexus	(-)	1C
Nabil and colleagues	2009	Series of cases	8 weeks	22	Baseline pain relief in 50%	Pain at the puncture site 81% and diarrhea 13%	1C
Pollitt and colleagues	2011	Case report	24 months	1	Total pain relief with the administration of phenol, in a patient who failed blocking technique with local anesthetic and pulsed radio frequency	(-)	1C
Bhatnagar and colleagues	2011	Series of cases	2 months	18	Basal pain relief in 80%	(-)	1C

scale. Repeated blocks in two patients led to further improvement. Follow-up depended on survival and was carried out for 14–120 days.

- In patients with incomplete relief of pain, residual somatic symptoms may be treated with either epidural injections of steroid or sacral nerve blocks.

Technique

- The stylet is removed from a standard 22-gauge, 3.5-in spinal needle, which is then manually bent about 1 in from its hub to form a 25°–30° angle. This maneuver facilitates positioning of the needle tip anterior to the concavity of the sacrum and coccyx.
- The needle is inserted through the skin wheal with its concavity oriented posteriorly, and, under fluoroscopic guidance, is directed anterior to the coccyx, closely approximating the anterior surface of the bone, until its tip is observed to have reached the sacrococcygeal junction.
- Retroperitoneal location of the needle is verified by observation of the spread of 2 mL of water-soluble contrast medium, which typically assumes a smooth margined configuration resembling an apostrophe.
- Four milliliters of 1% lidocaine or 0.25% bupivacaine is injected for diagnostic and prognostic purposes, or, alternatively, 4–6 mL 10% phenol is injected for therapeutic neurolytic blockade.

Perimedullar Block and Intraspinal Opioid Therapy

- Subarachnoid phenol saddle block is appropriate treatment for intractable perineal pain in the presence of urinary diversion and colostomy. It is performed with a spinal needle at the L5–S1 level with the patient seated and inclined backward.
- When the above conditions are not met, the subarachnoid route for neurolysis may be preferred because the spread of the lytic substance in this case is more predictable.
- Because motor paresis can be a complication, perimedullary (spinal or epidural) opioid therapy, with or without dilute concentrations of local anesthetic, is a preferable option. Chronic spinal infusion could be carried out through a variety of drug delivery systems ranging from a temporary, percutaneous, tunnelized, epidural catheter to a totally implanted system. Nevertheless, the limited availability and high cost of these implantable devices, as well as development of tolerance, are potential limiting factors.

Peripheral Nerve Block

- Blockade of paravertebral nerves may be considered when pain is referred from the bony pelvis.

- Peripheral neurolysis for the management of cancer pain is well described but seldom used, as most of the pain emanating from the pelvic structures is of sympathetic origin.

Pudendal Nerve Block

- The PN lies close to the internal pudendal artery and posterior to the SSp ligament.
- Successful block of the PN bilaterally provides analgesia to the lower third of the vagina and to the posterior two thirds of the vulva.
- A PN block can be performed:
  - Transvaginally, by puncturing the wall of the vagina at the juncture of the ischial spine and the SSp ligament to avoid unintentional needle placement into the rectum, bladder, bowel, or uterine artery.
  - Transgluteally, where the nerve is blocked medially to the ischiatic spine slightly below the ischiosacral ligament through a skin wheal and a 3.5-in, 22-gauge needle.
  - Through the buttock, puncturing the PN proximally before its passage through Alcock's canal at the intersection of a vertical line descending from the posterosuperior ischiatic spine and a transversal one (horizontal) crossing the sacrococcygeal joint. A neurostimulator attached to a shielded needle permits precise localization of the PN by reproducing dysesthesia in its distribution area.
- PN block with electromyographic studies of the pelvic floor can help differentiate neuralgia caused by nerve entrapment from other causes of perineal pain.

Neuromodulation (Sacral Nerve Stimulation)

Sacral stimulation has been used to successfully treat voiding dysfunction for several years. For instance, some patients suffering from IC have benefited from electrical modulation of the sacral nerves and report improvement in pain and urinary urgency. Recently, pain physicians have applied the technique for the treatment of CPP. The transforaminal approach consists of a trial stimulation in which an electrode is placed percutaneously into the S3 or S4 foramen in the area of the nerve roots. If the trial is successful, the patient is taken to the operating room, where the permanent lead is placed and tunneled subcutaneously to an implanted pulse generator. In an observational study of 10 patients undergoing sacral nerve stimulation for intractable pelvic pain, 9 reported a decrease in pain severity for at least 19 months. In another study, 11 patients were followed for 36 months after undergoing sacral stimulator placement; 9 experienced extended and significant reduction in their pelvic pain, and 2 failed the therapy soon after implantation. This failure was likely due to a false-positive result during the trial. These preliminary studies suggest that sacral stimulation may be helpful in reducing pelvic pain among properly chosen patients who undergo a successful stimulator trial.

Technique

Psychiatric comorbidities, substance misuse/abuse, and issues of secondary gain should be assessed prior to implementation. This examination is usually performed by a licensed psychologist. Test stimulation with a temporary lead is performed under fluoroscopic guidance. The lead is placed through the sacral hiatus and advanced in an anterograde fashion toward the sacral foramen or inserted through the low lumbar vertebrae and advanced retrograde toward the sacral foramen. The lead is then positioned with contacts placed inside the S3 or S4 foramen, and test stimulation is performed to ensure coverage over the intended pelvic region. A dressing is placed over the insertion site to anchor the lead as well as to prevent infection. A trial of stimulation is then performed on an outpatient basis for three to five days. If the patient reports a significant reduction in pain during the trial (typically considered at least a 50% reduction), a permanent stimulator implantation is offered. The implantation is performed in an operating room. During the surgery, the percutaneous leads are anchored to underlying fascia, tunneled underneath the skin, and attached to the pulse generator (battery), which is placed in a subcutaneous pocket. Several locations are suitable for placement of the pulse generator including the upper buttock or inferior to the last rib anteriorly.

Neuromodulation (SCS)

SCS has been used for the treatment of lumbosacral radicular pain after spine surgery, intractable cardiac ischemia, peripheral vascular disease, occipital neuralgia, and complex regional pain syndrome. There is emerging evidence that a midline dorsal column pathway exists that may mediate the perception of visceral pelvic pain; therefore, dorsal column stimulation may serve an effective means of treating CPP. For instance, Kapural and colleagues reported that six female patients with severe CPP undergoing dual-lead implantation with the lead tip between the levels of T11–12 described significant improvement in pain scores and activities of daily living during an average follow-up of 2.6 years. Although the study was retrospective and small, it provided a framework for other researchers to clarify the efficacy of SCS in visceral pelvic pain with randomized controlled trials.

CONCLUSION

- Chronic pelvic pain is a common complaint that is well defined and involves multiple mechanisms. Some of the conditions have clear management pathways but many do not. In these CPP syndromes, a holistic multidisciplinary team approach is required with active patient involvement.
- In the yet obscure world of pelvic pain, interventional techniques are helpful when properly designed in a comprehensive evaluation of the patient's psychological, physiologic, and sexual status.
- In the setting of nononcologic pain, these procedures have diagnostic, prognostic, and therapeutic value.
- Because the pelvis is complex neuroanatomically and neurophysiologically, pelvic pain may exhibit mixed characteristics of somatic, autonomic, visceral, and neuropathic origin. Underlying pathogenic pain mechanisms in CPP require a variety of treatment strategies including medications, physical restoration, behavioral medicine techniques, surgery, neuromodulation, and SHP and ganglion impar blocks/neurolysis. A thorough systematic evaluation with proper screening for coexisting diseases is critical to formulating a rational treatment plan. Furthermore, a multidisciplinary approach to patients with CPP aids in coordinating the assessments of primary care physicians and specialists in pain medicine, urology, gynecology, gastroenterology, physiotherapy, and psychology.
- The use of sympathetic blocks (either the hypogastric or the ganglion impar) seems promising in the setting of chronic pelvic pain, including pain caused by nonbacterial prostatitis and vulvar or clitoral pain.
- In the world of cancer pain, sympathetic blocks may also be used for diagnostic purposes and for predicting the efficacy of neurolytic techniques.

Bibliography

Amaranath I, Wexner SD. Caudal epidural block in the management of proctalgia fugax. *Am J Pain Manage.* 1994;4:153.

Anderson RU. Management of chronic prostatitis—chronic pelvic pain syndrome. *Urol Clin North Am.* 2002;29:235.

Baranowski AP, Johnson NS. A review of urogenital pain. *Pain Rev.* 1999;6:53.

Bensignor MF, Labbat LJ, Robert R, Ducrot P. Diagnostic and therapeutic pudendal nerve block for patients with perineal non-malignant pain. In: *8th World Congress on Pain.* Paris: IASP; 1996:56.

Bergeron S, Khalifé S, Glazer HI, et al. Surgical and behavioral treatments for vestibulodynia: two-and-one-half year follow-up and predictors of outcome. *Obstet Gynecol.* 2008;111: 159–166.

Bonica JJ. Cancer pain. In: Bonica JJ, ed. *Management of Pain.* Philadelphia: Lea & Febiger; 1990.

Cervero F. Sensory innervation of the viscera: peripheral basis of visceral pain. *Physiol Rev.* 1994;74:95–138.

Cervero F, Laird JM. Understanding the signaling and transmission of visceral nociceptive events. *J Neurobiol.* 2004;61: 45–54.

Chamberlain WE. The symphysis pubis in the roentgen examination of the sacroiliac joint. *Am J Roentgenol Radium Ther.* 1930;24:621.

Cohen SP, Chen Y, Neufeld NJ. Sacroiliac joint pain: a comprehensive review of epidemiology, diagnosis and treatment. *Expert Rev Neurother.* 2013;13:99–116.

Day M. Sympathetic blocks: the evidence. *Pain Pract.* 2008;8:98–109.

Death AB, Kirby RL, MacMillan CL. Pelvic ring mobility: assessment by stress radiography. *Arch Phys Med Rehabil.* 1982;63:204.

Drossman DA. Sexual and physical abuse in women with functional or organic gastrointestinal disorders. *Ann Intern Med.* 1990;113:828.

Duncan CH. A psychosomatic study of pelvic congestion. *Am J Obstet Gynecol.* 1952;64:1–12.

Edwards RD, Robertson IR, MacLean AB, Hemingway AP. Pelvic pain syndrome: successful treatment of a case by ovarian vein embolization [case report]. *Clin Radiol.* 1993; 47:429.

Everaert K, Devulder J, De Muynk M, et al. The pain cycle: implication for the diagnosis and treatment of pelvic pain syndromes. *Int Urogynecol J Pelvic Floor Dysfunct.* 2001;12:9–14.

Fall M, Baranowski AP, Elneil S, et al. EAU guidelines on chronic pelvic pain. *Eur Urol.* 2010;57:35–48.

Ghaly AF, Chien PW. Chronic pelvic pain: clinical dilemma or clinician's nightmare. *Sex Transm Infect.* 2000;76:419–425.

Grant SR, Salvati EP, Rubin RJ. Levator syndrome: an analysis of 316 cases. *Dis Colon Rectum.* 1975;18:161.

Greenman PE. Principles of diagnosis and treatment of pelvic girdle dysfunctions. In: Greenman PE, ed. *Principles of Manual Medicine.* Baltimore: Williams & Wilkins; 1991:225–232.

Grimaud JC, Bouvier M, Naudy B, et al. Manometric and radiologic investigations and biofeedback treatment of chronic idiopathic anal pain. *Dis Colon Rectum.* 1991;34:690.

Gunter J. Chronic pelvic pain: an integrated approach to diagnosis and treatment. *Obstet Gynecol Surv.* 2003;58:615–623.

Howard FM. Chronic pelvic pain. Clinical gynecologic series. An expert's view. *Obstetrics and Gynecology.* 2003;101:594–611.

Jänig W, Koltzenburg M. Pain arising from the urogenital tract. In: Maggi CA, ed. *Nervous Control of the Urogenital System.* London: Harwood Academic. 1993:525–578.

Kamm MA, Hoyle CHV, Burleigh DE, et al. Hereditary intestinal anal sphincter myopathy causing proctalgia fugax and constipation. *Gastroenterology.* 1991;100:809.

Kapural L, Narouze SN. Spinal cord stimulation is an effective treatment for the chronic intractable visceral pelvic pain. *Pain Med.* 2006;7:440–443.

Khan A, Ahmed M, Talati J. Seminal vesicle cystic dilatation masquerading as proctalgia fugax. *Br J Urol.* 1989;64:428.

Linley JE, Rose K, Ooi L. Understanding inflammatory pain: ion channels contributing to acute and chronic nociception. *Pflugers Arch.* 2010;459(5):657–669.

Marenco G, Lanoe Y, Perrigot M, et al. A new canal syndrome: compression of the pudendal nerve in Alcock's canal or perineal paralysis of cyclists [French]. *Presse Med.* 1987;16:399.

McGiveney JQ. The levator syndrome and its treatment. *South Med J.* 1965;58:505.

McMahon SB, Dmitrieva N, Koltzenburg M, et al. Visceral pain. *Br J Anaesth.* 2009;75:132–144.

Morales AJ, Murphy AA. Endoscopic treatment for endometriosis. *Obstet Gynecol Clin.* 1999;26:121.

Patt R, Plancarte R. Superior hypogastric plexus and ganglion impar. In: Hahn MB, McQuillan PM, Sheplock GJ, eds. *Regional Anesthesia: An Atlas of Anatomy and Techniques.* St. Louis: Mosby; 1996.

Patt RB. Peripheral neurolysis and the management of cancer pain. *Pain Digest.* 1992;2:30–37.

Patt RB. Therapeutic decision making for invasive procedures. In: Patt RB, ed. *Cancer Pain.* Philadelphia: Lippincott; 1993.

Patt RB, Plancarte R. Pelvic pain. In: Raj P, ed. *Pain Medicine. A Comprehensive Review.* St. Louis: Mosby; 1996:440–448.

Peters AA, Trimbos-Kemper GC, Admiraal C, Trimbos JB, Hermans J. A randomized clinical trial on the benefits of adhesiolysis in patients with pelvic adhesions and chronic pelvic pain. *Br J Obstet Gynaecol.* 1992;99:59.

Pezet S, McMahon SB. Neurotrophins: mediators and modulators of pain. *Annu Rev Neurosci.* 2006;29:507–538.

Plancarte R. Superior hypogastric plexus block: a very effective and underutilized diagnostic and therapeutic procedure. Paper presented at: Worldwide Pain Conference 2000; July 19, 2000; San Francisco, CA.

Plancarte R, Aldrete JA. Hypogastric plexus block: retroperitoneal approach. *Anesthesiology.* 1989;71:A739.

Plancarte R, Amescua C, Patt RB, Allende S. Presacral blockade of the ganglion of Walther (ganglion impar). *Anesthesiology.* 1990;73:A751.

Plancarte R, Amescua C, Py HRB, Aldrete JA. Superior hypogastric plexus block for pelvic cancer pain. *Anesthesiology.* 1990;73(2):236–239.

Plancarte R, de Leon-Casasola OA, El-Helaly M, Allende S, Lema MJ. Neurolytic superior hypogastric plexus block for chronic pelvic pain associated with cancer. *Reg Anesth.* 1997;22:562–568.

Plancarte R, González-Ortiz JC, Guajardo-Rosas J, Lee A. Ultrasonographic-assisted ganglion impar neurolysis. *Anesth Analg.* 2009;108(6):1995–1996.

Plancarte R, Guajardo J. Superior hypogastric plexus block and ganglion impar. *Tech Reg Anesth Pain Manag.* 2005;9:86–90.

Plancarte R, Guajardo J, Lee A. On the true origins of the Walther's ganglion blockade and more. *Pain Pract.* 2008;8:333–334.

Reginald PW, Adams J, Franks S, Wadsworth J, Beard RW. Medroxyprogesterone acetate in the treatment of pelvic pain due to venous congestion. *Br J Obstet Gynecol.* 1989;96:1148.

Rigor BM Sr. Pelvic cancer pain. *J Surg Oncol.* 2000;75:280.

Robert R, Prat-Pradal D, Labat JJ, et al. Anatomic basis of chronic perineal pain: role of the pudendal nerve. *Surg Radiol Anat.* 1998;20:93.

Schug SA, Saunders D, Kurowski I, Paech MJ. Neuraxial drug administration: a review of treatment options for anaesthesia and analgesia. *CNS Drugs.* 2006;20:917–933.

Shafik A. Pudendal canal syndrome: a new etiological factor in prostatodynia and its treatment by pudendal canal compression. *Pain Digest.* 1998;8:32.

Shafik A. Neuronal innervation of urethral and anal sphincters: surgical anatomy and clinical implications. *Curr Opin Obstet Gynecol.* 2000;12:387–398.

Shafik A. Pudendal canal syndrome: a cause of chronic pelvic pain. *Urology.* 2002;60:199.

Siegel S, Paszkiewicz E, Kirkpatrick C, et al. Sacral nerve stimulation in patients with chronic intractable pelvic pain. *J Urol.* 2001;166:1742–1745.

Simopoulos TT, Manchikanti L, Singh V, et al. A systematic evaluation of prevalence and diagnostic accuracy of sacroiliac joint interventions. *Pain Physician.* 2012;15:E305–E344.

Sinaki M, Merritt JL, Stilwell GK. Tension myalgia of the pelvic floor. *Mayo Clin Proc.* 1977;52:717.

Stearns L, Boortz-Marx R, Du Pen S, et al. Intrathecal drug delivery for the management of cancer pain: a multidisciplinary consensus of best clinical practices. *J Support Oncol.* 2005;3:399–408.

Stein A. *Heal Pelvic Pain: A Proven Stretching, Strengthening, and Nutrition Program for Relieving Pain, Incontinence, IBS, and Other Symptoms Without Surgery.* New York, NY: McGraw-Hill; 2009.

Stovall TG, Ling FW, Crawford DA. Hysterectomy for chronic pelvic pain of presumed uterine etiology. *Obstet Gynecol.* 1990;75:676.

Tetzschner T, Sorensen M, Lose G, et al. Pudendal nerve function during pregnancy and after delivery. *Int Urogynecol J Pelvic Floor Dysfunct.* 1997;8:66.

Thompson WG. Proctalgia fugax. *Dig Dis Sci.* 1981;26:1121.

Travell JG, Simons DG. *Myofascial Pain and Dysfunction: The Trigger Point Manual, Vol 2: The Lower Extremities.* Baltimore: Williams & Wilkins; 1992.

Van Goor H. Consequences and complications of peritoneal adhesions. *Colorectal Dis.* 2007;9(suppl 2):25–34.

Vleeming A, Schuenke MD, Masi AT, Carreiro JE, Danneels L, Willard FH. The sacroiliac joint: an overview of its anatomy, function and potential clinical implications. *J Anat.* 2012;221:537–567.

Wald A. Functional anorectal and pelvic pain. *Gastroenterol Clin North Am.* 2001;30:243.

Walling MK, Reiter RC, O'Hara MW, et al. Abuse history and chronic pain in women. I. Prevalences of sexual and physical abuse. *Obstet Gynecol.* 1994;84:193–199.

Whitehead WE, Wald A, Diamant NE, et al. Functional disorders of the anus and rectum. *Gut.* 1999;45(suppl 2):1155.

Zondervan KT, Yudkin PL, Vessey MP, et al. Prevalence and incidence in primary care of chronic pelvic pain in women: evidence from a national general practice database. *Br J Obstet Gynaecol.* 1999;106:1149.

37 THORACIC PAIN

P. Prithvi Raj, MD

INTRODUCTION

- Pain of the thoracic region is a frequently encountered complaint for specialists in pain management.
- Often generated from disorders of the viscera contained within the thoracic cavity.
- Diagnosis of these syndromes is difficult because the vague quality of the visceral pain makes it difficult to distinguish visceral pain from a referred pain that may coexist.
- The diagnostic dilemma is further complicated by the fact that efferent somatosensory and efferent visceral impulses of both the somatosensory and autonomic nervous systems impinge on the spinal cord at the same place, approximately within the levels of T1 to T7 (*viscerosomatic convergence*).
- Acute angina (heart T1 to T4) may, therefore, be experienced as epigastric discomfort, left shoulder or arm pain, left chest pain, or right-sided chest and arm pain.
- Although many acute thoracic pain syndromes exist, only the more chronic syndromes that are likely to be encountered in a pain center are discussed in this chapter.
- Table 37-1 lists some of the common acute pain states encountered in the thoracic region.
- Categorized as visceral, musculoskeletal, myofascial, neurogenic, and other.

VISCERAL PAIN

LUNGS AND TRACHEA

- Visceral afferent fibers from the trachea and bronchi are carried to the central nervous system (CNS) through afferent fibers of the vagus and upper thoracic sympathetic nerves (T2 to T7).
- Pain associated with the trachea and bronchi radiates to the sternum.
- The lung parenchyma and the visceral pleura are insensate and, thus, do not produce pain following surgery or trauma.
- The parietal pleura transmits pain along somatic nerves, including the brachial plexus (C8, T1), intercostal nerves (T1 to T12), and phrenic nerves (C3 to C5).
- Pain from the parietal pleura (eg, arising from carcinoma, pneumonia, or pleurisy) is often sharp,

TABLE 37-1   Thoracic Pain

VISCERAL	MUSCULOSKELETAL	NEUROGENIC	MISCELLANEOUS

Thorax	Bony origin
	  Rib/sternum
		Herpes zoster
		  Acute
		  Postherpetic neuralgia
			Vascular
			  Angina
			  Pulmonary infarct
			  Aortic

Lung/trachea
  Pneumonia
  Pleurisy
  Carcinoma (Pancoast)
	Costochondritis (Tietze's syndrome)
	Vertebrae
	  Disk disease
	  Facet syndrome
	  Compression fracture: osteoporosis (steroids)
	  Degenerative joint disease
	  Bone metastases		

Heart
  Myocarditis
  Mediastinitis
  Angina
	Soft tissue
	  Muscle ligaments
	  Breast
		Causalgia (CRPS)
		  Posttrauma
		  Postsurgery
			Infectious disease

Esophagus
  Carcinoma
  Esophagitis
	Posttrauma
	Postsurgery
		Myelopathies
		Demyelination
		Spinal cord injury
			Metastatic disease

piercing, and knifelike and is worsened by effort or deep respiration.

- Parietal pleural pain radiates to the supraclavicular region, the shoulder area, and the area supplied by the intercostal nerves.
- Although this pain may initially be confused with angina, angina is not exacerbated by coughing or deep respiration.

Pain Management

- Intermittent or continuous epidural blocks using local anesthetics and steroids alone or in combination may be used to block pain mediated by spinal nerve roots and autonomic visceral components.
- The use of transcutaneous electrical neural stimulation (TENS) and myofascial trigger point injections in spastic paraspinal muscle may help breathing and improve the patient's clinical condition.
- Pain associated with the trachea and bronchi because of carcinoma may improve after vagotomy.
- Pain associated with cancerous involvement of the visceral pleura and surrounding tissues should be treated with an aggressive multidisciplinary approach, including tricyclic antidepressants, narcotic analgesics, nerve-blocking techniques, psychological counseling, neuromodulatory techniques, and a strong emotional support system.

CARDIAC

- The visceral afferent fibers of the heart are transmitted through the vagus, the cervical ganglia (middle and inferior cervical nerves), and the upper five thoracic

ganglia (thoracic cardiac nerves), and enter the CNS at T1 to T5 (see Figure 37-1).
- Most cardiogenic pain is secondary to ischemia.
- Whether ischemia is due to coronary artery vasospasm, coronary atherosclerosis, or acute coronary arterial insufficiency, the symptoms may be similar: substernal, crushing, or epigastric pain—a feeling of tightness, constriction, and heaviness that may become progressively more severe or intense.
- The pain frequently radiates to the left sternal border, left shoulder, arm, and neck, and there may be an accompanying feeling of impending doom.
- Acute infectious processes, such as endocarditis and myocarditis, produce symptoms of pleuritic substernal or epigastric pain that may be lancinating or paroxysmal or that may become continuous and more severe.

Pain Management

- Acute treatment includes administration of oxygen, reduction of myocardial work through rest, and administration of coronary artery dilating agents, such as β-blockers, calcium channel-blocking drugs, nitrites, sedatives, antibiotics, and antiviral agents, as indicated.
- Coronary artery revascularization or balloon angioplasty may be indicated.
- The pain produced by these acute processes may require potent narcotic analgesics.
- Acute treatment is rarely given in the pain clinic setting, but it is imperative that myocardial ischemia be excluded as an etiology of chest pain before initiating any treatment involving chest pain.
- Chronic chest pain or referred sympathetic pain (shoulder–hand syndrome) may be treated by stellate

(A)

(B)

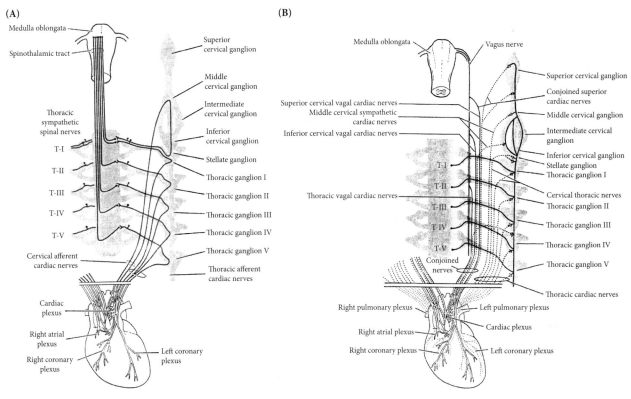

FIG. 37-1. Autonomic nerve supply to the heart. (A) Efferent nerve supply. (B) Afferent nerve supply.

ganglion block or by interruption of preganglionic sympathetic nerves T2 to T5.

- The possibility of cardiac causalgia following the onset of angina pectoris has been suggested.
- Cardiac causalgia is characterized by constant burning and chronic substernal chest discomfort.
- Hyperesthesia of the sternum and the chest wall over the painful area may be present.
- Although nitroglycerin and rest do not relieve the pain of cardiac causalgia, calcium channel-blocking drugs may be effective.
- The role of sympathetic nervous system blockade with respect to cardiac causalgia has not been fully evaluated.

ESOPHAGUS

- Visceral afferent fibers from the esophagus are carried through inferior cervical sympathetic nerves and the vagus (upper esophagus T2 to T5) and through thoracic cardiac sympathetic nerves and the stellate ganglion (lower esophagus T5 to T8) to the CNS.
- Pain from the upper esophagus radiates to the midsubsternal area, lower neck, lateral chest, and arms, whereas lower esophageal pain (esophagitis, spasm of the gastroesophageal junction) radiates to the area over the heart or epigastrium.

- Esophageal pain is paroxysmal, occurring with swallowing and radiating to the back at the level of the lesion.
- Pain associated with inflammation, acidic conditions, chemical irritation, mechanical irritation or dilation, and/or autonomic dysfunction may be relieved with antacids, histamine H_2-blocking drugs, misoprostol (Cytotec), metoclopramide hydrochloride (Reglan), or antiflatulents.
- Pain from esophageal cancer described as substernal, epigastric, and exacerbated by swallowing may be relieved by blocking spinal nerve roots T2 to T5 for upper esophageal lesions in combination with vagotomy or by blocking T5 to T8 for lower esophageal lesions.
- Management of esophageal pain is similar to other visceral structures of the thoracic region, such as the trachea, bronchi, and heart, based on their afferent and efferent innervations.

MUSCULOSKELETAL PAIN

- Thoracic musculoskeletal pain is a frequent complaint and may be related to trauma, postsurgical changes, infectious processes, degenerative changes, overuse phenomenon, or inflammatory processes.

- The site of the pain may involve the vertebrae, the bony thorax, and the soft tissue or musculoligamentous structures.

COSTOCHONDRITIS (TIETZE SYNDROME)

- Pain of the costochondral junctions along the anterior chest wall may follow blunt chest trauma; persistent coughing, as with chronic obstructive pulmonary disease or acute respiratory infection; overuse of the upper extremity (from activities such as washing windows and painting); or chest surgery.
- True Tietze syndrome is most frequently unilateral, involving the second and third costal cartilages (see Figure 37-2).
- This pain is described as mild to moderate over the anterior chest wall.
- If the pain is severe enough, the patient may confuse it with a myocardial infarction.
- Differential diagnosis includes underlying malignancy and sepsis.
- Tietze syndrome, which is often a diagnosis of exclusion, occurs in all age groups (including children) but is most frequently observed in persons younger than 40 years of age.
- Bulbous swellings that may persist for several months and point tenderness over the costochondral junctions are characteristic of Tietze syndrome.
- Exacerbations and remissions of the pain can remain localized or radiate to the arm and shoulder.

Pain Management

- Treatment may include local heat, nonsteroidal anti-inflammatory drugs (NSAIDs), local infiltration with a local anesthetic solution/steroid combination, intercostal nerve blocks, or electroacupuncture therapy.
- TENS may be useful until the irritative process or inflammatory reaction subsides.

COSTOCHONDRITIS

- Costochondritis presents as inflammation of multiple costochondral or costosternal articulations.
- It may radiate widely and mimic intrathoracic and intra-abdominal disease.
- Since multiple articulations are usually involved, local tenderness is elicited with palpation, which may reproduce the symptoms of the radiating pain.
- Costochondritis most frequently occurs in adults 40 years of age and older.
- Additional costochondral pain problems include trauma to the sternum and ribs, with subsequent fractures, dislocations, and separation of the ribs, cartilage, and sternum.

Pain Management

- Treatment is similar to that of Tietze syndrome once the diagnosis is made and other underlying causes of cardiac, gastrointestinal, and arthritic processes and myofascial strain have been ruled out.

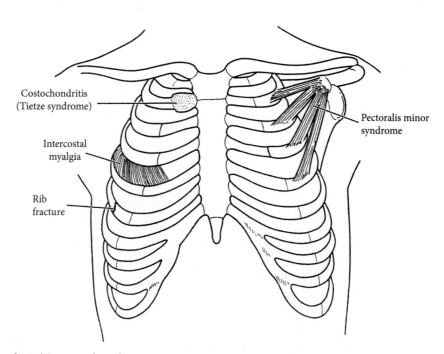

FIG. 37-2. Costochondritis (Tietze syndrome).

- Costochondral arthritis, osteoporosis, infection, and trauma or delayed healing following thoracic surgery can be a challenge to therapeutic interventions.
- TENS can be very helpful when the electrical signal is used in a crossed fashion over the area of pain.
- Electroacupuncture therapy is a useful adjunct.
- Periodic intercostal nerve blocks and thoracic epidural or intrapleural catheter techniques have been described.
- If permissible, local infiltration near the site of pain may be beneficial.

SLIPPING RIB SYNDROME (SOMETIMES CALLED NIP NERVE SYNDROME)

- A unique disorder encountered by the pain physician is slipping rib syndrome. It frequently occurs from a disarticulation of the inferior rib margins. Characteristically it presents as pain in the abdomen or lower thoracic anterior chest wall. It can occur idiopathically or after traumatic injury (abdominal surgery or blunt trauma).
- Clinical examination includes having the patient lie in the supine position. The operator's hands are placed on the upper quadrant and placed under the rib margin. Lifting upward one can feel the mobility of the distal rib. There is frequently a "click" or a snap that occurs as one elevates the distal rib. This snapping is associated with the patient's usual pain.
- Treatment frequently involves local injections of local anesthetics with steroids.

VERTEBRAL DISORDERS

- Painful disorders of the thoracic vertebrae may involve osteoporosis, compression fractures, thoracic facet syndrome, ankylosing spondylitis, postural abnormalities (scoliosis), or injuries involving forced or violent flexion or extension movement of the spine.
- Pain associated with fractures, infections, degenerative arthritic processes, metabolic bone disease, or primary or metastatic malignancies is also commonly encountered.
- Compression fractures of the thoracic vertebrae that are due to trauma, osteoporosis secondary to aging or corticosteroid use, and degenerative changes are common.
- Patients complain of encircling pain along the intercostal nerves, aggravated by twisting motions, coughing, or postural changes.
- In the acute setting, fractured vertebrae and ribs produce severe, constricting pain of the thorax, which may inhibit respiration.

- The pain is generally accompanied by severe muscle spasms of the intercostal and paraspinous muscles, inhibiting the patient from obtaining adequate sleep or movement.

Pain Management

- Treatment consists of local heat or ice, TENS, NSAIDs, and nonopioid and opioid analgesics.
- Nerve-blocking techniques, such as single-shot and continuous epidural blocks, single-level or multiple-level intercostal blocks, paravertebral somatic nerve blocks, and intrapleural catheter techniques, can also be used.

MYOFASCIAL PAIN

- The paravertebral muscles (eg, the longissimus thoracis and iliocostalis muscles) are a common source of thoracic pain.
- Pain can be reproduced by pressure on the trigger area and is often relieved by massage, vapocoolant spray, or the injection of a local anesthetic/steroid mixture.

POSTTHORACOTOMY PAIN

- Chronic pain after thoracotomy can be aggravated due to various etiologic mechanisms.
- Some authors suggest that surgical excision of intercostal nerves, designed to relieve pain, may result in late postoperative pain caused by neuroma formation. This technique has been condemned.
- Complications of chemically induced intercostal neuritis with the use of absolute alcohol resulted in a recommendation against the use of such agents.
- Many of the common causes of postthoracotomy pain are amenable to therapeutic interventions.

ENTRAPMENT OF NERVE FIBERS IN SCAR TISSUE

- In the thoracic region, one may encounter noxious input from cutaneous receptors of a mild to severe degree secondary to scar tissue formation or nerve entrapment in scar tissue.
- When nerve fibers are trapped in scar tissue, a light touch on the scar produces intense radiating pain, sometimes accompanied by burning pain from associated reflex sympathetic dystrophy.
- The pain can be described as dull and aching, with frequent bouts of sharp, shooting pain associated with particular movement.
- Localized pain can be aggravated by direct pressure on the scar itself, and one might find referred pain to

areas more closely associated with the scar tissue or more remote.

- Patients complain of exquisite tenderness over areas of the scar, hyperalgesia, and incapacitation.
- Injection of the scar with a local anesthetic agent is diagnostic.

Pain Management

- Repeated injection of a local anesthetic mixed with a steroid is likely to provide long-term relief.
- Ablation of irregular bundles of nerve element, such as neuromas, may prove beneficial, but neuroablative procedures may result in either less intense or more intense pain.
- It is suggested that neuromas found in scar tissue may give rise to the "viscerosensory reflex."
- It is thought that the internal viscera are connected embryologically to cutaneous manifestations throughout the entire body. By pressing on or moving the various connective tissue elements of the somatosensory areas served by the same neurologic tissue, one can produce visceral or autonomic symptoms.
- Thus, injection of a painful cutaneous scar may alleviate abdominal or thoracic visceral pain that may appear to be remote from the site itself.
- Several clinicians recommend cryoanalgesia of involved intercostal nerves at the time of surgery to prevent postthoracotomy pain and pulmonary complications; however, cryoanalgesia is not without possible complications, because secondary neuralgia may occur.
- Others have suggested the use of TENS for treatment of postthoracotomy pain.
- For acute postthoracotomy pain management, epidural narcotic infusions may be more effective than cryoanalgesic measures or TENS.

NEUROMA

- A palpable neuroma in the scar, loss of pinprick sensation over the skin, and elicitation of pain on palpation are diagnostic.
- Repeated injections of a local anesthetic/steroid mixture may relieve the pain.
- Persistent pain from a localized neuroma may respond well to neurolytic injection of phenol or to cryolysis.

SYMPATHETIC DYSTROPHY (ALSO KNOWN AS CRPS 1 OR CRPS 2)

- Burning pain associated with hyperpathia, decreased skin temperature over the area, and increased sweating characterize this syndrome.

- Pain is relieved by paravertebral sympathetic block, nerve root block, or epidural block of sympathetic fibers.
- This pain may also respond to the use of calcium channel-blocking drugs, blockers, antidepressants, anti-inflammatory medications, and neural stabilizing agents, such as fluphenazine.

MYOFASCIAL TRIGGER POINTS

- Tender trigger points located in the pectoral and anterior serratus muscles and accompanied by spasm in those muscles are a common source of anterior chest pain (see Figure 37-2).
- Pain is reproduced by pressure on the trigger point and relieved by local anesthetic injection or vapocoolant spray technique.
- The pain is not relieved by intercostal block because the pectoral muscles are innervated by the branches of the brachial plexus.
- TENS and physical therapy involving stretching exercises, deep massage, and passive and then active range-of-motion techniques are helpful in preventing recurrence.
- Myofascial trigger points can also be the source of postthoracotomy pain.
- They can be located by careful palpation of the paravertebral tissues.
- Local injections, TENS, and epidural blocks as well as local heat and ice, physical therapy, and anti-inflammatory agents may be helpful.

NEUROGENIC PAIN

- It is important to mention pain syndromes of the thorax, acute herpes zoster, and chronic postherpetic neuralgia.
- Additional pain syndromes in the thoracic region involving nerve tissue or damage to nerve tissue include causalgia and intercostal neuropathies following trauma, surgical intervention, or intraneural injection.
- Irritation of the intercostal nerves can also occur following osteoarthritis of the joint space and destruction or tumor invasion of the intercostal nerve, with resultant mechanical compression.
- Hematoma or infiltration neuritis and postinjection neuritis can affect the intercostal nerves.
- Lesions of the spinal cord, including myelopathies, demyelination, and spinal cord traumatic injuries, may also contribute to thoracic pain.
- Causalgia involving any of the thoracic somatic nerves, thoracic intercostal nerves, or the spinal cord itself may be present.

OTHER CAUSES OF PAIN

SURGICAL SCARS

- Painful scars can occur after thoracic surgery.
- They cause a characteristic pain syndrome that usually persists for at least two months after the procedure.
- A continuous aching or burning sensation often extends beyond the scar.
- In addition, there is sensory loss and absence or sweating along the scar.
- Temperature, touch, pressure, and emotional factors can exacerbate the pain.
- The appearance of the scar is not significant. Smooth scars can be painful, and indurated scars can be painless.
- Histologic examination shows a chaotic formation of neural elements; neuromas may be present.
- The pain has been attributed to imperfect nerve regeneration.

Pain Management

- TENS, analgesics, antidepressants, anticonvulsants, local infiltration of anesthetics and corticosteroids, and nerve blocks have been used with varying degrees of success.
- Many patients have undergone scar resection with no pain relief.
- Delayed chest pain may also occur as a result of sternal wire sutures.

PAIN AFTER BREAST SURGERY

- Chest pain may be felt after extensive breast surgery, such as radical mastectomy.
- Patients usually have a burning pain in the axilla and upper chest; this may radiate to the medial part of the arm.
- The pain probably is secondary to transection of the intercostobrachial nerve.
- Postmastectomy surgical pain rarely lasts longer than three months after surgery.
- Some patients may have chronic pain after mastectomy. This pain frequently is in a nonanatomic area on the anterior chest wall and is extremely sensitive to touch.

PSYCHIATRIC CAUSES

- Panic disorder, depression, and other psychiatric maladies also may be manifested as chest pain.

BIBLIOGRAPHY

Bradley LA, Scarinci IC, Richter JE. Pain threshold levels and coping strategies among patients who have chest pain and normal coronary arteries. *Med Clin North Am*. 1991;75:1189.

Brand DL, Beck JG, Wielgosz AT. Unexplained chest pain: future directions for research. *Med Clin North Am*. 1991;75:1209.

Calabro JJ, Jeghers H, Miller KA, et al. Classification of anterior chest wall syndrome (C). *JAMA*. 1980;243:1420.

Eagle KA. Medical decision making in patient with chest pain. *N Engl J Med*. 1991;324:1282.

Fam AG, Smythe HA. Musculoskeletal chest wall pain. *Can Med Assoc J*. 1985;133:379.

Fineman SP. Long-term post-thoracotomy cancer pain management with interpleural bupivacaine. *Anesth Analg*. 1989;68:694.

Glynn CJ, Lloyd JW, Bernard JDW. Cryoanalgesia in the management of pain after thoracotomy. *Thorax*. 1980;35:325.

Gough JD, Williams AB, Vaughan RS, et al. The control of post-thoracotomy pain: a comparative evaluation of thoracic epidural fentanyl infusions and cryoanalgesia. *Anaesthesia*. 1988;43:780.

Levy MH. Integration of pain management into comprehensive cancer care. *Cancer*. 1989;63:2329.

Maiwand O, Makey AR. Cryoanalgesia for relief of pain after thoracotomy. *Br Med J*. 1981;282:49.

Ramamurthy S. Pain in thoracic region. In: Raj PP, ed. *Practical Management of Pain*. Chicago: Year Book Medical; 1986:464.

Richter JE. Practical approach to the diagnosis of unexplained chest pain. *Med Clin North Am*. 1991;75:1203.

Roll M, Kollind M, Theorell T. Clinical symptoms in young adults with atypical chest pain attending the emergency department. *J Intern Med*. 1991;230:271.

Rooney SM, Subhash J, Melormack P. A comparison of pulmonary function tests for postthoracotomy pain using cryoanalgesia and transcutaneous nerve stimulation. *Ann Thorac Surg*. 1986;41:204.

Stubbing JF, Jellicoe JA. Transcutaneous electrical nerve stimulation after thoracotomy. *Anesthesia*. 1988;43:296.

38 ARTHRITIS

Hong Yang, MD, PhD
Zuhre Tutuncu, MD
Arthur Kavanaugh, MD

INTRODUCTION

- Musculoskeletal disorders affect 20%–45% of the population.
- Pain, one of the cardinal features of arthritis, is the result of the action of numerous inflammatory mediators and inflammatory cell-derived products on local nerves.

- Although pain is a subjective feeling, it is one of the criteria that are used in clinical practice to assess patients' overall functioning, disease activity, and response to therapy.
- Pain, soreness, aches, stiffness, swelling, weakness, and fatigue account for more than 95% of all initial musculoskeletal presentations.
- Chronic disability from musculoskeletal disorders affects 6.1%–10% of the population.
- The most common inflammatory and noninflammatory conditions in men and women, by age in approximate order of prevalence, are listed in Table 38-1.
- Arthritis is a general term that describes more than 100 conditions. Specific management of pain in arthritic

TABLE 38-1 Common Rheumatologic Conditions*

| AGE | MEN | | WOMEN | |
---	NONINFLAMMATORY	INFLAMMATORY	NONINFLAMMATORY	INFLAMMATORY
18–34	Injury/overuse†	Spondyloarthropathies	Injury/overuse	Gonoccocal arthritis
	Low back pain	Gonoccocal arthritis	Low back pain	RA
		Gout		SLE
35–65	Low back pain	Bursitis	Osteoporosis	Bursitis
	Injury/overuse	Gout	Low back pain	RA
	OA	Spondyloarthropathies	Injury/overuse	USP
	Entrapment syndromes‡	USP	Fibromyalgia	
			Entrapment syndromes	
			OA	
			Raynaud phenomenon	
>65	OA	Bursitis	Osteoporosis	Bursitis
	Low back pain	Gout	OA	USP
	Osteoporosis	USP	Fibromyalgia	RA
	Fracture	RA	Low back pain	Gout
		Pseudogout	Fracture	Pseudogout
		Polymyalgia rheumatica		Polymyalgia rheumatica
		Septic arthritis		Septic arthritis

*Conditions are listed in approximate order of prevalence.

†Injury/overuse includes fracture, soft tissue injuries, tendonitis, and nonarticular rheumatism.

‡Entrapment syndrome includes carpal tunnel and tarsal tunnel syndromes; spondyloarthropathies include ankylosing spondylitis, psoriatic arthritis, and Reiter syndrome.

RA, rheumatoid arthritis; SLE, systemic lupus erythematosus; OA, osteoarthritis; USP, undifferentiated seronegative polyarthritis.

TABLE 38-2 Specific Features That Are Useful in Distinguishing Inflammatory From Noninflammatory Conditions

	CHARACTERISTICS OF CONDITION	
FEATURE	INFLAMMATORY	NONINFLAMMATORY
Joint pain	Yes (with activity and rest)	Yes (with activity)
Joint swelling	Soft tissue	Bony (if present)
Local erythema	Sometimes	Absent
Local warmth	Sometimes	Absent
Morning stiffness	Prolonged (>60 min)	Variable (<60 min)
Systemic symptoms	Common	Rare
ESR, CRP	Increased	Normal for age
Hemoglobin	Normal or low	Normal
Serum albumin	Normal or low	Normal
Synovial fluid, WBCs/mm³	≥2000	<2000
Synovial fluid, % PMNs	≥75%	<75%

conditions requires differentiation of the type of arthritis. The primary goals of the patient's evaluation are to discern if the complaint is:

1. Inflammatory or noninflammatory
2. Articular or periarticular in origin
3. Acute or chronic
4. Monoarticular/oligoarticular or polyarticular

- Musculoskeletal conditions are often classified as having inflammatory or noninflammatory symptoms or signs that reflect the nature of the underlying pathologic process. Specific features that are useful in distinguishing inflammatory versus noninflammatory conditions are given in Table 38-2.

EVALUATION

- While evaluating the patient, the physician should determine whether the complaint originates from articular or periarticular structures.
- Periarticular structures include tendon, bursa, ligament, muscle, bone, fascia, nerve, or overlying skin. Periarticular joint pain is usually focal and pain is experienced on active motion in a few, specific planes.
- Pain in arthritic conditions is present on both active and passive motion of the joint in all planes, and it is diffuse and produces deep tenderness.
- On presentation, the clinician should also determine if the arthritis is acute or chronic, based on whether the complaint has been present six weeks or less (acute) or longer than six weeks (chronic).
- The extent of articular involvement is defined as monoarticular (one joint), oligoarticular or pauciarticular (two to four joints), or polyarticular (more than four

joints). These approaches can help the physician categorize the complaint as:

1. Acute inflammatory monoarthritis/oligoarthritis (eg, septic arthritis, gout, pseudogout, viral arthritis, Reiter syndrome, Lyme disease, acute rheumatic fever, hemarthrosis, palindromic rheumatism)
2. Chronic inflammatory monoarthritis/oligoarthritis (eg, tuberculous arthritis, fungal arthritis, psoriatic arthritis, spondyloarthropathy, pseudogout, sarcoidosis, juvenile chronic arthritis)
3. Acute noninflammatory monoarthritis/oligoarthritis (eg, mechanical derangement, trauma)
4. Chronic noninflammatory monoarthritis/oligoarthritis (eg, osteoarthritis [OA], osteonecrosis, neuropathic arthritis, hemarthrosis, pigmented villonodular synovitis, foreign body synovitis)
5. Acute inflammatory polyarthritis (eg, viral arthritis, septic arthritis, acute rheumatic fever, Reiter syndrome)
6. Chronic inflammatory polyarthritis (eg, rheumatoid arthritis [RA], psoriatic arthritis, enteropathic arthritis, crystal-induced arthritis, juvenile arthritis, Lyme disease, systemic lupus erythematosus [SLE], scleroderma, mixed connective tissue disease, polymyalgia rheumatica, polymyositis)

- Chronic noninflammatory polyarthritis (eg, OA, hemochromatosis)

OSTEOARTHRITIS

GENERAL

- OA is the most common noninflammatory arthritic condition.
- It typically affects the joints of the hand, spine, and weight-bearing joints (hips, knees).
- OA generally involves more than one joint but can also occur as monoarthritis.
- Approximately 12% of the adult population has symptomatic OA, characterized by joint pain, crepitus, stiffness after immobility, and limitation of motion. A greater percentage (eg, 37% or more of patients over 60 years of age) will have radiologic changes consistent with OA without significant associated symptoms.
- The clinical joint symptoms are associated with defects in the articular cartilage that lead to changes in the underlying bone.
- OA is either primary/idiopathic or secondary.

EVALUATION

- Secondary causes of OA include trauma, obesity, congenital disorders, metabolic disorders, neuropathic disorders, and hemophilia.

- Laboratory tests tend to be normal for age. Synovial fluid is usually amber, clear, and noninflammatory with normal viscosity.
- Typical radiographic changes include loss of joint space, subchondral sclerosis, bony cysts, and reactive osteophytes.
- Articular erosions and osteoporosis are rare.
- It is important to note that radiographic findings do not necessarily correlate with clinical symptoms.
- When possible, synovial fluid aspiration should be done to evaluate all patients with acute onset of arthritis. Synovial fluid analysis provides unique and valuable information.
- The primary goal of synovial fluid analysis is to discern whether a synovial effusion is noninflammatory, inflammatory, septic, or hemorrhagic. There are a few disorders for which the synovial fluid analysis is diagnostic, for example, infectious and crystal-induced arthritis.
- Arthrocentesis may be therapeutic as well as diagnostic. For tense effusions, in which intra-articular pressure is high, removing fluid relieves symptoms and may decrease joint damage.
- Importantly, if present, septic arthritis should be diagnosed immediately and it should be treated with appropriate intravenous antibiotics and intensive follow-up.

TREATMENT

- The goals of therapy in OA are to relieve pain, maintain function, protect articular structures, and educate the patient.
- As there is no medication that has been shown to stop or reverse the disease process underlying OA, education about the disease and the rationale for therapy helps patients adhere to therapy.
- Pharmacologic therapy in pain management include nonnarcotic analgesics, nonsteroidal anti-inflammatory drugs (NSAIDs), topical agents (eg, capsaicin, topical NSAIDs), analgesics targeting neurotransmission (eg, duloxetine), intra-articular corticosteroids, and intra-articular hyaluronic acid preparations.
- Intra-articular injections may provide temporary or sustained relief of pain.
- Chronic use of strong narcotics and oral corticosteroids should be discouraged.
- Modification of activities, exercise (biking, walking, swimming), weight loss, splinting, joint protection, ambulatory assistive devices, physical therapy, hydrotherapy, heat/cold application, and self-help programs are nonpharmacologic measures that can play a crucial role in improving range of motion and stability and in decreasing pain.

1. Acupuncture as an adjunctive therapy is inconclusive.
2. Needle lavage and arthroscopy with debridement or lavage are not recommended.
3. Arthroscopic partial meniscectomy was found to be no better than physical therapy alone for patient with OA and meniscus tear. It should be reserved for patients refractory to conservative treatments.
4. Realignment osteotomy is an option in active patients with symptomatic unicompartmental OA of the knee with malalignment.

- For those with advanced disease, joint replacement surgery may dramatically improve the quality of life. Surgery should be considered for patients who experience intractable/refractory pain, loss of function or mobility, and radiographic evidence of advanced degenerative disease in the joint.
- A survey of 440 practicing rheumatologists revealed the following preferences for initial treatment of OA of the knee: nonnarcotic analgesic, 37%; low-dose NSAIDs, 35%; high-dose NSAIDs, 13%; physical therapy, 10%; and intra-articular corticosteroids, 6%. If the initial treatment failed to curtail symptoms, the preferred second therapy was: intra-articular corticosteroid, 33%; high-dose NSAIDs, 30%; low-dose NSAIDs, 23%; physical therapy. 8%; and nonnarcotic analgesics, 5%.
  1. Current therapies mostly target pain and function with modest effectiveness. There is a large unmet need in OA for newer treatment options not only to control pain but also to slow down the structural progression of the disease.
  2. Newer therapies under study:
     - Tanezumab is a humanized monoclonal antibody that targets nerve growth factor. It is under study at present for the treatment of chronic pain. A phase III, placebo- and active-controlled study indicated tanezumab may be efficacious for the treatment of OA pain.
     - The Neydharting mud pack has a favorable effect on the clinical parameters, quality of life, and need for medications in patients with knee OA.
     - Bisphosphonates have some reported beneficial effects in treating OA. Significant reduction in numeric rating scale pain was observed in the first three years with bisphosphonate use.
     - Nuclear magnetic resonance (NMR) has been shown to stimulate repair processes and cartilage and to influence pain signaling. A one-year survey with multicenter data of more than 4500 patients with degenerative rheumatic diseases treated with therapeutic NMR showed improvement in their ability in functional parameters.

CHRONIC INFLAMMATORY ARTHRITIS

- Chronic inflammatory arthritis is an inflammatory articular condition that has persisted more than six weeks.
- If fewer than four joints are involved, the patient has chronic monoarthritis/oligoarthritis. Synovial fluid analysis should be considered in such conditions.
- If chronic tuberculosis or fungal arthritis is suspected, synovial biopsy may be indicated. Gout and pseudogout are the other conditions that might be considered with monoarthritis/oligoarthritis.
- Patients who present with chronic oligoarthritis or polyarthritis should be evaluated for other chronic inflammatory conditions including connective tissue diseases.
- Table 38-3 describes joint and extra-articular manifestations and laboratory findings, which, if present, may assist in the diagnosis of a specific chronic inflammatory arthritis.

RHEUMATOID ARTHRITIS

GENERAL

- Since RA is the most common type of chronic inflammatory arthritis, RA should be a major consideration in patients with symmetric inflammatory arthritis of more than six weeks in duration.

- RA is a chronic, systemic, inflammatory disorder of unknown etiology.
- The primary pathologic site in RA is the synovium, which is a thin layer surrounding joints. Synovial tissues become inflamed and proliferate, forming pannus, which in turn may invade bone, cartilage, and other articular and periarticular structures (eg, ligaments) leading to damage, deformities, and functional disability.
- RA affects approximately 1% of the population worldwide.
- Women are affected about three times more often than men.
- The peak onset is between 35 and 50 years of age.
- Diagnostic criteria for the classification of RA are summarized in Table 38-4.

EVALUATION

- No laboratory or diagnostic test by itself is diagnostic in RA.
- Rheumatoid factor (RF) is the test that is most closely associated with RA. It is present in 75%–85% of the patients with established RA. A newer test that provides similar information is the anti-citrullinated protein antibody (ACPA) test.
- Other laboratory tests that can be helpful in supporting the diagnosis of RA include synovial fluid analysis, measurement of acute phase reactants (erythrocyte

TABLE 38-3 Chronic Inflammatory Polyarthritis: Diagnosis

DIAGNOSIS	JOINT MANIFESTATIONS	EXTRA-ARTICULAR MANIFESTATIONS	LABORATORY FINDINGS
RA	Symmetric polyarthritis involving typical joints	Rheumatoid nodules, vasculitis, ocular, pulmonary lesions	Elevated RF* in ≥80% of patients
Spondyloarthropathy	Asymmetric oligoarthritis Inflammatory back pain Sacroiliitis	Typical skin rash Ocular involvement Genitourinary tract inflammation Bowel inflammation	Radiographic findings of sacroiliitis HLA-B27
Psoriatic arthritis	Asymmetric oligoarthritis Erosive peripheral arthritis (DIP and/or PIP joints) Spondylitis	Psoriatic skin lesions Nail changes	Negative RF in 80% of patients
Gout	Episodic monoarthritis/oligoarthritis	Tophi	Intra-articular MSU crystals in synovial fluid Elevated serum urate levels
CPPD	Episodic monoarthritis/oligoarthritis		Intra-articular calcium pyrophosphate crystals in synovial fluid
		Liver disease, DM, heart disease, hypogonadism if patient has hemachromatosis	PTH, TSH, calcium, phosphorous, magnesium, iron studies
Systemic lupus erythematosus	Nondeforming inflammatory arthritis	Malar rash, photosensitivity, alopecia, oral/genital sores, digital ulcers	ANA, other autoantibodies Hematologic abnormalities

*RF, rheumatoid factor; MSU, monosodium urate; ANA, antinuclear antibody; DIP, distal interphalangeal; PIP, proximal interphalangeal.

TABLE 38-4 Revised Criteria for the Classification of Rheumatoid Arthritis, ACR/EULAR 2010

Target population (who should be tested?): patients who:
1. Have at least one joint with definite clinical synovitis (swelling)
2. Have synovitis not better explained by another disease

Classification criteria for RA (score-based algorithm: add score of categories A–D; a score of ≥6/10 is needed for classification of a patient as having definite RA)

A. Joint involvement	
1 large joint	0
2–10 large joints	1
1–3 small joints (with or without involvement of large joints)	2
4–10 small joints (with or without involvement of large joints)	3
>10 joints (at least 1 small joint)	5
B. Serology (at least one test result is needed for classification)	
Negative RF *and* negative ACPA	0
Low-positive RF *or* low-positive ACPA	2
High-positive RF *or* high-positive ACPA	3
C. Acute-phase reactants (at least one test result is needed for classification)	
Normal CRP *and* normal ESR	0
Abnormal CRP *or* abnormal ESR	1
D. Duration of symptoms	
<6 weeks	0
≥6 weeks	1

sedimentation rate [ESR], C-reactive protein [CRP]), and complete blood count (CBC).

- Elevations in ESR and/or CRP levels provide a surrogate measure of inflammation and may be useful in gauging disease activity as well as the response to therapy.
- In RA, synovial fluid is expected to be inflammatory (Table 38-2).
- Early in the disease course plain radiographs may show only soft tissue swelling or joint effusion.
- Nearly 70% of patients developing bony erosions do so within the first two years of disease.
- Erosions may be seen in virtually any joint but are most common in the metacarpophalangeal (MCP), metatarsophalangeal (MTP), and wrist joints.

TREATMENT

- Although OA and RA are different arthritic conditions, pain management principles are similar.
- Goals of therapy in RA are to educate the patient, relieve pain, reduce inflammation, protect articular structures, control systemic involvement, and maintain function. Overall, the goal is remission, or as low a state of disease activity as possible for each individual.
- The approach to treatment of RA has changed dramatically over the past two decades.

- It is now recognized that the long-term prognosis for RA patients is poor and warrants the institution of aggressive therapy within the first few months of onset of RA.
- Most RA patients initially receive symptomatic treatment with NSAIDs.
- Low-dose corticosteroids (≤10 mg) are often introduced, particularly at the beginning of therapy or during flairs of disease activity.
- RA patients, especially those with aggressive disease, should receive disease-modifying drugs (DMARDs) or biologic agents early in the disease course.
- Methotrexate (with concomitant folate) is the most commonly used DMARD. Other DMARDs include hydroxychloroquine, sulfasalazine, and leflunomide. Biologic agents include tumor necrosis factor (TNF) inhibitors (infliximab, etanercept, adalimumab, golimumab, certolizumab pegol), an interleukin 1 inhibitor (anakinra), B-cell-targeted therapy (rituximab), an inhibitor of T-cell costimulation (abatacept), and an interleukin 6 inhibitor (tocilizumab).
- Altering disease progression with DMARDs and/or biologic agents has substantial impact on pain as well as other symptoms of disease.
- Some RA patients may receive intra-articular corticosteroid injections, for example, if one or two joints flare.
- Pain management is not limited to NSAIDs. Other types of analgesics are also prescribed.
- Ambulatory/assistive devices, orthotics/splints, physical/occupational therapy, exercise, rest, and self-help programs are nonpharmacologic agents that are helpful in treatment of pain and maintenance of functional status.

Do the benefits of opioid analgesics outweigh the risks in patients with persistent pain due to RA? *Bottom line:* Weak opioids (such as codeine and tramadol) may be effective in the short-term management of RA pain, but adverse effects are common and may outweigh the benefits; alternative analgesics should be considered first.

BIBLIOGRAPHY

Cush JJ, Kavanaugh AF, eds. *Rheumatology Diagnosis and Therapeutics*. Philadelphia: Lippincott Williams & Wilkins; 2000.

Ruddy S, Harris E, Sledge CB, eds. *Kelley's Textbook of Rheumatology*. Philadelphia: WB Saunders; 2001.

Whittle SL, Richards BL, Buchbinder R. Opioid analgesics for rheumatoid arthritis pain. *JAMA*. 2013;309(5):485–486. doi:10.1001/jama.2012.193412.

39 CANCER PAIN

Rodolfo Gebhardt, MD
T. Joel Berry, MD
Allen W. Burton, MD

EPIDEMIOLOGY

- The World Health Organization (WHO) estimates that by 2030, there will be 26 million new cases of cancer worldwide. As new treatments increase survival rates, cancer patients will live longer with pain from the disease and its treatment.
- Cancer pain and its undertreatment are epidemic. Approximately 59% of patients undergoing treatment for cancer and 64% of patients with advanced cancer have pain. Persistent pain is prevalent in 33% of patients who have completed curative anticancer therapy. On average, 43% of patients with cancer suffer from undertreated pain. Most (an estimated 70%) cancer pain is due to tumor involvement with soft tissue, viscera, nerves, or bone and due to structural changes in the body secondary to the tumor (eg, muscle spasm or imbalance).
- Up to 25% of cancer pain is due to cancer therapy, including chemotherapy, radiotherapy, immunotherapy, and/or surgery.
- Cancer pain can be categorized as: (1) pain caused by the cancer itself, (2) pain related to treatment, and (3) other pain, including osteoarthritis, degenerative disc disease, and diabetic neuropathy.
- The impact of cancer pain is multiplied by the interaction of pain and its treatments with other common cancer symptoms: fatigue, dyspnea, weakness, nausea, constipation, and impaired cognition.
- Nearly all cancer-related pain is associated with and magnified by psychologic and spiritual distress.

ASSESSMENT

- The patient with cancer requires a careful and detailed history and physical examination to elicit the true nature of the pain. In addition, if there are multiple pain complaints, then each pain issue needs to be considered separately.
- When compiling a pain history in a patient with cancer, the history must include the standard pain questions:
  - Location
  - Intensity
  - Quality
  - Duration/temporal pattern
  - Initiating factors
  - Radiating components
  - Previous therapy or treatments (pharmacologic and nonpharmacologic)
  - Associated psychologic components
  - Associated social/family components
  - Other chronic pain diagnoses and treatments
- Questions must also be asked about the cancer diagnosis, progression, and treatments because cancer treatments and metastasis can cause pain (eg, chemotherapy and radiotherapy can induce neuropathies; thoracotomy and mastectomy can lead to postoperative pain syndromes).
- Any new pain in a patient with cancer is assumed to be disease progression until proven otherwise.
- The physical examination should also be detailed, as specific sensory or motor exam findings may indicate tumor location (primary or metastatic).
- After the physical examination, imaging can confirm the diagnosis:
  - Plain films: fractures, visceral pathology
  - Bone scans: increased bone growth or destruction
  - Magnetic resonance imaging: evaluation of soft tissue pathology, especially spinal neoplastic disease
  - Computed tomography: bone pathology
  - Positron emission tomography–computed tomography (PET-CT)
  - Electromyography/nerve conduction studies

MANAGEMENT

TREATMENT GUIDELINES

- The most effective form of treatment of any cancer-related pain is treatment of the cancer itself, which in the majority of cases reduces or eliminates the pain. Early intervention is the key to preventing the development of posttherapy neuralgias as well as to helping the patient tolerate potentially difficult oncologic treatment protocols. Appropriately dosed opioids are the cornerstone of effective cancer pain management. Management of opioid-related side effects and the appropriate use of adjuvants and procedures complete the treatment armamentarium.
- The control of pain involves modifying the source of the pain, altering the central perception of pain, and blocking the transmission of the pain to the central nervous system. An individual care plan must be designed and implemented, and reassessed at regular intervals to ensure that both the quality and the quantity of a patient's life are optimized.
- Cancer pain can be treated effectively in 85%–95% of patients with an integrated program of systemic, pharmacologic, and anticancer therapy. The remaining

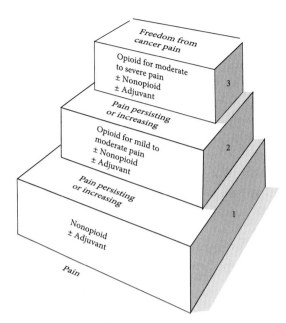

FIG. 39-1. WHO analgesic ladder for the treatment of cancer pain.

patients can be appropriately treated with invasive procedures.

- Several algorithms exist for the treatment of cancer-related pain. The first was WHO's analgesic ladder (Figure 39-1). A more detailed treatment guideline was later published by the National Cancer Care Network (NCCN). Use of a cancer pain treatment algorithm by oncologists improves cancer patients' symptom control.

- Although oversimplified, the basic tenets of the WHO analgesic ladder remain helpful in the treatment of cancer pain: begin with a nonopioid analgesic (aspirin, acetaminophen, nonsteroidal anti-inflammatory drugs [NSAIDs]) and increase to intermediate or stronger opioids and/or adjuvant medications as needed.

- Our group within the University of Texas MD Anderson Cancer Center has published a modified and condensed version of the NCCN guideline that fits on a pocket card (Figure 39-2). Our recommendation is to prescribe stronger opioids and adjuvants sooner and to reassess treatment frequently to deal with increased pain levels. One need not start on the bottom rung of the ladder. In cases of severe pain, it is sometimes appropriate to initiate strong opioids and/or adjuvant analgesics.

- The specifics of which opioid, starting dose, and adjuvants to use rest largely in the realm of the art of medicine; little comparative evidence exists that would permit us to recommend specific analgesic combinations and doses.

Cancer Pain

Guidelines Change Over Time—For Updates Refer to www.mdanderson.org

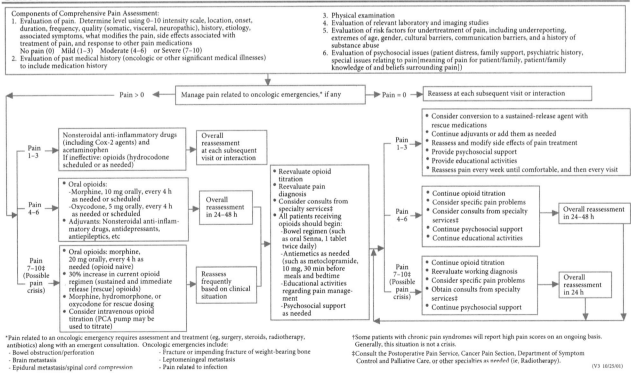

FIG. 39-2. MD Anderson cancer pain treatment guideline. Reproduced from Bruera E, Burton A, Cleeland C. Cancer Pain Guidelines. Houston: University of Texas MD Anderson Cancer Center; 2001.

TABLE 39-1   Common Nonopioid and Opioid Analgesics

MEDICATION CLASS	MEDICATION	ADULT STARTING DOSE
Nonopioids	Acetaminophen	325–650 mg PO q4–6h
	Tramadol	50–100 mg PO q6h
NSAIDs	Ibuprofen	400–800 mg PO q6–8h
	Salicylate	500–750 mg PO q8–12h
	Naproxen	250–500 mg PO q8–12h
	Ketorolac	15–30 mg IV q6–8h
COX-2-specific	Celecoxib	100–200 mg PO q12–24h
NSAIDs	Rofecoxib	12.5–25 mg PO q24h
	Valdecoxib	10–20 mg PO q24h
Short-acting opioids	Hydrocodone	5–10 mg PO q4h prn
	Morphine	10–30 mg PO q3–4h prn
	Oxycodone	5–10 mg PO q3–4h prn
	Hydromorphone	1–3 mg PO q3–4h prn
	Transmucosal fentanyl (Actiq)	200–400 µg TM q3–8h
Long-acting opioids	Morphine controlled-release	15 mg PO q12h
	Oxycodone controlled-release	10 mg PO q12h
	Transdermal fentanyl (Duragesic)	25 µg/h, replaced q72h
	Methadone	2.5–10 mg PO q8–12h

- In general, treatment intensity may be based on pain reported on a written or verbal numeric or facial expression pain intensity scale and on the patient's degree of opioid tolerance. On the analog/numeric pain scale, where 0 is no pain and 10 is the worst pain imaginable, pain scaled 1–3 corresponds to mild pain, 4–6 refers to moderate pain, and 7–10 signifies severe pain.
- Mild-to-moderate opioids include tramadol, codeine, and hydrocodone, and strong opioids include morphine, oxycodone, oxymorphone, fentanyl, hydromorphone, tapentadol, and methadone. Common nonopioid, adjuvants (coanalgesics), and opioid analgesics are described in Table 39-1.

SELECTING THE APPROPRIATE ANALGESIC DOSE

- The appropriate analgesic dose depends on the pain scale result and history of opioid therapy. The efficacy of the therapy should be periodically reassessed, with dosing adjusted as necessary.

Nonopioid Analgesics

- The nonopioid analgesics (WHO Step 1) are characterized by a ceiling effect, above which there is no additive affect. NSAIDs achieve analgesia mainly by decreasing circulating levels of inflammatory mediators released at the site of tissue injury—specifically by

inhibiting the enzyme cyclooxygenase (COX). COX catalyzes the conversion of arachidonic acid to prostaglandins and leukotrienes, which sensitizes nerves to painful stimuli. COX-2-specific NSAIDs produce analgesia and anti-inflammation activity equivalent to those of nonselective NSAIDs, without the COX-1 side effects of gastrointestinal toxicity and inhibition of platelet aggregation.

Weak to Moderate Opioids

- The so-called weak- to moderate-potency opioids (WHO Step 2) are frequently combined with an NSAID or acetaminophen to create a synergistic effect. The limitation of this combination therapy is that there is an analgesic ceiling associated with NSAIDs as well as a dose-dependent toxicity. It is at this step that we employ the analgesic adjuvants listed in Table 39-2. Such adjuvants treat concurrent symptoms that exacerbate pain, produce independent analgesia for specific types of pain, and increase the analgesic efficacy of opioids.
- Note that the following weak to moderate opioids are listed on the Drug Enforcement Agency's Schedule 3; thus, prescriptions may be phoned in, written for multiple refills, and written on standard prescription pads:
  ○ Acetaminophen with codeine is another commonly prescribed weak opioid.

TABLE 39-2   Adjuvant Analgesics

MEDICATION CLASS	MEDICATION	ADULT STARTING DOSE
Anticonvulsants	Gabapentin (Neurontin)	100–300 mg PO qhs, with dose escalations to 3600 mg/d divided tid
	Tiagabine (Gabitril)	2–4 mg PO q24h, with dose escalations to 56 mg/d divided bid to qid
Tricyclic antidepressants	Amitriptyline (Elavil)	10–25 mg PO every night
	Nortriptyline (Pamelor)	10–25 mg PO every morning
	Desipramine (Norpramin)	10–25 mg PO every morning
Selective serotonin reuptake inhibitors	Sertraline (Zoloft)	25–50 mg PO qd
	Paroxetine (Paxil)	10–20 mg PO qd
Psychostimulants	Dextroamphetamine (Dexedrine)	5–10 mg PO every morning and noon
	Methylphenidate (Ritalin)	5–10 mg PO every morning and noon
Bisphosphonates	Etidronate (Didronel)	5–10 mg/kg/d PO*,†
	Pamidronate (Aredia)	90 mg IV every month*,†

*Diener KM. Bisphosphonates for controlling pain from metastatic bone disease. *Am J Health Syst Pharm.* 1996;53:1917–1927.

†LaCivita CL. Pain management for bone metastases. *Am J Health Syst Pharm.* 1996;53:1907.

○ Tramadol is a weak μ agonist available as a sole agent or in combination with acetaminophen.

"Strong" Opioids

- The pure opioid agonists (WHO Step 3) do not have a ceiling effect and are dose-limited only by dose-dependent side effects. Opioid analgesics bind to the μ receptor. Investigators have identified multiple $μ_1$ receptors, and this genetic polymorphism may result in varying expression of these receptors in different patients, which would explain why some patients respond better to one opioid class than to another.
  - ○ Morphine, the gold standard of opioid analgesics, forms the basis by which all other classes of opioids are compared. Morphine is converted to morphine-3-glucuronide (M3G) and morphine-6-glucuronide (M6G) via glucuronyl transferase in the liver. M3G has low affinity for the opioid receptor but may be responsible for the neuroexcitatory toxic effects of morphine. M6G has potent opioid activity but is converted in a smaller quantity than other metabolites. Because these metabolites are renally excreted, they should be avoided in patients with renal impairment. Morphine is available in immediate- and controlled-release formulations. It is also available in parenteral and preservative-free formulations (suitable for neuraxial use).
  - ○ Oxycodone, which is potent when used as a sole agent, is also combined with acetaminophen or an NSAID, which limits the dose. It is currently available in immediate- and sustained-release oral preparations.
  - ○ Oxymorphone is a semisynthetic opioid and is about three times more potent than morphine. Because it avoids metabolism by the CYP450 system, drug–drug interactions are less likely to occur. Dose adjustment is not recommended in patients with hepatic dysfunction. However, oxymorphone dosing should be decreased in patients with renal impairment.
  - ○ Tapentadol is unique in that it is a μ-opioid receptor agonist, norepinephrine reuptake inhibitor, and serotonin reuptake inhibitor. Its multiple mechanisms of action allow for its use in a wide variety of pain conditions. Glucuronidation serves as the primary means of metabolism by converting tapentadol to an inactive metabolite.
  - ○ Hydromorphone is available in oral and parenteral formulations (including preservative-free formulations suitable for neuraxial use). The controlled-release formulation available in other countries will soon be sold in the United States.

TABLE 39-3 Transdermal Fentanyl Equivalency Ratio*

IV/SC MORPHINE (mg)	ORAL MORPHINE (mg)	TRANSDERMAL FENTANYL (μg/h)
20	60	25
40	120	50
60	180	75
80	240	100

*Data from Bruera E, Burton A, Cleeland C. *Cancer Pain Guidelines.* Houston: University of Texas MD Anderson Cancer Center; 2001.

- ○ Fentanyl is a semisynthetic opioid available in transdermal, parenteral, buccal, neuraxial, and transmucosal formulations that is useful in the management of severe cancer pain in the opioid-tolerant patient (Table 39-3). Transdermal and oral transmucosal fentanyl citrate (Actiq) are difficult to titrate and should be reserved for patients with chronic pain who have exhausted oral opioid options. The suggested equivalency ratio is 100:1 (oral morphine:fentanyl transdermal patch in milligrams per 24 h). It is important to prescribe breakthrough doses of another opioid with initiation of the patch. The patch dose should not be increased more frequently than every three days, and the increase should be based on the additional amount of breakthrough opioid required during a three-day period. When rotating a patient off the fentanyl patch, a new opioid should be started 12 h after removal of the patch. Breakthrough medication should be available during and after this critical period.
- ○ Methadone, a long-acting opioid available parenterally and orally, has the added benefit of creating an N-methyl-D-aspartate (NMDA) receptor antagonizing effect for cancer pain patients with neuropathic pain. Methadone has great utility when used cautiously in low doses and titrated upward carefully.

ROUTES OF ADMINISTRATION

- In patients not responding to oral medications (or unable to use their gastrointestinal tract), the other routes of administration are:
  - ○ Sublingual/transmucosal
  - ○ Rectal
  - ○ Intramuscular
  - ○ Subcutaneous
  - ○ Transdermal
  - ○ Transmucosal
  - ○ Parenteral
  - ○ Intracerebroventricular
  - ○ Epidural/subarachnoid

INCIDENT PAIN

- The appropriate interval for dosing depends on the opioid used and the route of administration, and dosing of short- or long-acting opioids should be scheduled at intervals that prevent breakthrough pain.
- Each incident dose should be approximately 10% of the total daily opioid dose.
- During imaging studies or procedural interventions for which a patient's positioning is not tolerated due to pain, fentanyl (transmucosal lozenge or buccal tablet) can be used for near immediate analgesic relief.
- Long-acting dosage forms of morphine sulfate (Oramorph) and oxycodone (OxyContin) are given every 8–12 h. Breakthrough doses of immediate-release products should always be prescribed in conjunction with these long-acting pharmaceuticals.

OPIOID SIDE EFFECTS

- The most common opioid side effects include nausea and vomiting, constipation, cognitive impairment, myoclonus, sedation, and respiratory depression. These side effects are generally self-limiting, except for constipation, which can be managed with a consistent regimen of bowel stimulants and laxatives.
- When starting a patient on opioids, we prophylactically administer ondansetron for nausea and Senokot S for constipation.
- Sedation can be managed by decreasing the dose of the opioid, rotating opioids, or adding a psychostimulant.

OPIOID ROTATION

- The long-term use of opioid analgesics may lead to opioid tolerance, but tolerance to a specific opioid does not predict tolerance to equianalgesic doses of other opioids—a finding referred to as "incomplete cross-tolerance." Table 39-4 presents the equianalgesic doses for opioid conversion. Due to incomplete cross-tolerance it is important to decrease the daily dose of a new opioid by 30%–50%.
- Methadone is unique in its nonlinear conversion ratios to morphine. The conversion ratio to morphine can range from 1:1 to 15:1. Because of its long half-life, methadone must be titrated upward slowly and with caution, using a short-acting opioid liberally until the methadone therapeutic dose is attained.

ANALGESIC ADJUVANTS: NEUROPATHIC PAIN

- Neuropathic pain can be caused by the direct invasion of tumor into nervous structures, by antineoplastic therapy, or by other cancer-related causes including:
  - Chemotherapy-induced peripheral neuropathies (ie, cisplatin, paclitaxel, and vincristine)
  - Radiotherapy-induced plexopathies (brachial, lumbar, and sacral)
  - Postherpetic neuralgia
- Up to 40% of cancer patients suffer from neuropathic pain. Many symptoms of neuropathic pain (ie, burning, lancing, electric shock-like allodynia and hyperalgesia) can be managed with adjuvant medications, including:
  - Antiepileptic drugs (gabapentin, pregabalin, and oxcarbazepine)
  - Heterocyclic antidepressants (amitriptyline, nortriptyline, and desipramine)
  - Serotonin–norepinephrine reuptake inhibitors (duloxetine and venlafaxine)

TABLE 39-4   Conversion Table for Opioids*

OPIOID	IV/SC OPIOID TO IV/SC MORPHINE	IV/SC MORPHINE TO IV/SC OPIOID	ORAL OPIOID TO ORAL MORPHINE	ORAL MORPHINE TO ORAL OPIOID
Hydromorphone	5	0.2	5	0.2
Meperidine	0.13	8	0.1	10
Levorphanol	5	2	5	0.2
Oxycodone	—	—	1.5	0.7
Hydrocodone	—	—	0.5	2

Oral morphine to IV/SC morphine: *divide by* 3; IV/SC morphine to oral morphine: *multiply by* 3

Example

To convert from hydromorphone 4 mg PO every 4 h plus two extra 2-mg doses of hydromorphone per day (4 mg) to oral morphine immediate-release (IR):

1. Total opioid amount: oral hydromorphone equals 28 mg/d
2. 28 mg × 5 = oral morphine 140 mg/d; 30% decrease = oral morphine 98 mg/d
3. New regimen: oral morphine IR 100 mg divided by 6 doses = oral morphine IR 15 mg every 4 h around the clock plus 7.5 mg every 2 h prn for breakthrough pain

*Data from Bruera E, Burton A, Cleeland C. *Cancer Pain Guidelines*. Houston: University of Texas MD Anderson Cancer Center; 2001.

○ Topical anesthetics (ie, lidocaine, lidoderm patch)
○ NMDA receptor antagonists (ie, dextromethorphan, methadone, and ketamine)

ANALGESIC ADJUVANTS: OTHER

- COX-2-specific NSAIDs produce analgesia and anti-inflammation activity equivalent to those of the non-selective NSAIDs, without the COX-1 side effects of gastrointestinal toxicity and inhibition of platelet aggregation.
- Any of the serotonin-specific reuptake inhibitors are useful in patients with situational depression.
- Low-dose benzodiazepines or butyrophenones (ie, haloperidol) are useful in treating anxiety.
- Low-dose heterocyclic antidepressants or the sedative-hypnotics (eg, zolpidem [Ambien] and zaleplon [Sonata]) are sometimes used to treat insomnia.
- For nausea, we optimize the bowel regimen and use ondansetron scheduled and as needed.
- For appetite stimulation, we use low-dose dronabinol (Marinol 2.5–5 mg twice daily).

INTERVENTIONAL PAIN MANAGEMENT

- When other analgesic measures have failed to provide adequate pain control or cause intolerable side effects, or when the risk:benefit ratio is highly favorable for a certain procedure, we use the following interventional techniques. The timing of the use of such modalities is controversial.
  ○ Neurolytic blocks (eg, celiac plexus block for pancreatic pain).
  ○ Neuraxial analgesia in the form of epidural Port-A-Cath or tunneled catheters, intrathecal tunneled catheters, intraventricular catheters, or implanted intrathecal catheter/pump systems. Several factors play a key role in patient selection for intrathecal therapy. One must consider a psychological evaluation, patient's comorbidities, prior medical regimens, oral medication side effects, discussion with patient's oncologist, and a successful intrathecal trial. After completion of the aforementioned factors, physicians can utilize intrathecal therapy for the treatment of cancer pain.
  ○ Vertebroplasty (for painful compression fractures or painful metastasis).
- We generally go to neuraxial techniques when the patient has poor analgesia or intolerable opioid side effects despite opioid rotation.
- Patients using neuraxial pain control methods must receive adequate follow-up to have their pumps refilled and/or dosage adjusted as needed. Frequently, drug combinations including local anesthetics and clonidine are useful in neuropathic pain states.
- Finally, in desperate situations where the pain is difficult to control, it may be appropriate to perform neurosurgical destructive procedures such as:
  ○ Anterolateral cordotomy (spinothalamic tractotomy)
  ○ Stereotactic mesencephalotomy
  ○ Midline myelotomy
  ○ Hypophysectomy
  ○ Dorsal root entry zone lesions

PALLIATIVE CARE

- Palliative care is the active, total care of patients whose disease is not responsive to curative treatments. Control of symptoms (including pain) and provision of psychological, social, and spiritual support are paramount. The goal of palliative care is to achieve the best possible quality of life for patients and their families. This growing area of medicine is often practiced in inpatient units, with a transitional approach that involves sending some patients home with home hospice care. This is a very patient-centered, multidisciplinary method of caring for a dying patient.

CONCLUSION

- As in other areas of pain management, the tenets of good cancer pain management are similar to those of any sound medical practice.
- Examine the patient carefully, set realistic treatment goals, and then administer medications and interventional treatments in concord with the patient and the oncologist.
- Remember to enlist the help of consultants with difficult cases (including specialists in physical medicine, hospice, and palliative care).

BIBLIOGRAPHY

Benedetti C, Brock C, Cleeland C, et al. NCCN practice guidelines for cancer pain. *Oncology.* 2000;11:135–150.

Benitez-Rosario MA, Salinas-Martin A, Aguirre-Jaime A, Perez-Mendez L, Feria M. Morphine–methadone opioid rotation in cancer patients: analysis of dose ratio predicting factors. *J Pain Symptom Manage.* 2009;37(6):1061–1068.

Bennett MI, Rayment C, Hjermstad M, et al. Prevalence and aetiology of neuropathic pain in cancer patients: a systematic review. *Pain.* 2012;153:359–365.

Boyle P, Levin BE, eds; IARC. *World Cancer Report.* Lyon: IARC Press; 2008.

Bruera E, Burton A, Cleeland C. *Cancer Pain Guidelines.* Houston: University of Texas MD Anderson Cancer Center; 2001.

Bruera E, Kim H. Cancer pain. *JAMA.* 2003;290(18):2476–2479.

Chamberloin K, Cottle M, Neville R, Tan J. Oral oxymorphone for pain management. *Ann Pharmacother.* 2004;1(7):1144–1152.

Chang HM. Cancer pain management. *Med Clin North Am.* 1999;83(3):711–736.

Cleeland CS, Gonin R, Hatfield AK, et al. Pain and its treatment in outpatients with metastatic cancer. *N Engl J Med.* 1994;330:592–596.

Deandrea S, Montanari M, Moja L, Apolone G. Prevalence of undertreatment in cancer pain. A review of published literature. *Ann Oncol.* 2008;19:1985–1991.

Deer TR, Smith HS, Burton AW, et al. Comprehensive consensus based guidelines on intrathecal drug delivery systems in the treatment of pain caused by cancer pain. *Pain Physician.* 2011;14:E283–E312.

DuPen SL, Du Pen AR, Polissar N, et al. Implementing guidelines for cancer pain management: results of a randomized controlled clinical trial. *J Clin Oncol.* 1999;17:361–370.

Hewitt DJ. The management of pain in the oncology patient. *Obstet Gynecol Clin.* 2001;28(4):819–846.

Levy MH. Drug therapy: pharmacologic treatment of cancer pain. *N Engl J Med.* 1996;335:1124–1132.

Lucas LK, Lipman AG. Recent advances in pharmacotherapy for cancer pain management. *Cancer Pract.* 2002;10(suppl 1):S14–S20.

Norton JA, Edwards AD. Pain in adults with cancer. In: *The Massachusetts General Hospital Handbook of Pain Management.* Philadelphia: Lippincott Williams & Wilkins; 2002; 453–469.

Parsons HA, de la Cruz M, El Osta B, et al. Methadone initiation and rotation in the outpatient setting for patients with cancer pain. *Cancer.* 2010;116:520–528.

Patrick DL, Engelberg RA, Curtis JR. Evaluating the quality of dying and death. *J Pain Symptom Manage.* 2001;22:717–726.

Portenoy RK. Treatment of cancer pain. *Lancet.* 2011;377:2236–2247.

Reddy SK, Shanti BF. Cancer pain: assessment and management. *Prim Care Cancer.* 2000;20:44–52.

Tzschentke TM, Christoph T, Kögel B, et al. (−)-(1R, 2R)-3-(3-Dimethylamino-1-ethyl-2-methyl-propyl)-phenol hydrochloride (tapentadol HCl): a novel μ-opioid receptor agonist/norepinephrine reuptake inhibitor with broad-spectrum analgesic properties. *J Pharmacol Exp Ther.* 2007;323:265–276.

van den Beuken-van Everdingen MH, de Rijke JM, Kessels AG, Schouten HC, van Kleef M, Patijn J. Prevalence of pain in patients with cancer: a systematic review of the past 40 years. *Ann Oncol.* 2007;18:1437–1449.

Walker PW, Palla S, Pei BL, et al. Switching from methadone to a different opioid: what is the equianalgesic dose ratio? *J Palliat Med.* 2008;11(8):1103–1108.

Walker SM, Goudas LM, Cousins MJ, et al. Combination spinal analgesic chemotherapy: a systemic review. *Anesth Analg.* 2002;95:674–715.

40 CENTRAL PAIN

Michael G. Byas-Smith, MD

BRAIN

ISCHEMIC INJURY

Description of Problem

- Central poststroke pain (CPSP) is a common ischemic-induced chronic pain syndrome. The injury may occur in a variety of regions in the brain including the brainstem, thalamus, and somatosensory cortex.
- The diagnosis of CPSP is made after identifying a definable brain lesion with imaging in concert with characteristic painful symptoms that do not result from peripheral disease. Keep in mind that patients may present with more than one foci of pain pathogenesis including central and peripheral combinations.
- The painful region may encompass a small area of the body but typically is in a large regional area of the body that does not follow a sclerotomal, myotomal, or dermatomal distribution.
- The onset of pain is variable including immediate and delayed. The duration of CPSP unfortunately may be intractable and effective treatments options that reliably eliminate symptoms are limited.
- No pain quality is pathognomonic for central pain, but constant burning, acute paroxysmal shooting, and aching sensations are common descriptions.
- The intensity of the pain is always extreme but in most cases quality of life is significantly impacted.
- Sleep disturbance, depression, and irritability frequently are significant findings.

Pathophysiology of Pain

- Most investigators agree that central CPSP is caused by perturbations of the somatosensory systems.
- Central pain is independent of abnormalities in muscle function, coordination, vision, hearing, vestibular functions, and higher cortical functions.
- Nonsensory symptoms are not necessary for the development of central pain.
- The two most widely discussed mechanisms for these sensory changes are the ectopic activity hypothesis and the neuroplastic change, synaptic reorganization hypothesis.
  - The mechanism for the ectopic activity involves the spontaneous or evoked discharge of neurons linked to the processing of somatosensory information. As a consequence of an imbalance in sensory neuronal

input and altered synaptic connections, the patient perceives discomfort.

○ The neuroplastic changes and hypersensitivity states which occur during and after nerve injury to the somatosensory system result from the activation of *N*-methyl-D-aspartate (NMDA) receptors by excitatory amino acids.

MULTIPLE SCLEROSIS (MS)

DESCRIPTION OF PROBLEM

- The body region involved in the ongoing pain virtually always displays thermal sensory abnormalities often with cold or tactile allodynia.
- Chronic pain in MS patients is a common finding and is believed to be from a central nervous system origin. Greater than 60% of patients with MS suffer chronic pain with at least 25% suffering from central pain mechanisms.
- Like other central pain syndromes, patients complain of a variety of different symptoms and body locations.
  ○ The qualities of pain include aching, burning, cutting, cramp-like sensations, prickling, and others.
  ○ The symptoms can be reported as being deep, superficial, or a combination of the two. The symptoms can be intermittent but the more severe cases involve constant nagging pain.
  ○ The location of the pain can vary but very commonly the patients will report symptoms in the lower extremities and patients will have pain involving multiple areas of the body upper extremities and lower extremities and truncal distribution of painful symptoms.
  ○ A trigeminal neuralgia and migraine-type headaches also commonly develop in patients with MS.

PATHOPHYSIOLOGY OF PAIN

- The diagnosis of central pain in MS is based partly on exclusion and partly on specific criteria.
  ○ Patients who have nontrigeminal central pain and duration of pain that is greater than six months and no other known causes or suspected source of peripheral generators of pain
  ○ This in combination with the diagnostic criteria for MS such as radiologic demonstrative lesions showing demyelination in the central nervous system
- Patients can present with a range of neurological disabilities but there has not been any evidence to suggest that severity of the neuromuscular symptoms correlates with the intensity and incidents of pain.

- The demyelinating plaques that characterize MS can occur throughout the central nervous system and are frequently found in the spinal cord.
- The central pain from MS is thought to be secondary to disruptions in the spinal thalamic track pathways.
- The lesions found in MS patients are thought to be the source of the ongoing pain, creating an imbalance and neuronal modulation of sensory information, particularly in regions involving pain and/or the involvement of abnormal discharges from sensory fibers and pathways native to the central nervous system.

SPINAL CORD

TRAUMATIC, ISCHEMIC INJURY

Description of Problem

- Painful sensations are common and troublesome sequelae of paraplegia and quadriplegia following a spinal cord injury.
- The incidence of pain in this population has been reported to be as high as 96%.
- The prevalence of severe debilitating pain is present in a smaller percentage of patients and often is resistant to a variety of therapeutic interventions.
- A number of classification schemes for the different types of painful syndromes have been devised over the years. In general, this schema divides the syndromes into categories related to symptoms occurring at the level of the injury below the cord injury and secondary to pathological changes that occur as a consequence of the trauma.
- Of these syndromes, the central dysesthetic pain is by far the more difficult to manage.
- Dysesthetic pain syndrome has been defined as the presence of pain caudad to the site of injury occurring for a period of time at least four weeks postinjury with the initial presentation of pain typically within the first year. The prevalence of dysesthetic pain is greatest in patients with incomplete quadriplegia with pain sensations commonly referred to the lower extremities and posterior trunk below the zone of injury.
- Using the McGill Pain Questionnaire the most commonly used descriptors of the sensations include cutting, burning, piercing, radiating, cruel, and nagging.

Pathophysiology of Pain

- The physiological hypothesis concerning this altered neurological state has not varied considerably over the past 50 years.
- These mechanisms include:
  ○ Loss of balance between different sensory channels

TABLE 40-1   Mechanism-directed Treatment Approach to Central Pain

SYMPTOM/SIGN	POSSIBLE MECHANISM	MODULATING TREATMENT
Spontaneous pain (paroxysms)	Ectopic activity	Anticonvulsants (gabapentin, lamotrigine, topiramate, carbamazepine, oxcarbazepine), antiarrythmics (lidocaine, mexiletine)
Spontaneous pain (burning, aching)	Sensitized nociceptors?	Tricyclic antidepressants (desipramine, amitriptyline), α_2-receptor agonists (clonidine), opioids (morphine, methadone), dorsal column simulation
Sympathetically maintained pain (burning, aching)	Pathological activity in sympathetic nervous system	α-Receptor antagonists (phentolamine, prazosin), α_2-receptor agonists (Zanaflex, clonidine), ganglionic blockade
Spatial and temporal summation	Progressive discharges in spinal neurons	NMDA receptor antagonists (ketamine, dextromethorphan, amantadine, memantine, methadone)
Thermal allodynia	Central neuroplastic changes due to unmasking of cold-sensitive cells	Tricyclic antidepressants (desipramine, amitriptyline), anticonvulsants (lamotrigine)
Dynamic mechanical allodynia	Neuroplastic changes, synaptic reorganization	NMDA receptor antagonists (ketamine, dextromethorphan, amantadine, memantine, methadone), anticonvulsant (gabapentin)
Static mechanical allodynia	Sensitization of C-nociceptors	Mexiletine, lamotrigine, carbamazepine, opioids
Punctate mechanical allodynia	Neuroplastic changes via Aδ fibers	Antiarrythmics (lidocaine, mexiletine), anticonvulsants (gabapentin, lamotrigine, topiramate, carbamazepine, oxcarbazepine)

○ Loss of spinal inhibitory mechanisms
○ The presence of pattern generators within the injured cord
- The bottom line is that a variety of abnormal electrophysiological and neurochemical abnormalities are potentially at play in any given patient.
- A variety of abnormal sensations are possible, some of which may be more responsive than others (Table 40-1).

CORD LESIONS/SYRINGOMYELIA

Description of Problem

- Syringomyelia is one of several cord lesions that commonly give rise to central pain.
- Its hallmark is the development of an expanding posttraumatic cyst with ascension of the motor and sensory levels, increasing motor disability, and development of new pain.
- Claimed incidences for syringomyelia vary between 1% and 3.2% using clinical criteria in the pre-MRI era and up to 59% using MRI.
- This disorder may take months to years to fully develop and as such is characteristically a late complication of cord injury.
- Patients with this problem usually complain of aching and burning pain at the level of the lesion, sometimes extending above and below the level of the lesion.
- Assessment of sensory and motor functions coupled with magnetic resonance imaging helps determine the diagnosis.
- Continuous escalation in pain intensity is the natural course of pain associated with syringomyelia.
- Surgical intervention to decompress the cyst may not bring the pain under control.

Pathophysiology of Pain

- Despite many hypotheses, the pathophysiology of syringomyelia is still not well understood.
- The advent of MRI techniques has greatly facilitated diagnosing the condition.
- The associated pain is presumably related to disturbances in the somatosensory apparatus of the cord and all the neurophysiological derangements are potentially involved (see Table 40-1).

TREATMENT APPROACHES FOR CENTRAL PAIN SYNDROMES

PHARMACOTHERAPY

Anticonvulsant Therapy

- The anticonvulsant medications have taken center stage in the management of neuropathic pain syndromes in general.
- With the exception of gabapentin and pregabalin, most anticonvulsant drugs presumably relieve neuropathic pain symptoms via sodium channel blockade.
- The newer seizure medications have a much better side effect profile compared with older-generation medications and provide similar levels of analgesia.
- Consequently, patients tolerate the higher doses of drug generally needed to achieve pain relief.
- Drugs such as gabapentin, lamotrigine, and topiramate are examples of drugs that have led the way to greater use of anticonvulsant for nerve injury pain.
- Older-generation drugs such as carbamazepine, phenytoin, and valproate acid are still used but usually as second- and third-line alternatives.
- Unfortunately there are no control studies involving the use of many of these medications in post-spinal

cord injury patients and other central pain syndromes, but the evidence is strong that nerve injury pain is responsive to this therapy.

- There is no clear rationale for choosing one medication over another as the initial treatment, but gabapentin has become the frontline anticonvulsant of choice in many practices throughout the world.

Antidepressant Drugs

- Prior to the advent of second-generation anticonvulsant drugs, tricyclic antidepressant drugs were the frontline, nonopioid treatment for control of central pain.
- It is rare that patients with central pain syndromes or neuropathic pain symptoms from peripheral origins are managed with a single agent.
- Polypharmacy is the method of the day and antidepressant medications should be included in the regimen.
- Parallel to the anticonvulsants, newer antidepressants with fewer side effects have been brought to the market but reports of better or equal analgesic potency in comparison to the older drugs have been slow to come.
- Consequently, amitriptyline, nortryptiline, and desipramine continue to be commonly prescribed for control of central pain.
- These agents are thought to modulate the somatosensory pathways by enhancing the descending inhibitory system.
- Some patients may benefit also from the positive mood-altering effects seen in the higher dose range.

Antiarrhythmic Drugs

- The oral anesthetic antiarrhythmic agents have been shown to be effective in management of neuropathic pain lesions in controlled studies but these drugs, that is, mexiletine, are not well tolerated and can be proarrhythmic in certain populations.
- Mexiletine should be the third or fourth choice when developing a treatment strategy.

Opioids

- There has been considerable controversy over the use of opioid analgesics for chronic management of neuropathic pain syndromes.
- Central pain syndromes tend to be refractory and require higher dosages to realize relief, and the opioids are no exception.
- A number of studies have shown the opioids to be effective in treating neuropathic pain syndromes but very few systematic studies exist.

- Opioid medications in comparison to other therapies including nonpharmacological approaches are rated highest in patient satisfaction among MS patients.
- Opioids have several potential analgesic sites of operation at the spinal cord and brain level of the central nervous system.
- Treatment decisions regarding the use of opioids are, for the most part, based on case reports and clinical experiences but the consensus among pain management specialists is that it is appropriate to use this class of medications chronically to control central pain.
- It is important to remember that patients with central pain syndromes typically will show greater resistance to analgesic therapy when compared with peripheral neuropathies.
- Opioids are the most commonly used medications in MS patients.

NMDA Receptor Antagonists

- Blockade of these receptors and secondary messenger systems can prevent and reverse these hypersensitivity states in animal preparations.
- While not as successful as the anticonvulsants, agents that possess NMDA receptor blocking (ketamine, dextromethorphan, memantine) effects have been utilized clinically with a modicum of success.

Intrathecal Analgesic Therapy

- Continuous infusion of intrathecal medications is used in select cases, particularly for spinal cord injury-induced central pain. Additional investigation is needed to validate any benefit.
- There are a variety of agents that produce acute and chronic relief of symptoms during intrathecal administration including congeners of morphine, baclofen, ziconitide, local anesthetics, and clonidine. Other agents are under investigation.
- Opioids continue to be the primary analgesic agent, but polypharmacy has become the standard approach to therapy.
- Baclofen targets spastic components of the pain while clonidine and ziconitide tend to be most efficacious when neuropathic pain continues to exist.

NEUROMODULATION

Transcutaneous Electrical Nerve Stimulation

- Nerve stimulation treatments have been studied for patients with pain from spinal cord injury.

- So-called TENS unit, or transcutaneous electrical nerve stimulation, has been shown to be effective in patients who experience pain at the level of injury.
- The technique is less effective below the site of injury. These conclusions are based on anecdotal reports in small case series but the therapy is fairly inexpensive and does not induce any significant risk to the patient at trial.

Dorsal Column Stimulation

- Implanted spinal cord stimulators have been used. The published data would suggest that this approach may not be indicated in that the results at this point have been disappointing. Additional study is needed.

Cortical Stimulation

- A variety of cortical stimulation techniques are available and used in clinical practice including deep brain stimulation, transcranial magnetic stimulation, and transcranial direct current stimulation.
- Anecdotal evidence shows efficacy for these techniques, but access to these approaches is limited and only utilized when more conservative techniques have been exhausted.

DORSAL ROOT ENTRY ZONE LESIONING

- The surgical treatments for spine cord lesions have been utilized for many years and are the most common neuroablative technique.
- Additional studies are needed to assess efficacy for this procedure and should be considered only when conservative approaches have been exhausted.

GAMMA KNIFE RADIAL SURGERY

- For severe cases, some institutions are using gamma knife radial surgery (GKS) for treatment of MS-associated trigeminal neuralgia. If successful, the technique will probably be expanded to other central pain disorders.

OTHER ALTERNATIVE APPROACHES TO THERAPY

- A variety of so-called alternative treatments have been studied for these patients including acupuncture, massage, relaxation, and chiropractic techniques.

- Because the traditional therapies have not proven to be effective for most of the patients with severe central pain disorders, a significant number of patients will seek out alternative approaches to controlling their symptoms.
- Cannabinoids are among a growing list of agents that are being tested for use in battling this difficult and debilitating disease. Further research is needed to elucidate the benefit of these therapies.

BIBLIOGRAPHY

Beric A. Central pain and dysesthesia syndrome. *Neurol Clin.* 1998;16:899–918.

Bodley R. Imaging in chronic spinal cord injury—indications and benefits. *Eur J Radiol.* 2002;42:13–53.

Canavero S, Bonicalzi V. Central pain syndrome: elucidation of genesis and treatment. *Expert Rev Neurother.* 2007;7(11): 1485–1497.

Canavero S, Bonicalzi V. *Central Pain Syndrome: Pathophysiology, Diagnosis, and Management.* 2nd ed. Cambridge: Cambridge University Press; 2011:268–283.

Cardenas DD, Turner JA, Warms CA, Marshall HM. Classification of chronic pain associated with spinal cord injuries. *Arch Phys Med Rehabil.* 2002;83:1708–1714.

Davidoff G, Roth E, Guarracini M, Sliwa J, Yarkony G. Function-limiting dysesthetic pain syndrome among traumatic spinal cord injury patients: a cross-sectional study. *Pain.* 1987; 29:39–48.

Foleya PL, Vesterinena HM, Lairdb BJ, et al. Prevalence and natural history of pain in adults with multiple sclerosis: systematic review and meta-analysis. *Pain.* 2013;154:632–642.

Loeser JD, Melzack R. Pain: an overview. *Lancet.* 1999;353:1607–1609.

Mehta S, Orenczuk K, McIntyre A, et al. Neuropathic pain post spinal cord injury part 2: systematic review of dorsal root entry zone procedure. *Top Spinal Cord Inj Rehabil.* 2013;19(1):78–86.

O'Donnell MJ, Diener H, Sacco RL, Panju AA, Vinisko R. Chronic pain syndromes after ischemic stroke: PRoFESS trial. *Stroke.* 2013;44:1238–1243.

Rogers CL, Shetter AG, Ponce FA, Fiedler JA, Smith KA, Speiser BL. Gamma knife radiosurgery for trigeminal neuralgia associated with multiple sclerosis. *J Neurosurg.* 2002;97:529–532.

Warms CA, Turner JA, Marshall HM, Cardenas DD: Treatments for chronic pain associated with spinal cord injuries: many are tried, few are helpful. *Clin J Pain.* 2002;18:154–163.

Wiesenfeld-Hallin Z, Aldskogius H, Grant G, Hao JX, Hokfelt T, Xu XJ. Central inhibitory dysfunctions: mechanisms and clinical implications. *Behav Brain Sci.* 1997;20:420–425.

41 COMPLEX REGIONAL PAIN SYNDROME

Paul J. Christo, MD, MBA
Brian G. Wilhelmi, MD, JD
Raimy R. Amasha, MD
Srinivasa N. Raja, MD

HISTORY

- In 1864, Dr Silas Mitchell and colleagues described a chronic pain syndrome with severe burning pain that followed injury to peripheral nerves from gunshot wounds sustained in the Civil War. Mitchell identified this condition as "causalgia" describing a constant burning pain.
- In 1900, Paul Sudeck described a troublesome painful condition in a limb, associated with swelling, stiffness, and vasomotor instability after trauma. He discovered acute patchy osteoporosis in the affected limb on x-ray imaging, a finding later termed "Sudeck's atrophy."
- Rene Leriche, a French surgeon, decades later connected the sympathetic nervous system (SNS) to causalgia by noting that sympathectomy provided pain relief in many of his patients. He termed the condition "reflex sympathetic dystrophy (RSD)."
- "RSD," however, is a misnomer as it implies a sole reflex mechanism caused by a hyperactive SNS.
- To incorporate new pathophysiologic evidence and establish uniform terminology and diagnostic criteria, the International Association for the Study of Pain (IASP) proposed taxonomy that grouped the disorders under the term "complex regional pain syndromes." Type I CRPS corresponds to RSD and occurs without an identifiable nerve lesion. Type II (previously "causalgia") results from a specific nerve injury.
- CRPS is a broad enough term to allow for sympathetically maintained pain (SMP) and sympathetically independent pain (SIP), both of which may contribute to a varying extent in the pain associated with CRPS types I and II.

EPIDEMIOLOGY

- CRPS may be triggered by a variety of insults, such as trauma, surgery, inflammation, stroke, nerve injury, and immobilization. Collectively, the evidence points to CRPS being a multifactorial disorder that is associated with an aberrant host response to tissue injury. No correlation exists between the severity of injury and the resulting painful syndrome.
- CRPS is a rare condition with an incidence between 5.46 and 26.2 cases per 100,000 person years and a prevalence of 20.7–26.2 per 100,000 persons.
- CRPS has been shown to disproportionately affect women over men by ratios ranging from 2.3–5 to 1.
- One study looked at 829 patients, 76% of whom were female, and found the age range from 9 to 85 years (median age 42) with only 12 patients younger than 14 years.
- CRPS in adults may have a predilection for the upper extremity, whereas CRPS in the pediatric population may have an increased predilection for the lower extremity. The clinical diagnosis of CRPS is not solely confined to the extremities. Patients with certain neoplasms of the lung, breast, central nervous system (CNS), and ovary, and patients suffering from stroke or myocardial infarction, may also exhibit signs and symptoms of CRPS.
- Psychological stressors and ineffective coping skills can negatively influence the natural history and severity of CRPS.
- New epidemiological tools including Web-based surveys and advocacy group websites may lead to improved epidemiological data gathering in the near future.

PATHOPHYSIOLOGIC MECHANISMS

- Both CRPS types I and II are hypothesized to be associated with neuronal injury as evidenced by the observations that CRPS I is also associated with posttraumatic focal minimal distal nerve injury affecting nociceptive small fibers as evidenced in recent literature.
- Injury results in abnormal response to neuropeptide release including substance P, glutamate, and bradykinin. These substances along with proinflammatory cytokines increase inflammation, peripheral nerve sensitization, and pain.
- The peripheral nervous system is eventually altered with fewer C-type and Aδ-type cutaneous afferent nerve fibers found within the affected region.
- Peripheral sensitization leads to CNS reorganization and altered nociception. "Windup" of wide-dynamic-range neurons is thought to be responsible for the allodynia and hyperalgesia experienced by patients. The generation of central sensitization and consequent activation of *N*-methyl-D-aspartate (NMDA) receptors may sustain this neuronal hyperexcitability following nerve injury. NMDA antagonists can attenuate the neurochemical cascade that leads to central sensitization and provide pain relief.

- SNS dysfunction has been implicated in the development of CRPS. A warm, red, and swollen affected limb has decreased levels of norepinephrine, which remain decreased even as the limb may become cold, cyanotic, and atrophic. This finding, along with the absence of changes in adrenoceptor density, suggests that a denervation supersensitivity of adrenergic receptors may play a role in the autonomic clinical features and the pain in some patients with CRPS. The SNS may play a role in the generation of pain as adrenergic receptors have been found on nociceptors.
- Systematic review of the literature suggests that CRPS is associated with the presence of a proinflammatory mediator in the blood, blister fluid, and CSF, with differing profiles in acute and chronic cases. In chronic CRPS patients, significant increases in TNF-α, bradykinin, interleukins, interferon-γ, monocyte chemoattractant protein-1 (MCP-1), and soluble receptor for advanced glycation end products (sRAGE) have been found in blood, skin blister fluid, and/or CSF.
- Compelling evidence supports an autoimmune component to CRPS. Serum studies have revealed the presence of autoantibodies reactive to autonomic nerve surface antigens. Treatment with IVIG has been reported to decrease pain, providing support for an autoimmune component to the disease.
- Abnormal nerve sprouting and C-fiber excitation by the SNS may explain the abnormal discharges observed in peripheral nerves following nerve damage.

CLINICAL MANIFESTATIONS

- Great heterogeneity of symptoms exists in patients suffering from CRPS. The diversity of presentation is thought to exist due to multiple causative pathologic mechanisms and an evolution of such processes over time.
- A triad of stages (acute, dystrophic, and trophic) based on progressive signs and symptoms in CRPS has been proposed; however, a prospective study of more than 800 patients with the diagnosis could not substantiate a sequential progression of the syndrome. In a study of 113 patients, cluster analysis revealed three subgroups based on homogeneity of signs, symptoms, and duration of CRPS. These subgroups did not differ in duration of CRPS, which argues against a chronologic progression of the disease. Despite a lack of clear chronologic progression, phenotypic subgroups may endure for research and treatment purposes.
- The signs and symptoms of CRPS reflect changes in the sensory, autonomic, and motor systems.
- Patients frequently describe burning and stinging pain, but other common pain descriptors include "aching, shooting, squeezing, and throbbing." Many report hyperesthesia to ordinary cutaneous stimuli such as contact with clothing or cool breezes.
- Patients often relate pain from nonpainful stimuli (allodynia) or exaggerated responses to mildly painful stimuli (hyperalgesia).
- Temperature changes in the environment may exacerbate the pain. Certain patients may even guard the affected region from cutaneous or thermal stimulation by wearing a glove or sock or exhibiting protective postures.
- Vasomotor disturbances in CRPS include temperature asymmetry and/or skin color changes. Patients may complain that an extremity feels warm and appears red or feels cool and looks dusky or gray.
- Sudomotor changes are seen as an asymmetry of either hyperhidrosis or dryness in the painful region.
- Patients may present with evidence of edema in the affected limb that appears shiny or smooth. Trophic disturbances in the affected limb may present as alteration in skin, nails, or hair pattern.
- If selective sympathetic blockade in the absence of somatic blockade relieves pain and/or allodynia, the patient is regarded as having a sympathetically maintained pain (SMP) component. If sympathetic blockade fails to alleviate the pain associated with CRPS, the syndrome is viewed as SIP. The results of sympathetic blockade need to be interpreted with caution, however, due to the potential for false-positive and false-negative results.
- Motor dysfunction may manifest as dystonia, muscle spasms, tremor, or weakness of the painful muscle groups. More severe cases, of CRPS, can cause muscle atrophy and contractures. Occasionally, patients report myoclonic movements or complain of myofascial pain in the affected region.
- The psychological, emotional, and social toll of CRPS is often disabling to the patient. Many patients experience depression, anxiety, and fear. No well-designed studies have connected these psychological symptoms to the cause or the result of the syndrome, however, and the psychological distress of CRPS is generally considered a result of chronic pain and disability.
- Substantial cost is associated with a CRPS diagnosis and treatment resulting from impaired job performance, unemployment, loss of income and financial difficulties. Patients making insufficient overall treatment progress or in whom comorbid psychiatric disorders/major ongoing life stressors are identified should additionally receive general cognitive–behavioral therapy to address these issues. The psychological component of treatment can work synergistically with medical and physical/occupational therapies to improve function and potentially increase return to the workforce.

DIAGNOSIS

- The IASP criteria, originally published in 1994, for diagnosis of CRPS do not list the number of signs and symptoms needed to make a diagnosis. An investigation of the internal and external validity of the IASP criteria led to the 2003 Budapest criteria.
- The Budapest criteria require a patient to display pain disproportionate to any inciting event (Table 41-1). The patient must additionally display at least one symptom in three of the following four categories: sensory (hyperesthesia, allodynia), vasomotor (temperature or skin color changes), sudomotor/edema (sweating or edema asymmetry in the affected limb), or motor/trophic (trophic changes or motor dysfunction); and at least one objective sign in two or more of the following categories: sensory (hyperalgesia or allodynia), vasomotor (temperature or skin color asymmetry), sudomotor/edema (edema or sweating abnormalities), or motor/trophic (weakness, tremor, dystonia; hair, nail, skin changes). There must not be a diagnosis that better explains the signs and symptoms.
- The fact that the somatosensory symptoms of CRPS type II extend beyond the course of the affected peripheral nerve distinguishes this syndrome from an isolated peripheral mononeuropathy.
- CRPS is a clinical diagnosis, but tests can aid in confirmation and ruling out other diagnosis.
- Testing can clarify the existence of SMP and autonomic dysfunction or can rule out conditions that mimic CRPS.

TABLE 41-1 Budapest Diagnostic Criteria for Complex Regional Pain Syndrome

1. Continuing pain, which is disproportionate to any inciting event
2. **Must report at least one symptom in three of the following four categories:**
   Sensory: Reports of hyperesthesia and/or allodynia
   Vasomotor: Reports of temperature asymmetry and/or skin color changes and/or skin color asymmetry
   Sudomotor/edema: Reports of edema and/or sweating changes and/or sweating asymmetry
   Motor/trophic: Reports of decreased range of motion and/or motor dysfunction (weakness, tremor, dystonia) and/or trophic changes (hair, nail, skin)
3. **Must display at least one sign at time of evaluation in two or more of the following categories:**
   Sensory: Evidence of hyperalgesia (to pinprick) and/or allodynia (to light touch and/or temperature sensation and/or deep somatic pressure and/or joint movement)
   Vasomotor: Evidence of temperature asymmetry (>1°C) and/or skin color changes and/or skin color asymmetry
   Sudomotor/edema: Evidence of edema and/or sweating changes and/or sweating asymmetry
   Motor/trophic: Evidence of decreased range of motion and/or motor dysfunction (weakness, tremor, dystonia) and/or trophic changes (hair, nail, skin)
4. There is no other diagnosis that better explains the signs and symptoms

- Vascular studies can rule out deep vein thrombosis or vascular insufficiency, EMG/NCT can rule out peripheral neuropathy, radiographs and MRI can rule out bone, disc, or soft tissue pathology, and blood testing can rule out infection, cellulitis, or rheumatologic disease.
- Outcome research has not supported the prognostic or therapeutic value of any diagnostic tests.
- Common test include those given in the next subsections.

THERMOGRAPHY

- Uses an infrared thermometer to detect cutaneous thermal changes in two extremities.
- A difference of 1.0°C is considered significant.

QUANTITATIVE SENSORY TESTS

- Measure the intensity of stimuli needed to produce sensations such as touch, vibration, warmth, coolness, and heat and cold pain thresholds.
- These tests are used to help detect sensory abnormalities related to hyperesthesia, hyperalgesia, allodynia, and temperature changes associated with neuropathic pain.

PLAIN RADIOGRAPHS

- Display a patchy osteopenia as soon as two to three weeks after the onset of CRPS.
- As the syndrome progresses, a ground-glass appearance to the bony anatomy reflects generalized osteopenia and cortical erosions.

TRIPLE-PHASE BONE SCINTIGRAPHY

- Intravenous administration of technetium (^{99m}Tc)-labeled diphosphonate or polyphosphate detects osseous abnormalities in the affected limb sooner than do plain films.
- The test is divided into three phases (angiographic images, regional blood pooling, and bony uptake of ^{99m}Tc).
- In CRPS patients, the third phase reveals an abnormally diffuse increased joint uptake affecting the painful extremity only.

SUDOMOTOR TESTING

- The resting sweat output test measures the sweat output of nonstimulated skin in both the painful and nonpainful limbs.

- The quantitative sudomotor axon reflex test measures the sweat output provoked by an electric current and then by cutaneous application of methacholine or acetylcholine.
- In CRPS patients, the latency after electric current stimulation and prolonged sweating is shorter in the affected extremity.

SYMPATHETIC BLOCKS

- Local anesthetic blockade of the sympathetic chain (stellate ganglion block for the upper extremity and lumbar sympathetic block for the lower extremity) is a potentially useful therapeutic tool, especially early in the disease. However, it is not useful as a diagnostic tool.
- A positive response (pain relief), while suggestive of CRPS, is not necessary for diagnosis. Patients with CRPS and SMP who experience symptomatic improvement following local anesthetic sympathetic blocks may benefit from having a series of blocks incorporated into their treatment regimen.
- Due to the risk of false-positive and false-negative tests associated with these procedures, a pharmacological sympathetic block with phentolamine can be used to diagnose a sympathetically maintained component of CRPS. Phentolamine is a nonspecific α-adrenergic receptor antagonist that is infused intravenously at 1 mg/kg over 10 min. A positive response (pain reduction) implies involvement of adrenergic mechanisms in the pain state.

TREATMENT

- Successful treatment of CRPS relies on an aggressive multidisciplinary approach that focuses on pain relief, physical rehabilitation, and control of psychological dysfunction.
- A trusting physician–patient relationship is vital to endure the frustrations of therapeutic trials with the potential for limited benefit or side effects.
- Patients who delay treatment for as little as six months following diagnosis demonstrate poorer long-term prognosis.

PHYSICAL THERAPY

- Expert consensus recommends physical therapy as integral to the treatment of CRPS. Despite this, no randomized controlled trials report a favorable impact on the natural history of CRPS.
- Treatment consists of progressive desensitization following adequate analgesia with techniques such as regional anesthesia or other pain medications.

Desensitization usually includes the use of heat, cold, vibration, massage, and contrast baths.
- Once the patient tolerates these interventions, isometric strengthening exercises are introduced.
- Finally, more aggressive treatment modalities that facilitate mobilization and resumption of activity in the affected limb are instituted: range of motion exercises, isotonic strengthening, and aerobic conditioning.
- Patients may require months to complete this process and also may experience a transient increase in their pain and swelling at the beginning of physiotherapy.
- An overarching principle in the management and treatment of CRPS is the use of interventional procedures to optimize the participation in physical therapy.

PSYCHOLOGICAL THERAPY

- Patients bear a high burden of psychological pathology including depression and anxiety, which contributes heavily to the disability associated with CRPS. Practitioners should at minimum describe the potential for psychological issues and evaluate for Axis I disorders.
- Expert consensus recommends psychotherapy aimed at improving coping skills, relaxation, and biofeedback for pain exacerbations.
- Cognitive–behavioral therapy is designed to refocus dysfunctional thought patterns concerning CRPS pain into patterns to facilitate rehabilitation.
- Mirror therapy, for example, includes exercising the unaffected arm while attending to its reflection in place of the concealed affected arm (multiple movements of the shoulder, elbow, wrist, and hand). Although firm conclusions could not be drawn regarding the efficacy of mirror therapy, there was good-quality evidence(level 2) that graded motor imagery plus medical management was more effective than standard physiotherapy plus medical management for upper or lower limb CRPS I.

PHARMACOTHERAPEUTIC AGENTS

- Few placebo-controlled trials have been performed to assess treatment efficacy in patients with CRPS. Pharmacological treatment is therefore based on studies involving CRPS and other chronic neuralgias.

Corticosteroids and Nonsteroidal Anti-inflammatory Drugs

- Randomized clinical trials have supported the treatment of the acute phase of CRPS with corticosteroids.
- Expert opinion states that nonsteroidal anti-inflammatory drugs (NSAIDs) can be effective in

some patients; however, clinical studies have not demonstrated significant benefit.

- Steroids may suppress CRPS-induced ectopic neural discharges and reduce the inflammatory component of the syndrome.
- Chronic use of steroids, however, is not recommended due to an unfavorable risk–benefit ratio.

Tricyclic Antidepressants

- This class of medication can reduce pain, alleviate depression, and facilitate sleep in patients with CRPS.
- Randomized controlled trials provide evidence that antidepressants treat neuropathic pain in patients with postherpetic neuralgia and diabetic neuropathy.
- The mechanism of action may relate to reuptake inhibition of norepinephrine and serotonin in the CNS. These neurotransmitters may promote the effects of the descending, antinociceptive pathways in the CNS.
- Selective serotonin reuptake inhibitors are less effective in treating neuropathic pain.
- Tricyclic antidepressants can produce cardiac conduction abnormalities, anticholinergic side effects, orthostatic hypotension, and sedation.

Cation Channel Blockers

- Anticonvulsants (gabapentin, carbamazepine, pregabalin) are effective in treating neuropathic pain associated with trigeminal neuralgia and diabetic neuropathy.
- One prospective trial has indicated that gabapentin may provide benefit in spontaneous and evoked pain. Another prospective trial demonstrated no change in pain symptoms, but reduction in sensory deficits.
- Anticonvulsants can produce somnolence, memory impairment, tremors, and ataxia depending on the drug utilized.

Opioids

- The long-term beneficial effects of opioids in neuropathic pain is uncertain. Therefore, opioids are added only when CRPS-related pain responds poorly to other drug therapies.
- If opioids are chosen for treatment, methadone may be selected due to its concomitant blockade of the NMDA receptor. Tramadol with its dual action on serotonin/norepinephrine reuptake and the mu receptor has proven effective in trials for peripheral neuropathy and may be of use in CRPS.

Topical Agents

- Lidocaine patches are useful in treating the allodynic component of CRPS in focal areas of pain.

- DMSO (50% for two months) is a free radical scavenging agent shown in one prospective trial to significantly reduce pain when compared with placebo.
- Capsaicin can produce analgesia in CRPS and peripheral neuropathy through its release and reuptake inhibition of substance P. Patients are often unable to tolerate the burning sensation associated with capsaicin treatment limiting its usefulness.

Other Drug Therapies

- Randomized controlled trials have not confirmed the efficacy of calcium channel blockers, bisphosphonates, oral α-adrenergic agents (prazosin, phenoxybenzamine), calcitonin, clonidine, or muscle relaxants. Studies, however, have yielded favorable evidence that the NMDA antagonist ketamine when given as an IV infusion for 4 h/d for a total of 10 days in patients with CRPS I and II positively correlated with a decrease in pain score. Other studies specifically looking at the S+ enantiomer of ketamine IV continuously for 4.2 days in patients with CRPS I also demonstrated a positive correlation with decrease in pain score.
- The efficacy of longer-term IV ketamine infusion has been substantiated with reports of patients 11 weeks post IV infusion with statistically significant reduction in pain scores. These notable differences were no longer significant at week 12. However, at present, there are insufficient data to draw definite conclusions regarding the neuropathic pain benefit.

SYMPATHETIC BLOCKS

- Sympathetic blockade with local anesthetics for diagnostic or therapeutic reasons has been used for many years as an integral component of the treatment plan for CRPS. The anecdotal literature suggests efficacy, but a systematic review (meta-analysis) revealed weak evidence for sympathetic blockade as a therapeutic modality because fewer than one third of patients obtained complete pain relief. Moreover, none of these studies permitted estimation of the duration of pain relief among those patients who responded to initial sympathetic blockade.
- Despite this finding, patients who derive meaningful relief from diagnostic sympathetic block (SMP) merit a series of frequent sympathetic ganglion blocks with local anesthetic for several weeks.
- Cervical or lumbar sympathetic blocks are performed intermittently or in series. Such blocks should spare both sensory and motor functions, thus permitting patients to participate in physical therapy and rehabilitation.

- Physical therapy is often initiated subsequent to the blocks to maximize the analgesic effects of the blockade.
- If relapses occur or if repetitive blocks produce temporary pain relief, surgical sympathectomy, radiofrequency lesioning, or chemical neurolysis can be considered.
- In patients who fail to respond to sympathetic blocks, epidural or somatic blocks (brachial or lumbar plexus) can facilitate the transition to physical therapy.

REGIONAL AND NEURAXIAL BLOCKADE

- Lumbar, brachial, or epidural local anesthetic injections also block the corresponding sympathetic nerves.
- Similar to sympathetic blocks, somatic blocks can be performed in series or intermittently.
- Great care must be taken to ensure proper range of motion during physical therapy given that affected limbs are anesthetized during regional or neuraxial anesthesia.

NEUROMODULATION AND NEURAXIAL THERAPY

- The mechanism of action of spinal cord stimulation (SCS) is incompletely understood but may involve inhibition of sympathetic function and changes in spinal or supraspinal GABA-mediated neurochemistry.
- Systemic clinical review of 1 RCT and 25 case series involving over 500 patients with implanted SCS in CRPS patients revealed 67% of patients had >50% reduction in pain as assessed on a visual analog scale.
- Two studies have evaluated the cost-effectiveness of SCS in CRPS. SCS was shown to be cost-effective when compared with physical therapy alone or conventional medical management.
- In carefully screened patients with CRPS and in the context of multidisciplinary treatment, SCS can improve health-related quality of life.
- Intrathecal baclofen has been useful in treating dystonia, improving functional use, and nociceptive flexor reflexes associated with CRPS.
- Epidural or intrathecal clonidine administered to CRPS patients reduces associated pain.

CONCLUSION

- While much remains unknown regarding the pathophysiology of CRPS, significant advancement in our understanding has been accomplished over the prior 10 years.

- Many authors wonder whether animal models for SMP can accurately depict the complexity of pain manifested in humans.
- The clinical criteria for CRPS have been refined to improve the sensitivity and specificity of diagnosis, yet further improvement on diagnostic accuracy remains.
- CRPS treatments are diverse, and no single treatment is uniformly effective.
- An aggressive multidisciplinary approach to the alleviation of pain and restoration of function that includes one or more modalities such as medications, sympathetic/somatic blockade, physical therapy, psychological intervention, neuromodulation, and neuraxial analgesia is recommended.

BIBLIOGRAPHY

Bruehl S, Chung OY. Psychological and behavioral aspects of complex regional pain syndrome management. *Clin J Pain.* 2006;22(5):430–437.

Capello ZJ, Kasden ML, Louis DS. Meta-analysis of imaging techniques for the diagnosis of complex regional pain syndrome type I. *J Hand Surg Am.* 2012;37(2):288–296.

Harden RN, Bruehl S, Perez RS, et al. Validation of proposed diagnostic criteria (the "Budapest criteria") for complex regional pain syndrome. *Pain.* 2010;150(2):268–274.

Harden RN, Oaklander AL, Burton AW, et al. Complex regional pain syndrome: practical diagnostic and treatment guidelines, 4th edition. *Pain Med.* 2013;14(2):180–229.

Harris EJ, Schimka KE, Carlson RM. Complex regional pain syndrome of the pediatric lower extremity: a retrospective review. *J Am Podiatr Med Assoc.* 2012;102(2):99–104.

Kahr D, Tschernatsch M, Schmitz K, et al. Autoantibodies in complex regional pain syndrome bind to a differentiation-dependent neuronal surface autoantigen. *Pain.* 2009;143(3): 246–251.

Kemler MA, Barendse GA, van Kleef M, et al. Spinal cord stimulation in patients with chronic reflex sympathetic dystrophy. *N Engl J Med.* 2000;343:618.

Lee BH, Scharff L, Sethna NF, et al. Physical therapy and cognitive-behavioral treatment for complex regional pain syndrome. *J Pediatr.* 2002;141(1):135–140.

Lohnberg JA, Altmaier EM. A review of psychosocial factors in complex regional pain syndrome. *J Clin Psychol Med Settings.* 2013;20:247–254 [Epub ahead of print].

Marinus J, Moseley GL, Birklein F, et al. Clinical features and pathophysiology of complex regional pain syndrome. *Lancet Neurol.* 2011;10(7):637–648.

O'Connell NE, Wand BM, McAuley J, et al. Interventions for treating pain and disability in adults with complex regional pain syndrome. *Cochrane Database Syst Rev.* 2013;4:CD009416.

Oaklander AL, Rissmiller JG, Gelmaan LB, et al. Evidence of focal small-fiber axonal degeneration in complex regional pain syndrome-I (reflex sympathetic dystrophy). *Pain.* 2006;120:235–243.

Parkitny L, McAuley JH, Di Pietro F, et al. Inflammation in complex regional pain syndrome: a systematic review and meta-analysis. *Neurology.* 2013;80(1):106–117.

Perez RS, Zollinger PE, Dijkstra PU, et al. CRPS task force: evidence based guidelines for complex regional pain syndrome type 1. *BMC Neurol.* 2010;10:20.

Raja SN, Grabow TS. Complex regional pain syndrome I (reflex sympathetic dystrophy). *Anesthesiology.* 2002;96:1254.

Rice ASC, Maton S; Postherpetic Neuralgia Study Group. Gabapentin in postherpetic neuralgia: a randomized, double blind, placebo controlled study. *Pain.* 2001;94:215.

Sharma A, Agarwal S, Broatch J, Raja SN. A web-based cross-sectional epidemiological survey of complex regional pain syndrome. *Reg Anesth Pain Med.* 2009;34(2):110–115.

Stanton-Hicks M, Janig W, Hassenbusch S, Haddox JD, Boas R, Wilson P. Reflex sympathetic dystrophy: changing concepts and taxonomy. *Pain.* 1995;63:127–133.

Turner JA, Loeser JD, Deyo RA, Sanders SB. Spinal cord stimulation for patients with failed back surgery syndrome or complex regional pain syndrome: a systemic review of effectiveness and complications. *Pain.* 2004;108(1–2):137–147.

van Hilten BJ, van de Beek WJ, Hoff JI, et al. Intrathecal baclofen for the treatment of dystonia in patients with reflex sympathetic dystrophy. *N Engl J Med.* 2000;343:625.

Veldman PH, Peynen HM, Arntz IE, Goris RJ. Signs and symptoms of reflex sympathetic dystrophy: prospective study of 829 patients. *Lancet.* 1993;342:1012–1016.

42 GERIATRIC PAIN

F. Michael Gloth III, MD, FACP, AGSF

THE SCOPE OF THE PROBLEM

- In no segment of our population is pain more prevalent and more challenging to treat than in our seniors.
- Studies indicate that as many as half of community-dwelling seniors suffer from pain that interferes with their ability to function normally. The prevalence of pain in nursing homes is an estimated 80%, with analgesics used in 40%–50% of residents.
- One of the greatest risk factors for having inadequately treated pain is simply being over 70 years of age.

REASONS FOR THE VULNERABILITY OF SENIORS TO PAIN

- Reasons for poor pain management include lack of physician training, inadequate pain assessment, and the reluctance of physicians to prescribe opioids.
- As most elderly patients take multiple medications for comorbid conditions, prescribing for the older adult in pain can be daunting.
- Pain has not been studied thoroughly in elderly subjects, and many studies have focused on threshold levels of mechanical, electrical, or thermal stimuli.
- With age, pain tolerance decreases, and pain complaints increase in frequency.
- Aging changes the dispersal of medications throughout the body, as well as blood flow to organs, protein binding, and body composition.
- Most analgesics are metabolized primarily by the liver and/or kidneys, and renal function typically declines with age, although routine indicators of renal function (eg, serum creatinine) may show little change.
- Factors that impede pain control include depression, secondary gain, anxiety, and mentally focusing on the pain.

ASSESSMENT

- A formal pain assessment, a prerequisite to adequate pain control, is a challenge in seniors.
- Many pain scales that lack optimal standardization in seniors and cannot be applied in the presence of common disabilities, such as visual or cognitive impairment.
- The Functional Pain Scale (see Figure 42-1), which has been standardized in an older population (inclusive of dementia subjects) for reliability, validity, and responsiveness, has three levels of assessment:
  - First, the patient rates pain as "tolerable" or "intolerable." (Intolerable pain should be considered an urgent matter requiring immediate further evaluation and intervention with frequent follow-up to ensure improvement into the "tolerable" range as rapidly as possible.)
  - Second, a functional component adjusts the score depending on whether a person can respond verbally.
  - Finally, the 0–5 scale allows rapid comparison with prior pain levels (responsiveness). Ideally all patients should reach a 0–2 level, preferably 0–1.

0 = No Pain

1 = Tolerable (and doesn't prevent any activities)

2 = Tolerable (but prevents some activities)

3 = Intolerable (but can use telephone, watch TV, or read)

4 = Intolerable (and can't use telephone, watch TV, or read)

5 = Intolerable (and unable to talk because of pain)

FIG. 42-1. The Functional Pain Scale. Responsiveness and validity data have been collected in a frail, elderly population.

- It may be difficult to determine the etiology of pain in seniors because their symptoms can differ from those of younger patients. For example, certain types of visceral pain may be less intense in seniors; thus, a "surgical abdomen" may present without leukocytosis or marked pain. In older patients, myocardial infarctions may be "silent," but a common complaint, like headache, may be due to a serious cause, like temporal arteritis, cervical osteoarthritis, depression, congestive heart failure, subdural hematoma, or electrolyte disturbance.
- After analysis of a patient's pain history and physical examination for obvious or subtle manifestations of a serious disease, an aggressive treatment plan should be initiated.

TREATMENT

- Curing the source of pain is ideal at any age, but aggressive palliation is appropriate in cases that lack a cure or while waiting for a cure to take effect.

NONPHARMACOLOGIC INTERVENTIONS

- In an older population with a high risk of adverse events, nonpharmacologic options should be considered first.
- At the outset nociception can be suppressed by chilling the area to reduce release of prostaglandins and other mediators that may sensitize C fibers, chilling or warming the area to encourage the release of endogenous opioids, and modifying the noxious response either centrally or peripherally.
- Transcutaneous electrical nerve stimulation, percutaneous electrical nerve stimulation, and acupuncture release endogenous opioids.
- Nerve blocks and tumor site radiation may be useful.
- Alternative or complementary medical interventions, such as relaxation techniques, biofeedback (particularly with vascular headaches), and hypnosis, are options. Because chronic pain patients may be using these therapies without oversight, it is useful to obtain a good history on *all* therapies being used.
- Physical therapy and occupational therapy offer a variety of modalities that improve pain relief.

PHARMACOLOGIC INTERVENTIONS

- When considering pharmacologic interventions in older adults, it may be necessary to emphasize safety before efficacy.
- Cost is another priority consideration.

- When, on hospitalization, pharmacologically noncompliant patients receive medications as prescribed, overmedication may occur and cause adverse events.
- Because of the potential for drug interactions, elimination of unnecessary medications is advisable.
- Doses may require adjustment to account for the altered pharmacokinetics and bioavailability in the elderly.
- More research is needed to determine if, in this population, it is safer or more effective to prescribe low doses of multiple analgesics with different mechanisms of action or to maximize doses of individual medications.

NONOPIOIDS

- Nonopioids, such as acetaminophen, are generally the first line of therapy for mild to moderate pain. Acetaminophen is usually well tolerated in the elderly but may be contraindicated in patients taking drugs metabolized through the liver or with hepatic disease.
- Cyclooxygenase 2 (COX-2) inhibitors have a better gastrointestinal (GI) safety profile than other nonselective, nonsteroidal anti-inflammatory drugs (NSAIDs). This does not mean that they are safe for an older adult population, however. COX-2 inhibitors as well as other NSAIDs have been associated with an increase in cardiovascular and renal risk (with the possible exception of naproxen).
- Some NSAIDs, for example, ibuprofen, inhibit the antiplatelet activity of aspirin, and it is not known if low-dose aspirin therapy obviates the GI safety of COX-2 agents.
- One option for NSAID use in older adults is the option of using a topical agent. Some, such as diclofenac gel 1%, have been associated with lower adverse events, perhaps due to far less systemic distribution. The drawback, of course, is that their effect is local as well.
- Many older patients, especially those who are homebound, take antiepileptic agents, or have fat malabsorption syndromes, are deficient in vitamin D. This deficiency is a potential cause of deep musculoskeletal pain or superficial light pressure pain. Vitamin D and calcium supplementation decrease rates of fracture and the attendant pain.
- Tricyclic antidepressants, some antiepileptic agents (eg, clonazepam, carbamazepine, gabapentin, and phenytoin), and mexiletine are recommended for neuropathic pain. As most of these agents are approved for other indications, selection may be predicated on using a single agent to combat multiple problems. Effective doses for pain are usually below those needed for the treatment of depression or seizures.
- Drugs approved by the Food and Drug Administration (FDA) for neuropathic pain include gabapentin, pregabalin, and duloxetine.

- Amitriptyline, imipramine, and anxiolytics, such as hydroxyzine, that are associated with anticholinergic effects should be avoided in seniors.

OPIOIDS

- Although addiction risk is low with opioids used for acute pain in patients who are not substance abusers (<0.1%), elderly patients may associate opioids with addiction, and this may be an issue even in the final days of life.
- To counteract constipation with opioid use, patients should consume adequate hydration and bulk fiber (so long as hydration is maintained) and should be as mobile as possible. A senna product is often helpful, and when chronic cathartics must be used, an agent such as sorbitol usually provides relief within days. Sorbitol is well tolerated, lacks long-term GI effects, and is relatively inexpensive. Patients may request reimbursable prescription lactulose, which carries a caution label for use in diabetics.
- Although more costly, other drugs, such as methylnaltrexone, directly affect opioid receptors and carry a specific indication for opioid-induced constipation. For most people, relief can be expected within the hour of administration.
- Some adverse events, such as pruritus, may be associated with receptor binding and may be remedied by using a more potent opioid.
- In the elderly, a short-acting opioid should be administered first, appropriate dosing established, and then a switch made to a controlled-release formulation.
- Regular dosing provides better pain relief with fewer narcotics than does intermittent dosing, which should be avoided.
- Inpatients should be told they may refuse a scheduled medication if they do not need it or are developing side effects, but nurses should inform the attending physicians immediately should this occur.
- Patients require close attention (for change in cognition, physical findings, and pain) during the first 24 hours after an opioid adjustment.
- Patient-controlled analgesia, with oral or parenteral agents, can lead to the best pain control with the least amount of opioid.
- Opioids may be started at doses too low for the elderly under the "start low and go slow" principle; thus, medication should be increased by 25%–100% when pain relief is inadequate. If patients metabolize opioids quickly and experience breakthrough pain after 8 hours of adequate pain relief, the dosing frequency should be increased to every 8 hours instead of increasing the dosage.
- A controlled-release morphine or oxycodone should never be prescribed more frequently than every 8 hours. If breakthrough pain occurs after 3–4 hours of relief, the amount of medication should be increased without changing the dosing schedule.
- The transdermal buprenorphine patch offers another option for older adults. As a schedule III agent it is easier to prescribe in the long-term care setting and lasts for an entire week.
- Older patients who metabolize medication slowly may get relief with less frequent dosing at surprisingly small quantities of opioids, such as 15–30 mg of controlled-release morphine every 24 hours.
- Greater amounts of analgesic may be necessary to initially bring pain under control, than to maintain control once the anxiety associated with inadequate pain control is eliminated.
- It would be catastrophic to crush long-acting, controlled-release agents for older patients who have difficulty swallowing pills.
- Use of short-acting opioids may facilitate tolerance and lead to higher opioid dosage requirements for adequate pain control.
- Meperidine has been associated with a host of adverse events in seniors and should be avoided either alone or in combination with a product such as hydroxyzine, which is anticholinergic and can be associated with orthostatic hypotension and confusion.
- Opioids that are antagonistic to the μ-receptor are less desirable, given the high prevalence of unrecognized and untreated depression in seniors who can benefit from the euphoric component that occurs with binding of the μ-receptor.
- The transdermal fentanyl patch may be useful when oral medication cannot be administered and subcutaneous or intraspinal routes are too cumbersome. In the older patient, however, these patches should be avoided as a first-line agent because age-related changes in body temperature and subcutaneous fat and water may cause fluctuation in absorption. Deaths have occurred in opioid-naive seniors using one 50 μg patch per hour. Thus, older patients should never be started on doses higher than 25 μg/h. In addition, the patient should be opioid tolerant, which is defined as taking at least 60 mg of oral morphine equivalent. Peak serum levels occur in 8–12 hours, and removal leaves a subcutaneous reservoir of active drug with a half-life of approximately 18 hours.
- In elderly patients, the route of administration is an important consideration because of age-related changes in skin integrity and GI absorption and motility.
- Terminally ill patients may present with symptoms resembling opioid toxicity that are really

manifestations of the dying process. Great care must be taken before ordering an opioid antagonist, such as naloxone, which can cause an agonizing withdrawal in patients who have used opioids for a prolonged period.

ADVERSE EVENTS

- Adverse drug reactions occur in elderly patients more than twice as often as in younger subjects and increase with the number of medications. Thus, an elderly patient taking six medications is 14 times more likely to have an adverse reaction than a younger one.
- Patients taking opioids, particularly older males with enlarged prostates, should be queried about urinary retention.
- Suspected adverse events should be evaluated thoroughly. Often, reactions may be misinterpreted as side effects from medication. For example, the exhausted sleep of a patient whose long-standing pain has finally been relieved may be mistaken as a side effect of morphine.
- Dementia occurs in approximately 5% of the population 65 years and older and in more than 20% after age 85. Disorientation often increases when a patient is moved to a different environment, such as a hospital. Previously undetected dementia may become manifest following an overnight hospitalization, even in the absence of infection or use of centrally acting medication.
- An older patient who demonstrates a mental status change while in the hospital must be carefully evaluated. Infections, such as pneumonia or those occurring in the urinary tract, may present solely as a change in mental status and improve rapidly with appropriate antibiotic therapy.

ADJUVANT ANALGESICS

- For refractory nonmalignant pain in the frail elderly, nonopioids can often be used to reduce the dosage in an opioid regimen.
- Analgesic adjuvants, such as NSAIDs and amphetamines, may improve opioid tolerance and pain resolution.
- The adjuvant use of agents such as nortriptyline, clonazepam, carbamazepine, phenytoin, gabapentin, tramadol, and mexiletine is beneficial for neuropathic pain.
- Antiepileptic medications are used to manage certain painful conditions, including trigeminal neuralgia (or glossopharyngeal neuralgia), which may occur frequently in elderly patients. Gabapentin is indicated for postherpetic neuralgia and may be effective when administered initially at 100 mg orally one to three times daily and increased by 300 mg/d as needed. Clonazepam, carbamazepine, or phenytoin may serve as an alternative. Some of the greatest concerns with antiepileptic agents are their propensity to disrupt balance and to interfere with vitamin D metabolism.

OTHER ISSUES AFFECTING SUCCESSFUL PAIN CONTROL

- The staff of multispecialty pain clinics or colleagues in other disciplines should be consulted whenever pain control is not achieved.

In some setting, for example skill nursing facilities, regulatory burden negatively impact pain control efforts. For example, in the nursing home (unlike the hospital), special schedule II prescriptions must be written and sent by FAX and by regular mail BEFORE a patient can be medicated for pain. This has done nothing to curb diversion, but has done much to make patients in that setting suffer, a direct result of overzealous regulation.

- The role of spirituality in pain control has not received adequate attention and may be important in seniors.
- Many of our frail, older patients do or will live in a nursing home or assisted living facility where the prevalence of inadequately controlled pain is high. Thus, quality assurance measures for these institutions should include evaluation and protocols for good pain management.

BIBLIOGRAPHY

AGS Panel on Persistent Pain in Older Persons. The management of persistent pain in older persons. *J Am Geriatr Soc.* 2002;50(6, Suppl):S205.

AGS Panel on the Pharmacological Management of Persistent Pain in Older Persons. Pharmacological management of persistent pain in older persons. *J Am Geriatr Soc.* 2009;57(8): 1331–1346.

Allcock N, McGarry J, Elkan R. Management of pain in older people within the nursing home: a preliminary study. *Health Soc Care Comm.* 2002;10(6):464–471.

American Geriatrics Society. 2012 Beers Criteria Update Expert Panel (Fick DM et al, Semla TP.) Updating the Beer's criteria for potentially inappropriate medication use in older adults. *J Am Geriatr Soc.* 2012;60(4):616–631.

Baraf HS, Gloth FM, Barthel HR, et al. Safety and efficacy of topical diclofenac sodium gel for knee osteoarthritis in elderly and younger patients: pooled data from three randomized, double-blind, parallel-group, placebo-controlled, multicentre trials. *Drug Aging*. 2011;28(1):27–40.

Bernabei R, Gambassi G, Lapane K, et al. Management of pain in the elderly patients with cancer. *J Am Med Assoc*. 1998;279(23):1877–1882.

Chamberlain BH, Cross K, Winston JL, et al. Methylnaltrexone treatment of opiod-induced constipation in patients with advanced illness. *J Pain Symptom Manag*. 2009;38(5):683–690.

Cleeland CS, Gonin R, Hatfield AK, et al. Pain and its treatment in outpatients with metastatic cancer. *N Engl J Med*. 1994;330:592.

Cleeland CS, Janjan NA, Scott CB, et al. Cancer pain management by radiotherapists: a survey of radiation therapy oncology group physicians. *Int J Radiat Oncol Biol Phys*. 2000;47(1):203–208.

Cusack BJ. Pharmacokinetics in older persons. *Am J Geriatr Pharmacother*. 2004;2(4):274–302.

Edwards RR, Fillingim RB. Age-associated differences in responses to noxious stimuli. *J Gerontol A Biol Sci Med Sci*. 2001;56(3):M180–M185.

Gibson SJ, Farrell M. A review of age differences in the neurophysiology of nociception and the perceptual experience of pain. *Clin J Pain*. 2004;20(4):227–239.

Gloth FM III. Geriatric pain: factors that limit pain relief and increase complications. *Geriatrics*. 2000;55(10):46.

Gloth FM III. Pain management in older adults: prevention and treatment. *J Am Geriatr Soc*. 2001;49:188.

Gloth FM III, Gundberg CM, Hollis BW, et al. The prevalence of vitamin D deficiency in a cohort of homebound elderly subjects compared to a normative matched population in the United States. *J Am Med Assoc*. 1995;274:1683.

Gloth FM III, Scheve AA, Stober CV, et al. The Functional Pain Scale (FPS): Reliability, validity, and responsiveness in a senior population. *J Am Med Dir Assoc*. 2001;2(3):110.

Gordon RS. Pain in the elderly. *J Am Med Assoc*. 1979;241:2491.

Harati Y, Gooch C, Swenson M, et al. Double-blind randomized trial of tramadol for the treatment of the pain of diabetic neuropathy. *Neurology*. 1998;50:1842.

Helme RD, Meliala A, Gibson SJ. Methodologic factors which contribute to variations in experimental pain threshold reported for older people. *Neurosci Lett*. 2004;361(1–3):144–146.

Hölmich P, Uhrskou P, Ulnits L, et al. Effectiveness of active physical training as treatment for longstanding adductor-related groin pain in athletes: randomised trial. *Lancet*. 1999;353:439.

Hyman SE, Cassem NH. Pain. In: Rubenstein E, Federman DD, eds. *Scientific American Medicine. Vol 11: Neurology*. New York: Scientific American; 1994:12.

Jones JS, Johnson K, McNinch M. Age as a risk factor for inadequate emergency department analgesia. *Am J Emerg Med*. 1996;14(2):157–160.

Jones SC. Relative thromboembolic risks associated with COX-2 inhibitors. *Ann Pharmacother*. 2005;39(7):1249–1259.

Kenshalo DR. Somesthetic sensitivity in young and elderly humans. *J Gerontol*. 1986;41(6):732–742.

Kienzler JL, Gold M. Systemic bioavailability of topical diclofenac sodium gel 1% versus oral diclofenac sodium in healthy volunteers. *J Clin Pharmacol*. 2010;50(1):50–61.

Konstantinopoulos PA, Lehmann DF. The cardiovascular toxicity of selective and nonselective cyclooxygenase inhibitors: comparisons, contrasts, and aspirin confounding. *J Clin Pharmacol*. 2005;45(7):742–750.

Lasco A, Catalano A, Benvenga S. Improvement of primary dysmenorrhea caused by a single oral dose of vitamin D: results of a randomized, double-blind, placebo-controlled study. *Arch Intern Med*. 2012;172(4):366–367.

Li G, Wang L, Shofer, JB, et al. Temporal relationship between depression and dementia: findings from a large community-based 15-year follow-up study. *Arch Gen Psychiatry*. 2011;68(9):970–977.

Mangoni AA, Jackson SHD. Age-related changes in pharmacokinetics and pharmacodynamics: basic principles and practical applications. *Br J Clin Pharmacol*. 2004; 57(1):6–14.

Marco CA, Schoenfeld CN, Keyl PM, et al. Abdominal pain in geriatric emergency patients: variables associated with adverse outcomes. *Acad Emerg Med*. 1998;5:1163.

Martin GM. Biology of aging. In: Goldman L et al, eds. *Cecil Medicine*. 23rd ed. Saunders, 2007;chap. 22.

Morellow CM, Leckband SG, Stoner CP, et al. Randomized double-blind study comparing the efficacy of gabapentin with amitriptyline on diabetic peripheral neuropathy pain. *Arch Intern Med*. 1999;159:1931.

Mouton CP, Bazaldua OV, Pierce B, et al. Common infections in older adults. *Am Fam Physician*. 2001;63(2):257–268.

Mukherjee D, Nissen SE, Topol EJ. Risk of cardiovascular events associated with selective COX-2 inhibitors. *J Am Med Assoc*. 2001;286(8):954–959.

Onder G, Pedone C, Landi F, et al. Adverse drug reactions as cause of hospital admissions: results from the Italian group of pharmacoepidemiology in the elderly (GIFA). *J Am Geriatr Soc*. 2002;50(12);1962–1968.

Parmelee PA, Katz IR, Lawton MP. The relation of pain to depression among institutionalized aged. *J Gerontol*. 1991;46:P15.

Pautex S, Herrmann FR, Le Lous P, et al. Improving pain management in elderly patients with dementia: validation of the Doloshort observational pain assessment scale. *Age Aging*. 2009;38(6):754–757.

Pitkala KH, Strandberg TE, Reijo ST. Management of nonmalignant pain in home-dwelling older people: a population-based survey. *J Am Geriatr Soc*. 2002;50:1861.

Plassman BL, Langa KM, Fisher GG, et al. Prevalence of dementia in the United States: the aging, demographics, and memory study. *Neuroepidemiology*. 2007;29(1–2):125–132.

Rahme E, Bardou M, Dasgupta K, et al. Hospitalization for gastrointestinal bleeding associated with non-steroidal anti-inflammatory drugs among elderly patients using low-dose aspirin: a retrospective cohort study. *Rheumatology*. 2007;46(2):265–272.

Rahme E, Nedjar H. Risks and benefits of COX-2 inhibitors vs non-selective NSAIDs: does their cardiovascular risk exceed their gastrointestinal benefit? A retrospective cohort study. *Rheumatology*. 2007;46(3):435–438.

Rich BA. Pain in society: ethical issues and public policy concerns. *Biobehav Approaches Pain*. 2009;515–528.

Schreuder F, Bernsen RMD, van der Wouden JC. Vitamin D supplementation for nonspecific musculoskeletal pain in non-western immigrants: A randomized controlled trial. *Ann Fam Med*. 2012;10(6):547–555.

Schumacher GA, Goodell H, Hardy JD, et al. Uniformity of the pain threshold in man. *Science.* 1940;92:110.

Sherman DE, Robillard E. Sensitivity to pain in the elderly. *Can Med Assoc J.* 1960;83:944.

Slatkin N, Thomas J, Lipman AG, et al. Methylnaltrexone for treatment of opioid-induced constipation in advanced illness patients. *J Support Oncol.* 2009;7(1):39–46.

Solomon DH, Schneeweiss S, Glynn RJ, et al. Relationship between selective cyclooxygenase-2 inhibitors and acute myocardial infarction in older adults. *Circulation.* 2004;109:2068–2073.

Stolee P, Hillier LM, Esbaugh J, et al. Instruments for the assessment of pain in older persons with cognitive impairment. *J Am Geriatr Soc.* 2005;53(2):319–326.

Thomas J, Karver S, Cooney GA, et al. Methylnaltrexone for opioid-induced constipation in advanced illness. *N Engl J Med.* 2008;358:2332–2343.

Turner NJ, Haward RA, Selby PJ. Cancer in old age-is it inadequately investigated and treated? *Brit Med J.* 1999;319(7205(1)):309–312.

Vadivelu N, Hines RL. Management of chronic pain in the elderly: focus on transdermal buprenorphine. *Clin Interv Aging.* 2008;3(3):421–430.

Zhang J, Ding EL, Song Y. Adverse effects of cyclooxygenase 2 inhibitors on renal and arrhythmia events. Meta-analysis of randomized trials. *J Am Med Assoc.* 2006;296(13):1619–1632.

43 MYOFASCIAL PAIN AND FIBROMYALGIA

Robert D. Gerwin, MD

INTRODUCTION

- Muscular pain may be one of the most common reasons for visits to physicians when one includes complaints associated with low back pain, neck and shoulder pain, arthritis, and tension headache in addition to primary myalgias.
- The prevalence of localized muscle pain is reported to be 20%, and that of widespread muscle pain, as high as 10%.

MYOFASCIAL PAIN SYNDROME

- Myofascial pain syndrome (MPS) may be acute or chronic, regional or widespread, but, in every case, it is associated with tenderness or pain localized to a linear or nodular hardening in a muscle that is called a "myofascial trigger point."

CLINICAL FEATURES

- Motor:
  - Taut (hardened) band of muscle that runs the length of the muscle
  - Twitch or local contraction of muscle band on mechanical stimulation
  - Restricted range of motion
  - Weakness
- Sensory:
  - Tenderness (allodynia, hypersensitivity) of the taut band (known as the myofascial trigger point or zone)
  - Referred pain
- Autonomic:
  - Skin temperature changes
  - Lacrimation
  - Piloerection (goose bumps)
- Viscerosomatic syndromes:
  - Cardiac
  - Esophageal–gastrointestinal–hepatic
  - Genitourinary
- MPS results from acute (eg, whiplash) or chronic (eg, repetitive strain syndromes) muscle overload or secondary to visceral pain with viscerosomatic convergence (eg, endometriosis or painful bladder).
- Muscle that is fatigued and/or eccentrically loaded is susceptible to injury.
- An abnormal motor end-plate mechanism is thought to cause taut bands that extend between myotendinous junctions.
- Injured or inflamed muscle rapidly leads to central sensitization, lowering the threshold to nociceptive and nonnociceptive stimulation and producing hypersensitivity, allodynia (the phenomenon of nonpainful stimulation being perceived as painful), and referred pain.
- MPS can persist long after the initial injury has resolved.
- Myofascial trigger zones may develop in the referred pain zone as well as in muscles that are agonists or antagonists of the muscle(s) that was initially injured.

CLINICAL PRESENTATION

- Pain generally occurs with activity but, in more severe cases, can be present at rest and interfere with sleep.
- Taut (hardened) bands shorten affected muscles and increase their diameter or cross-sectional bulk, which can result in nerve entrapment syndromes, such as the piriformis syndrome of the sciatic nerve, brachial plexus compressions in the interscalene compartment and the thoracic outlet, and median nerve compression by the pronater teres muscle. Entrapment by trigger points is usually intermittent compression, so

that electromyogram and nerve conduction studies are usually normal.

- Range of motion may be limited because of taut muscle bands or pain, and weakness may occur in affected muscles; the mechanism, thus, may involve central fatigue from persistently contracted taut bands within the muscle.
- Referred pain, a spinal cord and thalamic phenomenon, often occurs with or without pain in the primary trigger zone.
- Referred pain syndromes can be mistaken for other conditions (radiculopathy or viscerosomatic pain syndromes).
- Some typical myofascial pain syndromes are:
  - Piriformis syndrome (entrapment of the sciatic nerve)
  - Interscalene compartment syndrome (entrapment of the brachial plexus)
  - Thoracic outlet-like syndrome (entrapment of the brachial plexus between the clavicle and first rib)
  - Hyperabduction syndrome
  - Viscerosomatic syndromes (cardiac, gastrointestinal, hepatic, genitourinary)
  - Headaches (chronic tension type, with or without migraine)
  - Temporomandibular joint syndrome
  - "Frozen" shoulder or impaired shoulder mobility
- Mechanical stimulation of the primary trigger zone reproduces the pain, including referred pain.

DIAGNOSIS

- Identification of the primary trigger zone that reproduces the patient's pain is made by physical examination and reproduction of pain on palpation.
- A taut band of muscle is palpable and tender.
- Limited range of motion is a frequent and helpful sign, but motion may appear normal in hypermobile people.
- Referred pain may be elicited after 4–5 seconds.
- In the case of deep muscles like the multifidi, needling the muscle may be necessary to elicit the symptoms.
- Laboratory tests may identify coexisting, aggravating, or perpetuating conditions but do not support the clinical diagnosis of MPS.

TREATMENT

- Treatment is specific (treating the trigger point directly), general (treating pain and sleeplessness), and corrective (identifying and correcting the predisposing and perpetuating factors that may lead to and aggravate MPS) (Tables 43-1, 43-2, and 43-3).

TABLE 43-1   Treatment of MPS: Physical Modalities

Primary
   Local trigger point compression
   Local trigger point stretch
   Myofascial release
   Muscle play
   Therapeutic stretch
   Self-stretch
   Muscle reeducation
Adjunctive
   Intermittent cold
   Postisometric relaxation
   Strain–counterstrain
   Dry needling or injection (local anesthetic or botulinum toxin)
   Massage
   Ultrasound
   Electrical stimulation
   Acupuncture

- First, the clinician must inactivate the myofascial trigger point to relieve pain and restore normal function.
- Second, conditions that create and maintain trigger points, such as significant foot pronation, leg length inequality, and ergonomic stresses, must be corrected or eliminated.
- Inactivation of the trigger point is achieved manually or by needling the trigger point (Table 43-1). Most techniques compress and stretch the trigger point, followed by muscle reeducation and restoration of normal muscle sequencing during movement. Postisometric relaxation, reciprocal inhibition, and contract–relax techniques are all useful in stretching muscle.
- In hypermobile patients, therapeutic and self-stretching are relatively contraindicated, and treatment is directed locally to the trigger point.
- Ultrasound aids in the identification of trigger points for treatment, though this generally remains a research technique. Manual palpation to identify trigger points is much more efficient.
- Electrical stimulation reduces pain and allows manual treatment to proceed more comfortably.
- Cold Laser treatment is effective in eliminating trigger points.
- Strengthening to maintain improvement is reserved until muscle pain has been significantly reduced.

TABLE 43-2   Needling or Injection of the Trigger Point

Purpose
   Diagnostic
   Rapid relief of pain
   Facilitation of manual (physical) therapy
Medications
   Short-acting local anesthetics without epinephrine
   "Dry needling" with no drug (mechanical stimulation of the trigger point alone)
   Botulinum toxin

TABLE 43-3   Pharmacologic Treatment of MPS

Over-the-counter drugs
Nonsteroidal anti-inflammatory drugs
Antidepressant drugs (those that inhibit reuptake of serotonin and nor-
  epinephrine, like the tricyclic antidepressants and venlafaxine)
Muscle relaxants
Antispasticity drugs (tizanidine)
Anticonvulsants
Opioid analgesics (preferably long-acting, slow-release)
Botulinum toxin

Trigger Point Needling

- Trigger point needling or injection of a local anesthetic has been shown to be effective in relieving pain.
- Needling or injection confirms a diagnosis if the pain is relieved rapidly.
- Therapy is precise; the needle should enter the trigger zone and elicit a twitch response for best results. Outcome does not vary whatever the material injected or if only dry needling (no material injected) is done.
- The effect of needling or injection is often temporary, lasting days, and should be combined with manual (physical) therapy (Table 43-2).
- Lidocaine 0.25% has been shown to produce the least post-injection pain after trigger point injection and is extremely short-acting, an advantage should nerve block occur.
- Lidocaine 1% is more commonly used, however, because of its wide availability. 0.1 or 0.2 cc will inactivate a trigger point.
- Injection of 25 units of botulinum toxin type A or 1250 units of botulinum toxin type B into the trigger zone (except in head and neck muscles, where 5–10 units of botulinum toxin type A are injected) produces longer-lasting pain relief than does dry needling or the injection of local anesthetics. Open-label studies have shown promise in treating MPS with botulinum toxin, but one small, randomized, double-blind, placebo-controlled trial showed only a trend toward improvement of those injected a second time 6 weeks after the initial injection. A randomized, controlled study of the use of botulinum toxin type A in low back pain, however, showed significantly greater efficacy of the toxin compared with saline. Myofascial trigger points were definitely injected in that study.

Pharmacologic Treatment

- Pharmacologic treatment (Table 43-3) is directed toward pain relief and sleep improvement.
- Acetaminophen and aspirin provide short-term pain relief in mild pain states.
- NSAIDs are not used for any anti-inflammatory purpose in muscle but for their analgesic activity, including that against postinjection pain. If NSAIDs are used for a long period, the selective COX-2 inhibitors should be used.
- Some anticonvulsant drugs (carbamazepine, gabapentin, and pregabalin) are effective in the treatment of neuropathic pain. Other of the newer anticonvulsants (topiramate, lamotrigine) have had mixed results in trials of treatment of neuropathic pain. Nevertheless, anticonvulsant medications may reduce muscle pain and can be given a trial in patients with MPS.
- Tizanidine, an α_2-adrenergic agonist, is efficacious in the treatment of MPS. The major adverse effects are daytime drowsiness, dry mouth, and the possibility of an initial drop in blood pressure. The drug is started at a low dose of 1–2 mg at night and then titrated upward to effectiveness on a twice or three times daily schedule.
- Cyclobenzaprine, related to the tricyclic antidepressants, has garnered mixed reports about its efficacy in treating MPS and is not recommended except as adjunctive treatment.
- Carisoprodol is to be avoided because it is highly addictive.
- In one study, the benzodiazepine derivative clonazepam (start with 0.5 mg every night and titrate upward) was effective in treating MPS.
- Sleep disruption can be treated with melatonin (3 mg every night), drugs such as zolpidem (5–10 mg every night), or antidepressants such as trazodone (50–150 mg every night).
- Opioids are used strictly for pain relief. They can be liberating for someone who is disabled by pain, but they can cause physical dependence and, rarely, addiction; create constipation; and impair cognitive function. If considered for long-term use, only long-acting, slow-release forms should be used, such as controlled-release forms of morphine sulfate, oxycodone, methadone, and fentanyl. These drugs should be used only by physicians experienced in their management.
- Tramadol alone at 50–100 mg every 4–6 hours or with acetaminophen up to 800 mg/d can be used for pain of moderate intensity. *Caution*: Tramadol in combination with certain antidepressant drugs can lower the seizure threshold.

Other Treatment Options

- Acupuncture is useful for pain relief. In a form of acupuncture called "superficial dry needling," the needle is placed 2–3 mm under the skin over the trigger point. Relaxation of the trigger point can be seen. The usual manual treatment protocol follows (Table 43-1).
- When the clinician identifies depression or other emotional stress that might underlie and aggravate

the MPS, screening by a social worker, psychologist, or psychiatrist for psychologic treatment is in order.

- Psychologic treatment options for MPS include education, cognitive behavioral therapy, and antidepressants or anxiolytics when indicated.
- Activation of the limbic system can reinforce neck and shoulder trigger points. This is an outgrowth of cognitive-behavioral therapy.

Summary

- MPS patients are treated with manual inactivation of the trigger point (physical therapy, including trigger point compression, massage, local and therapeutic stretching, and self-stretching). *Warning:* Stretching should be done cautiously or not at all in hypermobile MPS individuals.
- Trigger points that do not release manually are needled or injected with local anesthetic. Botulinum toxin is used as a long-lasting trigger point injection in cases where needling or local anesthetic combined with physical therapy does not give long-term relief.
- Postural, ergonomic, mechanical (structural), hormonal, nutritional, and other medical precipitating and perpetuating factors are identified and corrected.
- Strengthening, including lumbar stabilization, is performed when pain levels are reduced enough to allow the patient to perform resistive and stabilizing exercises without an undue increase in pain.
- Counseling and cognitive-behavioral therapies are employed where warranted.
- Medications are used when necessary to treat symptoms:
  o Sleep disturbance: melatonin 3 mg every night, trazodone 50–150 mg every night, amitriptyline 25–50 mg every night, or zolpidem 5–10 mg every night.
  o Antispasticity drugs: tizanidine starting at 1–2 mg every night and titrating to effectiveness two or three times daily up to 8 mg three times daily can significantly reduce pain.
  o Muscle relaxants: cyclobenzaprine 10 mg three times daily or methylcarbamoyl 500–750 mg three times daily, for short-term use. Carisoprodol should be avoided.
- Analgesics are for short-term use, the type depending on the severity of the pain. For acute, severe pain, rapid-onset, short-duration opioids like oxycodone/APAP 5/325 and hydrocodone/APAP 5/500, every 4 hours as needed, are used. For pain that is sub-acute or for chronic severe pain, slow-release, long-acting opiates like controlled-release morphine sulfate and oxycodone, methadone, or fentanyl patch are used, starting at low doses and titrating upward to efficacy. For lesser pain tramadol starting at 50 mg two to four times

daily and titrating to effectiveness (50–100 mg every 4–6 h/d, maximum dose of 800 mg/d) or NSAIDs are used. For mild pain, over-the-counter preparations are satisfactory.

FIBROMYALGIA SYNDROME

- Fibromyalgia syndrome (FMS) is a chronic, widespread muscular pain syndrome that is the second most common disorder seen by rheumatologists.
- FMS is not a disease per se but rather is a chronic, widespread pain syndrome that can have multiple etiologies.

CLINICAL FEATURES

- Pain is related to neuroplastic changes of the central nervous system that result in general hypersensitivity to all types of stimuli through the unmasking of dormant synapses and reduction of central inhibition. There is also a component of pain caused by peripheral sources of pain. Myofascial trigger points have been shown to be an important source of pain in FMS.
- FMS patients have decreased serum serotonin levels and impaired central serotonin metabolism as well as elevated levels of cerebrospinal fluid substance P. They have low levels of insulin-like growth factor 1 and decreased function of the hypothalamic–pituitary–adrenal axis with low serum androgen levels that correlate with poor physical functioning and with pain.
- The hallmark of FMS is widespread muscular pain in three or four quadrants of the body (ie, upper and lower and right and left sides) of 3 or more months' duration.
- Pain is often accompanied by unusual fatigue and disturbed sleep.
- FMS occurs in about 3.5% of women and 0.5% of men and is more common with advancing age. It occurs in children as well as adults.
- FMS is comorbid with many other conditions, such as rheumatoid arthritis, systemic lupus erythematosus, Lyme disease, hepatitis, Sjögren's syndrome, and myofascial pain syndrome.

CLINICAL PRESENTATION

- Patients with FMS complain of widespread muscle pain that interferes with activity, fatigue out of proportion to any sleep disorder, and impaired sleep (they usually awaken feeling tired).
- FMS patients often have associated problems of depression, headache, joint pain, morning stiffness,

Raynaud's phenomenon, bladder irritability, irritable bowel syndrome, and painful intercourse.

- Many of these associated conditions are the result of myofascial trigger point syndromes that present in patients with FMS (eg, muscular headaches, morning stiffness, and pelvic floor or viscerosomatic pain syndromes).
- FMS patients complain of difficulty concentrating and of short-term memory impairment.
- Symptoms can be so severe they cause many to seek disability retirement.

DIAGNOSIS

- The diagnosis is based on the history of chronic, widespread pain and the presence of bilateral muscle tenderness (tender points) that affects the upper and lower halves of the body.
- The American College of Rheumatology (ACR) established criteria for the diagnosis of FMS to aid in the development of clinical studies, and these criteria have been adopted for clinical use. The presence of tenderness at 11 or more of 18 preselected sites has a diagnostic sensitivity of 88% and a specificity of 81%. Nine sites are examined bilaterally (Table 43-4). There need not be 11 or more tender points at any given examination in clinical practice, but, over time, muscle tenderness must be widespread, which the criteria ensure.
- The tender point examination is conducted by palpating muscle with a force sufficient to blanche the fingernail, approximately 4 kg pressure.
- In clinical practice, tenderness is not confined to the sites designated in the ACR criteria but must be present in a widespread distribution. Care should be taken when examining for tenderness to distinguish tender, taut muscle bands of myofascial trigger points so as not to confuse FMS with MPS.

Myofascial trigger points are commonly found in fibromyalgia patients. The referred pain from the trigger points can often explain the person's pain.

TABLE 43-4   Tender Point Sites for Fibromyalgia Examination

Suboccipital
Lower anterior cervical
Upper trapezius
Supraspinatus
Parasternal at second rib
Lateral epicondylar region
Anterior gluteal fold
Greater trochanter of the hip
Medial fat pad above the knee (vastus medialis)

TABLE 43-5   Differential Diagnoses for Fibromyalgia

Myofascial pain syndrome
Drug-induced: statin cholesterol-lowering drugs
Hypothyroidism
Iron deficiency
Vitamin B_{12} deficiency
Infections
Candidiasis
Parasitic
Bacterial (*Mycoplasma*)
Sleep apnea, restless leg syndrome
Myoadenylate deaminase deficiency

- The associated problems of joint stiffness, Raynaud's phenomenon, interstitial cystitis, and so on need not be present to diagnose FMS.
- Other causes of widespread, chronic muscle pain should be excluded (Table 43-5).
- Orthostatic hypotension is seen in many patients with FMS; blood pressure and pulse should be taken supine, immediately after standing, and 2 minutes after standing.
- Numerical rating scales for pain (0 = no pain, 10 = worst possible pain) are useful for assessing the degree of pain a patient is experiencing.
- The Fibromyalgia Impact Questionnaire assesses the impact of pain on a patient's life.
- A polysomnogram or sleep disorder consultation may be necessary to diagnose treatable sleep disturbances.

TREATMENT

Pharmacologic Treatment

- As with MPS, over-the-counter analgesics may be used to treat pain when necessary.
- Nonsteroidal, anti-inflammatory drugs.
- Muscle relaxants and antispasticity drugs (cyclobenzaprine 10 mg three times daily).
- Duloxetine and milnacipran are serotonin and norepinephrine reuptake inhibitor (SNRI) drugs that have been shown in randomized controlled trials to decrease the pain in fibromyalgia patients. Tricyclic antidepressants that inhibit the reuptake of serotonin and norepinephrine provide short-term improvement. Amitriptyline, at doses of 25–50 mg every night, has been the most thoroughly studied and has led to improvement for as long as 6 months. Tramadol may cause seizures when used with a variety of antidepressant drugs and, therefore, should either be avoided or be used with caution in association with amitriptyline. Fluoxetine at 20 mg daily and sertraline at 50 mg daily are also effective. Antidepressants improve sleep, fatigue, and pain but not the tender point count.

- Anticonvulsants reduce neuropathic pain and can be used nonspecifically in FMS. Pregabalin has been shown to be effective, and gabapentin is also commonly used.
- Antispasticity drugs (tizanidine starting at 1–2 mg every night, slowly titrating upward).
- Opiates.
- Nutritional supplements (S-adenosyl-L-methionine).
- Hormone therapy:
  o Growth hormone titrated to an insulin-like growth factor 1 (IGF-1) level of 250 mg/mL improves FMS after about 6 months of treatment at a cost of approximately $1000/mo. Symptoms recur after treatment is stopped. Growth hormone is not recommended for routine management.
  o When hypothyroidism coexists with FMS, thyroid supplementation may resolve FMS symptoms. No data support the use of other kinds of hormonal therapy.
- Some studies have found that S-adenosyl-L-methionine at 200 mg/d improves pain, fatigue, mood, and morning stiffness.

Low-dose propranolol (20 mg/d), but not high dose, has been shown to be effective in treating the orthostatic hypotension and tachycardia that is often seen in these patients.

PHYSICAL TREATMENT

- Graded aerobic exercise is the most effective form of physical therapy, in the short and long term (up to 4 years). Moderately intense aerobic exercise two or three times per week, with minimal eccentric muscle activity, improves physical functioning, cardiovascular fitness, and self-efficacy, but pain levels, tender point counts, mood and depression, and sleep and fatigue may not improve.
- Physical therapy otherwise is useful primarily to identify and treat coexistent problems, such as MPS, postural dysfunctions, and ergonomic stresses.
- Electrical stimulation.
- Acupuncture is an effective complementary therapy.

PSYCHOLOGIC TREATMENT

- Education.
- Teaching coping skills and relaxation training constitutes cognitive-behavioral therapy (educational content varied considerably among studies).
- Biofeedback, especially combined with exercise, improves function and reduces tender points.

- Hypnosis and meditation-based stress reduction each improve pain ratings and function and can reduce the number of tender points.
- Psychotherapy.

OTHER TREATMENT

Treatment of myofascial trigger points is effective in treatment of FMS pain.

- A multidisciplinary treatment program combining behavioral modification, education, and physical training is effective.
- Treatment of sleep disturbance is important and should include attention to sleep hygiene (darkened room, using the bed only for sleep and sexual intercourse) and medications to promote sleep, such as melatonin 3 mg before bedtime, trazodone 50–150 mg at bedtime, or a pharmaceutical such as zolpidem 5–10 mg at bedtime. Amitriptyline improves sleep.
- There is no evidence to support the use of magnesium or magnesium-malic supplements, DHEA, guaifenesin, corticosteroids, sex hormones, and herbal supplements.
- The associative disorders of headache, interstitial cystitis, irritable bowel syndrome, irritable bladder syndrome, dysmenorrhea, and dyspareunia should be treated symptomatically, but muscular (myofascial) causes of these conditions that can be treated specifically should be assessed.
- Trigger point injections are used to treat coexistent MPS, but injection of tender points with local anesthetics or with corticosteroids has no proven benefit in FMS.

SUMMARY

- Diagnosis is positive in identifying widespread muscle tenderness in a person with a history of chronic, widespread pain, and negative in excluding other causes of widespread myalgia.
- An antidepressant drug that inhibits uptake of both serotonin and norepinephrine, such as duloxetine at up to 60 mg/d, is used to relieve pain and improve sleep.
- Sleep is improved with trazodone 50–150 mg nightly, melatonin 3 mg nightly, or a drug such as zolpidem 5–10 mg nightly. A sleep consultation should be sought if the patient suffers a serious sleep disorder or significant daytime hypersomnia. Caffeine and other drugs that interfere with sleep, such as opiates, and sympathomimetic drugs such as nasal decongestants should be avoided.

- A moderately intensive aerobic exercise program that avoids excessive eccentric resistive exercise should be instituted.
- Pain is treated with a suitable analgesic if necessary.
- A multidisciplinary approach combining graded aerobic exercise, cognitive-behavioral therapy, and patient education should be used.
- Coexistent conditions (such as hypothyroidism, iron deficiency, and vitamin B_{12} deficiency) and comorbid MPS, ergonomic and postural stressors, and psychologic disorders are treated.
- Comorbid MPS is treated with trigger point injections or needling.
- Complementary/alternative methods of treatment, such as supplementation with S-adenosyl-L-methionine, use of acupuncture, and biofeedback, should be considered.

Bibliography

Affaitati G, Constantini R, Fabrizio A, et al. Effects of treating peripheral pain generators in fibromyalgia patients. *Eur J Pain.* 2011;15:61–69.

Affaitati G, Fabrizio A, Savini A, et al. A randomized, controlled study comparing a lidocaine patch, a placebo patch, and anesthetic injection for treatment of trigger points in patients with myofascial pain syndrome: evaluation of pain and somatic pain thresholds. *Clinical Therapeutics.* 2009; 31:708–720.

Alonso-Bianco C, Fernandez-de-las-Peñas C, Morales-Cahazas M, et al. Multiple active myofascial trigger points reproduce the overall spontaneous painpattern in women with fibromyalgia and are related to widespread mechanical hypersensitivity. *Clin J Pain.* 2011;27:401–413.

Bennet RM, Cook DM, Clark SR. Hypothalamic–pituitary–insulin-like growth factor axis dysfunction in patients with fibromyalgia. *J Rheumatol.* 1997;24:1384.

Burckhardt CS, Clark SR, et al. The fibromyalgia impact questionnaire: development and validation. *J Rheumatol.* 1991;18:728.

Burckhardt CS, Mannerkorpi K, Hedenberg L, et al. A randomized, controlled clinical trial of education and physical training for women with fibromyalgia. *J Rheumatol.* 1994;21:714.

Clark SR, Jones KD, Burckhardt CS, et al. Exercise for patients with fibromyalgia: risks versus benefits. *Curr Rheumatol Rep.* 2001;3:135.

Coderre TJ, Katz J, Vaccarino AL. Contribution of central neuroplasticity to pathological pain: review of clinical and experimental evidence. *Pain.* 1993;52:259.

Cummings TM, White AR. Needling therapies in the management of myofascial trigger point pain: a systematic review. *Arch Phys Med Rehabil.* 2001;82:986.

Dessein PH, Shipton EA, Joffe BI. Hyposecretion of adrenal androgens and the relation of serum adrenal steroids, serotonin and insulin-like growth factor-1 to clinical features in women with fibromyalgia. *Pain.* 1999;83:313.

Foster L, Clapp L, Erickson M, et al. Botulinum toxin A and chronic low back pain: a randomized, double blind study. *Neurology.* 2001;56:1290.

Ge HY, Wang Y, Fernandez-de-las-Peñas C, et al. Reproduction of overall spontaneous poan pattern by manual stimulation of active myofascial trigger points in fibromyalgia syndrome patients. *Arthritis Res Ther.* 2011March 22;13(2):R48.

Gowans SE, deHueck A, Voss S, et al. A randomized, controlled trial of exercise and education for individuals with fibromyalgia. *Arthritis Care Res.* 1999;12:120.

Kissel JT, Miller R. Muscle pain and fatigue. In: Schapira AHV, Griggs RC, eds. *Muscle Diseases.* Woburn, Mass: Butterworth–Heinemann; 1999:33.

Loscher WN, Nordlund MM. Central fatigue and motor cortical excitability during repeated shortening and lengthening actions. *Muscle Nerve.* 2002;25:864.

Mense S, Simons D. *Muscle Pain: Understanding Its Nature, Diagnosis, and Treatment.* Philadelphia, Pa: Lippincott Williams & Wilkins; 2001:158.

Newham DJ, McPhail G, Mills KR, et al. Ultrastructural changes after concentric and eccentric contractions of human muscle. *J Neurol Sci.* 1983;61:109.

Pillemer SR, Bradley LA, Crofford LJ. The neuroscience and endocrinology of fibromyalgia. *Arthritis Rheum.* 1997;40:1928.

Rowe PC, et al. Neurally mediated hypotension and chronic fatigue syndrome. *Am J Med.* 1998;105(3A):15S.

Russell IF. Neurochemical pathogenesis of fibromyalgia syndrome. *J Musculoskel Pain.* 1996;4:61.

Simons DG, Travell JG, Simons LS. *Myofascial Pain and Dysfunction: The Trigger Point Manual.* Vol 1. Baltimore, Md: Williams & Wilkins; 1999:19, 69.

Wolfe F, Smythe HA, Yunus MB, et al. The American College of Rheumatology 1990 criteria for the classification of fibromyalgia: report of the multicenter criteria committee. *Arthritis Rheum.* 1990;33:160.

44 PEDIATRIC PAIN

Robert S. Greenberg, MD

CHILDREN HAVE PAIN, TOO

- As it has in adults, pain has long been undertreated in children, but this neglect is no longer acceptable, and clinicians now realize the necessity of considering and treating pain and painful procedures in children.

HISTORICAL REASONS FOR THE UNDERTREATMENT OF PAIN IN CHILDREN

- Despite increasing awareness of the importance of treating pain as a disease, pain is still inadequately managed, even in adults. This problem may be more acute in children who lack the ability to demand relief from pain.

- Small children, especially preverbal infants, cry in reaction to discomfort (hunger, heat or cold, wet clothing, boredom, tiredness, frustration, presence of strangers) as well as to pain; therefore, it is easy to discount or misinterpret crying caused by pain. Astute caregivers, however, learn to distinguish the wails of prelanguage babies (he's sleepy, she's hungry) and either meet their needs or distract them from their discomfort.

- Fear/anxiety exacerbates pain; yet adults may fail to appreciate the level of fear/anxiety felt by a young child about to undergo even a minimally painful experience. This is especially true if the child does not understand what is happening or why it is happening—only that it hurts.

- If the caregiver who usually takes away his or her pain (or pangs) is involved in the painful procedure, the young child may experience anxiety-increasing confusion.

- Some adults have a cavalier attitude about children's pain. If the adult knows the child's pain will soon subside, the adult may believe it is not worth treating.

- Some adults believe that it is an important life lesson and part of "growing up" for a child to learn to bear pain.

- Adults generally shed tears only in response to emotional distress, while children shed tears readily for a host of reasons. Some adults believe that children, especially boys, should be taught never to cry.

- Sometimes adults think that a child's complaint of pain is merely a ruse. If a child says her or his stomach hurts on a school day, for example, the adult may think the child simply wants to stay home from school.

- These attitudes join with the limited ability of children to provide clinically relevant information about their pain and the persistence of misinformation about pain to hinder appropriate pain management in children.

- Thus, the "coming of age" of the recognition, definition, and management of pain in children is very recent.

NEED FOR A MULTIDISCIPLINARY APPROACH

- The multidisciplinary approach needed to achieve adequate pain management in adults with chronic pain may be even more important in children, and this multidisciplinary approach should involve parents or guardians whenever possible.

- In fact, achieving adequate pain management in children requires that the child/patient, patient's family, and medical professionals establish good lines of communication so they can educate each other about the problem and potential solutions.

- A multidisciplinary approach allows all involved to achieve clarity about the purpose of pain management and to set realistic goals.

FACTORS THAT MODULATE PEDIATRIC PAIN

CHILD-SPECIFIC FACTORS

- Age
- Sex
- Temperament
- Previous pain experience
- Family environment
- Cognitive/developmental level
- How well the child can interpret information about the cause and prognosis of pain
- Ability to identify pain triggers
- Expectations about treatment efficacy
- Knowledge and ability to execute practical drug and nondrug therapy
- Ability to recognize stress and knowledge about how to deal with it

BEHAVIORAL FACTORS

- Repertoire of distress responses
- Ability to accommodate drug and nondrug therapy
- Management and resolution of stressful situations
- Ability to participate in routine activities (home, school, sports, social)

EMOTIONAL FACTORS

- Anticipatory anxiety, which may heighten distress and accelerate/escalate the effect of the initiating factor
- Fear regarding an undiagnosed condition and/or continuing pain
- Situation-specific stress (home, school, sports, social)
- Frustration regarding disruption to activities that serve as positive reinforcers of life
- Underlying/inherent anxiety or depression

PAIN ASSESSMENT IN CHILDREN

OBJECTIVE/OBSERVATIONAL/BEHAVIORAL

- Enables the clinician to translate objective/observed aspects of the patient's condition into an interpretation of pain. This method is used for children who cannot perform a self-assessment.

TABLE 44-1 **The CHEOPS Scale**

PARAMETER	FINDING	POINTS
Cry	None	1
	Moaning	2
	Crying	2
	Screaming	3
Facial expression	Smiling	0
	Composed	1
	Grimace	2
Child verbal	Positive	0
	None	1
	Complaints other than pain	1
	Pain complaints	2
	Pain and nonpain complaints	2
Torso	Neutral	1
	Shifting	2
	Tense	2
	Shivering	2
	Upright	2
	Restrained	2
Touch	Not touching	1
	Reach	2
	Touch	2
	Grab	2
	Restrained	2
Legs	Neutral	1
	Squirming, kicking	2
	Drawn up, tensed	2
	Standing	2
	Restrained	2

- Special scales may be used for children with special problems (obtunded, mental retardation, physical disabilities, etc).
- CHEOPS (see Table 44-1):
  - This scale is suggested for children 1–5 years of age.
  - Sum of all six parameters: minimum score = 4; maximum score = 13.
- Self-report:
  - Enables the patient to translate his or her own sense of pain into an objective scale for others to record and follow.
  - The FACES method for providing self-reports of pain was developed for use in children (see Figure 44-1).
  - A visual analogue scale or numeric scale can also be used (see Figure 44-2).

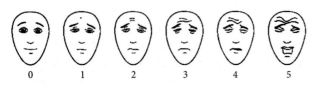

FIG. 44-1. When using the FACES scale, explain to the child that each face is for a person who feels happy because he has no pain (hurt) or sad because he has some or a lot of pain. Face 0 doesn't hurt at all.

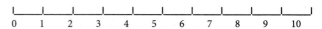

FIG. 44-2. When using a numeric scale, explain to the child that at one end of the line is a 0, which means that a person feels no pain (hurt). At the other end is a 10, which means the person feels the worst pain imaginable. The numbers 1 to 9 range from a very little pain to a whole lot. Ask the child to choose the number that best describes how well he or she is feeling. On this scale, a 10 is equivalent to a 5 on the FACES scale in Figure 44–1.

PAIN TREATMENT IN CHILDREN

NSAIDS

- Mode of action: inhibition of cyclo-oxygenase
- Used in the initial/basic treatment of most pediatric pain
- Can cause decreased platelet effect (especially aspirin) and bone reformation (ibuprofen, ketorolac, naproxen), so consider the benefit/risk if there is a history of gastrointestinal bleeding, airway or intracranial surgery, or bone fracture ("osteotomies" and spine)
- Should be used (if not contraindicated) for most pain as an adjunct to severe pain, for example, treatment with opioids to decrease overall opioid use (see Table 44-2).

OPIOIDS

- Opioids are commonly used to treat acute pain or sedation in children. Can use various routes (intravenous, intramuscular, subcutaneous, epidural, nasal, sublingual, transdermal, and oral).
- Chronic is controversial and should be limited to special cases (terminal, long term, or weaning).
- In the young child and infant, dosing is based on weight and titration to effect. Caution must be used in extremely young infants and obstructive sleep apnea regarding respiratory depression.
- Table 44-8 lists commonly used opioids and dosing.

ADJUVANT AGENTS

- These drugs, while some are associated with treatment of depression, have become recognized as effective adjuvants in many acute (and chronic) pain scenarios.
- Some of the most likely to be useful in acute pain management are listed in Table 44-3.

LOCAL ANESTHETICS

Pharmacology

- See Table 44-4.
- Amides (bupivacaine, lidocaine, etidocaine, ropivacaine, mepivacaine, prilocaine).

TABLE 44-2   **NSAIDs Used to Treat Pediatric Pain***

DRUG	AVAILABILITY	DOSING REGIMEN	CAVEATS
Acetaminophen	Drops: 100 mg/mL	15 mg/kg/dose PO q4h	Excellent analgesic base if given around the clock
Feverall	Elixir: 80, 120, 160, 325 mg/5 mL	30 mg/kg/first dose PR	
Liquiprin	Tablets: 120, 325, 500 mg	Max dose: 75 mg/kg/d or 4 g/d	Caution in renal and/or hepatic failure
Panadol	Chewable tabs: 80, 120, 160 mg		Caution in G6PD deficiency
Tempra	Caplets: 160, 325, 500 mg		
Tylenol	Rectal suppository: 80, 120, 325, 650 mg		
APAP			
Paracetamol			
Aspirin	Tablets: 81, 325, 650 mg	10–15 mg/kg PO q4h	Generally not used for pain, except for arthritic/chronic conditions
Anacin	Chewable tablets: 81 mg	Max dose: 4 g/d	
Bayer	Caplets: 80, 165, 625, 500, 650 mg		Caution: Reye's syndrome association, eg, contraindicated during viral syndrome
Buffered	Rectal suppository: 60, 120, 200, 325, 650 mg		
Empirin			
ASA			
Choline magnesium trisalicylate	Solution: 500 mg/mL	7.5–15 mg/kg PO q6h	Does not have much effect on platelets
	Tablets (scored): 500, 750, 1000 mg		Can be split bid
Trilisate			
Ibuprofen	Suspension: 100 mg/mL	4–10 mg/kg PO q6h	Excellent base analgesic if given around the clock, especially for musculoskeletal pain
Advil	Tablets: 200, 400, 600, 800 mg		
Motrin			May affect bone reformation
Medipren			
Nuprin			
Ketorolac	Injection: 15, 30 mg/mL	0.5 mg/kg IV (IM) or PO q6h	Keep well hydrated
Toradol	Tablets: 10 mg	Max total dose: 120 mg/kg/d	Caution if renal impaired or history of GI bleeding
		5-day maximum duration of therapy	May affect bone reformation
Naproxen	Suspension: 125 mg/mL	5 mg/kg PO q8–12h	May affect bone reformation
Aleve	Tablets: 200, 250, 375, 500 mg	Max total dose: 30 mg/kg/d	
Naprosyn			
Propacetamol Pro-Dalfalgan (not available in the United States)	Injection: reconstituted from powder, usually 10 mg/mL	30 mg/kg IV (over 20 min) q6h	Excellent postoperative analgesic base if given around the clock
		Max adult dose: 8 g/d	Caution in renal and/or hepatic failure
		2-day maximum duration of therapy	Caution in G6PD deficiency

*Paraphrased from Yaster et al.

TABLE 44-3   **Adjuvant Agents Used to Treat Pediatric Pain**

CLASS	DRUG (TRADE NAME)	DOSING REGIMEN	NOTES
Amphetamines (can be added as a means to counter the sedative and potentiate the analgesic effects of high-dose opiates)	Methylphenidate (Concerta, Ritalin, Ritalin-SR)	0.3 mg/kg/dose (2.5–5 mg/dose) PO with breakfast and lunch May increase in 5-mg intervals weekly unless side effects appear	Caution in hypertension, glaucoma, Tourette's syndrome
	Dextroamphetamine (Dexedrine)	5 mg PO q May increase in 5 mg intervals weekly unless side effects appear	
Antinarcoleptics	Modafinil (Provigil)	3–5 mg/kg PO qam (usually 100–200 mg/d)	Especially helpful when opioids cause severe sedation yet are still not completely analgesic, for example, sickle cell crises
Anticonvulsants	Gabapentin (Neurontin)	5 mg/kg or 300 mg PO qhs	A good option for neuropathies/chronic pain
		May increase to 300 qmg PO tid	
			Take time to work (2–3 weeks)
			May cause somnolence, dizziness, nystagmus

(Continued)

TABLE 44-3 Adjuvant Agents Used to Treat Pediatric Pain *(Continued)*

CLASS	DRUG (TRADE NAME)	DOSING REGIMEN	NOTES
Alpha agonists	Clonidine (Catapress)		Will also cause some sedation and lower blood pressure
	Tizanidine (Zanaflex)	Approx 50 μg/kg/dose PO q6–8h	Good to ameliorate the muscle spasm associated with orthopedic manipulation
			Less sedation and hypotension than with clonidine
Benzodiazepines	Diazepam (Valium)	0.1–0.2 mg/kg IV q2–6h (depending on needs) 0.2–0.3 mg/kg PO q4–6h	Used especially for muscle spasm/ spasticity which can cause severe pain postorthopedic/genitourinary procedures
			Can cause burning on IV injection. Long half-life in neonates
	Lorazepam (Ativan)	0.05–0.1 mg/kg IV q4–8h	Sometimes tolerated better than diazepam: less hypotension and sedation
		0.05–0.2 mg/kg PO q6–8h	See precautions for diazepam

- Esters (chloroprocaine, procaine, tetracaine, cocaine).
- pK_a = pH at which half of the drug is in ionized form.
- Generally, weak bases that exist in aqueous solutions in nonionized and ionized forms. Only the nonionized form can cross the nerve membrane to block the sodium channel from the inner membrane.
- Protein binding:
  ○ Bind to plasma proteins.
  ○ α_1-acid glycoproteins are the predominant protein-binding local anesthetics.
    ▪ Increased in inflammatory disease and cancer (less risk)
    ▪ Decreased in children <6 months of age (greater risk of free agent causing toxicity)
  ○ Lipid solubility: Highly lipid-soluble agents cross nerve membranes readily and may ascend along the nerve membrane.

Factors Affecting Neural Blockade

- Na^+ channel blockers
- Minimum effective blocking concentration
  ○ Fiber size/myelinization
  ○ pK_a

TABLE 44-4 Common Drugs Used in Pediatric Nerve Blocks

DRUG/TYPE OF BLOCK	PK_a	PROTEIN BINDING (%)	EQUI-EFFECTIVE CONCENTRATION	POTENCY	CONCEN-TRATION (%)	ONSET	DURATION (min)	MAXIMAL DOSES WITHOUT EPINEPHRINE (mg/kg)	MAXIMAL DOSES WITH EPINEPHRINE (mg/kg)
Chloroprocaine									
Infiltration	8.7	—	2	4	1–2	Rapid	30–45	8	10
Epidural					2–3	Rapid	30–60		
Procaine	8.9	6	2	1				7	8.5
Tetracaine	8.5	76	0.25	16	1	Slow	60–150		
Spinal									
Bupivacaine	8.1	96	0.25	16				2	3
Infiltration					0.25–0.5	Slow	90–360		
Peripheral					0.25–0.5	Slow	120–360		
Epidural					0.125–0.5	Slow	120–360		
Lidocaine	7.9	64	1	4				5	7
Infiltration					0.5–1.0	Rapid	30–60		
Topical					2–10	Rapid	30–60		
Peripheral					1.0–2.0	Rapid	30–90		
Epidural					0.3–2.0	Rapid	30–90		
Spinal					5.0	Rapid	30–90		
Mepivacaine	7.6	78	1	2				5	6
Infiltration					1.0	Slow	60–90		
Peripheral					1–1.5	Slow	60–120		
Epidural					1.5–2.0	Slow	60–120		
Prilocaine	7.9	55	1	3				5	7
Ropivacaine									
Epidural	8.1	94	0.2	14	0.2–0.5	Slow	60–240		

○ Acid–base
○ Local calcium concentration
○ Nerve stimulation rate
○ Local concentration effects
○ Temperature

Toxicity

- Peak absorption is site-dependent: intercostal, intratracheal > caudal/epidural > brachial plexus > distal peripheral > subcutaneous
- Total drug dose
- Clinical signs of toxicity:
  ○ Central nervous system: visual disturbance, tinnitus, anxiety, twitching, convulsions, cardiorespiratory depression, coma, death
  ○ Cardiovascular system: vasodilation, hypotension, ventricular dysrhythmias, myocardial depression, cardiovascular collapse
  ○ Respiratory system: respiratory arrest, hypoxia
  ○ Allergy: uncommon with amides, more likely vasovagal reaction; ester allergy more common, especially with patients allergic to *para*-aminobenzoic acid
  ○ Methemoglobinemia: associated with prilocaine, especially in newborns, for example, EMLA

Treatment Regimen

- Start with ABCs.
- Intravenous lipid emulsion
- Prolonged CPR (especially with bupivacaine) may be required.

Common Applications

Axial Blocks

- Caudal/lumbar/thoracic epidural
- Intrathecal/spinal anesthesia

Regional Blocks

- Head (infra-orbital, supraorbital, palantine, greater occipital)
- Upper limb (interscalene, supra/infra-clavicular, axillary)

- Trunk (intercostal)
- Abdomen (transversus abdominus plane [TAP], rectus abdominus)
- Lower limb (lumbar plexus, femoral, sciatic [infra-gluteal, popliteal], ankle)
- Bier/intravenous
- Field/transdermal

INTRAVENOUS PATIENT-CONTROLLED ANALGESIA

- As pain, especially acute, postoperative pain, is not of constant intensity, and the person who best knows the pain is the patient, patient-controlled analgesia systems have been well accepted, even in the pediatric population.
- In the situation where a child is too young or too sick (ie, debilitated) to provide his or her own initiation of drug dosing (pushing a button), a properly trained nurse or parent/guardian can intervene and provide the necessary dose of medication.

Principles of PCA

- Patient/parent/nurse-controlled analgesia systems all have similar elements.
  ○ Drug in a reservoir
  ○ Mechanized/computerized management of drug delivery
  ○ Means to deliver drug (intravenous line, subcutaneous access)
  ○ Programmed regimen to deliver drug
    ▪ Basal infusion = a continuous delivery of medication.
    ▪ Bolus infusion = dose of medication to be delivered on demand of the patient/parent/nurse.
    ▪ Lockout doses = maximum number of doses that can be delivered to a patient in a certain period (eg, doses/hour).
    ▪ Lockout time = minimum number of minutes that must transpire between doses.
- "Smart" PCA incorporating complex algorithms that adjust basal and bolus regimens.
- Drugs commonly used for PCA in the pediatric population are listed in Table 44-5.

TABLE 44-5 **Common Drugs/Starting Regimens for PCA**

DRUG	CONCENTRATION	BASAL (µg/kg/h)	BOLUS (µg/kg/dose)	LOCKOUT min	LOCKOUT doses/h	COMMENTS
Fentanyl	10 µg/mL	0.5	0.5	15	3	Commonly used for infants May have facial pruritus/blanching
Nalbuphine	1 mg/mL	20	20	8	5	May have a ceiling effect and fewer side effects
Morphine	1 mg/mL	20	20	8	5	May also be sedating
Hydromorphone	0.2 mg/mL	4	4	8	5	May have fewer side effects and be less sedating

Systematizing Management

- Protocol development, for example, perioperative management that provides anticipatory intervention (eg, preoperative use of multimodal techniques such as gabapentin, tizandine, and bisacodyl)
- Systemwide education
  - Parent/nurse/physician education
  - Observation/assessment
  - Management of side effects
  - Management of operational failures

EPIDURAL ANALGESIA

Principles of Regional Analgesia

- Anatomy/placement
  - The epidural potential space can be injected with a variety of medications from several access points along the patient's back: cervical, thoracic, lumbar, and caudal. Furthermore, in smaller children (<5 years of age), it is not difficult to enter the epidural space from the caudal site and then thread a catheter within the space to a higher level.
  - Use of specialty catheters (eg, Tsui stimulating catheter) to aid in identifying appropriate myotomal/dermatomal level of placement.
  - In larger children and adults, the lumbar or thoracic epidural space is entered from a puncture in the lower or upper back, respectively.
  - Nearly all epidural placements in children occur at the time of the surgical procedure, with the child asleep.

Diamond Theory

- Sympathetic, sensory, motor blockade:
  - Local anesthetics are the mainstay of axial analgesia in children (see above discussion of local anesthetics).
  - The three basic effects of local anesthetics placed in the epidural space are sympathetic blockade, diminution (or ablation) of the afferent pain signals to the brain, and blockade of outgoing, efferent, motor signals.

- The height (or cephalocaudal dimension) of the block depends on the volume of the agents injected relative to the point of injection. In contrast to intrathecal injections, the baricity of the agent and the position of the patient have little, if any, effect.
- Anesthesia versus analgesia: The density of the block, or the differential effect of the agents on sympathetic (always), sensory (usually), or motor (sometimes) pathways, depends on the amount of agent injected (concentration).
- Adjuvants: Pathways that contribute to postoperative pain can be affected by epidural injection of agents before, during, and/or after the operative procedure. In addition to local anesthetics, opiate agonists and α-agonists improve and augment effects while reducing the overall side effect profile.
  - Opiates (fentanyl, hydromorphone, morphine)
  - Clonidine

Common Drug Regimens

Single-shot Caudal

- With a 22-gauge needle (or angiocatheter), a single injection can be given for intra- and postoperative pain relief.
- This can be performed for common outpatient procedures such as herniorrhaphy and circumcision.

Epidural PCA

- Continuous epidural analgesia (with or without bolus, depending on the patient's ability to participate) can be provided via the caudal, lumbar, or even thoracic route.
- Doses are calculated based on the total dose allowed of local anesthetic using mg programming in the pump.
- Local anesthetics and additives used for epidural PCA are described in Tables 44-6 and 44-7.

Management of Side Effects

- Nausea/vomiting: ondansetron, diphenhydramine, droperidol, metoclopramide
- Itching: diphenhydramine, hydroxyzine, butorphanol, naloxone infusion

TABLE 44-6   Local Anesthetics Used for Epidural Anesthesia in the Pediatric Population

LOCAL ANESTHETIC	BASAL (mL/kg)	BOLUS (mL/kg)	LOCKOUT min	LOCKOUT doses/h	MAXIMUM DELIVERED (mg/kg/h)
Infant: lidocaine (2 mg/mL)	0.5	0	N/A	N/A	1
Child: lidocaine (3 mg/mL)	0.2	0.1	15	3	1.5
Bupivacaine (0.8 mg/mL)	0.2	0.1	15	2	0.32
Bupivacaine (1 mg/mL)	0.2	0.1	15	2	0.4
Ropivacaine (1.5 mg/mL)	0.2	0.1	15	2	0.6
Ropivacaine (2 mg/mL)	0.2	0.1	15	2	0.8

TABLE 44-7   Additives (Opiate and/or Clonidine) Used to Improve the Analgesic Effect of Epidural Analgesia (and May Permit Using a Lower Concentration)

DRUG GROUP	DRUG	CONCENTRATION	COMMENTS
Opiate	Fentanyl	1–2 µg/mL	Tends to stay in area of deposition
	Hydromorphone	10–20 µg/mL	May ascend up the spinal cord somewhat
	Morphine	10–20 µg/mL	Tends to ascend cephalad and is more likely to be associated with respiratory depression
Local anesthetic	Lidocaine	Infants: 1 mg/mL Children: 3 mg/mL	Serum levels may be monitored (keep ≤4 mcg/mL) to reduce risk of toxicity
	Max dose: 1.5 mg/kg/h		
		Older children: 5 mg/mL	
	Bupivacaine	0.0625%–0.125%	Gives a good differential block for postoperative analgesia at lower concentrations
	Max dose: 0.4 mg/kg/h		
	Ropivacaine	0.1%–0.2%	Less cardiac toxicity at equianalgesic concentrations
	Max dose: 0.8 mg/kg/h		
α-agonist	Clonidine	0.5–1 mg/mL	Potentiates both local anesthetic and opiate May be associated with some hypotension and sedation

TABLE 44-8   Common Oral Opiates Used to Treat Pediatric Pain

DRUG	WITH ACETAMINOPHEN	AVAILABILITY	DOSE
Hydrocodone	120 mg	Solution: 2.5 mg/5 mL	Based on hydrocodone 0.1 mg/kg q4h
Vicodin	500 mg	Tablet: 2.5 or 5 mg	
Hydromorphone		Tablet: 2, 4 mg	0.2 mg/kg q4h
Dilaudid		Rectal suppository: 3 mg	0.2 mg/kg q6h
Methadone		Solution: 5, 10 mg/5 mL	0.1 mg/kg q4h
Morphine		Solution: 10, 20, 100 mg/5 mL	0.3–0.5 mg/kg q4h
MS-Contin		Tablets: 10, 15, 30 mg	0.3–0.5 mg/kg q4h
		Extended release: 15, 30, 60, 100 mg	
Oxycodone		Solution: 1 mg/mL	0.1 mg/kg q4h
		Tablet: 5 mg	0.1 mg/kg q4h
Percoset	25 mg	5 mg	Based on acetaminophen
Tylox	500 mg	5 mg	
Oxycontin		Extended release: 10, 20, 40 mg	

- Constipation: Senokot
- Urinary retention: urinary catheter

Transition to Home

- Basal analgesia is converted to oral analgesia.
- Once the patient can tolerate eating some food, oral analgesics (eg, oral opioids, see Table 44-8) are given, the basal infusion is discontinued (leaving the bolus only for a while as a rescue), and then PCA is discontinued.

PRESCRIPTION FILLING

- It is best not to assume that every drug is available in every neighborhood pharmacy, especially the liquid forms of opiates.

FOLLOW-UP

- It is easy to neglect to follow up once patients have gone home. A simple call may reveal problems that can be solved by an experienced clinician.

BIBLIOGRAPHY

Schechter NL, Berde CB, Yaster M. *Pain in Infants, Children, and Adolescents.* Baltimore, Md: Lippincott Williams & Wilkins; 2003.

Yaster M, Cote CJ, Krane EJ, et al. *Pediatric Pain Management and Sedation Handbook.* Baltimore, Md: Mosby; 1997.

45 PERIPHERAL NEUROPATHY

Anand C. Thakur, MD

- Peripheral neuropathy: A large group of nerve disorders with multiple etiologies and presentations.
- Epidemiology: The presence of polyneuropathy is 2.4% in midlife but rises to 8% in patients greater than 55 years of age.
- Definition: Neuropathy is a disturbance of nerve structure or function.
- Peripheral neuropathy is divided into three subtypes:
  - Mononeuropathy: Usually caused by a single large nerve injury in the upper or lower extremity and/or cranial nerves. Mechanism of injury is usually compression, but may arise from many different entities.
  - Mononeuropathy multiplex: A situation in which two or more mononeuropathies evolve in close temporal sequence. Pain is the first symptom followed by sensory loss and weakness in the distribution of each single nerve. Mechanism of injury is related to infection, vasculitis, diabetes, paraneoplastic syndromes, ischemia, or connective tissue disorder.
  - Polyneuropathy: Involves multiple single nerve injury or multiple nerves injured at once.
- Comment etiology for peripheral neuropathies:
  - Metabolic: Liver disease, uremia, and porphyoria.
  - Endocrine: Diabetes, hyperthyroidism, and hypothyroidism.
  - Nutritional: Vitamin B deficiencies (B1, B2, B6, and B12), folic acid deficiency, gastric bypass surgery, alcohol abuse, pellagra, and beri beri.
  - Connective tissue disorders: SLE, rheumatoid arthritis, scleroderma, Sjögren's syndrome, and polyarteritis nodosa.
  - Inflammatory diseases: GBS, HIV, Lyme disease, CIDP, and leprosy.
  - Genetic: Charcot–Marie–Tooth disease, Fabry's disease, hereditary sensory neuropathy.
  - Toxic agents: Thallium, arsenic, cisplatin, and isoniazid.
  - Paraneoplastic syndrome: Carcinoma, lymphoma, and leukemia.
  - Amyloidosis, vasculitis, and sarcoidosis.

Abbreviations: GBS, Guillain–Barré syndrome; CIDP, chronic inflammatory demyelinating polyneuropathy; SLE, systemic lupus erythematosus.

- Pathophysiology:
  - Peripheral neuropathy falls under the umbrella of neuropathic pain, which is pain arising from abnormalities or dysfunction within the central or peripheral nervous system.
  - Peripheral neuropathies involve a single nerve or root, multiple individual nerves, and/or small fiber syndromes that do not conform to nondermatomal patterns.
  - Site of initial injury helps to better categorize neuropathic pain.
    - Peripheral: Painful peripheral polyneuropathies, focal entrapment neuropathies, traumatic neuropathies, and postsurgical syndromes (stump pain and phantom pain post-amputation and postthoracotomy syndrome).
    - Central: Traumatic brachial plexus avulsion, traumatic spinal cord injury, ischemic cerebral vascular injury, syringomyelia, and arachnoiditis.
    - Mixed: Complex regional pain syndrome (Type I—reflex sympathetic dystrophy) and (Type II—causalgia); acute herpetic and postherpetic neuralgia, meningioradiculopathies, and epidural/spinal cord compression.
- Peripheral mechanisms of nerve injury:
  - One third of all the cases of peripheral neuropathy develop in response to diabetes mellitus. The second most common cause is alcoholism. Further, still a large percentage of peripheral neuropathies are idiopathic.
  - Peripheral nerve injury involves trauma to the nerve fiber. There is an increased expression of sodium channels extending from the area of injury to the entire axon. The nerve becomes hypersensitive to ectopic stimuli. The neural membrane becomes unstable post-injury. The threshold response to chemical, mechanical, and thermal stimuli decreases. This increased expression of sodium channels on injured axons is the thought process behind the effect of sodium channel blockers and membrane stabilizing agents for the treatment of neuropathic pain and peripheral neuropathy.
  - Nerve injury causes the "inflammatory soup" in response to trauma. The release of inflammatory mediators leads to peripheral sensitization of the nerve endings.
  - The inflammatory soup consists of excitatory amino acids, hydrogen ions, potassium ions, nerve growth factors, catecholamines, serotonin, prostaglandins, cytokines, and bradykinins.
  - Another possible mechanism of peripheral neuropathy involves the sprouting of alpha adrenergic receptors in uninjured nerves and sympathetic fibers into the dorsal root ganglia of the injured nerve. Sympathetically mediated pain may occur in these situations. Sympathetic blockade or the application

alpha–adrenergic receptor antagonist (phentolamine) may help decrease the pain.

- Another possible mechanism with very limited support is ephaptic transmission in direct nerve to nerve coupling and contact. This form of communication involves electrical and chemical synapses. This bypasses the traditional routes of communication. This may lead to sympathetic efferents activating nociceptive afferents, thereby causing worsening sympathetic and neuropathic pain.

- Central mechanisms of peripheral nerve injury:
  - Peripheral nerve injury leads to decreased input into the central nervous system thereby inducing changes into the CNS. This is the mechanism that is proposed for diabetic neuropathy.
  - According to Wall and Melzack's gate theory, peripheral nerve injury/neuropathy can cause a loss of large A-beta fibers, thus resulting in a reduced nonnociceptive sensory input. This would allow for a lack of "gate" functioning, thus increasing the pain response.
  - Another mechanism of a centrally mediated response to peripheral neuropathy involves the death of dorsal horn interneurons in Rexed lamina II. These interneurons inhibit nociceptive transmission in the dorsal horn. Nerve injury allows for an influx of excitatory amino acids (EAA—glutamate and aspartate) which cause repeated firing of the dorsal horn interneurons, thus eventually leading to the cellular death of these dorsal horn interneurons. The inhibitory function of these interneurons is lost, pain transmission is left unabated.
  - Opioid and gamma–aminobutryic acid (GABA) receptors are downregulated post-experimental nerve injury. Both GABA and opioids are actively involved in inhibition of nociceptive transmission in the CNS. This allows for an imbalance in the excitatory and inhibitory pathways in the central nervous system.
  - In normal situations the C fibers localize to Rexed lamina II. A fibers predominate in all Rexed lamina except lamina II. After peripheral nerve injury in C fibers, A fibers sprout into lamina II. A fibers normally respond to mechanical nonnociceptive input. This sprouting mechanism allows for normally mechanical nonnociceptive input via peripheral A fibers to trigger interneurons in the pain pathway.
  - Central sensitization or "windup" phenomenon involves an increase in central nervous system input from injured peripheral afferents. This leads to a direct change in the central nervous system with a facilitated pathway of pain transmission. This

involves central nervous system neuronal changes such as a lower firing threshold, broadened nociceptive receptive fields, NMDA type glutamate receptor activation which leads to facilitated calcium transport, and spontaneously firing cells.

- "Phenotypic switching" post-peripheral nerve injury involves A-beta fibers, which normally do not release substance P, gaining the ability to release substance P thereby again creating a circumstance in which nonnociceptive input triggers the pain/nociceptive response.

- Common neurophysiologic elements in peripheral neuropathies:
  - Peripheral neuropathies commonly present a gradual sensory loss in a stocking–glove distribution. The longest nerve fibers are most easily injured. This is why the toes are most commonly affected first advancing to the more proximal legs. Disease progression involves the next longest fibers in the calves, proximal legs, fingers to the wrists, hands and forearms, and then chest.
  - Large sensory fiber loss involves a peripheral neuropathy in which there is usually a loss of vibration and joint position sense.
  - Small fiber peripheral neuropathy affects small myelinated and unmyelinated fibers causing a loss of pain, pinprick, and cold perception in a gradient fashion.
  - Light touch is carried by both large and small fibers and in most mononeuropathies there is both large and small fiber loss.
  - Polyneuropathies are usually symmetric. Mononeuropathies are usually asymmetric.
  - Acute onset neuropathies must be aggressively diagnosed and treated to find an underlying etiology. If left untreated or undiagnosed fatality may occur as in Guillain–Barré syndrome.

- Clinical features:
  - Along with a careful history and physical, a sensory and motor nerve length dependent pattern to help establish diagnoses of peripheral neuropathy.
  - Pain is often the most common presenting symptom for polyneuropathy. It is rarely present without other sensory abnormalities. Pain location and other symptoms are often the most important piece of historical information.
  - Peripheral neuropathies involve (1) baseline spontaneous pain and (2) evoked stimulus-dependent pain.
  - Evoked pain refers to an increase in pain following stimulation over and above the patient's baseline pain. It is an intense crescendo post-stimulation of the symptomatic area.

o Evoked pain and fear of evoked pain significantly restricted activities and functionality. Patients are less likely to engage in activities of all types that may induce pain.

o Evoked pain involves all abnormal responses to stimulation. Hyperalgesia involves a lowered nociceptive firing threshold. Hyperpathia involves a raised threshold with a delayed but explosive response status stimulation. Allodynia involves conscious pain experienced from nonnoxious stimuli.

o Small fiber polyneuropathies, as can develop with diabetes, start distally at the toes and progress proximally. There is a progression of findings that begin with small fibers (including pain) and move to larger fibers including loss of motor function. This can eventually lead to motor loss. Foot drop, gait disturbances, and severe functional losses happen over time.

o Power and deep tendon reflexes are usually preserved in patients with polyneuropathy.

o Sensory examination should include vibration testing, proprioception, light touch and special stimuli testing specifically light touch eliciting pain (allodynia), ice (temperature and abnormal lingering after sensations), single pinprick (sensory deficit or hyperpathia), and multiple pinpricks (summation pain—pain that goes more intense with repeated stimuli or lingering after sensations—common in polyneuropathy).

• Symptoms:
o Early: Distal numbness and tingling, distal neuropathic pain, gait imbalance, and toe weakness.
o Late features: Progression of numbness and tingling to proximal limbs, prominent neuropathic pain, easy tripping, worsening of gait, and frequent falls.

• Signs:
o Early signs: Distal sensory loss to cold, pinprick and/or vibration, reduction or loss of ankle reflex, Romberg sign, impaired tandem walking, and toe extensor weakness.
o Late signs: Distal loss of cold, pinprick, vibration, and joint position sense; loss of reflexes at ankles and knees; foot drop and inability to toe-and-heel walk.

• Abnormal sensations in neuropathic pain:
o Allodynia: A painful response to a usually nonnoxious stimuli (light touch is preceded as burning pain).
o Spontaneous pain: Burning, shooting, and lancinating.
o Paresthesias: Abnormal nonnoxious sensations that are spontaneous or evoked (tingling).
o Dysesthesias: Spontaneous or evoked pain that is abnormal (unpleasant tingling).
o Hyperalgesia: A normally noxious stimulus that produces an exaggerated painful response.

o Hyperpathia: A noxious or nonnoxious stimulus that produces an exaggerated painful response.

• Diagnosis:
o There are many current reviews detailing diagnosis and management of patients with painful peripheral neuropathy.
o Metabolic disorder, most commonly diabetes, is the most common cause of painful polyneuropathy.
o Neuropathy in diabetic patients ranges from 4% to 8% at initial presentation and increases to 15%–50% after 20–25 years.
o Some studies report an incidence of neuropathy painful and nonpainful up to 66%.
o The likelihood of neuropathy increases with the duration and disease.
o Incidence of painful neuropathy is 11.6% in insulin-dependent diabetes and 32.1% in non-insulin-dependent diabetes.
o There are many underlying causes to neuropathy or metabolic, nutritional, toxic, genetic, inflammatory, paraneoplastic, and connective tissue disorders. The underlying disease entity must first be established and managed.
o Evaluation of peripheral neuropathy involves a careful history and physical examination; electrodiagnostic testing and laboratory testing can reveal a cause in 76% of patients.
o Neurological examination in most peripheral neuropathies demonstrates a distal pattern of sensory loss from the toes to the more proximal legs, and with the progression of disease sensory loss travels from the fingertips to the wrists and forearms.
o This pattern is usually called a stocking and glove loss of sensation. This sensory loss is gradual in nature. It is not commonly abrupt.
o Sensory loss patterns are commonly symmetric. Asymmetric findings usually imply a superimposed process such as radiculopathy of a single or multiple roots, a plexopathy, spinal cord process, or a brainstem or cerebral cortex lesion.
o Injury to large sensory fibers results in loss of vibration and joint position sense.
o Injury to small fibers, myelinated and unmyelinated, will result in loss of pain pinprick and cold sensation.
o Light touch is carried by both small and large fibers. Most neuropathies involve both large and small fibers.
o In neuropathies strength is lost in a similar fashion to sensory examination, but later in the course of disease.
o After careful history and physical, laboratory assessment is necessary. Standard testing involves serum

electrolytes, creatinine, blood urea nitrogen, standard rheumatological screens, thyroid function tests, and chest x-ray.

○ If the above studies are essentially normal, further testing can involve serum protein electrophoresis (to rule out paraneoplastic syndromes, multiple myeloma, and paraproteinemias); HIV antibody testing, Lyme titers, skeletal survey (to rule out tumor and multiple myeloma); vitamin B1, P2, B6, B12, niacin, and folate levels; lumbar puncture (to rule out Guillain-Barré and multiple sclerosis); testing for toxic substances; and nerve biopsy.

○ Electrodiagnostic studies EMG (electromyography) and NCV (nerve conduction velocity) are an extension of the neurological exam.

○ Mononeuropathies and mononeuropathy multiplex are often easily diagnosed by EMG and NCV.

○ Electromyography distinguishes demyelinating diseases (reduction in nerve conduction velocities) from axonal damage (sitting reduction in amplitude of evoked responses) and neuropathy.

○ Unfortunately, electrodiagnostic testing does not reveal small fiber polyneuropathies.

○ Quantitative sensory testing (QST) is a more sensitive method of demonstrating small fiber neuropathies and injury. Threshold responds to heat, painful heat, cold, and painful cold stimuli allows assessment of small fiber damage.

○ Thermography has minimal value in the assessment of peripheral neuropathies.

• Management:

○ After the established diagnosis or etiology of the specific peripheral neuropathy, the goals such as symptomatic pain control, enhanced function (increase activity, concentration and socialization), reduced impairments (improved sleep and appetite), elimination of pain, and cure are not realistic treatment endpoints.

○ Pain control involves a multidisciplinary approach with rational polypharmacy with agents that act at multiple receptor subtypes.

○ Nerve injury causes increased sodium channel expression on injured peripheral nerves. Sodium channel antagonists: carbamazepine, oxcarbazepine, tricyclic antidepressants, and topical lidocaine.

○ Local anesthetics and antiarrhythmics have been recognized to suppress ectopic impulses in experimental nerve injury and have been used for peripheral neuropathic pain.

○ Sympatholytic agents have been mentioned for both the diagnosis and treatment of peripheral neuropathic pain. Nerve injury causes expression of alpha adrenergic receptors. Intravenous phentolamine infusion analgesia is a possible predictor of response to regional sympathetic ganglionic blockade and also possibly oral and transdermal sympatholytic agents. Clonidine, an alpha2-adrenergic agonist, has been postulated to help with neuropathic pain.

○ Calcium channel antagonists such as gabapentin and oxcarbazepine exert their effect by blocking the central sensitization that is mediated by calcium ion influx.

○ Descending inhibition of the pain pathway from the cerebral cortex to the dorsal horn of the spinal cord is augmented by opioids, tricyclic antidepressants, and tramadol. The use of opioids for the long-term treatment of noncancer neuropathic pain is controversial.

○ SSRIs are effective in controlling depression and anxiety but have little effect on pain in nondepressed patients. Fluoxetine (Prozac) blocks the presynaptic reuptake of serotonin. It has a benign side effect profile. Paroxetine (Paxil) has demonstrated benefit in diabetic neuropathy where fluoxetine did not.

○ Tricyclic antidepressants remain the mainstay of pharmacological treatment for peripheral neuropathic pain. Antidepressants and anticonvulsants also have analgesic properties. One must always be aware of the FDA indication for these medications and off-label and on-label uses.

○ Peripheral and systemic corticosteroids have had both empiric and anecdotal data to support its use. Perineural injection of corticosteroids have a potential membrane-stabilizing effect and reduce to spontaneous ectopic discharge seen in injured nerves and neuromas. There may also be a transient suppressive effect on C-fiber transmission.

○ Patients usually require a compliant therapy with agents from different classes, pain coping strategies, relaxation training, biofeedback, supportive psychotherapy, regular exercise, and increased social function.

BIBLIOGRAPHY

American Academy of Neurology, Therapeutics and Technology Assessment Subacute Committee, assessment: thermography in neurological practice. *Neurology.* 1990;40:523–525.

Benzon HT, et al. *Essentials of Pain Medicine and Regional Anesthesia* (Chapter 53). 2005:418–425.

Calcutt NA. Potential mechanisms of neuropathic pain and diabetes. *Int Rev Neurobiol.* 2002;58:205–228.

Devor M, Gorvin-Lippman R, Raber P. Corticosteroids suppress ectopic neural discharge originating in experimental neuromas. *Pain.* 1985;22:127–137.

Devor M, Wall P, Catalan N. Systemic lidocaine silences ectopic neuroma and DRG discharge without blocking nerve conduction. *Pain.* 1992;48:261–268.

Donofrio P. *Textbook of Peripheral Neuropathy* (Chapter 1). 2012:1–7.

Dyck PEJ, Kratz KM, Karnes JL, et al. The prevalence by stage severity of various types of diabetic neuropathy, retinopathy and nephropathy in a population based cold report: The Rochester diabetic neuropathy study. *Neurology.* 1993;43:817–824.

Dyck PJ, Oviatt KF, Lambert EH. Intensive evaluation of referred unclassified neuropathies yields improved diagnosis. *Ann Neurol.* 1981;10:222–226

Elliott KJ. Taxonomy and mechanisms of neuropathic pain. *Semin neurol.* 1994;14:195–205.

England JD, Asbury AK. Peripheral neuropathy. *Lancet.* 2004;363:2151–2161.

Feldman EL, Russell JW, Sullivan KA, et al. New insights into the pathogenesis of diabetic neuropathy. *Curr Opin Neurol.* 1999;12:553–563.

Fields HL, Rowbotham MC. Multiple mechanisms of neuropathic pain: a clinical perspective. In: Gebhart GF, Hammond DL, Jensen TS. eds. *Proceedings of the Seventh Ruled Congress on Pain.* Seattle, WA: IASP Progress; 1994:437–454.

Galer B, Harle J, Rowbotham M. Response to intravenous lidocaine infusion predicts subsequent response to oral mexiletine: a prospective study. *J Pain Sympt Manage.* 1996;12:161–167.

Galer BS. Painful polyneuropathy: diabetes, pathophysiology, and management. *Semin Neurol.* 1994;14:237–246.

Galer DBS. Neuropathic pain of peripheral origin: advances and pharmacologic treatment. *Neurology.* 1995;45(Suppl 9):S17–S25.

Johansson A, Bennett G. Effect of local methylprednisolone on pain in a nerve injury model. *Reg Anesth.* 1997;22: 59–65.

Martyn CN, Hughes RAC. Epidemiology of peripheral neuropathy. *Journal Neurol Neurosurg Psychiatry.* 1997; 62:310–318.

Mersky H, Bogduk N (eds). *Classification of Chronic Pain: Description of Chronic Pain Syndromes and Definition of Pain Terms.* Seattle, WA: IASP Press; 1994.

Portenoy RK. Chronic opioid therapy for chronic nonmalignant pain: from models to practice. *APS.* 1992;J1:285–288.

Raja SN, Treede RD, Davis KD, Campbell J. Systemic α adrenergic blockade with phentolamine: a diagnostic test for sympathetically mediated pain. *Anesthesiology.* 1991;74:691–698.

Ross MA. Neuropathies associated with diabetes. *Med Clin North Am.* 1993;77:111–124.

Thomas PK. Diabetic neuropathy: models, mechanisms and mayhem. *Can J Neurol Sci.* 1992;19:1.

Verrotti A, Giuva T, Morgese G, et al. No new transients in the etiopathogenesis of diabetic peripheral neuropathy. *J Child Neurol.* 2001;16:389–394.

Woolf CJ, Mannion RJ. Neuropathic pain: aetiology, symptoms, mechanisms, and management. *Lancet.* 1999;353:1959–1964.

Ziegler D, Gries FA, Spuler M, et al. The epidemiology of diabetic neuropathy. *J Diabetes Complicat.* 1992;6:49–57.

46 PHANTOM LIMB PAIN

Steven R. Hanling, MD
Ralph E. Tuttle, DO

NOMENCLATURE

- Residual Limb Pain (RLP) is a localized painful nociception in the residual limb following amputation.
- Phantom Limb Pain (PLP) is defined as pain perceived to be emanating from the absent limb.
- Phantom Limb Sensations (PLS) are any input other than pain that is perceived to originate in the missing limb.
- Phantom Complex (aka Phantom Limb Syndrome) is defined as the presence of all three amputated-related symptoms. It may be a useful term in discussion with patients as the three elements are frequently difficult to distinguish as separate entities by patients.

HISTORY

- Symptoms of PLP were first reported in the 16th century by the French military surgeon Ambroise Pare (1552) who described "faux sentiments," or phantom limb sensations, and "la douleur es parties amputees," what is now defined as phantom limb pain. Pare postulated both peripheral and central etiologies, which are still being refined.
- The term "Phantom Limb" was coined in 1871 by civil war surgeon Silas Weir Mitchell.
- The existence of PLP has been questioned as recently as the 1980s and amputees who sought treatment were frequently misperceived as being mentally disturbed. A survey of military amputees (majority Vietnamese) revealed a 85% prevalence rate. 61% discussed their symptoms with their physicians, but only 17% received any form of treatment.

EPIDEMIOLOGY

- Current studies have found as high as 77% of patients experience symptoms of PLP after amputation. Eighty-two percent of those who suffered have expressed symptoms to their physician with 68% receiving some form of treatment.
- The prevalence of PLP following amputation is approximately 72% with possibly higher incidence in those with a history of preexisting pain. In 75% of cases, the onset of PLP symptoms immediately follows limb amputation, but in some patients symptom onset can be delayed for up to several weeks.

- In a 2009 survey of amputees, 74.5% reported phantom limb pain, 45.2% endorsed stump pain, and 35.5% had a combination of both types of pain. 14.8% reported no residual pain symptoms.

MECHANISM(S) OF PLP

- Multifactorial Mechanism—Peripheral and Central—not fully elucidated (Figure 46-1)
- Peripheral
  - Neuroma sprouting and sensitization (considered primary mechanism until 1990s). Amputation-associated influx of chemical mediators leads to *sensitization* of remnant nerve endings via mechanisms such as upregulation of voltage-gated Na and Ca channels and can allow for transmission of nonpain stimulus as a painful stimulus or *ectopic firing*. This can occur due to signaling changes in peripheral nerves and formation of *ephapses* (lateral and nonsynaptic nerve connections) between damaged nerve fibers and demyelinated pain nerve fibers.
- Neuraxial (Spinal)
  - Sustained or intense activation of peripheral nociceptors during and after an amputation can lead to *central sensitization* (prolonged synaptic excitability) and *wind up* (increasing output with a repeated stimuli) in the dorsal root ganglion.
  - Persistent increased stimulus to the Dorsal Root Ganglion (DRG) may result in *decreased inhibitory pain pathway tone* and associated increased ectopic nerve firing as well as production of substance P by A-beta fibers (substance P is normally produced in A-delta and C pain-related nerve fibers).
  - In animal models, peripheral nerve injury can induce glial cell proliferation and sympathetic sprouting into the DRG. This *sympathetic-sensory coupling* may help account for subjective increases in pain with emotion and explain the occasionally successful treatment of phantom limb pain with adrenergic blocking agents.
- Central (Supraspinal)
  - *Somatosensory cortical reorganization* is thought to be the neural correlate of phantom limb pain. Early evidence for this theory was based on a primate study mapping cortical changes after digit amputations with the aid of electrodes. Subsequent human studies, based on magnetoencephalography (MEG) and blood oxygen level–dependent functional magnetic resonance imaging (fMRI), found ingrowth of the homuncular representation of the body into areas previously representing the amputated limb.
  - In studies comparing amputees with phantom limb pain versus those without phantom limb pain, all patients who experienced some cortical reorganization but greater ingrowth (ie, neuroplasticity) showed some correlation with the incidence of phantom limb pain.

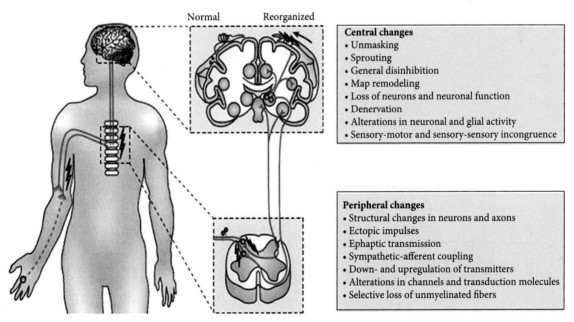

FIG. 46-1. Possible sites involved in the pathophysiology behind phantom pain. (Reproduced, with permission, from Flor H, Nikolajsen L, Staehelin Jensen T. Phantom limb pain: a case of maladaptive CNS plasticity. *Nature Rev Neurosci.* November 2006;7:873–881.)

CLINICAL MANIFESTATIONS

- Referred Sensations: Somatosensory cortical reorganization (Figure 46-2) helps explain why patients with amputations may induce phantom limb sensation and/or pain when they touch an area of the body whose cortical representation now overlaps the area previously represented the amputated limb. In the upper extremity this can occur with light touch to the corner of the lips. In lower extremity amputations, patients may experience this same phenomenon with bowel movements or urination. It is important for patients to understand that these phenomena are normal and that the occurrence of phantom limb sensation is not an indicator of future phantom pain.
- Patients can be reticent to discuss symptoms of phantom limb sensation and phantom limb pain for fear of being branded as having a psychiatric condition. They often question the validity of their symptoms and this can induce unnecessary levels of anxiety and distress. It can be helpful to discuss with patients that phantom limb sensation is a normal phenomenon following amputation. Phantom limb pain, however is a pathologic condition. Some patients note phantom limb sensation to be helpful in their progression to independent ambulation.
- Patients suffering from PLP at times note the phantom limb feels like it was in the position of the original injury.

TREATMENTS

- PLP treatments vary widely. A review of the literature demonstrates greater than 40 different methods of treatment for PLP. This variation likely mirrors the complexity of the pathophysiology of phantom limb pain. In general the current literature is mixed in terms of both methodological quality and durability of effect for both preventative therapies and treatment modalities.
- Preventative efforts should focus on achieving excellent pain control throughout the perioperative period starting at least 24 hours prior to surgery. Although evidence on the "best" means to achieve this pain control is mixed, the common theme seen in the literature is the correlation between preamputation pain and the severity of subsequent phantom limb pain.
- Although a recent study showed perioperative epidurals, started 48 hours preoperatively and continued 48 hours postoperatively, decreased PLP at 6 months, similar results occurred in the group that utilized IV PCA in the preoperative period. Several other well-designed studies have not found a distinct advantage of epidurals in reducing the incidence or severity of PLP.
- There are currently no disease modify drugs for any of the components of phantom limb complex. Current medication treatments focus on symptom management in order to decrease suffering and increase patient function. Broad treatment categories include pharmacologic, physical medicine and rehabilitation, complementary alternative medicine (CAM), and interventional treatments.
- The only medication to show significantly durable effects (≥ 1 year) is calcitonin provided during the first postamputation week if symptoms occurred. However, this study had only nine patients and a follow-on study of calcitonin treatment for chronic PLP did not prove effective.
- Gabapentin results are mixed with a study involving administration for 30 days after amputation having no effect on the incidence or severity of PLP and study on gabapentin for existing phantom limb pain reported as positive when measured at 6 weeks.

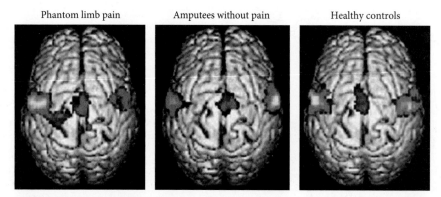

Phantom limb pain   Amputees without pain   Healthy controls

FIG. 46-2. Functional MRI comparing changes in the somatosensory and motor areas between healthy patients, amputees without phantom limb pain, and amputees with phantom limb pain. The imaging denotes extension of the cortical representation of the mouth region into the regions of the hands and arm, *only in patients with phantom limb pain*. (Reproduced, with permission, from Flor H, Nikolajsen L, Staehelin Jensen T. Phantom limb pain: a case of maladaptive CNS plasticity. *Nature Rev Neurosci.* November 2006:7:873–881.)

- Ketamine, but not memantine, has shown efficacy in pain reduction but the effect was measured at less then 72 hours in each case, making it difficult to interpret its ability to provide durable relief.
- Small case series on treatment of peripheral nerves by prolonged ambulatory continuous peripheral nerve block (CPNB), pulsed radiofrequency ablation, or peripheral nerve stimulation (PNS) shows the possibility of treatment for intractable PLP. An initial positive response to local anesthetic block at the inciting nerve or neuroma is crucial in predicting potential benefit.
- A case series of four patients treated with Spinal Cord Stimulation (SCS) for PLP has been reported; however, the number of patients treated in this study were low and the durability of effect has not been properly evaluated. Other reports suffer from small numbers, heterogeneous study populations, and outcome measures.
- Outcomes related to surgical revision of amputation-related neuromas are not uniformly successful, which seems consistent with the multifactorial nature of persistent phantom pain. A notable caveat to that statement is that surgical revision of clinically significant postamputation heterotopic ossification (HO) (prevalence rate up to 65%) is associated with a low recurrence rate, decreased limb pain, and increased functioning with prosthetic limbs.
- Deep Brain Stimulation (DBS) and Motor Cortex Stimulation (MCS) have been utilized to target structures such as the thalamus, periaqueductal gray, and the motor cortex to yield significant improvements in pain severity, analgesic use, and improved quality of life. Specific results with phantom limb pain are still too limited to make these mainstream recommendations in light of their associated risk. Transcranial Magnetic Simulation (TMS), a proven modality in the treatment of depression, has limited results in pain, but if treatment effects can be prolonged it may offer a noninvasive alternative to MCS.
- Mirror therapy, first reported in 1996 by Dr. Ramachandran, consists of patients focusing on the mirror image of their intact limb and viewing the virtual image of the missing limb "moving" in the mirror in response to their motor commands. Dr. Ramachandran and others have noted an association with an inability to move a person's phantom limb or "paralyzed phantom limb" associated with PLP—especially when the phantom limb sticks in the position of injury. A subsequent randomized controlled trial has shown promising results for this non-invasive, inexpensive therapy, although all the studies on this topic are limited by small numbers of patients. Overall mirror therapy, mental imagery, and graded motor imagery techniques often require persistent

and prolonged application with varying degrees of durability. However these procedures are easily learned and administered by patients, and are noninvasive, inexpensive, and of minimal risk. This combination of attributes makes them logical to be tried before high-dose medications and invasive procedures and makes them beneficial for patients in remote areas of the world with constrained healthcare assets. (ie, land mine victims).
- Psychological modalities such as Cognitive Behavioral Therapy (CBT) have not been directly evaluated for effects on PLP but have shown benefits in other types of pain. Because PLP is not often found in isolation, and CBT is another noninvasive and economical treatment, it should be considered before high-dose medications and invasive procedures.

CONCLUSION

- Phantom limb pain is a frequently occurring phenomenon in amputees who present with a normal psychological profile. It should not be assumed that such pain is a psychosomatic manifestation related to the loss of a limb. However, it is true that symptoms are frequently triggered and exacerbated by psychological factors in a manner not unlike other pain syndromes. The effect is most likely mediated via the sympathetic nervous system and by an increase in peripheral muscle tension.
- Currently there is no one treatment that can be considered uniformly efficacious and durable for a majority of patients. Therefore, treatments should focus on the restoration of function and relief of pain through multimodal and interdisciplinary care. Medications should be dosed based on their efficacy for other known indications such as neuropathic pain to avoid unnecessary complications. The risk benefit of utilizing procedural treatments must be weighed carefully as well with consideration given to the use of CAM modalities that although unproven specifically for PLP and appear to have a much better risk profile than many of our other treatments.
- Future efforts need to focus on large-scale studies to validate risk factors and treatment options. Genomics studies have started and may offer clues to more effective treatments. Ultimately, PLP research must start to bridge the gap between treatments and prevention of PLP in surgically amputated patients. A case series on preemptive mirror therapy to prevent PLP in patients receiving amputation after failed attempts at limb preservation shows potential and a larger scale trail to include pre- and postamputation fMRI is underway.

BIBLIOGRAPHY

Beaumont G, Mercier C, Michon P-E, et al. Decreasing phantom limb pain through observation of action and imagery: a case series. *Pain Med.* 2011;12(2):289–299.

Bittar RG, Otero S, Carter H, et al. Deep brain stimulation for phantom limb pain. *J Cln Neurosci.* 2005;12(4):399–404.

Bone M, Critchley P, Buggy DJ. Gabapentin in postamputation phantom limb pain: a randomized, double-blind, placebo-controlled, cross-over study. *Reg Anesth Pain Med.* 2002;27(5):481–486.

Borghi B, D'Addabbo M, White PF, et al. The use of prolonged peripheral neural blockade after lower extremity amputation: the effect on symptoms associated with phantom limb syndrome. *Anesth Analg.* 2010 Nov;111(5):1308–15.

Cohen S, Hsu E. Postamputation pain: epidemiology, mechanisms, and treatment. *J Pain Res.* 2013:121.

Eichenberger U, Neff F, Svetcic G, et al. Chronic phantom limb pain: the effects of calcitonin, ketamine, and their combination on pain and sensory thresholds. *Anesth Analg.* 2008;106(4):1265–1273.

Flor H. Phantom-limb pain: characteristics, causes, and treatment. *The Lancet Neurology.* 2002;1(3):182–189.

Flor H. Phantom limb pain. In: Basbaum AI, Bushnell MC, eds. *Science of Pain.* Academic Press; 2009:699–706.

Flor H, Elbert T, Knecht S, et al. Phantom-limb pain as a perceptual correlate of cortical reorganization following arm amputation. *Nature.* 1995;375(6531):482–484.

Forsberg JA, Pepek JM, Wagner S, et al. Heterotopic ossification in high-energy wartime extremity injuries: prevalence and risk factors. *Journal Bone Joint Surg.* 2009;91(5):1084–1091.

Halbert J, Crotty M, Cameron ID. Evidence for the optimal management of acute and chronic phantom pain: a systematic review. 2002; Available from: http://journals.lww.com/clinicalpain/Abstract/2002/03000/Evidence_for_the_Optimal_Management_of_Acute_and.3.aspx

Hanling SR, Wallace SC, Hollenbeck KJ, et al. Preamputation mirror therapy may prevent development of phantom limb pain: a case series. *Anesth Analg.* 2010;110(2):611–614.

Ilfeld BM, Bertram TM, Hanling S, et al. Treating intractable phantom limb pain with ambulatory continuous peripheral nerve blocks: a pilot study. *Pain Med.* 2013;14(6):935–942.

Jaeger H, Maier C. Calcitonin in phantom limb pain: a double-blind study. *Pain.* 1992;48(1):21–27.

Karanikolas M, Aretha D, Tsolakis I, et al. Optimized perioperative analgesia reduces chronic phantom limb pain intensity, prevalence, and frequency: a prospective, randomized, clinical trial. *Anesthesiology.* 2011;14(5):1144–1154.

Keil G. So-called initial description of phantom pain by Ambroise Paré. ["Chose digne d'admiration et quasi incredible": the 'douleur ès parties mortes et amputées']. 1990.

Kern U, Busch V, Rockland M, et al. Prevalence and risk factors of phantom limb pain and phantom limb sensations in Germany: a nationwide field survey. *Schmerz.* 2009;23(5):479–488.

Ketz AK. The experience of phantom limb pain in patients with combat-related traumatic amputations. *Arch Phys Med Rehabil.* 2008;89(6):1127–1132.

Knotkova H, Cruciani RA, Tronnier VM, et al. Current and future options for the management of phantom-limb pain. *J Pain Res.* 2012:39–49.

Lambert AW, Dashfield AK, Cosgrove C, et al. Randomized prospective study comparing preoperative epidural and intraoperative perineural analgesia for the prevention of postoperative stump and phantom limb pain following major amputation. *Reg Anesth Pain Med.* 2001;26(4):316–321.

MacIver K, Lloyd DM, Kelly S, et al. Phantom limb pain, cortical reorganization and the therapeutic effect of mental imagery. *Brain.* 2008;131(Pt 8):2181–2191.

Nikolajsen L, Finnerup NB, Kramp S, et al. A randomized study of the effects of gabapentin on postamputation pain. *Anesthesiology.* 2006;105(5):1008–1015.

Nikolajsen L, Hansen CL, Nielsen J, et al. The effect of ketamine on phantom pain: a central neuropathic disorder maintained by peripheral input. *Pain.* 1996;67(1):69–77.

Nikolajsen L, Jensen TS. Phantom limb pain. *Br J Anaesth.* 2001;87(1):107–116.

Pinzur MS, Garla PGN, Pluth T, et al. Continuous postoperative infusion of a regional anesthetic after an amputation of the lower extremity. *A Randomized Clinical Trial.* 2009:1–6.

Potter BK, Burns TC, Lacap AP, et al. Heterotopic ossification following traumatic and combat-related amputations: prevalence, risk factors, and preliminary results of excision. *J Bone Joint Surg.* 2007;89(3):476–486.

Ramachandran VS, Hirstein W. The perception of phantom limbs. The D. O. Hebb lecture. *Brain.* 1998;121(Pt 9):1603–1630.

Rathmell JP, Kehlet H. Do we have the tools to prevent phantom limb pain? *Anesthesiology.* 2011;114(5):1021–1024.

Rauck RL, Kapural L, Cohen SP, et al. Peripheral nerve stimulation for the treatment of postamputation pain—a case report. *Pain Pract.* 2012;12(8):649–655.

Richardson C, Glenn S, Nurmikko T, et al. Incidence of phantom phenomena including phantom limb pain 6 months after major lower limb amputation in patients with peripheral vascular disease. *Clin J Pain.* 2006;22(4):353–358.

Sherman RA, Sherman CJ. Prevalence and characteristics of chronic phantom limb pain among American veterans. Results of a trial survey. *Am J Phys Med.* 1983;62(5):227–238.

Shinder V, Govrin-Lippmann R, Cohen S, et al. Structural basis of sympathetic-sensory coupling in rat and human dorsal root ganglia following peripheral nerve injury. *J Neurocytol.* 1999;28(9):743–761.

Viswanathan A, Phan PC, Burton AW. Use of spinal cord stimulation in the treatment of phantom limb pain: case series and review of the literature. *Pain Pract.* 2010;10(5):479–484.

West M, Wu H. Pulsed radiofrequency ablation for residual and phantom limb pain: a case series. *Pain Pract.* 2010;10(5):485–491.

Woolf CJ. Central sensitization: implications for the diagnosis and treatment of pain. *Pain.* 2011;152(3 Suppl):S2–S15.

47 POSTHERPETIC NEURALGIA

Annie Philip, MBBS
Rajbala Thakur, MBBS

DEFINITION

- Postherpetic neuralgia (PHN), the most common painful sequelae of acute herpes zoster, is defined as a persistent, unilateral dermatomal pain lasting for more than 120 days after the onset of zoster rash.

EPIDEMIOLOGY/RISK FACTORS

- PHN is the third most common cause of neuropathic pain in the USA.
- Incidence and prevalence of PHN varies with age, developing in about 9%–34% of individuals with herpes zoster, depending on the definition used. The incidence may be as high as 47% in persons older than 60 years of age; however, the precise figures differ greatly depending on whether the patients studied are in the community or are part of clinical trials.

MAJOR RISK FACTORS FOR DEVELOPING PHN

- Older age
- Greater acute pain during herpes zoster
- Greater severity of rash
- Prodromal pain

MINOR RISK FACTORS

- Female gender
- Greater sensory abnormalities in the affected dermatomes
- Polyneuropathy
- Psychosocial variables
- Opthalmic distribution

PATHOGENESIS

- Sensory sensitization and deafferentation are the most important pathophysiological mechanisms involved in the development of PHN.
- Reactivation of latent virus followed by its replication causes inflammatory neural damage in the involved sensory ganglion, dorsal horn, and peripheral nerve, inducing a cycle of peripheral as well as central sensitization that results in ongoing chronic pain.

- Severity of neural damage correlates with the severity of acute syndrome and subsequent PHN.
- Sensitized and irritated nociceptors and DRG cells maintain the peripheral sensitization and also result in central sensitization. The primary neurotransmitter in this process is glutamate which activates the NMDA receptor.
- Deafferentation, resulting from excitotoxicity, cell death, and central plasticity, is another important mechanism. In PHN there may be a complete loss of both large and small diameter sensory afferent fibers. This loss of peripheral input results in the development of spontaneous discharges in the deafferentated central neurons and leads to intrinsic changes in the CNS. This produces constant pain in addition to severe mechanical allodynia in the area of sensory loss.

CLINICAL MANIFESTATION OF PHN

- PHN most often occurs as a continuum of acute herpes pain, but can occur after a lapse of months to years following an acute episode of zoster.
- The pain can extend beyond the dermatome of the initial rash and is precipitated as well as exacerbated by immunosuppression, stress, or a surgical procedure.

Thoracic dermatomes are the most commonly affected dermatomes (Table 47-1).

- Patients often describe PHN pain as a constant, burning, throbbing, or episodic sharp electric shock–like sensation.
- Allodynia, an excessively painful response to an innocuous stimulus, is a common symptom of PHN, and may be the most debilitating symptom associated with this disorder. Tactile allodynia can be so severe that patients with truncal PHN are not able to tolerate the sensation of clothing against the affected skin site.
- Pruritis with or without pain may be present.
- Skin can exhibit scarring, discoloration, hypoesthesia, hyperesthesia, hyperalgesia, and paraesthesias.

TABLE 47-1 **Dermatomal Distribution of Herpes Zoster and PHN**

- Thoracic: 50%
- Cranial: 10%–20% ophthalmic division of trigeminal nerve and other cranial nerves
- Cervical: 10%–20%
- Lumbar: 10%–20%
- Sacral: 2%–8%
- Generalized: <1%

- Musculoskeletal signs and symptoms may consist of painful muscle spasm, trigger points, weakness or paralysis of local muscle, and reduced range of joint motion.

DIAGNOSIS of PHN is based primarily on clinical findings.

TREATMENT OF PHN

- Management of PHN is a challenging task for the clinician and frustrating and often debilitating for the patient. A multimodal, individualized therapeutic approach is optimal. A modified World Health Organization (WHO) analgesic ladder can be used as a first line tool to help guide the therapy See Figure 47-1.
- Pharmacotherapy is the mainstay of management and includes topical medications, antiepileptics, antidepressants, opioids, and NMDA antagonists. Adjuvant modalities including TENS unit, acupuncture and behavioral cognitive therapy, invasive interventions with neuraxial analgesia, peripheral somatic nerve blocks, sympathetic blocks, spinal cord stimulation, ablative procedures, and surgical intervention have a minimal role in the management of PHN pain.

PHARMACOTHERAPY

Topical Medications

- **Lidocaine Patch 5%:** The FDA approved for the treatment of PHN. The patch is efficacious in the treatment of patients with clinical evidence of allodynia. Lidocaine is a sodium channel blocker and it inhibits ectopic discharge in damaged nociceptors. A randomized, controlled crossover trial showed that lidocaine patch was strongly preferred by PHN patients over a vehicle patch (78.1% vs. 9.4%). Lidocaine gel is also efficacious in PHN patients with allodynia and this should be considered if lidocaine patches are not available, affordable, or their application is problematic.
- **Capsaicin:** This compound works by depleting algogenic peptides, namely substance P, from peripheral nociceptors resulting in pain relief. High-dose capsaicin patch 8% was approved by the FDA in 2009 for the treatment of PHN. This patch is applied under medical supervision. To avoid discomfort, the affected area is prepared with topical local anesthetic cream for 30–45 minutes prior to application of the patch. The patient may also need additional analgesics before and after treatment. Up to four patches can be used concurrently. Two randomized, double-blind placebo-controlled studies in patients with neuropathic pain 6 weeks after application of high-dose capsaicin patch showed 2–12 week reduction in pain intensity by 30% compared with 0.04% capsaicin cream.

In addition over-the-counter capsaicin preparations including 0.025% and 0.075% Capsaicin cream and 0.025% patch are available and may be somewhat useful in PHN. Initial application causes worsening of the burning sensation but repeated application results in desensitization of the unmyelinated epidermal nerve fibers.

- **Other Topical Treatments:** A number of compounded preparations, including mixtures of analgesics and adjuvant medications, are occasionally used in clinical practice with a varying degree of success.
- **Systemic Medications:** Anticonvulsants are the first line agents used for the treatment of PHN because of

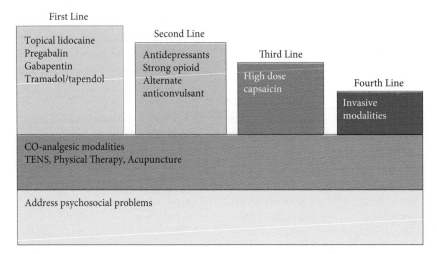

FIG. 47-1. Recommended analgesic ladder for PHN.

their excellent safety profile as compared to the tricyclic antidepressants. They are especially useful in reducing the lancinating component of neuropathic pain.

Gabapentinoids

- These medication bind to the alpha-2 delta subunit of the L-type calcium channel, stabilizing the cell membrane. This effect inhibits the release of glutamate, an excitatory neurotransmitter implicated in central sensitization. Side effects include somnolence, dizziness, visual disturbances, balance problems, and peripheral edema. These medications are eliminated via the kidneys; hence, dosage adjustments need to be done in case of renal insufficiency.
- **Gabapentin** is rapidly absorbed after oral administration. Absorption of this medication is mediated partially by co-transport mechanism in the gut that becomes saturated at higher doses. The bioavailability of gabapentin at a dose of 300 mg is 60% but this falls to 40% with 600 mg dose. The efficacious dose for gabapentin is 1800–3600 mg/d in three divided doses. Two large randomized controlled trials showed that the use of gabapentin resulted in statistically significant reduction in pain ratings, as well as improvement in sleep, mood, and quality of life at daily dose between 1800 and 3600 mg.

  Extended release gabapentin is said to be independent of the gut co-transport mechanism with possible reduced incidence of side effects. It was not found to be more effective than placebo when given 1800 mg once daily, but another randomized double-blinded placebo-controlled study in PHN showed that this formulation was more effective than placebo in twice daily dosing (600 mg AM and 1200 mg PM).
- **Pregabalin** has a similar efficacy profile to gabapentin but may have the advantage of more convenient dosing and a faster titration to an effective dose. Pregabalin is efficacious at a dose of 150–600 mg/d in two divided doses. This was shown to provide superior pain relief compared to placebo.
- Other anticonvulsants like valproic acid, carbamazepine, and topiramite are used rarely in clinical practice.

Antidepressants

- These medications have a number of postulated mechanisms of action that may explain their analgesic effects in PHN. These include inhibition of reuptake of norepinephrine and serotonin, modulation of opioid receptors, sodium channel blockade, NMDA, and histamine receptor antagonism. Side effects include orthostatic hypotension, sedation, constipation,

urinary retention, weight gain, blurred vision, palpitation, and QT prolongation.
- **Tricyclic Antidepressants:** These medications should be started at a low dose, typically 25 mg at night, and titrated slowly to a target dose of 75–100 mg/d in a single evening dose. In elderly or frail individuals, these agents can be started using a 10 mg evening dose. In a prospective, randomized, double-blind, crossover comparison study, 6 weeks of therapy with amitriptyline (12.5 mg–150 mg/d), lorazepam (0.5 mg–6 mg/d), or an inactive placebo, amitriptyline was found to be significantly more effective. Nortriptyline and desipramine might be equally effective and better tolerated than amitriptyline.
- **Selective Serotonin and Norepinephrine Reuptake Inhibitors (SNRIs):** Duloxetine and Venlafaxine have not been studied in PHN but have shown beneficial effects in the treatment of peripheral neuropathy and diabetic neuropathy related pain. Effective dose of Cymbalta is 60–120 mg/d and Effexor 75–225 mg/d.

Opioid Analgesics

- Opioid medications have an important role in the treatment of PHN but are prescribed as a second or third line agent. They can be used as single agents but mostly used as a part of combination therapy. When these medications are used for chronic pain, discuss and monitor for opioid tolerance, physical dependence, opioid abuse (relatively rare in elderly population), opioid-induced hyperalgesia, hypogonadism, and immune suppression. Few of the opioid medications have been studied and found effective in the management of PHN.
- **Oxycodone:** Analgesic efficacy of oral oxycodone was evaluated in a double-blind crossover trial in which it was shown to result in significant reduction in allodynia, steady pain, and spontaneous paroxysmal pain. Oxycodone treatment resulted in superior scores of global effectiveness, disability reduction, and patient preference compared to placebo.
- ***Combination Therapy:*** One recent study has demonstrated that the combination of gabapentin and morphine was superior to either of these medication used alone in relieving PHN. However, another recent study failed to show that oxycodone/pregabalin combination was superior to pregabalin/placebo.
- ***NMDA Antagonists:*** NMDA receptor is thought to play an important role in central sensitization and maintenance of chronic pain states including PHN. Ketamine is the most common among this group that includes Dextromethorphan and memantine: Common side effects for this class of medication include hypertension, tachyrythmias, hallucianations,

and other CNS side effects. In clinical practice ketamine can be used as outpatient infusion therapy, a part of the topical compounded creams or compounded oral preparations. In a double-blind crossover study between IV ketamine (0.15 mg/kg) and IV morphine (0.075 mg/kg) ketamine reduced allodynia and abnormal heat pain sensation. Dextromethorphan and memantine have been studied but did not show any benefit in decreasing pain due to PHN.

INVASIVE INTERVENTIONS

- In clinical practice, invasive interventions are usually reserved as a second or third line treatment option in cases where more conservative treatments have been exhausted.
- **Sympathetic Nerve Blocks:** Sympathetic nerve blocks like stellate ganglion blocks for craniofacial involvement and lumbar sympathetic blocks for lower extremity pain are used both in acute herpes zoster pain and PHN. Retrospective data revealed effectiveness in 41%–50% of patients with PHN, but no long-term benefit was observed.
- **Neuraxial Blockade:** In clinical practice, epidural local anesthetics with or without steroids are used for management of refractory PHN. Scant data exists to support the routine use of epidural or intrathecal analgesia in management of PHN. In a double-blind, randomized, controlled clinical trial, intrathecal use of methylprednisolone was shown to be effective in intractable PHN, but these results have not been replicated. Moreover, concern regarding the association between this therapy and development of arachnoiditis precludes its routine use.
- **Peripheral Nerve Blocks:** Intercostal nerve blocks have been reported to provide longlasting pain relief in patients with thoracic PHN.
- **Cryoablation:** In small study, considerable benefit was reported in 11 out of 14 patients who had undergone cryotherapy to the intercostal nerve for thoracic PHN. Currently, radio frequency ablation has replaced cryoablation as a modality for similar clinical indications in pain management.
- **Spinal Cord Stimulation:** Effects of spinal cord stimulation therapy was studied prospectively in a case series of 28 patients—4 with herpes zoster and 24 with PHN. Long-term pain relief was obtained in 82% of the patients with PHN.

ALTERNATIVE MODALITIES

- **TENS (transcutaneous electrical nerve stimulation):** There are few case series that show beneficial effects

with the use of this therapy, but other studies have failed to show benefit.
- **Psychological Interventions:** PHN affects the overall quality of life, although the effect of cognitive behavioral therapy has not been specifically studied in PHN.
- **Acupuncture:** A single, randomized, controlled trial of auricular and body acupuncture was performed in 62 patients with PHN. There was *no difference in pain* relief in the treatment and placebo group.
- *Surgical Intervention*: Multiple interventions including thalamic stimulation, anterolateral cordotomy, and Dorsal Root Entry Zone (DREZ) lesioning are described in the literature. Given a high risk–benefit ratio, these approaches are not recommended.

PREVENTION OF PHN

- Prevention of PHN is closely tied to prevention of herpes zoster. See Table 47-2.
- Early initiation of antiviral therapy reduces the viral damage and pain associated with herpes zoster and incidence and severity of PHN.
- Small dose of tricyclic antidepressant, amitriptyline, is the one studied, but nortriptyline could be as effective and better tolerated.
- Aggressive pain control in the acute zoster phase.
- Gabapentin has been shown to be efficacious for PHN prevention in animal studies.
- Corticosteroids and invasive interventions have no proven role in prevention of PHN.

KEY POINTS

- PHN is the most common complication following an acute episode of PHN and is defined as the persistence of pain 120 days after the onset of rash.
- Biggest risk for developing PHN is older age.
- First line of treatment is pharmacotherapy including topical lidocaine, anticonvulsants, antidepressants, and opioids.

TABLE 47-2 **Prevention of Herpes Zoster and PHN**

- Childhood primary varicella vaccination is important in preventing the occurrence of chicken pox, hence subsequent episodes of herpes zoster and PHN
- Zoster vaccination for immunocompetent adults >60 years of age has been shown to be helpful in reducing the incidence of herpes zoster, decreasing the severity of PHN and overall Burden of Illness
- The United States Centers for Disease Control and Prevention recommends administration of varicella-zoster immune globulin (VZIG) to immunocompromised seronegative persons with recent exposure to patients with chicken pox or zoster.

- Invasive treatments are only considered for patients who have failed medical therapy due to risk of complication and no strong data supporting this therapy.

Bibliography

Bennett GJ. Hypothesis on the pathogenesis of herpes zoster-associated pain. *Ann Neurol.* 1994;35(Suppl):S38–S41.

Bowsher D. The effects of pre-emptive treatment of postherpetic neuralgia with amitryptiline: a randomized, double-blind, placebo-controlled trial. *J Pain Symptom Manage.* 1997;13:327–331.

Derry S, Sven-Rice A, Cole P, et al. Topical capsaicin (high concentration) for chronic neuropathic pain in adults. *Cochrane Database Syst Rev.* 2013;2:CD007393.

Doi K, Nikai T, Sakura S, et al. Intercostal nerve block with 5% tetracaine for chronic pain syndromes. *J Clin Anesth.* 2002;14(1):39–41.

Dworkin RH, Schmader KE. Treatment and prevention of postherpetic neuralgia. *Clin Infect Dis.* 2003;36:877–882.

Eide PK, Jorum E, et al. Relief of PHN with the NMDA receptor antagonist ketamine: a double blind, crossover comparison with morphine and placebo.

Fields HL, Rowbotham M, Baron R. Postherpetic neuralgia: irritable nociceptors and deafferentation. *Neurobiol Dis.* 1998;5:209–227.

Frampton JE, Foster RH. Pregabalin in the treatment of PHN. *Drugs.* 2005;65:111–118.

Galer BS, Rowbotham MC, Perander J. Topical lidocaine patch relieves postherpetic neuralgia more effectively than a vehicle topical patch: results of an enriched enrollment study. *Pain.* 1999;80:533–538.

George T, Lewith JF, Machin D. Acupuncture compared with placebo in PHN. *Pain.* 1983;361–268.

Harke H, Gretenkort P, Ladleif HU, et al. Spinal cord stimulation in PHN and in acute herpes zoster pain. *Anes Analg.* 2002;94(3):694–700.

Irving G, Jensen M, Cramer M, et al. Efficacy and tolerability of gastric retentive gabapentin for the treatment of PHN: results of a double-blind, randomized, placebo-controlled clinical trial. *Clin J Pain.* 2009;25(3):185–192.

Jackson JL, Gibbons R, Meyer G, et al. The effect of treating herpes zoster with oral acyclovir in preventing postherpetic neuralgia: a meta-analysis. *Arch Intern Med.* 1997;157:909–912.

Kotani N, Kushikata T, Hashimoto H, et al. Intrathecal methylprednisolone acetate for intractable PHN. *N Eng J Med.* 2000;343:1514–1519.

Kumar V, Krone K, Mathieu A. Neuraxial and sympathetic blocks in herpes zoster and PHN: an appraisal of current evidence. *Reg Anesth Pain Med.* 2004;29:454–461.

Kuraishi Y, Takasaki I, Nojima H, et al. Effects of the suppression of acute herpetic pain by gabapentin and amitriptyline on the incidence of delayed postherpetic pain in mice. *Life Sci.* 2004;74(21):2619–2626.

Max MB, Schafer SC, Culnane M, et al. Amitriptyline, but not lorazepam, relieves PHN. *Neurology.* 1988;38:1427.

Oxman MN, Levin MJ, Johnson GR, et al. For the Shingles Prevention Study Group. A vaccine to prevent herpes zoster and postherpetic neuralgia in older adults. *N Engl J Med.* 2005;352:2271–2284.

Rice ASC, Maton S. PHN Study Group. Gabapentin in PHN: a randomized, double blind, placebo controlled study. *Pain.* 2001;94:215–224.

Rowbotham MC, Harden N, Stacey B, et al. Gabapentin for the treatment of PHN. A randomized controlled trial. *J Am Med Assoc.* 1998;280:1837–1842.

Volpi A, Gross G, Hercogova J, et al. Current management of herpes zoster: the European view. *Am J Clin Dermatology.* 2005; 6:317–325.

Watson CP, Babul N. Efficacy of oxycodone in neuropathic pain. A randomized trial in PHN. *Neurology.* 1998;50:1837–1841.

Weaver B. The burden of herpes zoster and postherpetic neuralgia in the United States. *J Am Osteopath Assoc.* 2007;107(Suppl S2–S7):117.

Zin, Nissen LM, O'Callaghan JP, et al. A randomized, controlled trial of oxycodone versus placebo in patients with postherpetic neuralgia and diabetic peripheral neuropathy treated with pregabalin. *J Pain.* 2010, 26:462–471.

48   POSTSURGICAL PAIN SYNDROMES

Harold J. Gelfand, MD
Christopher L. Wu, MD

INTRODUCTION

- Extent of the problem:
  1. A survey conducted in pain clinics in Scotland and Northern England, 20% of patients believed their operation was a cause of their chronic pain and half of these attributed their pain entirely to the surgical procedure.
  2. A review of the literature found the incidence of postoperative chronic pain to be:
     a. 30%–50% following amputation
     b. 20%–30% following breast surgery
     c. 30%–40% following thoracotomy
     d. 30%–50% following open coronary artery bypass
     e. 10% following inguinal hernia repair
     f. 10% following cesarean section
  3. Epidemiology is difficult to define because of the lack of randomized controlled trials and varying methodology and definitions for chronic pain.
     a. Is the time scale 3, 6, or 12 months?
     b. Does postoperative pain refer only to new-onset symptoms or can it be a progression of preoperative symptoms?

c. Efforts have been made to standardize the definitions and methodologies for the study of chronic pain.

- The International Association for the Study of Pain (IASP) defines postoperative chronic pain syndrome as:
  1. Pain that develops after a surgical procedure
  2. Pain of at least 2 months' duration
  3. Exclusion of other causes of the pain
  4. Exclusion of preexisting pain
- Mechanisms:
  1. Neuropathic pain can develop after tissue trauma from surgical procedures.
  2. Inflammation from tissue injury results in peripheral and central sensitization.
  3. After peripheral nerve injury, changes such as sprouting, spontaneous activity in nerve endings, and peripheral sensitization occur.
  4. Combined with the loss of somatosensory input from distal nerves, the increased activity from damaged nerves leads to the central sensitization that, in turn, leads to spontaneous pain and hyperalgesia.
  5. The glia and astrocytes also contribute to the development of central sensitization.
- Preoperative catastrophizing and anxiety are associated with significantly higher incidence of chronic postoperative pain.
- Multiple factors from genetic and psychological to tissue injury and regeneration contribute to acute pain, central sensitization, and the development of chronic postsurgical pain.
- General anesthesia or administration of opioids does not prevent the processes leading to central and peripheral sensitization.
- Animal studies have shown that preemptive analgesia reduces chronic postoperative pain behaviors beyond the perioperative period. However, human studies have had mixed results.

POSTAMPUTATION PAIN SYNDROME

- Pain after limb amputation is the best studied postoperative syndrome. This pain is broadly categorized as residual limb pain (stump pain), residual sensation, or phantom limb pain.

CHARACTERISTICS

- Residual limb pain is characterized by paresthesias and hyperalgesia in the stump and caused by numerous possible mechanisms to include neuroma formation, sympathetic dysfunction, or abnormal stump tissues (eg, scars or heterotopic ossification). Residual sensation is nonnoxious afferent input referred to the amputated or deafferented limb. Amputation is not a requisite for the development of residual sensation.

- Phantom limb sensation and pain are central phenomena often explained by Melzack's neuromatrix theory, which holds that a matrix exists for each body part and this matrix persists in the absence of the body part. Even after loss of the limb, therefore, the "pain memory" may continue.
- In these patients, modulation takes place at the somatosensory cortex, subcortex, and thalamus. These changes may occur prior to amputation in patients with extensive loss of limb function.
- Peripheral and spinal cord neuroplastic changes also contribute to amputation pain.
- Almost all patients experience phantom sensations, and the phantom limb may seem to resemble the amputated limb in shape and function.
- Eventually, phantom limb sensations may fade.
- Telescoping occurs when the distal phantom limb sensation approaches the stump and eventually is perceived within the stump.
- Both residual limb and phantom limb pain may be episodic.
- Some reports describe the pain intensity as mild. Others describe it as severe in as many as 40% of patients.
- The duration of phantom pain episodes ranges from more than 15 hours a day in approximately 25% of patients to less than 1 hour in 20%.
- Approximately 25% of patients report 20 or more days of phantom pain per month, but half may have pain 5 days or less a month.
- Phantom pain can occur after removal of body parts other than limbs, including the rectum, breast, tongue, teeth, and genitals.

INCIDENCE

- The incidence of postamputation pain ranges from 30% to 83% (see Table 48-1). Lower estimates tend to come from older studies that relied on patients' request for pain medicine to determine incidence.
- A survey conducted on military traumatic amputees from Vietnam and Operation Enduring Freedom/Operation Iraqi Freedom found that phantom pain was experienced in 72.2% and 76%, respectively, and residual limb pain was experienced in 48.3% and 62.9%, respectively.
- Phantom limb pain occurs less often in children and in those missing a limb as a result of congenital limb deficiency.
- The incidence of stump pain ranges from 5% to 62%.
- Residual limb pain persists in 5% to 10% of patients.
- Phantom pain occurs in 30% to 83% of patients.

TABLE 48-1   **Incidence of Postamputation Pain**

STUDY	RESIDUAL LIMB PAIN INCIDENCE (%)	PHANTOM PAIN INCIDENCE (%)
Finch et al.	18	30
Sherman et al.	—	78
Jensen et al.	—	59–65
Pohjolainen.	5	53
Krane and Heller	—	83
Nikolajsen et al.	—	55–81
Wartan et al.	57	55
Fisher and Hanspal	—	31
Nikolajsen et al.	—	59–79
Kooijman et al.	49	51
Fraser et al.	—	69
Gallagher et al.	48	69
Reiber et al.	48–63	72–76

- Phantom limb pain begins usually within 3 weeks of amputation.
- The frequency of painful episodes decreases in the first year but prevalence does not change.
- Half of individuals with phantom limb pain report no change in the intensity of their pain over time.
- Residual limb pain exists in 66% of patients with phantom limb pain and in half of those without phantom pain.
- The pain is often perceived to exist in the same location as the now-phantom limb.

RISK FACTORS

- Increased pain preoperatively increases the probability of postoperative phantom limb pain at 3-month follow-up by 33%–72%. The most significant predictor of chronic postamputation pain is the presence of preamputation pain in the affected limb.
- Postoperative residual limb pain is associated with phantom pain.
- Nonpainful phantom paresthesias also correlate with the presence of phantom pain.
- Pain may be more common after amputation for cancer than for trauma.
- No known associations exist with age, sex, site of amputation, ethnicity, or educational level.
- The effect of intraoperative anesthetic or surgical technique on postamputation pain is unknown.
- Other factors that may influence this pain include genetic predisposition, gender (female > male), upper extremity, anxiety, attention/distraction, urination/defecation, weather changes, and stump manipulation.

PREVENTION AND TREATMENT

- Treatment modalities are mostly based on extrapolation from clinical trials for other neuropathic pain syndromes as there are few clinical trials on the treatment of postamputation syndrome.
- Prolonged preoperative and postoperative treatment of pain with regional anesthesia may decrease the risk of phantom and residual limb pain, but the data are equivocal.
- It is recognized that pain management in the perioperative period is critical to blunt the development of postamputation pain syndrome, but specific protocols are lacking. However, initiation of analgesia prior to amputation surgery has been shown to favorably impact the development of phantom limb pain.
- The outcomes for surgical alleviation of postamputation syndrome are mixed; however, recent studies have shown improvement following peripheral nerve reconstruction and heterotopic ossification excision.
- Opioids may provide pain relief, perhaps because of cortical reorganization.
- Pain treatment may include calcitonin (100–200 IU up to five times a day), antidepressant drugs, anticonvulsant drugs, nonsteroidal anti-inflammatory drugs, tramadol, transcutaneous electrical nerve stimulation, deep brain stimulation, motor cortex stimulation, spinal cord stimulation, acupuncture, hypnosis, mirror therapy, or biofeedback. Case reports describe the use of continuous peripheral blockade for treatment of this pain.
- Ketamine may reduce spinal sensitization via N-methyl-D-aspartate receptor antagonism.
- Phentolamine and dexmedetomidine infusions may alleviate chronic phantom limb pain through inhibition of sympathetically mediated pain transmission.
- Intravenous lidocaine infusion can help with residual limb pain but not with phantom limb pain.
- Some investigators suggest that if pain treatment starts early, the success rate will be higher (80%–90%) than if it is started later (30%).
- Dorsal root entry zone lesions, cordotomy, thalamotomy, and sympathectomy provide short-term relief.
- Functional prostheses and rehabilitation may help.

POSTTHORACOTOMY PAIN SYNDROME

CHARACTERISTICS

- Manifests as an aching or burning pain along the thoracotomy scar that may persist months after surgery.
- Pain is usually related to intercostal nerve injury from either rib resection or retraction.
- Occurs in the first weeks after surgery.
- If the occurrence of pain is delayed in patients with cancer, tumor recurrence must be excluded.

- Intensity varies: 80% rate pain as 4 or less on the 11-point numeric rating scale.
- Although pain is often severe at 1 month, it usually subsides by 1 year.
- The pain is severe in 3%–5% at 1 year.

INCIDENCE

- May exceed 50% (see Table 48-2).
- Prevalence varies between 5% and 67%.
- Incidence, prevalence, and intensity decrease with time.

RISK FACTORS

- Preoperative pain and pain in the immediate postoperative period.
- The severity of postoperative pain (36% of patients with minor postoperative pain develop postthoracotomy pain syndrome (PTPS) vs. 56% of patients with moderate-to-severe acute postoperative pain).
- Pain in the immediate postoperative period may be the only factor that predicts PTPS.
- May be related to the patient's preoperative pain state.
- The incidence at 1 month and 1 year is increased in females versus males.
- Malignancy is not associated with an increased incidence of pain.
- May be associated with nerve dysfunction (as demonstrated by a loss of superficial abdominal reflex).
- Does not appear to be decreased by video assistance during thoracoscopic procedures.

PREVENTION AND TREATMENT

- Perioperative management recommendations for thoracotomy are found at the Procedure Specific

Postoperative Pain Management (PROSPECT) project website. It makes the following recommendations:
1. Preoperative: thoracic epidural with local anesthetic and opioid as a bolus and continued as an infusion or paravertebral block with bolus and infusion. If epidural or paravertebral is not possible, single bolus intrathecal opioid.
2. Intraoperative: thoracic epidural, paravertebral, or intercostal blocks with bolus (pre- or postoperatively) and infusion of local anesthetic.
3. Postoperative: thoracic epidural with local anesthetic and opioid infusion, paravertebral block with local anesthetic infusion, or intercostals block with local anesthetic infusion. Systemic nonsteroidal anti-inflammatory agents, COX-2 inhibitors, opioid patient–controlled analgesia, oral opioid, and acetaminophen.

- Intraoperative and postoperative use of epidural analgesia with local anesthetics decreases PTPS significantly compared with postoperative use of intravenous opiates.
- No significant difference in PTPS occurs with use of postoperative patient-controlled epidural analgesia versus postoperative intravenous analgesia.

POSTMASTECTOMY PAIN SYNDROME

CHARACTERISTICS

- Can involve chest wall, breast, scar, and arm/shoulder pain as well as phantom breast sensations or pain.
- The mechanism is probably nerve damage from surgery, radiation, chemotherapy, or tumor recurrence or a combination thereof.
- Onset is within the first weeks following a surgical procedure. Pain from recurrent cancer or radiation can take up to 5 years to develop.
- Women with postmastectomy pain syndrome (PMPS) are often misdiagnosed and undertreated, and have poor pain control.

INCIDENCE

- Up to 50% after surgery for cancer but varies by type of pain.
- Breast or chest wall pain incidence at 3 weeks is 35% and decreases to 23% at 1 year. In the same period, hyperesthesia decreases from 38% to 13%.
- The prevalence stays at 30% over a 6-year period.
- Arm pain incidence is stable between 3 and 15 months (55% vs. 51%).
- The incidence of phantom breast pain is approximately 13% at 3 weeks and 17% at 6 years.

TABLE 48-2 Incidence of Postthoracotomy Pain

STUDY	CHRONIC PAIN INCIDENCE (%)
Dajczman et al.	54
Kalso et al.	44
Landreneau et al.	22–44
Bertrand et al.	61–63
Perttunen et al.	61
Obata et al.	33–67
Hu et al.	41
Senturk et al.	62
Ochroch et al.	21
Maguire et al.	21–57
Wildgaard K	25–33

RISK FACTORS

- Preoperative breast pain may be a risk factor for postoperative phantom breast pain, although this suggestion is controversial.
- Preoperative depression and anxiety are associated but not statistically significant risk factors.
- Mastectomy with reconstruction (incidence 49%) is more likely than mastectomy alone (31%) or elective breast reduction (22%) to lead to PMPS.
- Reconstruction with prosthesis implantation has the highest risk of chronic pain (53%).
- A large retrospective trial found that chronic pain is more common after breast-conserving surgery compared with radical surgery, but this finding was not replicated in small, prospective trials.
- Axillary dissection increases the risk of chronic arm pain.
- The severity of acute postoperative pain and level of analgesic requirements predict chronic pain in the breast and ipsilateral arm.
- Postoperative radiation therapy is a risk factor for chronic pain and possibly for phantom sensations.
- Altered sensation in the intercostobrachial nerve is associated with neuralgia.

TREATMENT

- Preliminary evidence suggests that preemptive analgesia using regional anesthetic techniques and botulinum toxin injection at tissue expander sites may decrease the incidence.
- Can be treated using antidepressants, anticonvulsants, acupuncture, transcutaneous nerve stimulation, biofeedback, hypnosis, and other complementary medicine techniques.
- One randomized study found pain relief with topical capsaicin.

POSTCHOLECYSTECTOMY CHRONIC PAIN

CHARACTERISTICS

- Postcholecystectomy chronic pain syndrome (PCPS) involves poorly characterized and multifactoral abdominal pain.
- Symptoms include:
  1. Indigestion
  2. Noncolicky pain
  3. Dull or mild abdominal pain
  4. Severe abdominal pain
  5. Scar pain

INCIDENCE

- Varies from 3% to 56%

MECHANISMS

- Sphincter of Oddi dysfunction
- Bile duct stones
- Ulcer
- Colonic dysfunction
- Scar pain

RISK FACTORS

- Risk factors include:
  1. Psychologic vulnerability
  2. Female
  3. Long-standing preoperative pain
- Risk is decreased with classic "gallbladder attack symptoms."
- Surgical approach (laparoscopic vs. open) is not a factor.
- Pain at 6 weeks predicts pain at 1 year.
- It is unknown if neuraxial or regional anesthesia can decrease the risk.

POSTINGUINAL HERNIA CHRONIC PAIN

CHARACTERISTICS

- Pulling, tearing, or sharp pain of moderate to severe intensity adjacent to a scar from inguinal hernia repair
- May be neuropathic or somatic
- May lead to difficulty in walking or lead to sexual dysfunction

INCIDENCE

- Varies from "rare" to more than 30%.
- One large study found an incidence of 28.7% for pain at 1 year and functional impairment in half of the patients with pain.
- Technique affects incidence: Open repair was associated with a 63% incidence of chronic pain versus an 11%–15% incidence with laparoscopic repair.

MECHANISMS

- Ischemic: secondary to tension in the operative site or tight closure of the deep or superficial inguinal ring with edema formation.
- Nerve trauma during dissection with neuroma formation and secondary neuropathy.

RISK FACTORS

- Risk factors include:
  1. Ambulatory surgery
  2. Age less than 40 years
  3. Preoperative pain
  4. Pain in the immediate postoperative period
  5. Poor outlook
  6. Mesh repair
- Increased pain at 1 and 4 weeks postoperatively correlates with higher rates of moderate to severe pain at 12 months.
- Recurrent hernia repair has a fourfold higher incidence of moderate-to-severe pain.
- Lower incidences are reported for procedures performed at dedicated hernia centers.
- It is unknown if neuraxial or regional anesthesia can decrease the risk.

TREATMENT

- Recent international guidelines on the prevention and treatment of chronic postinguinal hernia repair pain recommends that the named nerves be protected if possible or else completely resected and aggressive perioperative analgesia be performed.
- A recent meta-analysis found that preemptive ilioinguinal nerve excision decreased the incidence of chronic postinguinal hernia repair pain.
- Triple neurectomy or directed neurectomy may alleviate chronic postinguinal hernia repair pain.

CHRONIC POSTPARTUM PAIN

CHARACTERISTICS

- Chronic pelvic pain: nonmenstrual pain in the lower abdomen persisting for at least 6 months
- Chronic cesarean delivery pain: abdominal wound scar pain persisting more than 3 months
- Chronic vaginal and perineal pain: marked by pain leading to difficulty with ambulation, micturition, defecation, and dyspareunia

INCIDENCE

- Chronic vaginal and perineal pain occurs in nearly 20% of parturients and persists for over a year in 10%–18%.

- Chronic pain following cesarean section occurs in 18%–20% of parturients.
- Other studies have found combined incidences as low as 1%–8% of patients.

MECHANISMS

- Macro and micro tissue injury.
- Scaring of the introitus.
- Episiotomy.
- Hormonally induced increase in cervical and uterine sensory afferents.
- Release of inflammatory substances.
- Direct nerve injury and traction on the ilioinguinal and iliohypogastric nerves following cesarean section.
- Endogenous oxytocin secretion in the postpartum period may confer protection against the development of chronic pain following childbirth.

RISK FACTORS

- Preexisting chronic pain and severity and duration of acute pain postoperatively are the most significant risk factors.
- Other risk factors:
  1. Depression
  2. Anxiety
  3. Chronic disease
  4. Genetic predisposition
  5. General anesthesia
  6. Emergency cesarean section
  7. Repeat surgery
  8. Length of incision
  9. Uterine exteriorization
  10. Closure of peritoneum
- Peripartum depression increases the acute pain experienced by parturients and places them at greater risk for chronic pain.
- Epidural anesthesia and method of delivery are not associated with the development of chronic postpartum pain.

TREATMENT

- Address preexisting chronic pain and psychological disorders.
- Interventions such as intrathecal clonidine, intravenous ketamine, and gabapentin or pregabalin may reduce the incidence of chronic postpartum pain.
- Chronic vaginal/perineal pain may respond to botulinum toxin injection, bupivacaine/steroid injection, and surgical interventions.

POSTSTERNOTOMY

CHARACTERISTICS

- Sharp, aching burning, lancing, or heavy pain at the surgical site.
- Pain may also be reported in the head, neck, shoulder, intrascapular, arms, and legs.

INCIDENCE

- Chronic poststernotomy pain incidence has been reported to be between 27% and 39%.

MECHANISM

- Pain is due to bone fracture, incomplete healing, osteomyelitis, sternocostal chondritis, costal fracture, intercostal nerve injury, brachial plexus injury, or nerve entrapment caused by sternal wires.

RISK FACTORS

- Risk factors include emergent surgery, repeat sternotomy, female gender, younger age, increased New York Heart Association class, and severe pain on postoperative day 3.
- Saphenous vein grafts may lead to chronic leg pain.
- Some studies implicate internal mammary artery harvest.

TREATMENT

- Optimal pain management improves patient functional outcome, decreased morbidity, and may aid in the reduction in the incidence of chronic poststernotomy pain.
- Thoracic epidural, primary opioid postoperative analgesia, and use of gabapentinoids have not shown any impact on the incidence of chronic poststernotomy pain.
- Gabapentanoids and diclofenac have been shown to effectively treat chronic poststernotomy pain.
- There is little evidence supporting chronic opioid use for chronic poststernotomy pain.
- Intercostal nerve blocks, RF ablation of the dorsal root ganglion, epidural injections, spinal cord stimulators, or peripheral nerve stimulators may be attempted to treat chronic poststernotomy pain.

CONCLUSION

- Preoperative pain increases the risk for postoperative pain. This may be related to modulation of the peripheral and central nervous system.
- Structural changes or alterations of inhibitory and facilitatory mechanisms maintain the pain state.
- Peripheral factors include neuroma formation in surgically cut nerves with spontaneous and abnormally induced activity. A neuroma can lead to hyperalgesia, allodynia, and chronic pain.
- Acute postoperative pain is another contributor.
- The trauma of surgery may lead to sensitization and subsequent peripheral/central changes that cause chronic pain.
- Psychological vulnerability and genetic predisposition are implicated in numerous studies on the development of chronic pain.
- Treatment options have been inadequately studied.
- Traditional treatments, such as opiates, anti-inflammatory drugs, anticonvulsants, and other non-opiate analgesics, are the primary therapies.

BIBLIOGRAPHY

Alfieri S, Amid PK, Campanelli G, et al. International guidelines for prevention and management of post-operative chronic pain following inguinal hernia surgery. *Hernia.* 2011;15: 239–249.

Alves Nogueira Fabro E, Bergmann A, do Amaral E, et al. Post-mastectomy pain syndrome: incidence and risks. *Breast.* 2012 June;21(3):321–325.

Andreae MH, Andreae DA. Local anesthetics and regional anesthesia for preventing chronic pain after surgery. *Cochrane Database Syst Rev.* 2012;10:1–94.

Bay-Nielsen M, Perkins FM, Kehlet H. Pain and functional impairment 1 year after inguinal herniorrhaphy: A nationwide questionnaire study. *Ann Surg.* 2001;233:1.

Bertrand PC, Regnard JF, Spaggiari L, et al. Immediate and long-term results after surgical treatment of primary spontaneous pneumothorax by VATS. *Ann Thorac Surg.* 1996;61:1641–1645.

Bisgaard T, Rosenberg J, Kehlet H. From acute to chronic pain after laparoscopic cholecystectomy: a prospective follow-up analysis. *Scand J Gastroenterol.* 2005;40:1358–1364.

Biyik I, Gülcüler M, Karabiga M, et al. Efficacy of gabapentin versus diclofenac in the treatment of chest pain and paresthesia in patients with sternotomy. *Anadolu Kardiyol Derg.* 2009;9:390–396.

Bjelland EK, Stuge B, Engdahl B, et al. The effect of emotional distress on persistent pelvic girdle pain after delivery: a longitudinal population study. *BJOG.* 2013;120:32–40.

Borghi B, D'Addabbo M, White PF, et al. The use of prolonged peripheral neural blockade after lower extremity amputation:

the effect on symptoms associated with phantom limb syndrome. *Anesth Analg.* 2010;111:1308–1315.

Bruce J, Drury N, Poobalan AS, et al. The prevalence of chronic chest and leg pain following cardiac surgery: a historical cohort study. *Pain.* 2003;104:265–273.

Buchheit T, Pyati S. Prevention of chronic pain after surgical nerve injury: amputation and thoracotomy. *Surg Clin N Am.* 2012;92:393–407.

Burckard G, Sycha T, Lieba-Samal D, et al. The pattern and time course of somatosensory changes in the UVB sunburn model reveal the presence of peripheral and central sensitization. *Pain.* 2013;154:586–597.

Callesen T, Bech K, Kehlet H. Prospective study of chronic pain after groin hernia repair. *Br J Surg.* 1999;86:1528.

Condon RE. Groin pain after hernia repair. *Ann Surg.* 2001;233:8.

Dajczman E, Gordon A, Kreisman H, et al. Long-term postthoracotomy pain. *Chest.* 1991;99:270.

Dickinson KJ, Thomas M, Fawole AS, et al. Predicting chronic post-operative pain following laparoscopic inguinal hernia repair. *Hernia.* 2008;12:597–601.

Doumouchtsis SK, Boama V, Gorti M, et al. Prospective evaluation of combined local bupivacaine and steroid injections for the management of chronic vaginal and perineal pain. *Arch Gynecol Obstet.* 2011;284:681–685.

Eisenach JC, Pan PH, Smiley R, et al. Severity of acute pain after childbirth, but not type of delivery, predicts persistent pain and postpartum depression. *Pain.* 2008;140:87–94.

Eisenach JC, Pan P, Smiley RM, et al. Resolution of pain after childbirth. *Anesthesiology.* 2013;118:143–151.

Finch DR, Macdougal M, Tibbs DJ, et al. Amputation for vascular disease: the experience of a peripheral vascular unit. *Br J Surg.* 1980;67:233.

Fisher K, Hanspal RS. Phantom pain, anxiety, depression, and their relation in consecutive patients with amputated limbs: case reports. *Br Med J.* 1998;316:903.

Fraser CM, Halligan PW, Robertson IH, et al. Characteristics of phantom limb phenomena in upper limb amputees. *Prosthet Orthot Int.* 2001;25:235.

Gallagher P, Allen D, Maclachlan M. Phantom limb pain and residual limb pain following lower limb amputation: a descriptive analysis. *Disabil Rehab.* 2001;23:522.

Gotoda Y, Kambara N, Sakai T, et al. The morbidity, time course and predictive factors for persistent post-thoracotomy pain. *Eur J Pain.* 2001;5:89.

Grusser SM, Winter C, Schaefer M, et al. Perceptual phenomena after unilateral arm amputation: a pre–post-surgical comparison. *Neurosci Lett.* 2001;302:13.

Gutierrez S, Liu B, Hayashida K, et al. Reversal of peripheral nerve injury-induced hypersensitivity in the postpartum period: role of spinal oxytocin. *Anesthesiology.* 2013;118:152–159.

Hanley MA, Jensen MP, Smith DG, et al. Preamputation pain and acute pain predict chronic pain after lower extremity amputation. *J Pain.* 2007;8:102–109.

Hinrichs-Rocker A, Schulz K, Jarvinen I, et al. Psychosocial predictors and correlates for chronic post-surgical pain (CPSP)—a systematic review. *Eur J Pain.* 2009;13:719–730.

Hsu E, Cohen SP. Postamputation pain: epidemiology, mechanisms, and treatment. *J Pain Res.* 2013;6:121–136.

Hu JS, Lui PW, Wang H, et al. Thoracic epidural analgesia with morphine does not prevent postthoracotomy pain syndrome: a survey of 159 patients. *Acta Anaesthesiol Sin.* 2000;38:195.

Huse E, Larbig W, Flor H, et al. The effect of opioids on phantom limb pain and cortical reorganization. *Pain.* 2001;90:47.

Ikeda H, Kiritoshi T, Murase K. Contribution of microglia and astrocytes to the central sensitization, inflammatory, and neutopathic pain in the juvenile rat. *Molecular Pain.* 2012;8:43.

Jensen MK, Andersen C. Can chronic poststernotomy pain after cardiac valve replacement be reduced using thoracic epidural analgesia? *Acta Anaesthesiol Scand.* 2004;48:871–874.

Jensen TS, Krebs B, Nielsen J, et al. Immediate and long-term phantom limb pain in amputees: incidence, clinical characteristics and relation-ship to pre-amputation limb pain. *Pain.* 1985;21:267.

Johner A, Faulds J, Wiseman SM. Planned ilioinguinal nerve excision for prevention of chronic pain after inguinal hernia repair: a meta-analysis. *Surgery.* 2011;150:534–541.

Kainu JP, Sarvela J, Tiippana E, et al. Persistent pain after caesarean section and vaginal birth: a cohort study. *Int J Obstet Anesth.* 2010;19(1):4–9.

Kalso E, Mennander S, Tasmuth T, et al. Chronic post-sternotomy pain. *Acta Anaesthesiol Scand.* 2001;45:935.

Kalso E, Perttunen K, Kaasinen S. Pain after thoracic surgery. *Acta Anaesthesiol Scand.* 1992;36:96.

Karanikolas M, Aretha D, Tsolakis I, et al. Optimized perioperative analgesia reduces chronic phantom limb pain intensity, prevalence, and frequency: a prospective, randomized clinical trial. *Anesthesiology.* 2011;114:1144–1154.

Katz J, Clarke H, Seltzer Z. Preventive analgesia: quo vadimus? *Anesth Analg.* 2011;113:1242–1253.

Katz J, Cohen L. Preventative analgesia is associated with reduced pain disability 3 weeks but not 6 months after major gynecologic surgery by laparotomy. *Anesthesiology.* 2004;101:169–174.

Katz J, Jackson M, Kavanagh B, et al. Acute pain after thoracic surgery predicts long term post-thoracotomy pain. *Clin J Pain.* 1996;12:50.

Kehlet H. Prospect Working Group. Procedure specific postoperative pain management 2011; *Thoracotomy.* Available at: www.postoppain.org. Accessed June 1, 2013.

Kehlet H, Jensen TS, Woolf CJ. Persistent postsurgical pain: risk factors and prevention. *Lancet.* 2006;367:1618–1625.

Kline CM, Lucas CE, Ledgerwood AM. Directed neurectomy for treatment of chronic postsurgical neuropathic pain. *Am J Surg.* 2013;205:246–249.

Knotkova H, Cruciani RA, Tronnier VM, et al. Current and future options for the management of phantom-limb pain. *J Pain Res.* 2012;5:39–49.

Kojima KY, Kitahara M, Matoba M, et al. Survey on recognition of post-mastectomy pain syndrome by breast specialist physician and present status of treatment in Japan, *Breast Cancer.* Published online; May 30, 2012: http://link.springer.com.ezproxy.welch.jhmi.edu/article/10.1007/s12282-012-0376-8/fulltext.html

Kooijman CM, Dijkstra PU, Geertzen JH, et al. Phantom pain and phantom sensations in upper limb amputees: an epidemiological study. *Pain.* 2000;87:33.

Kosharskyy B, Almonte W, Shaparin N, et al. Intravenous infusions in chronic pain management. *Pain Physician.* 2013;16:231–249.

Krane EJ, Heller LB. The prevalence of phantom limb sensation and pain in pediatric amputees. *J Pain Symptom Manage.* 1995;10:21.

Lahtinen P, Kokki H, Hynynen M. Pain after cardiac surgery: a prospective cohort study of 1-year incidence and intensity. *Anesthesiology.* 2006;105:794–800.

Landau R, Bollag L, Ortner C. Chronic pain after childbirth. *Int J Obstet Anesth.* 2013;22:133–45.

Landreneau RJ, Mack MJ, Hazelrigg SR, et al. Prevalence of chronic pain after pulmonary resection by thoracotomy or video-assisted thoracic surgery. *J Thorac Cardiovasc Surg.* 1994;107:1079.

Latremoliere A, Woolf CJ. Central sensitization: a generator of pain hypersensitivity by central neural plasticity. *J Pain.* 2009;10:895–926.

Lierz P, Schroegendorfer K, Choi S, et al. Continuous blockade of brachial plexus with ropivicaine in phantom pain: a case report. *Pain.* 1998;78:135.

Lou HY, Kong JF. The effects of prenatal maternal depressive symptoms on pain scores in the early postpartum period. *J Obstet Gynaecol.* 2012;32:764–766.

Macarthur AJ, Macarthur C, Weeks SK. Is epidural anesthesia in labor associated with chronic low back pain? A prospective cohort study. *Anesth Analg.* 1997;85:1066–1070.

Macdonald L, Bruce J, Scott NW, et al. Long-term follow-up of breast cancer survivors with post-mastectomy pain syndrome. *Br J Cancer.* 2005;92:225–230.

Macrae WA. Chronic pain after surgery. *Br J Anaesth.* 2001; 87:88.

Maguire MF, Ravenscroft A, Beggs D, et al. A questionnaire study investigating the prevalence of the neuropathic component of chronic pain after thoracic surgery. *Eur J Cardiothorac Surg.* 2006;29:800–805.

Mazzeffi M, Khelemsky Y. Poststernotomy pain: a clinical review. *J Cardiothorac Vasc Anesth.* 2011;25:1163–1178.

Meyerson J, Thelin S, Gordh T, Karlsten R. The incidence of chronic post-sternotomy pain after cardiac surgery—a prospective study. *Acta Anaesthesiol Scand.* 2001;45:940–944.

Nienhuijs S, Staal E, Strobbe L, et al. Chronic pain after mesh repair of inguinal hernia: a systematic review. *Am J Surg.* 2007;194:394–400.

Nikolajsen L, Ilkjaer S, Christensen JH, et al. Randomised trial of epidural bupivacaine and morphine in prevention of stump and phantom pain in lower-limb amputation. *Lancet.* 1997;350:1353.

Nikolajsen L, Ilkjaer S, Jensen TS. Effect of preoperative extradural bupivacaine and morphine on stump sensation in lower limb amputees. *Br J Anaesth.* 1998;81:348.

Nikolajsen L, Jensen TS. Phantom limb pain. *Br J Anaesth.* 2001;87:107.

Nikolajsen L. Postamputation pain: studies on mechanisms. *Dan Med J.* 2012, October;59:B4527.

Obata H, Saito S, Fujita N, et al. Epidural block with mepivicaine before surgery reduces long-term post-thoracotomy pain. *Can J Anaesth.* 1999;46:1127.

Ochroch EA, Gottschalk A, Augostides J, et al. Long-term pain and activity during recovery from major thoracotomy using thoracic epidural analgesia. *Anesthesiology.* 2002;97:1234.

Paterson LQ, Davis SN, Khalifé S, et al. Persistent genital and pelvic pain after childbirth. *J Sex Med.* 2009;6(1):215–221.

Perkins F, Kehlet H. Chronic pain as an outcome of surgery. *Anesthesiology.* 2000;93:1123.

Pertunen K, Tasmuth T, Kalso E. Chronic pain after thoracic surgery: a follow-up study. *Acta Anaesthesiol Scand.* 1999;43:563.

Pohjolainen T. A clinical evaluation of stumps in lower limb amputees. *Prosthet Orthot Int.* 1991;15:178.

Poobalan AS, Bruce J, King PM, et al. Chronic pain and quality of life following open inguinal hernia repair. *Br J Surg.* 2001;88:1122.

Poobalan AS, Bruce J, Smith WC, et al. A review of chronic pain after inguinal herniorrhaphy. *Clin J Pain.* 2003;19:48–54.

Poobalan AS, Bruce J, Smith WCS, et al. A review of chronic pain after inguinal herniorrhaphy. *Clin J Pain.* 2003;19:48–54.

Powell R, Johnston M, Smith WC, et al. Psychological risk factors for chronic post-surgical pain after inguinal hernia repair surgery: a prospective cohort study. *Eur J Pain.* 2012;16:600–610.

Reiber GE, McFarland LV, Hubbard S, et al. Service members and veterans with major traumatic limb loss from Vietnam war and OIF/OEF conflicts: survey methods, participants, and summary findings. *J Rehab Res Dev.* 2010;47:275–298.

Rork JF, Berde CB, Goldstein RD. Regional anesthesia approaches to pain management in pediatric palliative care: a review of current knowledge. *J Pain Symptom Manage.* 2013;46(6):859–873. Available online March 29, 2013 ahead of print.

Rothgangel AS, Braun SM, Beurskens AJ, et al. The clinical aspects of mirror therapy in rehabilitation: a systematic review of the literature. *Int J Rehab Res.* 2011;34:1–13.

Russell R, Dundas R, Reynolds F. Long term backache after childbirth: prospective search for causative factors. *Br Med J.* 1996;312(7043):1384–1388.

Senturk M, Ozcan PE, Talu GK, et al. The effects of three different analgesia techniques on long-term postthoracotomy pain. *Anesth Analg.* 2002;94:11.

Sherman RA, Sherman CJ, Parker L. Chronic phantom and stump pain among American veterans: results of a survey. *Pain.* 1984;18:83.

Theunissen M, Peters ML, Bruce J, et al. Preoperative anxiety and catastrophizing, a systematic review and meta-analysis of the association with chronic postsurgical pain. *Clin J Pain.* 2012;28:819–841

Vadivelu N, Schreck M, Lopez J, et al. Pain after mastectomy and breast reconstruction. *Am Surg.* 2008;74:285–296.

van Gulik L, Janssen LI, Ahlers SJ, et al. Risk factors for chronic thoracic pain after cardiac surgery via sternotomy. *Eur J Cardiothorac Surg.* 2011;40(6):1309–1313.

van Leersum NJ, van Leersum RL, Verwey HF, et al. Pain symptoms accompanying chronic poststernotomy pain: a pilot study. *Pain Med.* 2010;11:1628–1634.

VanDenKerkhof EG, Peters ML, Bruce J. Chronic pain after surgery. Time for standardization? A framework to establish core risk factor and outcome domains for epidemilological studies. *Clin J Pain.* 2013;29:2–8.

Wallace MS, Wallace AM, Lee J, et al. Pain after breast surgery: a survey of 282 women. *Pain.* 1996;66:195.

Wartan SW, Hamann W, Wedley JR, et al. Phantom pain and sensation among British veteran amputees. *Br J Anaesth.* 1997;78:652.

Wildgaard K, Ravn J, Nikolajsen L, et al. Consequences of persistent pain after lung cancer surgery: a nationwide questionnaire study. *Acta Anaesthesiol Scand.* 2011;55:60–68.

Wu CL, Tella P, Staats PS, et al. Analgesic effects of intravenous lidocaine and morphine on postamputation pain: a randomized double-blind, active placebo-controlled, crossover trial. *Anesthesiology.* 2002; 96:841–848.

49 MANAGING PAIN DURING PREGNANCY AND LACTATION

Amol Patwardhan, MD
James P. Rathmell, MD
Christopher M. Viscomi, MD
Ira M. Bernstein, MD

INTRODUCTION

- Pain occurs during pregnancy in nearly all women.
- Even during the course of an otherwise uncomplicated pregnancy, common musculoskeletal conditions can cause severe pain.
- Patients who have had long-standing painful disorders will enter pregnancy and present management challenges.

USE OF MEDICATIONS DURING PREGNANCY

- Medical management of the pregnant patient should begin with attempts to minimize the use of all medications and utilize nonpharmacologic therapies whenever possible.
- When opting for drug therapy, the clinician must consider any potential for harm to the mother, the fetus, and the course of pregnancy.
- With the exception of large polar molecules (such as heparin and insulin), nearly all medications will reach the fetus to some degree.
- The most critical period for minimizing maternal drug exposure is during early development—from conception through the tenth menstrual week of pregnancy (the tenth week following start of the last menstrual cycle). Drug exposure prior to organogenesis (prior to the fourth menstrual week) usually causes an all-or-none effect: the embryo either does not survive or develops without abnormalities. Drug effects later in pregnancy typically lead to single- or multiple-organ involvement, developmental syndromes, or intrauterine growth retardation.
- The U.S. Food and Drug Administration (FDA) has developed a five category labeling system for all approved drugs in the United States (Table 49-1). This labeling system rates the potential risk for teratogenic or embryotoxic effects based on available scientific and clinical evidence.

USE OF MEDICATIONS IN THE BREAST-FEEDING MOTHER

- High lipid solubility, low molecular weight, minimal protein binding, and the deionized state all facilitate excretion of medications into breast milk. The neonatal dose of most medications obtained through breast feeding is 1%–2% of the maternal dose.
- Only small amounts of colostrum are excreted during the first few postpartum days, thus early breast feeding poses little risk to the infant whose mother received medications during the delivery period.
- The majority of breast milk is synthesized and excreted during and immediately following breast feeding. Taking medications after breast feeding or during times when the infant has the longest interval between feedings and avoidance of long-acting medications will minimize drug transfer via breast milk.
- The American Academy of Pediatrics (AAP) has categorized medications in relation to the safety of maternal ingestion by breast-feeding mothers (Table 49-2). AAP recommends drugs and lactation database at http://toxnet.nlm.nih.gov/cgi-bin/sis/htmlgen?LACT for up to date information on these mediations.
- In general, AAP believes benefits of breast feeding outweigh the risk of exposure to most therapeutic agents.

MEDICATIONS COMMONLY USED IN PAIN MANAGEMENT

NONSTEROIDAL ANTI-INFLAMMATORY DRUGS (NSAIDS)

- Aspirin remains the prototypical NSAID and is the most thoroughly studied of this class of medication. First trimester exposure to aspirin does not pose appreciable teratogenic risk. Prostaglandins appear to trigger labor and the aspirin-induced inhibition of prostaglandin synthesis may result in prolonged gestation and protracted labor.
- Aspirin has well-known platelet-inhibiting properties and, theoretically, may increase the risk of peripartum hemorrhage.

TABLE 49-1   **FDA Pregnancy Risk Classification Categories for Medications Used in Pain Management**

FDA CLASSIFICATION	DEFINITION	EXAMPLES
Category A	Controlled human studies indicate no apparent risk to fetus. The possibility of harm to the fetus seems remote.	Multivitamins
Category B	Animal studies do not indicate a fetal risk or animal studies do indicate a teratogenic risk but well-controlled human studies have failed to demonstrate a risk.	Acetaminophen Ibuprofen, naproxen, oxycodone Lidocaine
Category C	Studies indicate teratogenic or embryocidal risk in animals, but no controlled studies have been done in women or there are no controlled studies in animals or humans.	Aspirin, ketorolac Caffeine Codeine, propoxyphene fentanyl, hydrocodone, methadone, meperidine, morphine, oxymorphone, butorphanol, nalbuphine bupronorphine, Tramadol Gabapentin, pregabalin Mexiletine Nifedipine Propranolol, metoprolol Sumatriptan Duloxetine, fluoxetine, amitriptyline Dexamethasone, prednisolone
Category D	Positive evidence of human fetal risk, but in certain circumstances, the benefits of the drug may outweigh the risks involved.	Imipramine Diazepam Phenobarbital Phenytoin Valproic acid Paroxetine
Category X	Positive evidence of significant fetal risk, and the risk clearly outweighs any possible benefit.	Ergotamine

FDA, Food and Drug Administration.

All opioid analgesics are FDA Risk Category D if used for prolonged periods or in large doses near term.

- Neonatal platelet function is inhibited for up to five days after delivery in aspirin treated mothers. Although low-dose aspirin therapy (60–80 mg/d) has not been associated with maternal or neonatal complications, higher doses appear to increase the risk of intracranial hemorrhage in neonates born prior to 35 weeks gestation.
- Circulating prostaglandins modulate the patency of the fetal ductus arteriosus. NSAIDs have been used therapeutically in neonates with persistent fetal

TABLE 49-2   **Classification of Maternal Medication Use During Pregnancy**

CLASSIFICATION	DEFINITION	EXAMPLES
Category 1	Medications that should not be consumed during lactation. Strong evidence exists that serious adverse effects on the infant are likely with maternal ingestion of these medications during lactation.	Ergotamine
Category 2	Drug whose infant effects in humans are unknown, but caution is urged.	Amitriptyline, desipramine, doxepin, fluoxetine, imipramine, trazodone Diazepam, lorazepam, midazolam
Category 3	Medications compatible with breast feeding.	Carbamazepine, phenytoin, valproate Atenolol, propranolol, diltiazem Codeine, fentanyl, methadone, morphine, propoxyphene Butorphanol Lidocaine, mexiletine Acetaminophen Ibuprofen, indomethacin, ketorolac, naproxen Caffeine

Adapted from Committee on Drugs, American Academy of Pediatrics. The transfer of drugs and other chemicals into human milk. *Pediatrics.* 2001;108:3 and revision published in *Pediatrics* August 2013.

circulation to induce closure of the ductus arteriosus via inhibition of prostaglandin synthesis. In utero, patency of the ductus arteriosus is essential for normal fetal circulation.

- Indomethacin has shown promise for the treatment of premature labor, but its use has been linked to antenatal narrowing and closure of the fetal ductus arteriosus.

- Neither ibuprofen nor naproxen has been linked to congenital defects. Use of ibuprofen and naproxen during pregnancy may result in reversible oligohydramnios (reflecting diminished fetal urine output) and mild constriction of the fetal ductus arteriosus.

- In a large series of NSAID use during pregnancy, naproxen and ibuprofen were most frequently used during the first and second trimesters because many patients stopped therapy once pregnancy was recognized and many of the rheumatic conditions remitted later in pregnancy. There was no significant difference in pregnancy outcome (duration of pregnancy and labor, vaginal delivery rate, maternal bleeding requiring transfusion, or incidence of congenital anomalies) or the health status of offspring at long-term follow-up (ranging from 6 months to 14 years). The authors concluded that NSAID therapy limited to periods of active rheumatic disease until weeks 34–36 did not adversely affect the neonate.

- In breast-feeding women, salicylate transport into breast milk is limited by its highly ionized state and high degree of protein binding. Caution should still be exercised if more than occasional or short-term aspirin use is contemplated during lactation as neonates have very slow elimination of salicylates. Both ibuprofen and naproxen are also minimally transported into breast milk, and are considered compatible with breast feeding; these agents are generally better tolerated than indomethacin.

- Acetaminophen provides similar analgesia without the anti-inflammatory effects seen with NSAIDs. Acetaminophen has no known teratogenic properties, does not inhibit prostaglandin synthesis or platelet function, and is hepatotoxic only in extreme overdosage. If persistent pain demands use of a mild analgesic during pregnancy, acetaminophen appears to be a safe and effective first choice agent. However, it should be noted that a recent study published in *JAMA Pediatrics* has suggested that maternal exposure to acetaminophen is associated with increased risk of ADHD in children. Larger studies are needed to confirm these findings.

- Acetaminophen does enter breast milk, although maximal neonatal ingestion would be less than 2% of a maternal dose and it is considered compatible with breast feeding.

OPIOID ANALGESICS

- Much of our present knowledge about the effects of chronic opioid exposure during pregnancy comes from studies of opioid-abusing patients. Pregnancy outcomes in studies of drug-abusing mothers must be interpreted with caution when attempting to establish the risks of a prescribed narcotic regimen in the pregnant patient with pain.

- Most studies suggest that methadone maintenance is associated with longer gestation and increased birth weight when compared with outcomes of untreated opioid abusers. However, both methadone-maintained and untreated opioid-abusing pregnant women deliver infants with lower birth weights and smaller head circumference than do drug-free controls. No increase in congenital defects has been observed in offspring of methadone consuming patients.

- Neonatal abstinence syndrome occurs in between 30% and 90% of infants exposed to either heroin or methadone in utero. Neonatal withdrawal symptoms may be more frequent if the maternal daily methadone dose exceed 20 mg. The majority of infants that will have symptomatic narcotic withdrawal are symptomatic by 48 hours postpartum, but there are reports of withdrawal symptoms beginning 7–14 days postpartum.

- Methadone levels in breast milk appear sufficient to prevent opioid withdrawal symptoms in the breast-fed infant. The American Academy of Pediatrics considers methadone doses of up to 20 mg/d to be compatible with breast feeding.

- Recognition of infants at risk for neonatal abstinence syndrome and institution of appropriate supportive and medical therapy typically result in little short-term consequence to the infant.

- There is no evidence to suggest a relationship between exposure to any of the opioid agonists or agonist-antagonists during pregnancy and large categories of major or minor malformations.

- The most extensive data are available for codeine and propoxyphene. No evidence was found for either agent to suggest a relationship to large categories of major or minor malformations.

- There are substantial data demonstrating no congenital anomalies associated with hydrocodone, meperidine, methadone, morphine, or oxycodone use during pregnancy.

- There are few reported exposures to other opioids, but there have been no reports linking the use of fentanyl, hydromorphone, oxymorphone, butorphanol, or nalbuphine with congenital defects.

- Postoperative analgesia for most pregnant women undergoing nonobstetric surgery can be readily provided using narcotic analgesics. Fentanyl, morphine, and hydromorphone are all safe and effective alternatives when a potent opioid is needed for parenteral administration. There are a range of safe and effective oral analgesics: For mild pain, acetaminophen alone or in combination with hydrocodone is a good alternative; for moderate pain, oxycodone alone or in combination with acetaminophen is effective; more severe pain may require morphine or hydromorphone, both of which are available for oral administration.

- Opioids are excreted into breast milk. Pharmacokinetic analysis has demonstrated that breast milk concentrations of codeine and morphine are equal to or somewhat greater than maternal plasma concentrations. The American Academy of Pediatrics considers use of many opioid analgesics including codeine, fentanyl, methadone, morphine, and propoxyphene to be compatible with breast feeding.
- Limited studies exist regarding safety of bupronorphine in pregnancy and breast feeding. However, more and more women are now treated with Suboxone. Bupronorphine is classified in category C in FDA pregnancy risk classification. Bupronorphine's high affinity with mu opioid receptor can pose a challenge in treating labor pain since other full opioid agonists are less effective. In such scenario, either bupronorphine can be divided in small doses to reduce its occupancy at the receptor or discontinued entirely and substituting it with a full agonist at adequate doses. Bupronorphine is excreted in breast milk and its concentration is similar to that in plasma. However, due to poor oral bioavailability of bupronorphine, it has little effect on neonatal abstinence syndrome.

LOCAL ANESTHETICS

- Few studies have focused on the potential teratogenicity of local anesthetics. Lidocaine and bupivacaine do not appear to pose significant developmental risk to the fetus. Only mepivacaine has any suggestion of teratogenicity; however, the number of patient exposures is inadequate to draw conclusions.
- Neither lidocaine nor bupivacaine appears in measurable quantities in the breast milk after epidural local anesthetic administration during labor. Intravenous infusion of high doses (2–4 mg/min) of lidocaine for suppression of cardiac arrhythmias led to minimal levels in breast milk. Based on these observations, continuous epidural infusion of dilute local anesthetic solutions for postoperative analgesia should result in only small quantities of drug actually reaching the fetus. The American Academy of Pediatrics considers local anesthetics to be safe for use in the nursing mother.

STEROIDS

- Most corticosteroids cross the placenta, although prednisone and prednisolone are inactivated by the placenta. Fetal serum concentrations of prednisone are less than 10% of maternal levels. No increase in malformations has been seen among patients exposed to corticosteroids during their first trimester of pregnancy. The use of corticosteroids during a limited trial of epidural steroid therapy in the pregnant patient probably poses minimal fetal risk.
- In the mother who is breast feeding, less than 1% of a maternal prednisone dose appears in the nursing infant over the next three days. This amount of steroid exposure is unlikely to impact infant endogenous cortisol secretion.

BENZODIAZEPINES

- First trimester exposure to benzodiazepines may be associated with an increased risk of congenital malformations. Diazepam may be associated with cleft lip/palate as well as congenital inguinal hernia. Benzodiazepine use immediately before delivery also risks fetal hypothermia, hyperbilirubinemia, and respiratory depression.
- In the breast-feeding mother, diazepam and its metabolite desmethyldiazepam can be detected in infant serum for up to 10 days after a single maternal dose. This is due to the slower metabolism in neonates compared to adults. Infants who are nursing from mothers receiving diazepam may show sedation and poor feeding. It appears most prudent to avoid any use of benzodiazepines during organogenesis, near the time of delivery, and during lactation.

ANTIDEPRESSANTS

- Antidepressants are often employed in the management of migraine headaches, as well as for analgesic and antidepressant purposes in chronic pain states.
- Although there are case reports of human neonatal limb deformities after maternal amitriptyline and imipramine use, large human population studies have not revealed association with any congenital malformation with the possible exception of cardiovascular defects after maternal imipramine use. There are no reports linking maternal desipramine use with congenital defects. Withdrawal syndromes have been reported in neonates born to mothers using nortriptyline, imipramine, and desipramine with symptoms including irritability, colic, tachypnea, and urinary retention.

- Amitriptyline, nortriptyline, and desipramine are all excreted into human milk. Amitriptyline, nortriptyline, desipramine, clomipramine, and sertraline were not found in quantifiable amounts in nurslings and that no adverse effects were reported. The American Academy of Pediatrics considers antidepressants to have unknown risk during lactation.
- Limited information available so far regarding the use of duloxetine and milnacipran do not indicate any adverse effect on the fetus when the drugs are consumed during pregnancy.

ANTICONVULSANTS

- Most data regarding the fetal risk of major malformation in women taking anticonvulsants is derived from the treatment of epilepsy. Among epileptic women receiving phenytoin, carbamazepine, or valproic acid, the risk of a congenital defect was approximately 5%, or twice that of the general population. Neural tube defects and, to a lesser extent, cardiac abnormalities predominate in the offspring of women taking carbamazepine and valproic acid and can be detected during routine prenatal screening (elevated α-fetoprotein level).
- The fetal hydantoin syndrome has been associated with phenytoin, carbamazepine, and valproate use during pregnancy; the syndrome consists of variable dysmorphic features including microcephaly, mental deficiency, and craniofacial abnormalities. The appearance of this syndrome may be predicted by either fetal genetic screening or by measuring amniocyte levels of the enzyme responsible for phenytoin metabolism.
- While anticonvulsants have teratogenic risk, epilepsy itself may be partially responsible for fetal malformations. Perhaps pregnant women taking anticonvulsants for chronic pain may have a lower risk of fetal malformations than those taking the same medications for seizure control.
- Patients contemplating childbearing who are receiving anticonvulsants should have their pharmacologic therapy critically evaluated. Those taking anticonvulsants for neuropathic pain should strongly consider discontinuation during pregnancy, particularly during the first trimester. Consultation with a perinatologist is recommended if continued use of anticonvulsants during pregnancy is being considered. Frequent monitoring of serum anticonvulsant levels and folate supplementation should be initiated, while maternal α-fetoprotein screening may be considered to detect fetal neural tube defects.
- Gabapentin and pregabalin are newer anticonvulsants that have been commonly used for treatment of neuropathic pain syndromes. Data available so far on gabapentin does not indicate any significant risk to either fetus or the neonate when the mother uses these medications regularly. Enough data does not exist for pregabalin.
- The use of anticonvulsants during lactation does not seem to be harmful to infants. Phenytoin, carbamazepine, and valproic acid appear in small amounts in breast milk, but no adverse effects have been noted. Limited data suggest no adverse effect of gabapentin in infants of lactating mothers consuming the medication.

ERGOT ALKALOIDS

- Ergotamine can have significant therapeutic efficacy in the episodic treatment of migraine headaches. However, even low doses of ergotamine are associated with significant teratogenic risk, while higher doses have caused uterine contractions and abortions.
- During lactation, ergot alkaloids are associated with neonatal convulsions and severe gastrointestinal disturbances.

CAFFEINE

- Caffeine is often used in combination analgesics for the management of vascular headaches. There are no identifiable risks with moderate caffeine ingestion ($100\,mg/m^2$, a dose similar to that found in two cups of brewed coffee), while ingestion of more than $300\,mg/d$ was associated with decreased birth weight. Caffeine ingestion combined with tobacco use increases the risk of delivering a low-birth-weight infant.
- Moderate ingestion of caffeine during lactation (up to two cups of coffee per day) does not appear to affect the infant. Breast milk usually contains less than 1% of the maternal dose of caffeine, with peak breast milk levels appearing 1 hour after maternal ingestion. Excessive caffeine use may cause increased wakefulness and irritability in the infant.

EVALUATION AND TREATMENT OF PAIN DURING PREGNANCY

- Severe pain during pregnancy most often arises from an extreme form of one of the more common musculoskeletal pain syndromes of pregnancy.
- Back pain and migraine headaches during pregnancy are also common problems that are encountered in practice.

MUSCULOSKELETAL CONSIDERATIONS IN PREGNANCY

Abdominal Wall and Ligamentous Pain

- Pain in the abdomen brings a pregnant woman to the obstetrician early. In most cases, the problem is not serious and the majority of cases can be diagnosed by physical examination alone. One of the most common causes of abdominal pain early in pregnancy is miscarriage and presents with abdominal pain and vaginal bleeding. Unruptured ectopic pregnancy and ovarian torsion may present with vague hypogastric pain and suprapubic tenderness. Once these conditions requiring the immediate attention of an obstetrician are ruled out, myofascial causes of abdominal pain should be considered.

- The round ligaments stretch as the uterus rises in the abdomen. If the pull is too rapid, small hematomas may develop in the ligaments (Figure 49-1). This usually begins at 16–20 weeks gestation with pain and tenderness localized over the round ligament which radiates to the pubic tubercle. Treatment is bed rest and local warmth along with oral analgesics in more severe cases.

- Less common is abdominal pain arising from hematoma formation within the sheath of the rectus abdominus muscle (Figure 49-2). As the uterus expands, the muscles of the abdominal wall become greatly

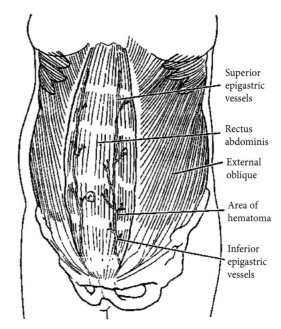

FIG. 49-2. Stretch of the abdominal wall in pregnancy can lead to tearing of the rectus abdominis muscle or inferior epigastric veins and formation of a painful hematoma within the rectus sheath. Pain is well localized and can be severe, often starting after a bout of coughing or sneezing. (Adapted with permission from Chamberlain G. ABC of antenatal care: abdominal pain in pregnancy. *British Med J.* 1991;302:1390.)

overstretched. Severe pain localized to a single segment of the muscle often follows a bout of sneezing. Diagnosis of rectus hematoma is made when localized pain is exacerbated by tightening the abdominal muscles (raising the head in the supine position). Ultrasonography can be helpful in confirming the diagnosis. Conservative management with bed rest, local heat, and mild analgesics is often all that is needed.

Hip Pain

- Two relatively rare conditions, osteonecrosis and transient osteoporosis of the hip, both occur with somewhat greater frequency during pregnancy. While the exact etiology is not known, high levels of estrogen and progesterone in the maternal circulation and increased interosseous pressure may contribute to the development of osteonecrosis.

- Transient osteoporosis of the hip is a rare disorder characterized by pain and limitation of motion of the hip and osteopenia of the femoral head. Both conditions present with hip pain during the third trimester, which may be either sudden or gradual in onset.

- Osteoporosis is easily identified with plain radiography demonstrating osteopenia of the femoral head with preservation of the joint space. Osteonecrosis

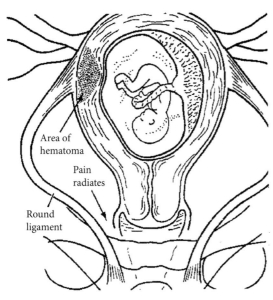

FIG. 49-1. Abdominal pain arising from stretch and hematoma formation in the round ligament typically presents between 16 and 20 weeks gestation with pain and tenderness over the round ligament which radiates to the pubic symphysis. (Adapted with permission from Chamberlain G. ABC of antenatal care: abdominal pain in pregnancy. *British Med J.* 1991;302:1390.)

is best evaluated with magnetic resonance imaging which will demonstrate changes before they appear on plain radiographs.

- Both conditions are managed symptomatically during pregnancy. Limited weight-bearing is essential in transient osteoporosis of the hip to avoid fracture of the femoral neck.

Posterior Pelvic Pain or Pelvic Girdle Pain

- The hormonal changes which occur during pregnancy lead to widening and increased mobility of the sacro-iliac synchondroses and the symphysis pubis as early as the tenth to twelfth week of pregnancy. This type of pain is described by a large group of pregnant women and is located in the posterior part of the pelvis distal and lateral to the lumbosacral junction.
- Relaxin, a hormone released by corpus luteum, softens the ligaments around the pelvic joints and this increased mechanical instability may contribute to pelvic girdle and back pain in pregnant patients.
- Many terms have been used in the literature to describe this type of pain including "sacroiliac dysfunction," "pelvic girdle relaxation," "pelvic girdle pain," and even "sacroiliac joint pain." The pain radiates to the posterior part of the thigh and may extend below the knee leading to misinterpretation as sciatica. The pain is less specific than sciatica in distribution and does not extend to the ankle or foot. Differentiating between back and posterior pelvic problems is a challenge.

Back Pain

- Back pain occurs at some time during pregnancy in about half of women and is so common that it is often looked upon as a normal part of pregnancy. The lumbar lordosis becomes markedly accentuated during pregnancy and may contribute to the development of low-back pain. Endocrine changes during pregnancy may also play a role in the development of back pain.
- Although radicular symptoms often accompany low-back pain during pregnancy, herniated nucleus pulposus (HNP) has an incidence of only 1:10,000. Pregnant women do not have an increased prevalence of lumbar intervertebral disc abnormalities. Direct pressure of the fetus on the lumbosacral nerves has been postulated as the cause of radicular symptoms.
- Back pain during pregnancy assumes one of three common patterns (Figure 49-3): pain localized to the sacroiliac area that increases as pregnancy progresses (also termed posterior pelvic pain) or pain localized to either the mid-thoracic area (high-back) or the lumbar area (low-back) that either decreases or does not change during the course of pregnancy. True

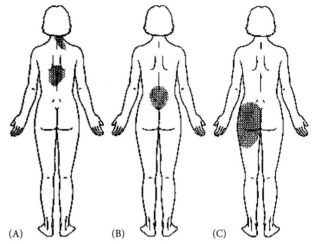

FIG. 49-3. Three types of pain were reported by a group of 855 women studied between 12 menstrual weeks of pregnancy and delivery. A, forty-nine percent of women reported back pain at some point during pregnancy, high-back pain by 10%; B, low-back pain by 40%; C, sacroiliac pain by 50%. (Adapted with permission from Ostgaard HC, Andersson GBJ, Karlsson K. Prevalence of back pain in pregnancy. *Spine.* 1991;16:549.)

sciatica with a dermatomal distribution occurs in only 1% of pregnant women.

- Evaluation begins with a thorough history which will often point the clinician to other causes. Patients with both preterm labor and premature rupture of membranes may present with low-back pain accompanied by uterine contractions and changes in the cervical os. Urologic disorders including hydronephrosis, pyelonephritis, and renal calculi may also present with low-back discomfort. Major morphologic changes occur in the collecting system of pregnant women including dilation of the calices, renal pelves, and the ureters.
- Physical examination should include complete back and neurologic evaluations. Particular attention should be directed toward the pelvis and sacroiliac joints during examination. Posterior pelvic pain (sacroiliac dysfunction) can often be distinguished from other causes of low-back pain based on physical examination. Positive straight leg raise (typical low-back pain with or without radiation to the ipsilateral lower extremity) during physical examination is consistent with either sacroiliac subluxation or herniated nucleus pulposus. Unilateral loss of knee or ankle reflex or presence of sensory or motor deficit is suggestive of lumbar nerve root compression.
- Pregnancy is not an absolute contraindication to radiographic evaluation. No detectable growth or mental abnormalities have been associated with fetal exposure to less than 10 rads—the dose received during a typical three-view spinal series typically does not exceed 1.5 rads. Plain radiographs will contribute vital

information primarily when fracture, dislocation, and destructive lesions of the bone are suspected.

- Magnetic resonance imaging (MRI) has revolutionized diagnostic imaging during pregnancy proving effective and reliable in the diagnosis of both infections and neoplasms. Although MRI appears to be safe during pregnancy, there are no long-term studies examining the safety of fetal exposure to intense magnetic fields during gestation. Practical guidelines for use of radiographic studies in the evaluation of the pregnant patients are given in Table 49-3.

- Few of the commonly used strategies to prevent low-back pain during pregnancy are universally effective. The American College of Obstetricians and Gynecologists recommends specific muscular conditioning exercises to promote good posture and prevent low-back pain during pregnancy.

- Reassurance and simple changes in the patient's activity level will often suffice to reduce symptoms to a tolerable level.

- If pain remains poorly controlled, referral to a physical therapist for evaluation and instruction in body

TABLE 49-3 Guidelines for Use of Neurodiagnostic Imaging in the Pregnant Patient

- Determine the necessity of a radiologic examination and the risks involved.
- If possible, perform the examination only during the first 10 days post-menses or, if the patient is pregnant, delay the examination until the third trimester or preferably postpartum.
- Determine the most efficacious use of radiation for the problem.
- Use magnetic resonance imaging if possible.
- Avoid direct exposure to the abdomen and pelvis.
- Avoid contrast agents.
- Do not avoid radiologic testing purely for the sake of pregnancy. Remember, you are responsible for providing the best possible care for the patient. The risk to the pregnant patient of not having an indicated radiologic examination is also an indirect risk to the fetus.
- If significant exposure is incurred by a pregnant patient, have a radiation biologist (usually stationed in the radiology department) review the radiology examination history carefully so that an accurate dose estimate can be ascertained.
- The decision to terminate pregnancy due to excessive radiation exposure is an extremely complex issue. Because any increased risk of malformations is considered to be negligible unless radiation doses exceed 0.1–0.15 Gy (10–15 rads), the amount of exposure that an embryo or fetus would likely receive from diagnostic procedures is well below the level for which a therapeutic abortion should be considered.
- Consent forms are neither required nor recommended. The patient should be informed verbally that any radiologic examinations ordered during pregnancy are considered necessary for her medical care. She should also be informed that the risks to the fetus from computed tomography/plain films are very low and that there are no known risks to humans of magnetic resonance imaging. Having the patient sign a consent increases the perceived risks and adds needlessly to her concerns during and after the examination.

Adapted with permission from Schwartz RB. Neurodiagnostic imaging of the pregnant patient. In: Devinsky O, Feldmann E, Mainline B, eds. *Neurological Complications of Pregnancy*. New York: Raven Press; 1994:243–248.

mechanics and low-back exercises may be beneficial. Aquatic exercise programs can be particularly helpful to the parturient and offer the added benefit of reducing the effects of gravity on the mother's musculoskeletal system. Massage and the surface application of heat or ice may also be useful.

- Mechanical support devices may help reduce symptoms of back pain and sacroiliac dysfunction. Widely available devices include a nonelastic trochanteric belt designed to support the abdomen and the use of a wedge-shaped pillow designed to support the abdomen of a pregnant while sleeping on her side.

- While the incidence of herniated nucleus pulposus during pregnancy is low, radicular symptoms are common and often accompany sacroiliac subluxation and myofascial pain syndromes. While the risk to the fetus following a single dose of epidural corticosteroid appears to be low, epidural steroids should be reserved for the parturient with the new onset of signs (unilateral loss of deep tendon reflex; sensory/motor change in a dermatomal distribution) and symptoms consistent with lumbar nerve root compression.

- Acetaminophen is the first analgesic to consider for management of minor back pain. While NSAIDs are the cornerstone of the pharmacologic management of back pain in nonpregnant individuals, their use during pregnancy remains controversial. Severe back pain may require treatment with narcotics and necessitate hospital admission for parenteral administration of opioid analgesics. Progressive ambulation over several days using the assistance and instruction of a skilled physical therapist is usually successful. Short courses of oral or parenteral opioids appear to add little risk to the fetus.

MIGRAINE HEADACHE DURING PREGNANCY

- Nearly 25% of women suffer from migraine headaches with the peak incidence during childbearing years. Migraines occur more often during menstruation, which has been attributed to a sudden decline in estrogen levels. During pregnancy, a sustained 50- to 100-fold increase in estradiol occurs. Indeed, 70% of women report improvement or remission of migraines during pregnancy.

- Migraine headaches rarely begin during pregnancy. Initial presentation of headaches during pregnancy should initiate a thorough search for potentially serious causes. The literature is replete with reports of intracranial pathology which mimicked migraines during pregnancy including strokes, pseudotumor cerebri, tumors, aneurysms, arteriovenous malformations, and cerebral venous thrombosis. Metabolic causes of headache during pregnancy include drug use, most notably, cocaine, anti-phospholipid antibody syndrome, and choriocarcinoma.

- Patients who present with their first severe headache during pregnancy should receive a complete neurologic examination and should be strongly considered for MRI, toxicology screen, and serum coagulation profiles. In the patient who presents with sudden onset of the "worst headache of my life," a subarachnoid hemorrhage should be ruled out. Progressively worsening headaches in the setting of sudden weight gain should suggest preeclampsia or pseudotumor cerebri. The triad of elevated blood pressure, proteinuria, and peripheral edema points toward preeclampsia; hyperreflexia and elevated serum uric acid are also found in patients with preeclampsia.

- For those pregnant women with a history of migraines prior to pregnancy and a normal neurologic examination, the therapeutic challenge is to achieve control of the headaches while minimizing risk to the fetus. Nonpharmacologic techniques, including relaxation, biofeedback, and elimination of certain foods often suffice for treatment.

- If pharmacologic therapy appears warranted, acetaminophen with or without caffeine is safe and effective. The short-term use of mild opioid analgesics like hydrocodone, alone or in combination with acetaminophen, also appears to carry little risk. When oral analgesics prove ineffective, hospital admission and administration of parenteral opioids may be required.

CONCLUSIONS

- Many physicians find themselves apprehensive about treating pain in pregnant patients. Evaluation and treatment are limited by the relative contraindication of radiography in the workup and the risks associated with pharmacologic therapy during pregnancy.

- Familiarity with common pain problems as well as the maternal and fetal risks of pain medications can allow the pain practitioner to help women achieve a more comfortable pregnancy.

- A single health care provider should be designated to coordinate specialist evaluations and integrate their suggestions into a single, integrated plan of care.

BIBLIOGRAPHY

American Academy of Pediatrics Committee on Drugs. The transfer of drugs and other chemicals into human milk. *Pediatrics*. 1994;93:137–150; Revisions in 2001 and 2013.

Briggs GG, Freeman RK, Yaffe SJ. *Drugs in Pregnancy and Lactation*. Baltimore, Md: Williams and Wilkins; 1990.

Chamberlain G. ABC of antenatal care: abdominal pain in pregnancy. *British Med J.* 1991;302:1390.

Fujii H, Goel A, Bernard N, et al. Pregnancy outcomes following gabapentin use: results of a prospective comparative cohort study. *Neurology*. 2013 April 23;80(17):1565–1570

Jones H. Treatment of opioid-dependent pregnant women: clinical and research issues. *J Subst Abuse Treat*. 2008;35(3):245–259

Liew Z, et al. Acetaminophen use during pregnancy, behavioral problems, and hyperkinetic disorders. *JAMA Pediatr*. 2014;168(9):865–866.

MacEvilly M, Buggy D. Back pain and pregnancy: a review. *Pain*. 1996;64:405–414.

Niebyl JR. Nonanesthetic drugs during pregnancy and lactation. In: Chestnut DH, ed., *Obstetric Anesthesia: Principles and Practice*. St. Louis, Mo: Mosby;1994:229–240.

Rathmell JP, Viscomi CM, Ashburn MA. Acute and chronic pain management in the pregnant patient. *Anesth Analg*. 1997;85:1074–1087.

Rathmell JP, Viscomi CM, Bernstein IM. Pain management during pregnancy and lactation. In: Raj PP, ed., *Practical Management of Pain*. 3rd ed. St. Louis, Mo: Mosby;2000:196–211.

Rungee JL. Low back pain during pregnancy. *Orthopedics*. 1993;16:1339–1344.

Schwartz RB. Neurodiagnostic imaging of the pregnant patient. In: Devinsky O, Feldmann E, Mainline B, eds., *Neurological Complications of Pregnancy*. New York: Raven Press;1994:243–248.

Silverstein SD. Headaches and women: treatment of the pregnant and lactating migraineur. *Headache*. 1993;33:533–540.

50 SICKLE CELL ANEMIA

Richard Payne, MD

INTRODUCTION—THE BASICS

- Sickle cell anemia was identified in the United States in 1910 by Herrick, who observed sickle-shaped red blood cells (RBCs) in an anemic black medical student in Chicago.

- Sickle cell anemia is an inherited autosomal dominant disorder, resulting from a single amino acid substitution in which valine replaces glutamic acid in the β-globin chain. In the homozygous type, both β-globin chains have the mutation (HbSS), and when RBCs are placed in an environment of decreased oxygen tension, they assume a sickled shape and impair the microcirculation. About 4% of African-Americans have the HbSS genotype.
  ○ People with sickle cell trait have one abnormal β-globin chain and one normal β-globin chain, and have no disease manifestations (except in rare

circumstances in which they are exposed to extreme physical exertion such as military exercises or competitive athletics).
  ○ Variants of the homozygous sickle cell genotype produce such as HbS-β thalassemia, and HbSC disease, may still produce sickling, but generally there are less severe manifestations.
- Fetal hemoglobin (HbF; the β-globin chain in adult hemoglobin is replaced by a γ chain) persists into the first months of life and inhibits blood from sickling when it constitutes >20% of the total hemoglobin.
- Hydroxyurea, which increases the production of HbF, is reserved for patients with severe disease and, compared with placebo, reduces the number of (1) vaso-occlusive crisis (VOC) episodes (including the time to first and second VOC), (2) acute chest syndromes, and (3) transfusions.

CLINICAL MANIFESTATIONS OF DISEASE

- The sickle hemoglobinopathy causes a hemolytic anemia and impairment of blood flow in the micro-circulation, leading to painful end-organ dysfunction, infection, stroke, and a plethora of other symptoms and signs.
  ○ The mortality of sickle cell disease in young children (<10 years of age) has been decreased by as much as 68% because of better comprehensive care, including the use of prophylactic antibiotics, better pain management, and in some cases the use of HLA sibling-match bone marrow transplantation.
  ○ General treatment strategies have many goals, including management of acute and chronic pain, prevention and treatment of infection, prevention of stroke, and management of end-organ damage and pulmonary hypertension. (Table 50-1).
  ○ Pain is a cardinal feature of sickle cell disease; however, the timing, severity, and frequency of painful episodes vary greatly.
- In general, approximately 20% of patients have pain rarely; 60% have one or two episodes each year, and 20% have more than two episodes per month and are considered severely affected.
- The classic VOC is a relatively unpredictable ischemic event that occurs when rigid sickled cells obstruct blood vessels. Table 50-2 lists the factors that influence the frequency of VOCs.
- Pain can be severe and is usually present in the bone, chest, and abdomen.
- Children may experience sickle cell dactylitis, most likely caused when avascular necrosis of the marrow produces swelling in the dorsal surfaces of the hands and feet. Repetitive splenic infarction in children

TABLE 50-1   Clinical Manifestations of Sickle Cell Disease

Acute painful episodes—so-called "vaso-occlusive crises"
- First symptom in about 25% of patients
- Most common reason to seek medical attention
- Most have no clear precipitant
- 50% of patients have associated signs—fever, swelling, etc.
- 1/3 patients have >6 pain-related hospitalizations/year
- No reliable "confirmatory" laboratory test or biomarker

Neurological complications—24% of patients have stroke by age 45
- Chronic transfusion therapy may help
- Hydroxyurea does not prevent stroke
- Maybe indication for bone marrow transplant
- Epilepsy two to three times more common in sickle cell disease

Multi-organ failure—may lead to death
- Timely exchange transfusions may reverse effects

Infection (sepsis, meningitis, pneumonia, osteomyelitis)
- Major cause of morbidity and death
- Asplenia major contributing factor

Renal failure—occurs in about 20% of patients
- **Pulmonary complications**—low oxygen tension in pulmonary arteries predisposes to sickling
  - Acute chest syndrome—chest wall pain, pneumonia, pulmonary infarcts in oxygen desaturation. Often occurs during acute painful episode. May be fatal.

Leg ulcers—more common in HbSS; often bilateral. May become super-infected

Other complications
- Cardiac
- Priapism
- Hepatobiliary
- Retinopathy

Data from Vichinsky EP. Overview of the clinical manifestations of sickle cell disease. Available at: http://uptdodate.com/contents/overview-of-the-clinical-manifestations-of-sickle-cell-disease.

produces recurrent abdominal pain and, eventually, an autosplenectomy.
- Other manifestations of the disease include aplastic and megaloblastic crises, sequestration crises (ie, sudden massive pooling of RBCs, especially in the spleen), hemolytic crises, osteomyelitis (especially *Salmonella typhimurium*), priapism, renal failure, jaundice and hepatomegaly, ischemic leg ulceration, stroke, and a host of other ischemic manifestations in every organ.
- The acute chest syndrome, an important variant of VOC, manifests as chest pain, with or without fever, in association with a pulmonary infiltrate.

TABLE 50-2   Factors Influencing the Frequency of Vaso-occlusive Crises

Increase frequency
- Cold weather
- Young adult males (15–25 years old)
- Pregnancy (especially third trimester)

Decrease frequency
- Presence of α-thalassemia
- Elevated HbF levels (>30% total hemoglobin)
- RBC membrane polymorphisms (inhibit aggregation to vascular endothelium)

TABLE 50-3   Causes of Death in Patients with Sickle Cell Anemia

Causes of death
- Pulmonary fat embolism
- Acute multi-organ system failure
- Acute chest syndrome
- Renal failure
- Seizures

Factors associated with risk of early death
- Persistent leukocytosis
- Depressed HbF levels

TABLE 50-4   Some Nonselective and COX-2-Selective NSAIDs Used to Manage Sickle Cell Pain

DRUG TYPE	NAME/BRAND	TYPICAL STARTING DOSE
Acetaminophen	Tylenol and others	650 mg q4h PO
Aspirin	Multiple	650 mg q4h PO
Ibuprofen	Motrin and others	200–800 mg q6h PO
Choline–magnesium trisalicylate	Trilisate	1000–1500 mg tid PO
Diclofenac sodium	Voltaren	50–75 mg q8-12 PO
Naproxen	Naprosyn	250–750 mg q12h PO
Naproxen sodium	Anaprox	275 mg q12h PO
Meloxicam	Mobic	7.5 mg PO daily
Ketorolac	Toradol	10 mg q4–6h PO (not to exceed 10 d)
Ketorolac		60 mg (initial), then 30 mg q6h IV or IM (not to exceed 5 d)
Celecoxib*	Celebrex	200 mg bid

*Selective for COX-2 isoenzyme.

- The acute chest syndrome may be caused by lung infarction or rib infarction with associated pleuritis and chest splinting and is associated with a higher mortality than other forms of VOC, particularly in children placed on intravenous opioid infusions who are not carefully monitored.
- The most common causes of death for sickle cell patients are listed in Table 50-3.
- Appropriate management of the acute chest syndrome includes the judicious use of opioids and aggressive respiratory treatments, especially the use of incentive spirometry.

"ROUTINE" MANAGEMENT OF VASO-OCCLUSIVE CRISES

- Standard treatment approaches to the management of a VOC episode include intravenous hydration, oxygen inhalation, and parenteral analgesics (opioids and nonopioids).
- Some experts assert that routine intravenous hydration is unnecessary in the absence of clinically apparent dehydration.
- The use of oxygen therapy is even more controversial in a controlled clinical trial in which patients were randomized to inhalation of 50% oxygen or room air, the duration of severe pain, the consumption of analgesics, and the length of hospitalization did not differ, even though the oxygen-treated group had a reduction in reversibly sickled cells.

GUIDELINES FOR ANALGESIC USE

- Tables 50-4 and 50-5 summarize information on the use of analgesics. The principles of pharmacologic management of acute and chronic sickle cell pain are similar to those for the management of pain in any group of patients with a serious, potentially life-limiting medical disorder.
- Bone pain is a particularly prominent feature of VOC and other forms of sickle cell pain; therefore, nonselective and COX-2-selective nonsteroidal anti-inflammatory drugs (NSAIDs) are used commonly as single agents or in combination with other analgesics, especially opioids (Tables 50-4 and 50-5).
- Although widely used, meperidine is associated with signs of central nervous system excitability, including seizures, related to accumulation of the normeperidine metabolite. Given the effects of sickle cell disease on kidney function, these patients are vulnerable to this toxic effect of meperidine, which should not be a first-line opioid for the treatment of acute or chronic pain.
- Emergency department guidelines for the treatment of sickle cell pain emphasize the need to evaluate patients quickly to assess and treat infections and treat pain aggressively. Some institutions have established day treatment hospitals for sickle cell patients so that pain management can be achieved efficiently by a group of clinicians who know the patient best. The Joint Committee on Accreditation of Healthcare Organization (JCAHO) now has standards for the assessment and management of sickle cell–related pain, and there are now published guidelines for the management of sickle cell–related pain (Table 50-6).

SUBSTANCE ABUSE CONCERNS

- The prevalence of substance abuse disorders in sickle cell patients appears to be grossly exaggerated, especially if one considers iatrogenic substance abuse.
- One study demonstrated that hematologists and emergency department physicians estimated that approximately 25% of adult sickle cell patients are addicted to illegal substances, when the published prevalence of addiction is actually much lower: no addiction found in 600 adults; "addiction" in 3 and "dependence" in 7

TABLE 50-5 Commonly Used Opioids for Moderate-to-Severe Pain

	USUAL STARTING DOSE	COMMENT
WHO STEP I/II OPIOIDS		

Codeine (with aspirin or acetaminophen)
  Tylenol #2 (15 mg codeine)
  Tylenol #3 (30 mg codeine)
  Tylenol #4 (60 mg codeine)
	60 mg q3–4h PO	• Fixed combination with aspirin or acetaminophen = DEA schedule III; single entity = DEA II
		• Usually 250 mg aspirin or acetaminophen/tablet
		• Take care not to reach toxic doses of aspirin and acetaminophen

Hydrocodone (with aspirin or acetaminophen)	10 mg q3–4h PO	• Same as for codeine
Lorcet, Lortab, Vicodin, etc.		• Vicodin Extra Strength has 750 mg acetaminophen/tablet

Oxycodone
  Roxicodone (single entity)
  Percocet, Percodan, Tylox, etc.
	10 mg q3–4h PO	• Available in controlled-release formulation (as single entity)

Tramadol
  Ultram (single entity)
  Ultracet (tramadol + ibuprofen)
	50 mg qid PO	• Although a μ-opioid agonist, it is not scheduled as an opioid
		• Also, blocks catecholamine reuptake
		• Nausea common side effect
		• Seizures may occur in doses >400 mg/d

WHO STEP II/III OPIOIDS		
Morphine Immediate release (MSIR)	30 mg q3–4h PO 10 mg q3–4h IV	• Standard by which all other opioids are compared • MSIR is a preferred rescue analgesic for controlled-release preparations • Morphine is also available as suppository
Sustained release (MS Contin, Oramorph, Kadian, Avinza)	30 mg q12h PO	• Some clinicians do not view MS Contin and Oramorph as therapeutically interchangeable • MS Contin available in 15, 30, 60, 100, and 200 mg tablets • Oramorph available in 15, 30, 60, and 100 mg tablets only • Oramorph ER is an extended release formulation that is "crush-resistant"*

Oxcodone
  Immediate release
  Sustained-release (OxyContin)
	5–10 mg q3-4h PO
	10–20 mg q 12h PO
		• Twice as potent as morphine
		• New Oxecta formulation is more difficult to crush
		• OxyContin has been reformulated into a more tamper-resistant preparation

Hydromorphone Dilaudid, others	8–12 mg q 24h PO	• OROS formulation (Exalgo) delivers hydromorphone over 24 hours and is "tamper-deterrent" • IR formulation is available as suppository
Fentanyl Duragesic (transdermal)	25–50 μg/h q 72h	• Available in intravenous and transdermal formulations • Transdermal formulation should not be used as primary therapy for acute painful episodes
Sublimaze, others		
Methadone	5–10 mg q6–8h PO	• Very stigmatized because of use to treat heroin addiction. Careful titration to avoid overdose because of long plasma half-life
Dolophine, others	2–5 mg q6–8h IV	

*Moorman-Li R, Motycka CA, Inge LD, et al. A review of abuse-deterrent opioids for chronic nonmalignant pain. *P&T*. 2012;37:412.

TABLE 50-6 Adjunctive Pharmacotherapies for Acute and Chronic Sickle Cell–related Pain

DRUG TYPE	NAME/BRAND	NOTES
Corticosteroids	Methylprednisolone	15 mg/kg (max dose 1000 mg) One study showed reduction in inpatient analgesics use during acute painful episode
Stimulants	Methylphenidate	No controlled trials in sickle cell pain May have intrinsic analgesic effects and can counteract somnolence produced by other meds

of 101 patients; and drug abuse "suspected" in 9 and "definite" in 5 of 114.

• The term *pseudo-addiction* has been used to describe drug-seeking behavior in patients who are provoked by inadequate control of pain. Sickle cell patients are at great risk for displaying "pseudo-addiction" behavior when their pain is inadequately controlled.
  ○ Morphine, oxymorphone, hydromorphone, and oxycodone are now available in formulations for oral administration that are more tamper resistant than older preparations and should be used, especially if a dual diagnosis of chronic pain and substance abuse is made.

BIBLIOGRAPHY

Ballas SK, Delengowski A. Pain measurement in hospitalized adults with sickle cell painful episodes. *Ann Clin Lab Sci.* 1993;23:358.

Baum KF, Dunn DT, Maude GH, et al. The painful crises of homozygous sickle cell disease: a study of risk factors. *Arch Intern Med.* 1987;147:1231.

Beutler E. The sickle cell disease and related disorders. In: Beutler E, Lictman MA, Coller BS, et al., eds. *Williams' Hematology.* 5th ed. New York: McGraw-Hill; 1995:616.

Brozovic M, Davies SC, Yardumian A, et al. Pain relief in sickle cell crisis. *Lancet.* 1986;2:624.

Charache S, Terrin ML, Moore RD, et al. Effect of hydroxyurea on the frequency of painful crises in sickle cell anemia. *N Engl J Med.* 1995;332:1317.

Cole TB, Spinkle RK, Smith SJ, et al. Intravenous narcotic therapy for children with severe sickle cell pain crises. *Am J Child.* 1986;140:1255.

Conley CL. Sickle-cell anemia: the first molecular disease. In: Wintrobe MM, ed. *Blood, Pure and Eloquent.* New York: McGraw-Hill; 1980:319.

Herrick JB. Peculiar elongated and sickle-shaped red corpuscles in a case of severe anemia. *Arch Intern Med.* 1910;6:517.

Ingram VM. Gene mutations in human hemoglobin: the chemical difference between normal and sickle cell haemoglobin. *Nature.* 1957;180:326.

Noguchi CT, Rodger GP, Serjeant G, et al. Levels of fetal hemoglobin necessary for treatment of sickle cell disease. *N Engl J Med.* 1988;318:96.

Platt OS, Brambilla DJ, Rosse WF, et al. Mortality in sickle cell disease: life expectancy and risk factors for early death. *N Engl J Med.* 1994;330:1639.

Portenoy RK, Payne R. Acute and chronic pain. In: Lowinson JH, Ruiz P, Millman RB, et al. eds. *Substance Abuse: A Comprehensive Textbook.* Baltimore, Md: Williams & Wilkins; 1992:691.

Rees DC, Olujohungbe AD, Parker NE, et al. Guidelines for the management of the acute painful crises in sickle cell disease. *Br J Haematol.* 2003;120:744.

Rucknagel DL, Kalinyak KA, Gelfand MJ. Rib infarcts and acute chest syndrome in sickle cell diseases. *Lancet.* 1991;337:831.

Shapiro BS, Benjamin LJ, Payne R, et al. Sickle cell-related pain: perceptions of medical practitioners. *J Pain Symptom Manage.* 1997;14:168.

Taliaferro WH, Huck JG. The inheritance of sickle-cell anemia in man. *Genetics.* 1923;8:594.

Vichinsky EP. (n.d.). Overview of the clinical manifestations of sickle cell disease. Available at: http://uptodate.com/contents/overview-of-the-clincal-manifestations-of-sickle-cell-disease. Accessed August 30, 2013.

Vichinsky EP. (n.d.). Overview of the management of sickle cell disease. Available at: http://uptodate.com/contents/overeiew-of-the-management-of-sickle-cell-disesase. Accessed August 30, 2013.

Vichinsky EP, Johnson PR, Lubin RB. Multidisciplinary approach to pain management in sickle cell disease. *Am J Pediatr Hematol Oncol.* 1982;4:328.

Weissman DE, Haddox JD. Opioid pseudo-addiction: an iatrogenic syndrome. *Pain.* 1989;36:363.

Zipursky A, Robieux IC, Brown, EJ, et al. Oxygen therapy in sickle cell disease. *Am J Pediatr Hematol Oncol.* 1992;14:222.

51 SPASTICITY

Michael Saulino, MD, PhD
Leonard Kamen, DO

DEFINITIONS

- Spasticity is the manifestation of hyperactive tone (hypertonia) signifying that the muscle stretch monosynaptic reflex has become isolated from supraspinal inhibitory modulation.
- Tone is a dynamic quality of motion expected by the nervous system in order to comfortably perform optimal functional activities.
- Tone can be excessively rigid representing a co-contracture in two or more opposing muscles or profoundly weak (flaccid).
- This functionally disrupting combination of weakness (negative sign) and/or rigidity (positive sign) is characterized as the upper motor neuron syndrome (UMNS).
- From a physiological perspective, spasticity represents a velocity-dependent resistance to passive stretch relative to the torque placed through the joint and associated soft tissues.
- Spasticity may be associated with the perception of pain.
- Disorders of proprioception, spatial orientation, and abnormal pain perception can be demonstrated in the UMNS.
- Table 51-1 lists etiology and common characteristics of the UMNS.

ASSESSMENT

- Spasticity, much like pain, has both a subjective and objective quality.
- To adequately measure the individual impact of spastic activity requires full assessment of medical etiology, co-morbidities, stretch reflex examination, passive/active range of motion, and functional impairment.
- Assessment by multiple disciplines may provide the most cohesive picture of the profound effect that spasticity has on the individual and caretakers (see Table 51-2).

TABLE 51-1   Etiologies of Spasticity

CAUSE	LOCATION	DISTRIBUTION	PAIN CHARACTERISTICS
Vascular Thrombosis/Hemorrhage Embolic	Brain, SC	Hemiparesis Paraparesis Tetraparesis	Central pain, post stroke shoulder-hand, myalgias, arthralgias
Multiple sclerosis	Brain, SC	Hemiparesis Paraparesis Tetraparesis	Peripheral dysesthesias, central pain
Spinal cord injury	SC	Paraparesis Tetraparesis	Deafferentation pain, heterotopic bone pain
Cerebral palsy	Brain	Monoparesis Hemiparesis Paraparesis Tetraparesis	Nocioceptive, mechanical pain, arthralgia
Traumatic brain injury	Brain	Monoparesis Hemiparesis Tetraparesis	Central pain, heterotopic bone pain
Myelopathy Syringomyelia Syringobulbia	Cervical and thoracic SC	Paraparesis Tetraparesis	Dysesthetic/central pain
Tumors Abscess Infection	Brain, SC	Monoparesis Hemiparesis Paraparesis Tetraparesis	Dysesthetic pain
Parkinson's disease	Brain	Tetraparesis	Axial pain/dysesthesias

TABLE 51-2   Essential Caregivers for Person with Spasticity

HEALTH CARE PROVIDER	RESPONSIBILITY
Medical Rehabilitation Specialist	Identifies etiology and initiates medical spasticity management. Modifies and monitors care
Physical Therapist	Applies physical treatment strategies Addresses the impact of spasticity on mobility
Occupational Therapist	Addresses the impact of spasticity on self-care skills, integrates functional activities
Psycho /social services	Assessment/treatment of coping skills, evaluation of environmental needs for clients with spasticity
Nursing/ancillary providers	Attends to acute care needs and prevention of secondary complications in patients with spasticity

TABLE 51-3   Modified Ashworth Scale (MAS)

MAS VALUE	DESCRIPTION
0	No increase in muscle tone
1	Slight increase in tone, manifested by catch and release, minimal resistance at end range of motion (ROM)
1+	Slight increase in tone, catch followed by minimal resistance throughout (<1/2) remainder of ROM
2	More marked increase in tone through ROM, affected parts easily moved
3	Considerable increase in tone, passive ROM difficult
4	Affected part(s) rigid in flexion and extension

- Clinical management requires measures that can portray changes in response to treatments. The Modified Ashworth Scale (MAS) has been validated and broadly applied (see Table 51-3).

EPIDEMIOLOGY

- Etiologies of spasticity are heterogeneous.
- This syndrome is usually seen in conditions that involve damage to the portion of the brain or spinal cord (SC) that controls voluntary movement.
- Spasticity can be associated with SC injuries, multiple sclerosis, cerebral palsy, stroke, and traumatic or anoxic brain injury, as well as some metabolic/degenerative diseases like adrenoleukodystrophy, amyotrophic lateral sclerosis, hereditary spastic paraparesis, stiff-person syndrome, and phenylketonuria.
- Although spasticity is known to be a common condition, the incidence and prevalence of spasticity is difficult to determine.
- The estimated incidence of spasticity for the most common etiologies is shown in Table 51-4.

TABLE 51-4   Prevalence of Spasticity in the United States

CONDITION	PREVALENCE	REASONABLE PROPORTION EXPERIENCING SPASTICITY	TOTAL SPASTIC PATIENTS
Cerebral palsy	750,000	50%	375,000
Multiple sclerosis	400,000	60%	240,000
Cerebrovascular accident (CVA)	7,000,000	20%	1,400,000
Traumatic brain injury	1,500,000	33%	500,000
SC injury	200,000	50%	100,000
Total			2,615,000

TREATMENT PROTOCOLS

- Developing realistic expectations for treatment remains the cornerstone of any management protocol.
- Nonmedication treatments are essential and require orchestration within the context of comprehensive care (see Table 51-5).
- Initial interventions may include removal of noxious stimuli such as a clogged catheter or relief of constipation, which may significantly alter spastic tone throughout the body.
- Skin breakdown or irritation, dental problems, or an ill-fitting brace can be promoted by and amplify spasticity.
- Physical and occupational therapists are crucial to both patients and caretakers in finding tone reduction techniques by proper positioning and seating system recommendations.
- Passive and active stretching, balance, and transfer training that engages extensor hypertonicity to assist performance of a stand pivot transfer may be incorporated.

ORAL MEDICATIONS

- Best suited for global or multisite muscle overactivity.
- Advantages: relatively easy without the need for specialized technical expertise, noninvasive, generic, and generally inexpensive, not controlled or scheduled, utility as a breakthrough strategy and secondary indications (pain, insomnia, epilepsy mood disorders).
- Disadvantages: tolerability (especially in patients with acquired cerebral injury), adverse effects (AEs) (sedation, drowsiness, lethargy and impairment in cognitive processing), poor choices for focal or regional spasticity, short half-life.

TABLE 51-5   Nonpharmacologic Treatment Options

MODALITY	PROPOSED MECHANISM	PRACTICAL APPLICATION
Muscle cooling	Increase in γ motorneuron excitability increase CNS inhibition Increase CNS inhibition	Ice stroking cooling garments
Superficial heat	Increase blood flow inhibit nocioception in SC	Moist heating by hydrocollator, infrared, diathermy or paraffin
Deep heat	Increase nerve conduction, gating stretch sensitive channels	Ultrasound continuous vs. pulsed
Stretching/ passive ROM	Production of actin and myosin Decrease stretch reflex.	Manual Serial casting Brace/splint
Neurofacilitation techniques	Retraining brain maps, neuroplasticity	Task-specific/oriented therapy, constraint-induced therapy

TABLE 51-6   Oral Medication Options for Spasticity

DRUG	ACTION	SIDE EFFECTS
Baclofen	Presynaptic GABA-B receptor agonist	Sedation, weakness, seizure, withdrawal
Dantrolene	Decrease the release of calcium from the sarcoplasmic reticulum of skeletal muscle	Weakness, hepatotoxity
Tizanidine	α-2 adrenergic receptor agonist	Orthostasis, sedation, dry mouth, drowsiness, dizziness, fatigue, and hepatotoxity
Clonidine	α-2 adrenergic receptor agonist	Hypotension, orthostasis
Diazepam	Stimulation of GABA-A receptor	Sedation, tolerance, cognitive impairment, withdrawal

- Classic six oral medications for spasticity: baclofen, diazepam, dantrolene, clonidine, and tizanidine (see Table 51-6).
- Skeletal muscle relaxants (methocarbamol, cyclobenzaprine, etc.) generally not indicated for spasticity.

NEUROLYTIC PROCEDURES

- Chemodenervation techniques have evolved over the last century (see Table 51-7).
- 20%–40% ethyl alcohol produces profound anesthesia and reduces spasticity by muscle fiber and nervous tissue destruction.
- Almost immediately affected by electrical stimulation (ES)-guided injections of aqueous phenol (3%–7%) directly over the selected motor nerve or motor end plates.
- AEs: injection site pain, necrosis, vascular injury, phlebitis, skin injury, painful peripheral neuropathy, and weakness in contiguous muscles.
- Botulinum toxin (BT) A and B strains are available from several manufactures in the United States (see Table 51-8).
- The mechanism of action is inhibition of the binding of acetylcholine prior to release at peripheral neuromuscular junctions.
- Weakening of muscle contracture is partial and clinical effects last approximately 90 days before sprouting of new terminal neuromuscular junctions are established.
- AEs: excessive weakness in targeted muscles, distant spread to nontargeted muscles, dysphagia, xerostomia, flu-like symptoms, respiratory distress, and injection site pain.
- Injections are spaced at least 90 days apart to prevent the potential for antibody formation.

TABLE 51-7 **Overview of Neurolytic Agents**

NEUROLYTIC AGENT	MECHANISM	INJECTION TECHNIQUE	AEs	ONSET	DURATION
Ethyl alcohol 20%–40%	Nervous and tissue destruction	EMG ES	Inj ection site pain, dysesthesias	<1 hour	2–36 months
Phenol 3%–7%	Nervous and tissue destruction	EMG ES	Injection site pain, dysesthesias	<1 hour	2–36 months
BT	Presynaptic block of Acetylcholine	Palpation EMG ES Ultrasound	Weakness, dysphagia, respiratory	Days	3–6 months

TABLE 51-8 **Commercial Botulinum Toxins Available in the United States**

SCIENTIFIC NAME	COMMERCIAL PRODUCT	STRAIN OF BOTULINUM
Onabotulinumtoxin A	Botox	A
Incobotulinumtoxin A	Xeomin	A
Abobotulinumtoxin A	Dysport	A
Rimabotulinumtoxin B	Myobloc	B

ITB THERAPY

- Intrathecal baclofen therapy (ITB) infusion exerts its therapeutic effect by delivering baclofen directly into the cerebrospinal fluid (CSF), thus affording enhanced distribution of this agent to target neurons in the SC.
- Patients can be considered candidates for ITB therapy when:
  - Spasticity is poorly controlled despite maximal therapy with other modalities;
  - Spasticity is poorly controlled because of limited patient tolerance of other modalities;
  - Adjustable spasticity reduction afforded by a programmable variable flow pump would be advantageous.

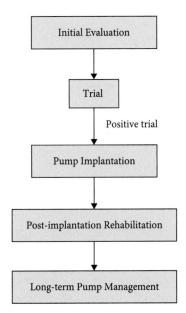

FIG. 51-1. Algorithm for ITB therapy.

- Algorithm for treatment (see Figure 51-1).
- AEs: excessive hypotonia, nausea, headache, dizziness, bowel and bladder changes, respiratory depression, increased thromboembolic risk, withdrawal, and overdose.

NEUROSURGICAL MANAGEMENT

- The primary focus is on interrupting the stretch reflex or attempting to increase inhibitory influence on motor pathways.
- Peripheral procedures: rhizotomy, neurectomy.
- Central procedures: cordotomy, myelotomy, DREZotomy.
- Intraoperative electromyography (EMG) assessment and aggressive postoperative rehabilitation are considered the standard of care.
- AEs: increase weakness, atrophy, sensory loss, dysesthesias, sexual, bowel or bladder dysfunction, spinal deformity, infection, dysesthesias, hemorrhage, and CSF leakage.

ORTHOPEDIC MANAGEMENT

- Goals: correction of musculoskeletal misalignments, deformities, and contractures.
- Four categories: musculotendinous lengthenings, tendon transfers, osteotomies, and arthrodeses.
- Lengthening can be done by three techniques: Z-type splitting and gliding method, lengthening release through the musculotendinous junction, and recession of the tendon at its insertion with resuturing to proximal soft tissues or bone.
- Tendon transfers attempt to utilize increased muscle tone by moving a muscle tendon unit with spasticity to antagonist group that possesses excessive weakness.
- Osteotomies attempt to correct the bony malalignment, but also to position the surrounding muscles in a more efficient biomechanical position.
- Arthrodesis is used when dynamic correction of certain deformities is not likely to be successful.

BIBLIOGRAPHY

Bohannon RW, Smith MB. Interrater reliability of a modified ashworth scale of muscle spasticity. *Phys Ther.* 1987, February;67(2):206–207.

Elovic EP, Esquenazi A, Alter KE, et al. Chemodenervation and nerve blocks in the diagnosis and management of spasticity and muscle overactivity. *PM R.* 2009, September 1;1(9):842–851.

Esquenazi A, Mayer N, Lee S, et al. Patient registry of outcomes in spasticity care. *Am J Phys Med Rehabil.* 2012;91(9):729–746.

Francisco GE, Saulino MF, Yablon SA, et al. Intrathecal baclofen therapy: an update. 2009, September 1;1(9):852–858.

Gracies JM. Pathophysiology of impairment in patients with spasticity and use of stretch as a treatment of spastic hypertonia. *Phys Med Rehabil Clin N Am.* 2001, November;12(4):747,68, vi.

Halpern R, Gillard P, Graham GD, et al. Adherence associated with oral medications in the treatment of spasticity. *PM&R.* 2013, May 3.

Kamen L, Henney HR, III, Runyan JD. A practical overview of tizanidine use for spasticity secondary to multiple sclerosis, stroke, and spinal cord injury. *Curr Med Res Opin.* 2008, February;24(2):425–439.

Lance JW. What is spasticity? *Lancet.* 1990, March 10;335(8689):606.

Lapeyre E, Kuks JB, Meijler WJ. Spasticity: revisiting the role and the individual value of several pharmacological treatments. *NeuroRehabilitation.* 2010;27(2):193–200.

Lechner HE, Frotzler A, Eser P. Relationship between self- and clinically rated spasticity in spinal cord injury. *Arch Phys Med Rehabil.* 2006, January;87(1):15–19.

Lundstrom E, Terent A, Borg J. Prevalence of disabling spasticity 1 year after first-ever stroke. *Eur J Neurol.* 2008 June;15(6):533–539.

Lynn AK, Turner M, Chambers HG. Surgical management of spasticity in persons with cerebral palsy. *PM&R.* 2009, September;1(9):834–838.

Mandigo CE, Anderson RC. Management of childhood spasticity: a neurosurgical perspective. *Pediatr Ann.* 2006, May; 35(5):354–362.

Mayer NH, Herman RM. Phenomenology of muscle overactivity in the upper motor neuron syndrome. *Eura Medicophys.* 2004, June;40(2):85–110.

Maynard FM, Karunas RS, Waring WP, III. Epidemiology of spasticity following traumatic spinal cord injury. *Arch Phys Med Rehabil.* 1990, July;71(8):566–569.

Meythaler JM. Concept of spastic hypertonia. *Phys Med Rehabil Clin N Am.* 2001, November;12(4):725,32, v.

O'Brien DF, Park TS. A review of orthopedic surgeries after selective dorsal rhizotomy. *Neurosurg Focus.* 2006, August 15;21(2):e2.

Patwardhan RV, Minagar A, Kelley RE, et al. Neurosurgical treatment of multiple sclerosis. *Neurol Res.* 2006, April; 28(3):320–325.

Phadke CP, Balasubramanian CK, Ismail F, et al. Revisiting physiologic and psychologic triggers that increase spasticity. *Am J Phys Med Rehabil.* 2013, April;92(4):357–369.

Rizzo MA, Hadjimichael OC, Preiningerova J, et al. Prevalence and treatment of spasticity reported by multiple sclerosis patients. *Mult Scler.* 2004, October;10(5):589–595.

Saulino M. The use of intrathecal baclofen in pain management. *Pain Management.* 2012, November 1; 2013, March; 2(6):603–608.

Saval A, Chiodo AE. Intrathecal baclofen for spasticity management: a comparative analysis of spasticity of spinal vs cortical origin. *J Spinal Cord Med.* 2010;33(1):16–21.

Sheean G, McGuire JR. Spastic hypertonia and movement disorders: pathophysiology, clinical presentation, and quantification. *PM&R.* 2009, September;1(9):827–833.

Smyth MD, Peacock WJ. The surgical treatment of spasticity. *Muscle Nerve.* 2000, February;23(2):153–163.

Tafti MA, Cramer SC, Gupta R. Orthopaedic management of the upper extremity of stroke patients. *J Am Acad Orthop Surg.* 2008, August;16(8):462–470.

Watanabe TK. Role of oral medications in spasticity management. 2009, September 1;1(9):839–841.

Wedekind C, Lippert-Gruner M. Long-term outcome in severe traumatic brain injury is significantly influenced by brainstem involvement. *Brain Inj.* 2005, August 20;19(9):681–684.

Wheeler A, Smith HS. Botulinum toxins: mechanisms of action, antinociception and clinical applications. *Toxicology.* 2013;306:124–146.

Yeargin-Allsopp M, Van Naarden Braun K, Doernberg NS, et al. Prevalence of cerebral palsy in 8-year-old children in three areas of the United States in 2002: a multisite collaboration. *Pediatrics.* 2008, March;121(3):547–554.

52 SUBSTANCE ABUSE

Matthew A. Ruehle, BA
Steven D. Passik, PhD
Kenneth L. Kirsh, PhD

INTRODUCTION

- The United States is facing two distinct, though interrelated public health crises—chronic pain and drug abuse.
- Illicit drug use and use of nonprescribed medications are steadily increasing in the United States.
- Treatment with opioids needs to be risk-stratified, with delivery tailored based on individual risk—one size does not fit all.
- Responsible management of pain and potential substance abuse requires a diverse set of measures and approaches, including (but not limited to): risk assessments, treatment agreements, urine drug tests, prescription monitoring programs, and referral to addiction specialists. No one facet of care is sufficient or complete; they must be used with one another.
- In diverse patient populations with chronic pain issues, a history of drug abuse presents a constellation

of stigmatizing psychosocial issues that can complicate the management of the underlying disease and undermine therapy.

- The interface between the therapeutic use of potentially abusable drugs and the abuse of these drugs is complex and must be understood to optimize pain management.
- Nonopioid options should be exhausted before opioid trials begin with most patients who have a history of substance abuse and those at high risk for substance abuse.
- Past drug abuse and other risk factors are more important when assessing risk than simply exposure to a drug of abuse.
- Chronic pain patients can be adequately and successfully treated only when addiction problems are noted by staff, and these patients' special needs are addressed.

RISK ASSESSMENT AND STRATIFICATION

- Risk assessment should be ongoing throughout patient care, not just an initial screening.
- Expectations should be clearly written in a treatment agreement that the patient signs.
- Use a standardized risk assessment (ORT, SOAPP, etc.) to help evaluate an individual patient's level of risk for medication abuse.
- Obtain personal history of drug abuse or misuse.
- Utilize laboratory urine drug testing (UDT) to verify patient medication use and test for nonprescribed medications and illicit substances.
- Consult local Prescription Monitoring Program (PMP) to detect possible "doctor shopping."

DEFINITION OF ADDICTION IN CHRONIC PAIN

- Definitions of addiction that include phenomena related to physical dependence or tolerance cannot be the model terminology for medically ill populations who receive potentially abusable drugs for legitimate medical purposes.
- A more appropriate definition of addiction notes that it is a chronic disorder characterized by "the compulsive use of a substance resulting in physical, psychological or social harm to the user, and continued use despite that harm."
- Any appropriate definition of addiction must include the concepts of loss of control over drug use, compulsive drug use, and continued use despite known harm.

TABLE 52-1 Differential Diagnosis of Aberrant Drug-Taking Attitudes and Behavior

Addiction
Pseudoaddiction (inadequate analgesic)
Other psychiatric diagnoses
Encephalopathy
Borderline personality disorder
Depression
Anxiety
Criminal intent

- The concept of "aberrant drug-related behavior" is a useful component of definitions of abuse and addiction and recognizes the broad range of behavior that may be considered problematic by prescribers.
- If drug-taking behavior in a medical patient can be characterized as aberrant, a "differential diagnosis" for this behavior can be explored (see Table 52-1).

PSYCHIATRIC COMPLICATIONS

- Impulsive drug use may indicate the existence of another psychiatric disorder, diagnosis of which may have therapeutic implications.
- Patients with a borderline personality disorder can express fear and rage through aberrant drug-taking and may behave impulsively and self-destructively during pain therapy. One of the more worrisome aberrant drug-related behaviors, forging a prescription for a controlled substance, can be an impulsive expression of fear of abandonment and may have little to do with true substance abuse in a borderline patient.
- Patients who self-medicate for anxiety, panic, depression, or even periodic dysphoria and loneliness can present with aberrant drug-taking behaviors.
- Careful diagnosis and treatment of psychiatric problems can at times obviate the need for such self-medication with opioids.

DETERMINING ABERRANCY OF BEHAVIOR

- In assessing the differential diagnosis for drug-related behavior, it is useful to consider the degree of aberrancy (see Table 52-2).
- The less aberrant behaviors (eg, aggressively complaining about the need for medications) are more likely to reflect untreated distress of some type, rather than addiction-related concerns.
- Highly aberrant behaviors (such as injection of an oral formulation) are more likely to reflect true addiction.

TABLE 52-2   Examples of Behaviors Indicative of Aberrancy at Both Ends of the Continuum

BEHAVIORS *LESS* INDICATIVE OF ABERRANCY	BEHAVIORS *MORE* INDICATIVE OF ABERRANCY
Drug hoarding during periods of reduced symptoms	Prescription forgery
Acquisition of similar drugs from other medical sources	Concurrent abuse of related illicit drugs
Aggressive complaining about the need for higher doses	Recurrent prescription losses
Unapproved use of the drug to treat another symptom	Selling prescription drugs
Unsanctioned dose escalation one or two times	Multiple unsanctioned dose escalations
Reporting psychic effects not intended by the clinician	Stealing or borrowing another patient's drugs
Requesting specific drugs	Obtaining prescription drugs from nonmedical sources

Although empirical studies are needed to validate this conceptualization, it may be a useful model when evaluating aberrant behavior.

NEED FOR A TAILORED APPROACH

- The differential between patients with no history of substance abuse and those who have a prior history of addiction has created a need for tailoring appropriate opioid management to the individual patient.
- Weigh both the patient's pain syndrome and risk of abuse when selecting a medication
- Considering both the type of medication, and the patient's personal risk level, tailor individual care to an appropriate level of monitoring. Suggestions on how to tailor care based on an individual's risk are given in Table 52-3.

ASSESSMENT: THE 4 As APPROACH

- The 4 As (Analgesia, Activities of daily living, Adverse events, and Aberrant drug-taking behaviors) are the clinical domains that need to be monitored during opioid-prescribing (see Table 52-4).

TABLE 52-3   Aspects of Patient Care to Tailor Approaches to Individual Risk

Risk level of medication prescribed
Strictness of treatment agreement
Amount of medication per prescription
Frequency of urine drug testing
Recommendation of pain-related psychotherapy and/or addiction assessment
Frequency of PMP consultation
Availability of medication "rescues"

TABLE 52-4   The 4 As of Outcome of Pain Management

OUTCOME AREA	EXPLANATION
Analgesia	This refers to the actual amount of relief experienced by the chosen opioid therapy.
	The most obvious A, but it should not be considered the only important part of opioid therapy.
Activities of daily living	This refers to whether or not the patient on opioid therapy has become more active as a result of opioid therapy.
	The domains of interest include physical, social, emotional, and family-functioning as well as improved sleep.
Adverse side effects	This refers to finding out whether or not the opioid therapy chosen has intolerable side effects for the patient.
	Typical adverse effects to screen for include constipation, nausea, sedation, and mental clouding.
Aberrant drug-related behaviors	This may be better referred to as "ambiguous noncompliance behaviors."
	In essence, this refers to whether or not the patient is engaging in socially undesirable behaviors with the opioid therapy that may or may not be indicative of addiction.
	Problem behaviors include self-escalating dose, hoarding medications, seeking out multiple providers for prescriptions, prescription forgery, and stealing prescription drugs.

Analgesia

- Improvement in pain control needs to be documented when prescribing opioid therapy.
- However, analgesia is not necessarily the most important outcome of pain management.
- An alternate view is how much relief it takes for patients to feel that their life is meaningfully changed so they can work toward the attainment of their goals.

Activities of Daily Living

- "Activities of daily living" refers to quality-of-life and function.
- Patients must understand that they must comply with all their recommended treatment options to improve their chances of returning to work, avocations, and social activities.

Adverse Events

- Patients must also be made aware of the adverse side effects inherent in the treatment of their pain condition with opioids and other medications.
- Side effects must be aggressively managed so that they do not overshadow the potential benefits of drug therapy.
- The most common side effects of opioid analgesics include constipation, sedation, nausea and vomiting,

dry mouth, respiratory depression, confusion, urinary retention, and itching.

Aberrant Drug-taking Behavior

- Patients must be educated through consent forms or contracts, or other means, about the parameters of acceptable drug taking.
- Even overall good outcome in every other domain might not constitute satisfactory treatment if the patient is not compliant with the contract in worrisome ways.
- Dispensing pain medicine in a highly structured fashion may become necessary for some patients who are in violation or constantly on the fringes of appropriate drug-taking.

Utilizing Risk Stratification in Practice

- Good opioid pain treatment in any patient follows two key rules:
  - The clinician must maintain an open and thoughtful attitude toward self-reports of pain.
  - The decision to use an opioid must be followed by skill in titration that focuses on balancing analgesia and side effects.
- Connecting with the patient and forming a therapeutic bond can often improve the reliability of self-report if trust can be maintained by both parties.
- Pain reports should be followed by nonjudgmental, interested, and concerned assessment that both recognizes them as a cry of distress and helps the patient articulate what she or he most needs help with.
- Titration should be aimed at and continued until effect or toxicity, bearing in mind that many patients may become tolerant and/or require very large doses of opioids for pain control. Recognition of the limited data on high dose-opiate therapy supports a cautious attitude.

URINE DRUG TESTING (UDT)

- UDT can be very useful for diagnosing potential abuse and for monitoring patients with a history of abuse.
- Use UDT to monitor adherence to medication plan; specifically to ensure that the patient is taking medications as prescribed, not taking nonprescribed controlled substances, and not using illicit drugs.
- In-office immunoassay testing can be useful for immediate results, but the high cut-off concentrations, cross-relativity, inability to identify individual medications and/or metabolites, and in some cases susceptibility to adulteration necessitate the use of laboratory testing.
- Quantitative laboratory testing can be used to identify specific medication types and to avoid potential false-positive or false-negative results seen with much less accurate immunoassay tests.
- Liquid chromatography, tandem mass spectrometry (LC/MS/MS) or gas chromatography, and mass spectrometry (GC/MS) are the preferred methods of quantitative testing.
- Specimen validity testing (SVT) should be ordered as medically necessary for patients in whom the possibility of adulteration, dilution, or substitution of the specimen is a concern. SVT is a clinically important constellation of tests (pH, specific gravity, creatinine) used to monitor the patient's adherence to the procedures, intent, and spirit of UDT collection, used by clinicians to assess not only the results of the specific UDT but also adherence to substance abuse treatments, parameters of the pain agreement, and the maintenance of sobriety. These tests constitute a check on behavior crucial to patients with an external locus of control (highly prevalent personality traits in those with pain and addiction). Clinicians can educate patients in advance about SVT so that they know that feedback is provided on these behaviors thus helping them reconsider engaging in them and recognizing their consequences. In the end, the term "specimen validity testing" will probably give way to new terminology that better captures these important clinical and behavioral issues and will be recognized as a misnomer.

PRESCRIPTION MONITORING PROGRAMS (PMPs)

- PMPs are designed to allow physicians to assess if patients are receiving prescriptions from multiple physicians, called "doctor shopping," which is a strong indication of abuse and/or diversion.
- There are currently 47 states with active PMPs. Each state has unique regulations, be sure to check the regulations in the state where you practice. Keep in mind that some states require PMP consultation before any prescription is written.
- PMPs are updated in almost real-time, which will allow physicians to identify potential doctor shopping quickly and efficiently.
- It is estimated that 3%–5% of schedule II prescriptions could be due to "doctor shopping," which represents thousands of prescriptions per year.

PATIENT MANAGEMENT

- A written contract between the treatment team and the patient helps provide structure for the treatment plan, establishes clear expectations of the roles played by both parties, and outlines the consequences of aberrant drug taking.

- The inclusion of scheduled and random urine drug tests in the contract can be useful in maximizing treatment compliance. Expectations regarding attendance of clinic visits and management of the supply of medications should also be stated.
- The amount of drug dispensed per prescription should be limited and refills made contingent on clinic attendance.
- Family members and friends should be involved in the treatment to help bolster social support and functioning. Becoming familiar with the family may help the treatment team identify family members who are drug abusers and who may potentially divert the patient's medications.

OPTIMIZING DRUG THERAPY FOR SUBSTANCE ABUSERS WITH PAIN

- For known substance abusers, nonopioid options should be exhausted before opioid trials begin with most patients with a history of substance abuse and those at high risk for substance abuse
- Optimal drug therapy for substance abusers with pain first employs the basic principles of good pain treatment with consideration of the unique pharmacologic needs of addicts and then adds the psychosocial, recovery, and additional structures necessary to attempt to maximize the likelihood of a good outcome (see Figure 52-1).
- Substance abusers are complex patients with two distinct diseases. Treatment of one with the assumption that it is most important and will "take care" of the other is a common mistake that results in additional suffering for the patient from either or both illnesses.
- Drug addicts are often alexithymic (many are unable to describe distress as other than "good" or "bad"), and this trait often leads to global distress in the face of negative emotions associated with pain and chronic illness.
- Drug selection in such patients is often limited to sustained-release delivery to avoid feeding into compulsive pill popping and/or use of opioids in the service of chemical coping.
- Use of a drug with a relatively low street value is recommended for patients who are battling for recovery but maintain unavoidable contact with the addiction subculture.
- Substance abusers often need structure, psychiatric input, and drug treatments that decentralize pain medication from their coping

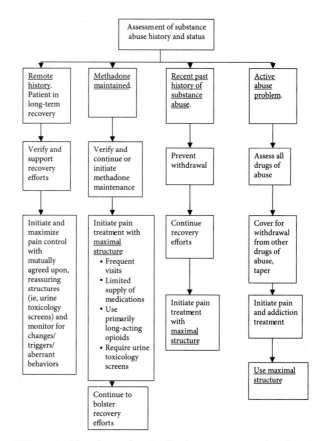

FIG. 52-1. Flowchart of optimal pain management for chronic pain patients with substance abuse issues.

INPATIENT MANAGEMENT

- Inpatient management of patients with active substance abuse problems includes and expands on the guidelines for outpatient settings.
- First, the patient's drug use should be discussed openly and the patient reassured that steps will be taken to avoid adverse events, such as drug withdrawal.
- In certain situations, such as for preoperative patients, patients should be admitted several days in advance when possible for stabilization of the drug regimen.
- It is important to provide the patient with a private room near the nurses' station to aid in monitoring the patient and to discourage attempts to leave the hospital for the purchase of illicit drugs.
- Visitors should be required to check in with nursing staff prior to visitation.
- Daily urine specimens should be collected for random toxicology analysis, and pain and symptom management frequently reassessed.
- Open and honest communication between the clinician and the patient reassures the patient that these guidelines were established in his or her best interest.

PATIENTS IN RECOVERY

- Pain management with patients in recovery presents a unique challenge.
- Due to fear of ostracism from some programs (eg, Alcoholics Anonymous), some patients may be leery of taking opioids. Thus, the first choice should be to explore nonopioid therapies with these patients, which may require referral to a pain center.
- Alternative therapies may include the use of nonopioid or adjuvant analgesics, cognitive therapies, electrical stimulation, neural blockade, or acupuncture.
- If opioids are prescribed, it is necessary to structure opioid use with opioid management contracts, random urine toxicology screens, and occasional pill counts. If possible, attempts should be made to include the patient's recovery program sponsor to garner his or her cooperation and aid in successful monitoring of the condition.
- Requiring the patient to document attendance at a 12-step program should be considered as a condition for ongoing prescribing.

BIBLIOGRAPHY

Bruera E, Moyano J, Seifert L, et al. The frequency of alcoholism among patients with pain due to terminal cancer. *J Pain Symptom Manage.* 1995;10:599.

Bruera E, Moyano J, Seifert L, et al. The frequency of alcoholism among patients with pain due to terminal cancer. *J Pain Symptom Manage.* 1995;10:599.

Handelsman L, Stein JA, Bernstein DP, et al. A latent variable analysis of coexisting emotional deficits in substance abusers: Alexithymia, hostility, and PTSD. *Addict Behav.* 2000;25:423.

Hay J, Passik SD. The cancer patient with borderline personality disorder: suggestions for symptom-focused management in the medical setting. *Psychooncology.* 2000;9:91.

Heit HA, Gourlay DL. Urine drug testing in pain medicine. *J Pain Symptom Manage.* 2004; 27:260.

Manchikanti L, Singh A. Therapeutic Opioids: a ten-year perspective on the complexities and complications of the escalating use, abuse, and nonmedical use of opioids. *Pain Physician.* 2008; 11:63.

Parrino M. *State Methadone Treatment Guidelines.* Washington, DC. TIPS 1 DHHS publication (SMA) 93–1991.

Passik SD, Weinreb HJ. Managing chronic nonmalignant pain: overcoming obstacles to the use of opioids. *Adv Ther.* 2000;17:70.

PMP Alliance. The alliances of states with prescription monitoring programs. Available at: http://www.pmpalliance.org/. Accessed September 26, 2013.

Rinaldi RC, Steindler EM, Wilford BB, et al. Clarification and standardization of substance abuse terminology. *J Am Med Assoc.* 1988;259:555.

53 BIOPSYCHOSOCIAL FACTORS IN PAIN MEDICINE

Martin D. Cheatle, PhD
Rollin M. Gallagher, MD, MPH

INTRODUCTION

- Approximately 30% of the American population suffers from chronic pain and this number continues to rise. Chronic, poorly controlled pain causes individual suffering and contributes to morbidity, mortality, and disability and the economic and societal costs of chronic pain are staggering.
- The 2011 Institute of Medicine (IOM) report "Relieving Pain in America: A Blueprint for Transforming Prevention, Care, Education, and Research" estimated the annual cost of chronic pain in the United States to be $560 to over $600 billion, including health care costs ($261–300 billion) and lost productivity ($297–336 billion).
- The IOM report outlined guiding principles to improve pain care, including effective pain management is a "moral imperative"; pain should be considered a disease with distinct pathology; there is a need for interdisciplinary treatment approaches; there is a need for pain education and training in all disciplines and training in interdisciplinary pain management; and there is a need for research to develop new and more effective treatments.
- Patients with chronic pain are complex and commonly have multiple medical and psychological comorbidities, including depression and anxiety. This requires a comprehensive assessment and interdisciplinary disciplinary treatment.
- A strictly biomedical approach is frequently ineffective, as psychosocial factors and neurobehavioral mechanisms play a significant role in the manifestation and maintenance of chronic pain as well as in the transition of acute to chronic pain. There is persuasive scientific and clinical evidence regarding the strong relationship between the pain experience and mood states.
- This chapter will provide an overview of the relationship between pain and common comorbid major psychiatric disorders, the assessment of these disorders in the pain population, and pharmacologic and psychological treatment strategies.

PAIN AND DEPRESSION

- Depression commonly co-occurs in patients with chronic pain. There have been a number of studies that demonstrated a strong association between depression and pain, revealing that patients with pain are more likely to be depressed than patients without pain.

- The prevalence of depression in chronic pain varies depending on the population site sampled. Bair et al. discovered based on a Medline database search that the rate of depression in pain patients ranged from 85% in dental clinics specializing in chronic facial pain to 52% in pain clinics, 27% in primary care clinics, and 18% in population-based settings. Another study surveyed a community sample and found that the prevalence of pain was 21.9%, with 35% of these pain sufferers acknowledging that they experienced concomitant depression.
- Several explanatory models have been postulated regarding the relationship between pain and depression, including that pain is a symptom of untreated depression and that the stress of coping with chronic pain and related physical and psychosocial functional impairments and disability causes or contributes to the development of depression, with persuasive evidence supporting the latter hypothesis. For example, the presence of any physical symptom increased the likelihood of a diagnosis of a mood or anxiety disorder in a sample of primary care patients by as much as threefold.
- Phenomenologically, depression plays an important role in the experience of chronic pain and is one factor along with somatization that is implicated in the process of transition from acute to chronic low back pain.
- Depressed pain patients tend to report higher levels of pain, greater disability, and pain related-interference and display more pain behavior than the nondepressed patients with pain.
- The impact of mood on pain and functionality appears independent of health care access. A prospective study involving 228 well insured, elderly residents of a retirement community who underwent semiannual evaluations of pain, depression, physical impairment, and health care utilization revealed that:
  - Pain and depression were commonly comorbid.
  - Increasing depression was associated with increasing pain-related impairment.
  - Even mild, subclinical depression can increase health care utilization.
- In summary, mood disorders are highly prevalent in the chronic pain population. Underdiagnosing and undertreating of co-occurring mood disorders can complicate recovery and contribute to poor quality of life.

MANAGING DEPRESSION IN PAIN PATIENTS

SCREENING FOR DEPRESSION

- Since the risk of developing depression is high in patients with chronic pain, clinicians should routinely screen for depression during treatment, especially if there is a significant change in pain intensity, functionality, or disability or an additional life stressor occurs such as loss of work or family roles, relationship issues, etc.
- There are a number of validated self-report screening tools for depression. The Beck Depression Inventory and the Profile of Mood States are two measures of depression that have been recommended by an expert consensus group on measuring emotional functioning in chronic pain.
- Other validated measures include:
  - Beck Depression Inventory-Fast Screen for Medical Patients
  - Zung Self-Rating Depression Scale
  - Center for Epidemiologic Studies Depression Scale
  - Patient Health Questionnaire (PHQ-9, PHQ-2).
- In choosing a depression-screening tool, consider brevity and ease of interpretation, particularly in a busy clinic setting.

DIAGNOSING A DEPRESSIVE DISORDER

- Patients with chronic pain may underreport symptoms of depression as they may be fearful that their pain will not be taken seriously or they are embarrassed by having to acknowledge a psychological disorder.
- The clinician may want to reduce a response bias by first exploring during the routine review of symptoms if they are experiencing any symptoms of depression such as sleep disturbance, suppressed libido, depressed mood, loss of interest or pleasure (anhedonia), low energy (anergia), change in appetite, and/or having pain in multiple sites.
- Additional history gathering should solicit information on:
  - Co-occurring medical disorders
  - Past psychiatric disorder
  - Family history of psychiatric disorders
  - Treatments for psychiatric disorders and response to treatment
  - History of marital/relationship discord (martial/relationship satisfaction and significant others response to patients pain are related to depressive symptoms)
  - General health condition
  - Substance use disorders—past and current
  - Health habits (cigarette use, caffeine consumption, exercise)
  - Psychological development, coping skills, and response to previous stressful life events
  - Mental status
  - Selective physical and laboratory examination as indicated.

- If a depressive disorder is present, differential diagnoses include major depressive disorder (single episode or recurrent), persistent depressive disorder (dysthymia), substance or medication-induced depressive disorder, or depressive disorder due to another medical condition.

EVALUATING PATIENT SAFETY: SUICIDE AND VIOLENCE

Suicidal Ideation and Chronic Pain

- Suicidal ideation and behavior are quite prevalent in the pain population and since pain and depression have several shared features, the presence of pain may obscure the detection and treatment of depression, placing these already vulnerable patients at increased risk for suicide.
- Tang and Crane completed a systematic review of the pain and suicide literature, which revealed that the risk of successful suicide doubled in the chronic pain population as compared to nonpain controls and that one of the main risk factors was comorbid depression. Other risk factors included family history of suicide, previous suicide attempt, female gender, and pain severity.
- The issue of pain, depression, and suicide is particularly relevant in the military veteran population where pain, depression, and posttraumatic stress are common, particularly in Veterans exposed to combat, and a recent study found that military veterans are twice as likely to commit suicide as nonveterans.
- The assessment of suicide risk should consider:
  - Presence of suicidal ideation
  - If the patient has a plan for committing suicide and whether the plans are vague or specific
  - The means to carry out a plan (such as a lethal amount of prescribed medications) or a gun
  - Previous history of plans or attempts
  - Lack of support from family
  - Coping abilities.
- Clinics should develop an action plan if a patient is identified as being suicidal. This plan should include contact numbers of local emergency departments and mental health crisis centers.
- A properly trained professional to assess risk and arrange appropriate management should evaluate all patients identified as suicidal.

Violence and Chronic Pain

- Pain clinicians should be aware that individuals with chronic pain who are engaged in active treatment have higher rates of violent ideation than do samples of community controls, and that the presence of depression increases risk.
- Other risk factors for violent ideation include job dissatisfaction, unemployment, workers' compensation, work rehabilitation programs, litigation, and when physicians diagnose or imply malingering.
- If opioids are being reduced or discontinued especially as a result of aberrant drug-related behavior the clinician should be cognizant of escalating agitation.
- At initial evaluation and when there is a treatment setback, the physician should ask the patients if they are experiencing angry outbursts or angry thoughts and, if so, whether they can control these events.
- As in the case of suicidal ideation, there should be an action plan to deal with patients who become agitated or threatening to the clinician or staff members.

PHARMACOLOGIC MANAGEMENT OF DEPRESSION

- Commonly prescribed antidepressants are classified in Table 53-1.
- Although no single drug is most effective in depression, dual-action antidepressants with noradrenergic and serotonergic reuptake inhibition may provide the most effective treatment and may also be effective for neuropathic pain.
- More than 80% of depressed patients respond to at least one medication, although individual antidepressants are effective in only 50%–60% of patients. Thus, when one does not work, a switch should be made to another with a different profile (eg, if an SSRI, try buproprion or an SNRI), or combination therapy (eg, SSRI with buproprion).
- Factors to consider in selecting an antidepressant include prior response, family history of a response, anticipated side effects, efficacy, remission rates, dosing simplicity (promotes adherence), adherence, and cost (if a patient cannot afford his or her expensive prescription antidepressant, the patient is likely to discontinue the drug).
- Anxiety and insomnia do not necessarily predict a better response to medications that have an enhanced sedative effect.
- The patient should be followed closely for a response to pharmaceuticals and the dose titrated upward if the patient does not respond in several weeks.
- The patient's attitude toward antidepressants should be assessed, as many patients may feel stigmatized by being prescribed an antidepressant.
- The clinician should confirm if the patient is in fact taking the medication.
- Educating patients and their families (if possible) about the benefits of the drug and the risk of relapse helps promote adherence.

TABLE 53-1   Medications for Depression

Tricyclics and Tetracyclics
Tertiary amine tricyclics
    Amitriptyline
    Clomipramine*
    Doxepine
    Imipramine
    Trimipramine
Secondary amine tricyclics
    Desipramine
    Nortriptyline
    Protriptyline
Tetracyclics
    Amoxapine
    Maprotiline
Selective Serotonin Reuptake Inhibitors (SSRIs)
    Citalopram
    Escitalopram
    Fluoxetine
    Fluvoxamine*
    Paroxetine
Dopamine–Norepinephrine Reuptake Inhibitors
    Bupropion
Serotonin–Norepinephrine Reuptake Inhibitors (SNRIs)
    Venlafaxine
    Duloxetine†
Serotonin Modulators
    Nefazodone
    Trazadone
Norepinephrine–Serotonin Modulator
    mirtazapine
Monoamine Oxidase Inhibitors (MAOIs)
Irreversible, nonselective
    Isocarboxazide
    Phenelzine
    Tranylcypromine
Reversible MAOI-A
    Moclobemide*
Selective Noradrenaline
Reuptake Inhibitor
    Reboxetine†

*Approved for treatment of obsessive–compulsive disorder (OCD) only.
†Not available in the United States.

ANTIDEPRESSANTS AS ANALGESICS

- Antidepressants have been an important component of an effective pharmacotherapy regimen for treating pain.
- Certain antidepressants reduce pain by a variety of mechanisms but mostly by enhancing the descending inhibitory pathways by increasing the availability of serotonin and norepinephrine in the synaptic cleft.
- There is persuasive evidence that tricyclic antidepressants are effective in reducing pain in low back pain, neuropathic pain disorders, headaches, and fibromyalgia.
- Serotonin-Norepinephrine reuptake inhibitors have been demonstrated to reduce pain in several painful conditions, including diabetic neuropathy and other neuropathies, chronic low back pain, and fibromyalgia and may reduce the frequency and severity of migraines.
- Selective serotonin reuptake inhibitors are less effective in providing analgesia but are better tolerated than tricyclic antidepressants (TCAs).
- In addition to any analgesic effect from antidepressants, pain perception can be altered by the beneficial effects of antidepressants on mood and sleep.

Tricyclic and Tetracyclic Antidepressants

- When prescribing TCAs, *the potential for a lethal overdose* and *the possibility of inducing a manic episode* in patients with or without history of mania must always be considered.
- Data from a number of controlled trials indicate that TCAs are effective analgesics.
- Amitriptyline is the most thoroughly studied, although desipramine, imipramine, clomipramine, nortriptyline, and doxepin have also been well studied.
- TCAs may also be efficacious as preemptive analgesia and for potentiating opioids for the treatment of post-operative pain.
- Evidence of the pain-relieving efficacy of the tetracyclics maprotiline and amoxapine is limited. Maprotiline is more effective than paroxetine but is not superior to TCAs.
- Given that all TCAs and tetracyclic antidepressants are equally effective in treating depression and that most TCAs are efficacious in pain disorders, the choice of antidepressant is often influenced by the side-effect profile:
  - Anticholinergic effects are common, though patients may develop tolerance, and include dry mouth, constipation, blurred vision, and urinary retention. Amitriptyline, imipramine, trimipramine, and doxepin are the most anticholinergic drugs; amoxapine, maprotiline, and nortriptyline are less anticholinergic; and desipramine is the least anticholinergic. Most experienced pain clinicians prescribe desipramine or nortriptyline because of their lower side-effect profile, the latter in lower doses (starting at 10–25 mg HS) because of its increased potency.
  - Sedation may be a welcome side effect in patients with sleep disturbances. Amitriptyline, doxepin, and trimipramine are most sedating; desipramine and protriptyline are the least sedating.
  - Autonomic effects due to α_1-adrenergic blockade result in orthostatic hypotension and are least to most likely to occur with amitriptyline, doxepine, clomipramine, amoxapine, and nortriptyline, in that order.
  - Cardiac effects, including tachycardia, prolonged QT intervals, and depressed ST segments on ECGs,

contraindicate TCAs and tetracyclics in patients with prolonged conduction times. In patients with a history of cardiac disease, these drugs should be initiated at low doses, with gradual increase and monitoring of cardiac function.

- The side effect burden and risk of untoward reaction with TCAs increases with patient age, and they should be used with caution in patients over the age of 50.
- Newer antidepressants (SSRIs, SNRIs) are generally less toxic in cases of overdose, but do not reduce the overall risk of suicide.

Selective Serotonin Reuptake Inhibitors

- Since fluoxetine was introduced in 1988, the SSRIs fluoxetine, fluvoxamine, sertraline, paroxetine, and citalopram have captured more than 50% of the US prescription antidepressant market owing to their favorable side-effect profile.
- Because of good efficacy rates and dosing simplicity, many patients with pain and depression receive SSRIs as initial treatment.
- Although the newer SSRIs can cost more than TCAs, the total cost of treatment is usually similar for patients who start with SSRIs and those who begin with TCAs but cannot tolerate them and must make additional office visits to switch to SSRIs.
- Although the antidepressant effects of SSRIs are not superior to those of TCAs and MAOIs, the more favorable side-effect profile and overdose safety of SSRIs often make them the first-choice treatment of depression.
- The SSRIs differ primarily in their half-lives. At two to three days, fluoxetine has the longest, and its active metabolite has a half-life of seven to nine days. The half-lives of other SSRIs are approximately 20 hours.
- Because all SSRIs are metabolized in the liver by the cytochrome P450 isoenzyme, clinicians should be careful about drug interactions. Citalopram is least affected by cytochrome P isoenzymes.
- The most common side effects of SSRIs include agitation, anxiety, sleep disturbance, tremor, sexual dysfunction, and headache.
- Citalopram (Celexa) has been reported to have a lesser rate of sexual side effects than other SSRIs.
- A novel multimodal antidepressant vortioxetine was recently approved for use in major depression. It is a variant of the older SSRIs and is theoretically a serotonin modulator and stimulator and also seems to have less sexual side effects.
- Rarely have SSRIs been associated with extrapyramidal-like symptoms, arthralgias, lymphandenopathy, inappropriate antidiuretic syndrome, agranulocytosis, and hypoglycemia.

- The interaction of SSRIs with MAOIs, other antidepressants, or higher doses of the analgesic tramadol causes the central serotonin syndrome manifested by abdominal pain, diarrhea, sweating, fever, tachycardia, elevated mood, hypertension, altered mental state, delirium, myoclonus, increased motor activity, irritability, and hostility. Severe manifestation of this syndrome can include hyperemia, cardiovascular shock, and death.
- SSRIs have no α-adrenergic antagonistic effect and are essentially devoid of the Type 1A antiarrhythmic effect of tricyclics; therefore, SSRIs rarely are associated with orthostatic hypotension.

Analgesic Effects of SSRIs

- A recent review of the literature revealed that five studies compared SSRIs to placebo in treatment of neuropathically mediated pain and that SSRIs were more effective in relieving pain than placebo. Fluoxetine was superior to citalopram and paroxetine in reducing fibromyalgia pain but there was no evidence to support the use of SSRIs in low back pain, pain from rheumatoid arthritis, osteoarthritis, or migraines.
- Studies comparing SSRIs with TCAs obtained consistently superior analgesia with TCAs.
- In 2000, Sindrup and Jensen identified all placebo-controlled drug trials involving treatment of pain in polyneuropathy and determined that the number of patients needed to treat to obtain one patient with more than 50% pain relief was 2.6 for tricyclics, 6.7 for SSRIs, 2.5 for anticonvulsant sodium channel blockers, 4.1 for gabapentin, and 3.4 for tramadol.

Dopamine–Norepinephrine Reuptake Inhibitors

- Bupropion (Wellbutrin) was synthesized in 1966 and emerged as an antidepressant without anticholinergic or cardiac effects. An increased incidence of drug-induced seizures in bulimic nondepressed subjects in one study, however, delayed its marketing. Subsequent studies of depressed patients did not replicate this finding, and the drug was reintroduced in 1989.
- Bupropion is as effective for depression as other antidepressants but is unique in that it is much less likely to cause sexual dysfunction.
- Because it blocks norepinephrine reuptake, bupropion has the potential for being an analgesic antidepressant, although this remains to be determined conclusively.
- In an open-label study, bupropion significantly reduced pain at eight weeks, and a double-blind, placebo-controlled, crossover trial showed that

150–300 mg bupropion was effective and well tolerated for the treatment of neuropathic pain. Because of its lower incidence of sexual side effects, it is often the preferred choice for a first-line medication for neuropathic pain, particularly when accompanied by depression.

- In approximately 5% of the patients consuming 450–600 mg/d, bupropion causes the adverse effects of delusions, hallucinations, and the risk of seizures because of its potentiating effects on the dopaminergic system.

Serotonin–Norepinephrine Reuptake Inhibitors

- There are several SNRI antidepressants on the market, including venlafaxine, duloxetine, levomilnacipran, and desvenlafaxine.
- The SNRIs venlafaxine and duloxetine block reuptake as effectively as TCAs without causing the undesirable side effects associated with those agents.
- Venlafaxine has a faster-than-usual onset of action and demonstrated efficacy in seriously depressed patients. Venlafaxine is generally well tolerated, and its side effects include nausea (37%), somnolence (23%), dry mouth (22%), and dizziness (22%). The most worrisome adverse effect is increased blood pressure, particularly in patients receiving more than 300 mg/d.
- Venlafaxine has an analgesic effect independent of its antidepressant effect. For example, in healthy volunteers venlafaxine increased the thresholds of pain tolerance to electrical sural nerve stimulation and of pain increase, indicating a potential analgesic effect for clinical neuropathic pain.
- A number of case reports validate venlafaxine's efficacy in pain disorders, but controlled studies are lacking.
- Venlafaxine is as effective as TCAs in reducing the number of migraine episodes and in providing migraine prophylaxis but is better tolerated having less adverse effects.
- The norepinephrine reuptake-inhibiting properties of venlafaxine, particularly at higher doses, along with its structural similarity to tramadol, an analgesic with both opioid agonist and monoaminergic activity, makes it a promising antidepressant for patients with chronic pain. In fact, norepinephrine reuptake inhibition may be crucial for relief of diabetic and postherpetic neuralgia pain.
- Duloxetine, with the same advantages of venlafaxine and an easier dosing schedule, has been approved for treatment of major depressive disorder, generalized anxiety disorder, and several pain disorders, including diabetic neuropathy, fibromyalgia, and chronic low back pain.

Serotonin Modulators

- The structurally related antidepressants trazodone and nefazodone are unrelated to the TCAs, MAOIs, or SSRIs.
- Trazodone has distinctive sedating properties and in lower doses is used to treat insomnia in both pain and depression.
- Nefazodone is an effective antidepressant. Its half-life of 2–4 hours calls for twice-daily doses. The sale of nefazodone under its original trade name, Serzone, was discontinued in the United States and Canada due to rare cases of hepatotoxicity, liver failure, and even death, but generic formulations are still available in the United States.
- No studies in humans have examined the analgesic effects of nefazodone, but in animal studies it produced an analgesic effect at the Mu1 and Mu2 receptors.
- The notable adverse reactions of nefazodone include hepatotoxicity, a drop in blood pressure, and drug interactions with triazolam (Halcion), alprazolam (Xanax), terfenadine/pseudoephedrine (Seldane), astemizole (Hismanal), and cisapride (Propulsid) due to its inhibition of cytochrome P450.

Norepinephrine–Serotonin Modulator

- The antidepressant mirtazapine (Remeron) antagonizes the central presynaptic α_2-adrenergic receptors, resulting in a potentiation of central noradrenergic and serotonergic transmission.
- Mirtazapine is an effective antidepressant, yet it lacks the anticholinergic effects of the TCAs and the anxiogenic effects of some SSRIs.
- Because of its broad neurotransmitter profile, mirtazapine has the potential to be an analgesic antidepressant, but this requires more investigation.
- Mirtazapine causes somnolence and is often used for treating insomnia, which is quite common in depressed individuals and pain patients but could be an adverse effect for some patients.
- Other adverse effects associated with mirtazapine include increased appetite with weight gain, which may be welcome in cancer but less so in patients with joint pain; increased serum cholesterol; and (among 0.3% of patients) agranulocytosis and neutropenia.

Monoamine Oxidase Inhibitors

- There are a number of FDA-approved MAOIs, including phenelzine (Nardil), tranylcypromine (Parnate), isocarboxazid (Marplan), and selegiline (Emsam), which is also available as a transdermal patch.
- MAOIs' mechanism of action is to inhibit the enzyme monoamine oxidase, which increases the availability of serotonin, norepinephrine, and dopamine.

- MAOIs may be effective for panic disorder with agoraphobia, posttraumatic stress disorder (PTSD), eating disorders, social phobia, and atypical depression characterized by hypersomnia, hyperphagia, anxiety, and the absence of vegetative symptoms; however, these medications are generally not used because of their potential toxicity (see below).
- MAOIs are typically prescribed only when the patient has been refractory to all other classes of antidepressants.
- Animal studies supporting the analgesic effects of MAOIs have not been replicated in pain patients.
- The side effects of MAOIs and the potential for precipitating a toxic central serotonin syndrome when combined with other medications and certain foods limit their use to treatment-resistant depression.
- A tyramine-induced hypertensive crisis in patients taking MAOIs can be life-threatening. Other side effects include orthostatic hypertension, weight gain, edema, sexual dysfunction, and insomnia.

Anticonvulsants

- Anticonvulsants have been used in pain management since the 1960s, very soon after they revolutionized the medical management of epilepsy.
- Anticonvulsants have an established role in the treatment of chronic neuropathic pain, especially when patients complain of shooting sensations or when the pain is lancinating or burning.
- The precise mechanism of action of anticonvulsants remains uncertain, but they may enhance γ-aminobutyric acid inhibition, voltage-gated calcium channel blockers, or sodium channel blockers.
- Gabapentin, topiramate, pregabalin, and lamotrigine all have efficacy in one or more neuropathic pain conditions. Older anticonvulsants, such as phenytoin, clonazepam (a benzodiazepine), and valproic acid, have not shown efficacy for pain in clinical studies and, because of their problematic toxicity, are generally not used, with the exception of carbamazepine, which is effective in trigeminal neuralgia.
- Many anticonvulsants have mood-stabilizing properties, but no controlled study supports the utility of mood-stabilizing agents as therapy in depression.
- The anticonvulsants lamotrigine and gabapentin may have antimanic and antidepressant activity.
- Gabapentin and pregabalin seem to be safe and well tolerated and have a favorable side effect profile, virtual absence of drug interactions although pregabalin produces equal efficacy in neuropathic pain disorders but at a lower dose and an easier dosing schedule.
- Lamotrigine requires careful dosing and close monitoring because it can cause a potentially severe skin rash. Many clinicians appear to be adding lamotrigine to the treatment regimens of bipolar patients with complex, treatment-resistant forms of illness and there is evidence that lamotrigine is more effective in preventing depressive relapse but less so on mania.
- A double-blind study found lamotrigine (50 or 200 mg/d) effective in treating depression in patients with bipolar disorder, and a placebo-controlled study found it effective and safe in relieving the pain associated with diabetic neuropathy.

PSYCHOTHERAPEUTIC TECHNIQUES

- The successful treatment of complex chronic pain patients relies upon a multidimensional, biopsychosocial approach employing rational psychopharmacologic treatment of the psychiatric comorbidities associated with chronic pain in concert with psychotherapeutic interventions targeting both pain coping and mood.
- The psychotherapeutic techniques used in treating chronic pain patients include:
  - Pain education
  - Supportive psychotherapy to strengthen patients' coping strategies
  - Cognitive behavioral therapy (CBT), which focuses on patients' maladaptive cognitions along with behavioral techniques, such as relaxation therapy and assertiveness training
  - Operant Behavioral therapy, based on behavior theory and social learning theory
  - Acceptance and Commitment Therapy (ACT), a form of CBT that focuses on a process of psychological flexibility and is an extension of operant theory
  - Dynamic psychotherapy, where the relationship with the therapist provides the context for the corrective emotional experience
  - Family therapy and couples therapy, which address the fact that chronic pain is not experienced in isolation and can cause disruption in the family and that family members can help either reinforce or extinguish a patient's aberrant, pain-prone behavior
  - Group therapy, which can be educational and/or psychotherapeutic.
- Categorization of these strategies as distinct entities is useful for heuristic purposes only. In clinical practice, psychiatrists/psychotherapists individualize a combination of approaches to match their patients' needs.

Cognitive Behavioral Therapy

- CBT is based on the theory that irrational beliefs, dysfunctional thoughts, and distorted attitudes toward the self, the environment, and the future perpetuate depression. Put simply, beliefs and thoughts affect emotions and lead to behavior/choices. When ones thoughts and beliefs are irrational and dysfunctional, this can lead to anxiety and/or depression, which can lead to poor choices/behavior thus reinforcing the dysfunctional thoughts.

- The process of CBT is to reduce depression by challenging these irrational beliefs and attitudes and replacing them with rational thoughts.
- CBT can guide patients to recognize that emotional responses to life are greatly influenced by their thoughts and that they can exercise control over the disruption produced by an unavoidable life event or chronic illness.
- Clinical studies have demonstrated the efficacy of CBT in treating mild to moderate depression.
- Patients with chronic pain often acquire maladaptive thought patterns (catastrophizing) and behaviors (kinesiophobia) contributing to fear/avoidance, promoting deconditioning, depression, and additional suffering.
- The goal of CBT is to help patients reconceptualize their view of pain and their role in healing and to promote being proactive in their health care rather than reactive and passive.
- The process of CBT is to acquire specific skills (relaxation therapy, cognitive restructuring, effective communication); consolidate and rehearse the new skills, maintain the new behaviors and utilize relapse prevention skills.
- CBT has been found effective in improving mood and function in a variety of pain disorders.
- Several investigators recommend providing CBT early in the course of illness to increase patients' confidence in managing symptoms and in their ability to reduce their health care utilization.

Operant Behavioral Therapy

- Operant behavioral therapy is based on the principles of operant conditioning and uses contingency management or operant conditioning to increase activity, reduce reinforcing pain-related behaviors, and minimizing pain-contingent medication use.

Acceptance and Commitment Therapy

- Acceptance and Commitment Therapy (ACT) is a form of CBT that is a directive and experiential type of therapy based on rational frame theory. The goal of ACT is to experience life mindfully and reinforce psychological flexibility.
- The core processes of ACT include:
  - Contact with the present moment

  - Self-as-context
  - Defusion
  - Acceptance
  - Values
  - Committed action.
- There are five randomized control trials on the use of ACT in chronic pain demonstrating efficacy.

Psychodynamic Psychotherapy

- Psychodynamic psychotherapy includes all psychotherapeutic interventions that share a basis in psychodynamic theories about the cause of psychological vulnerabilities.
- This form of psychotherapy is most often long term and has goals beyond immediate symptom relief and has not been studied extensively in chronic pain.

PAIN, ANXIETY DISORDERS, OCD, AND PTSD

- Anxiety disorders are the most common form of mental illness in the United States. In the pain population, studies have revealed the presence of anxiety disorders ranging from 30% to 60%.
- Severe, acute pain activates stress-related noradrenergic systems in the brain and is often accompanied by cognitive–emotional reactions, such as fear and anxiety, which to some degree are contextually determined. For example, pain in childbirth usually does not evoke fear or anxiety, whereas pain associated with traumatic injury, with uncertain outcome, often does.
- The association of pain, anxiety, and depression may have a common neurochemical substrate in the serotonergic systems. Anxiety disorders, along with depression and substance abuse, are the most common comorbid conditions in patients with chronic pain.
- Patients commonly experience anxiety because of the stress of living with pain, which can include loss of job causing financial problems, change in family roles, and diminished functionality.
- The stress of severe trauma, for example, incurred in battle or a motor vehicle accident, may lead to a driving phobia or PTSD, which can be comorbid with injury-related pain.
- The presence of comorbid obsessive–compulsive disorder (OCD) with chronic pain can make both conditions worse if the patient has to undertake compulsive motoric acts (like cleaning rituals) to control the anxiety associated with the obsession.
- These disorders can complicate a pain disorder both from their central and peripheral effects, and vice versa based on two demonstrated mechanisms. First, the neurotransmitters implicated in panic disorders

and phobic disorders, norepinephrine, serotonin, and γ-aminobutyric acid are implicated in pain modulation. Second, sympathetic arousal activated by stress and anxiety will increase neuronal firing of injured nerves in neuropathic pain.

- Consider also the challenges posed by a chronic pain patient whose pain management and pacing of activities are thwarted by (1) the compulsive cleaning rituals seen in OCD; (2) PTSD from a combat, rape, or motor vehicle accident; or (3) generalized anxiety or panic attacks further complicating disability.

- Other medical conditions can present with anxiety, such as neurologic disorders (cerebral neoplasm, cerebrovascular accident), systemic conditions (hypoxia, hypoglycemia, cardiac arrhythmias, anemia), endocrine disturbances (thyroid, pituitary, parathyroid), and deficiency states (B_{12}, pellagra) must be excluded by physical exam and appropriate laboratory tests, including imaging studies.

- It is also important to rule out anxiety secondary to prescription medication adverse effects, illicit drugs, toxins, and psychoactive substance abuse.

- In DSM-5, anxiety disorders include:
  - Selective mutism
  - Separation anxiety disorder
  - Specific phobias
  - Social anxiety disorder
  - Panic disorder
  - Agoraphobia
  - Generalized anxiety disorder.

- New in DSM-5 OCD is a separate section called Obsessive–Compulsive and related disorders and PTSD is under Trauma and Stressor-related disorders.

OBSESSIVE–COMPULSIVE DISORDER

- An estimated 1%–2% of individuals suffer from OCD. An obsession is a recurrent and intrusive thought, feeling, idea, or sensation, and a compulsion is a conscious, standardized, recurring pattern of behavior. People with this disorder recognize that their reactions to these thoughts and acts are irrational and disproportionate.

- In pain patients with OCD, the challenge is that they tend to view success and failure as all or nothing. A 30% improvement in pain may not be enough as it is not 100% relief. It is important to consistently establish and reiterate the realistic goals of treatment.

- The generally accepted hypothesis is that OCD involves abnormal serotonergic function regulation (although both serotonergic and nonserotonergic antidepressants effectively treat depression, only serotonergic drugs effectively treat OCD).

- Fluoxetine, fluvoxamine, sertraline, and paroxetine are all approved for the treatment of OCD, and high doses may be necessary, such as 80 mg/d fluoxetine. Of the TCAs, clomipramine is the most selective for serotonin reuptake and was the first FDA-approved drug for OCD. It is limited by its typical TCA side-effect profile.

- In OCD, operant behavioral therapy may be as effective as pharmacotherapy and may provide longer-lasting beneficial effects. The principal behavioral approaches in OCD are exposure and response prevention. Desensitization, thought stopping, flooding, and aversive conditioning have also been used.

- The best outcome in OCD occurs in patients provided with both pharmacotherapy and behavior therapy.

POSTTRAUMATIC STRESS DISORDER

- PTSD results when an individual is exposed to a traumatic event which is re-experienced persistently through intrusive thoughts, disturbing dreams of the event, dissociative flashbacks, and intense psychological and or physiological reaction to internal or external cues causing avoidance of stimuli associated with the event and persistent symptoms of increased arousal.

- Prevalence of PTSD in adults is approximately 3.5%. Ten to 20% of patients seen in primary care have PTSD and the cost of medical care is twice that of patients without PTSD.

- Chronic pain is common in patients with PTSD and it has been estimated that up to 30% of patients seen in pain clinics exhibit signs and symptoms of PTSD.

- It has been postulated the PTSD has a direct influence on depression severity, whereas depression has a direct influence on pain.

- Other theories of the mechanisms of pain and PTSD include anxiety sensitivity or a tendency to misinterpret anxiety symptoms as signs of harm causing an amplification of both emotional and physical sensations associated with pain. Additionally, it has been suggested that the comorbidity of pain and PTSD arises out of the overlap of common cognitive, affective, and behavioral symptoms (eg, avoidance, attentional biases, depression, and anxiety).

- The treatment of PTSD requires that clinicians first develop a therapeutic rapport with the patient allowing the patient to feel comfortable to tell their story of trauma.

- Education is important to explain to survivors and their families the nature of PTSD and responses to stress and how hypervigilance associated with PTSD can increase pain.

- Pharmacologically, antidepressants such as amitriptyline, imipramine, and phenelzine may be beneficial in treating chronic PTSD. Also, SSRIs such as fluoxetine and sertraline often act rapidly to modulate affect, memory, and impulses in PTSD, both protecting against their overwhelming intensity and loosening excessive inhibitions.
- Reports of uncontrolled studies with small samples suggest a benefit with paroxetine, citalopram hydrochloride, fluvoxamine, nefazodone hydrochloride, trazodone hydrochloride, bupropion hydrochloride, and mirtazapine.
- Non-SSRI drugs are considered second-line or augmentative treatment, and trazodone has been suggested for managing insomnia in PTSD.
- Prazosin has been proven in clinical trials to relieve the nightmares and sleep disorder associated with PTSD, and is now being used widely for that indication.
- Psychotherapy for PTSD includes exposure-based treatments where patients extinguish their unrealistic fears through repeatedly re-experiencing their traumatic event through imaginal exposure and in vivo to safe situations that typically trigger traumatic recollections.
- Other treatments for PTSD involve cognitive approaches similar to CBT for depressive disorders and other anxiety disorders, EMDR (Eye Movement, Desensitization, and Reprocessing) where patients engage in imaginal exposure to the original trauma while simultaneously performing saccadic eye movements, and Acceptance and Commitment Therapy.

GENERALIZED ANXIETY DISORDER

- Generalized anxiety disorder (GAD) is characterized by excessive worrying even about small issues that is difficult to control and is associated with somatic symptoms, such as muscle tension, irritability, difficulty sleeping, and restlessness.
- FDA–approved agents for the treatment of GAD include the benzodiazepines and buspirone.
- Although well-controlled data are lacking, long-term benzodiazepine use may be associated with tolerance, abuse, and dependence, and use in patients with a known or suspected substance use disorder is contraindicated.
- Buspirone is effective in the treatment of GAD and avoids the disadvantages associated with benzodiazepines, but it has a slower onset of action—typically one to three weeks.
- TCAs, SSRIs, trazodone, and nefazodone have been evaluated in GAD, but data are extremely limited and, in some studies, complicated by the inclusion of patients with major depression.

- Among the newer antidepressants, both venlafaxine extended-release (XR) and duloxetine have been approved for use in GAD.
- Psychotherapeutic interventions for GAD include CBT, operant behavioral therapy, and hypnosis.

ESTABLISHING AND MAINTAINING A THERAPEUTIC ALLIANCE

"The patient, though conscious that his condition is perilous, may recover his health simply through his contentment with the goodness of the physician."

Hippocrates

- Creating a therapeutic alliance with a patient suffering from chronic pain and concomitant psychiatric disorders and, if possible, the patient's family is critical in enhancing adherence to both pharmacologic and nonpharmacologic treatments and maximizing a positive treatment outcome.
- The first step in developing an effective and trusting relationship is to validate that the patient's pain is real and that having to endure pain causes significant suffering.
- The next step is an open discussion about the patient's past treatment experiences and fears and the patient's expectations of treatment response (for example, an antidepressant will completely resolve depressive symptoms).
- Last is patient education about the painful condition, the goals of treatment, the rationale for treatment choices, and the clinician's expectations of the patient's responsibilities for record keeping, adherence, and follow-up.
- Successfully titrating medications to their therapeutic potential requires that the clinician and patient communicate effectively about potential side effects, toxicity, drug interactions, and therapeutic targets. Establishing a therapeutic alliance will also help mitigate the fears and stigma of engaging in psychotherapy.
- Engendering ongoing trust in this relationship is critical when dealing with matters of safety, such as toxicity, suicide, and violence.

EDUCATING THE PATIENT AND THE PATIENT'S FAMILY

- Every patient and, when possible, appropriate family members should receive ongoing education about the relationship between pain and co-occurring psychiatric disorders, frequently reassuring the patient and their families that depression and anxiety are very common in individuals who suffer from chronic pain.

- Uninformed family members may discourage patients from taking psychotropic medication because they fear side effects or addiction or attending psychotherapy or may reinforce pain behaviors and disability.
- Topics of discussion can include the biopsychosocial model of pain care, the rational use of medications, the impact of pain on mood, anxiety, activities, and relationships.
- Encouraging patients to be involved in support groups can help patients maintain treatment gains.

TREATMENT ADHERENCE

- One of the most frustrating aspects of clinical practice is patient nonadherence to therapeutic interventions.
- Adherence behaviors include:
  ○ Continuing a prescribed treatment program
  ○ Keeping appointments
  ○ Taking medications as prescribed
  ○ Performance of home-based treatment programs (eg, exercises, meditation)
  ○ Avoidance of risky health behaviors.
- Successful treatment of pain and concomitant psychiatric disorders requires close adherence to treatment plans for long or indefinite durations to ensure full remission and prevent relapse or recurrence.
- Enhancing adherence includes promoting a cooperative, mutual participating patient-clinician relationship and cultivating and maintaining open communication particularly about adverse effects of treatment regimens and patient expectations from treatment.
- Treatment regimens should be simplified if possible (eg, use of long-acting medications if possible, avoiding divided doses, etc.)
- Behavioral techniques to improve adherence includes:
  ○ Self-monitoring (eg, use of journals, calendars)
  ○ Goal setting (setting realistic goals and measures of success)
  ○ Corrective feedback (mail or e-mail reminders, feedback, and encouragement at each office visit)
  ○ Contracting.
- In the early stages of treatment, clinicians must base interventions to enhance treatment adherence on the understanding that patients with pain and psychiatric disorders may be poorly motivated and unduly pessimistic about their chance of recovery.

CONCLUSION

- Pain activates emotions, and, in certain situations, emotions activate pain; thus, emotions and pain are inextricably intertwined in the phenomenology of chronic pain disorders.

- Emotions and pain share common neuroanatomic and neurophysiologic substrates.
- Managing unhealthy emotional responses to pain and the consequences of pain is part and parcel of the pain clinician's daily work. To treat pain without managing emotions or to treat emotions without treating pain is usually futile, dooming the patient to chronic suffering and the clinician to chronic frustration.
- To manage most patients with chronic pain effectively, clinicians must identify, diagnose, and treat common comorbidities, such as uncomplicated depression.
- Due to the high prevalence of comorbid depression and anxiety, easy access to mental health professionals with experience in treating pain and comorbidities is critical to success in a chronic pain practice.
- The clinician must assure the patient that such referrals are common and expected in pain treatment, and the patient must understand that this is critical to the success of any pain treatment program.
- In the case of comorbidities, the clinician should communicate a willingness to follow up the patient's emotional symptoms and psychosocial functioning with an interest equal to that expressed in the outcome of treatment of the pain symptoms.
- The clinician should educate the patient without a current psychiatric disorder about the frequency of comorbidities and encourage that patient to report the onset of depression or anxiety immediately. Attempt to mitigate concerns about the stigma of being labeled with a mental disorder.
- Because many pharmaceutical and psychotherapeutic strategies exist with a strong foundation of research support, clinicians should prescribe with confidence in achieving a response and with the realistic goal of attaining depression remission and effective control of many anxiety symptoms and disorders.
- Developing and maintaining a positive, trusting therapeutic alliance with the patient is the key to long-term success.

BIBLIOGRAPHY

Bair MJ, Robinson RL, Katon W, et al. Depression and pain comorbidity: a literature review. *Arch Intern Med.* 2003;163(20):2433–2445.

Bruns D, Disorbio M. Hostility and violent ideation: physical rehabilitation patient and community samples. *Pain Med.* 2000;1:131–139.

Cano A, Weisberg J, Gallagher RM. Marital satisfaction and pain severity mediate the association between negative spouse responses to pain and depressive symptoms in a chronic pain patient sample. *Pain Med.* 2000;1:35–43.

Centers for Disease Control and Prevention. Web-based injury statistics query and reporting system: leading causes of death reports. Available at: http://www.cdc.gov/injury/wisqars/leading_causes_death.html. Accessed September 15, 2013.

Cheatle MD. Depression, chronic pain, and suicide by overdose: on the edge. *Pain Med.* 2011, June;12(Suppl 2):S43–S48.

Dharmshaktu P, Tayal V, Kalra BS. Efficacy of antidepressants as analgesics: a review. *J Clin Pharmacol.* 2012, January;52(1): 6–17.

Dohrenwend B, Marbach J, Raphael K, et al. Why is depression co-morbid with chronic facial pain? A family study test of alternative hypotheses. *Pain.* 1999;83:183–192.

Gallagher RM. Integrating medical and behavioral treatment in chronic pain management. *Med Clin North Am.* 1999;83:823–849.

Gallagher RM, Mossey J. Inadequate pain care for elders: the need for a primary care–pain medicine community collaboration. *Pain Med.* 2002;3:180.

Gerrits MM, Oppen PV, van Marwijk HW, et al. Pain and the onset of depressive and anxiety disorders. *Pain.* 2014;155(1):53–59.

IOM (Institute of Medicine). *Relieving Pain in America: A Blueprint for Transforming Prevention, Care, Education, and Research.* Washington, DC: The National Academies Press; 2011.

Kroenke K, Spitzer RL, Williams JB, et al. Physical symptoms in primary care: predictors of psychiatric disorders and functional impairment. *Arch Fam Med.* 1994;3:774–779.

Magni G, Marchetti M, Moreschi C, et al. Chronic musculoskeletal pain and depressive symptoms in the National Health and Nutrition Examination, I: epidemiologic follow-up study. *Pain.* 1993; 53(2):163–168.

Miller LR, Cano A. Comorbid chronic pain and depression: who is at risk? *J Pain.* 2009;10(6):619–627.

Mossey J, Gallagher RM, Tirumalasetti F. The effects of pain and depression on physical functioning in elderly residents of a continuing care retirement community. *Pain Med.* 2000;1:340–350.

Picus T, Burton AK, Vogel S, et al. A systematic review of psychological factors as predictors of chronicity/disability in prospective cohorts of low back pain. *Spine.* 2002;27:E109–E120.

Rome H, Rome J. Limbically augmented pain syndrome (LAPS): kindling, corticolimbic sensitization, and the convergence of affective and sensory symptoms in chronic pain disorders. *Pain Med.* 2000;1:7–23.

Sindrup SH, Jensen TS. Efficacy of pharmacological treatments of neuropathic pain: an update and effect related to mechanism of drug action. *Pain.* 1999;83:389–400.

Tang NK, Crane C. Suicidality in chronic pain: a review of the prevalence, risk factors and psychological links. *Psychol Med.* 2006;36(5):575–586.

Tsang AM, Von Korff S, Lee J, et al. Common chronic pain conditions in developed and developing countries: gender and age differences and comorbidity with depression-anxiety disorders. *J Pain.* 2008;9(10):883–891.

54 GENERAL PRINCIPLES OF INTERVENTIONAL PAIN THERAPIES

Richard L. Rauck, MD

OVERALL CONSIDERATIONS

- Informed consent is essential before any procedure is undertaken. (See below for a detailed discussion of the important aspects of informed consent.)
- Practitioners should understand the difference between procedures with respect to expectation of therapeutic benefit versus desired diagnostic information.
- Practitioners should have the requisite training and skill set to perform intended interventional procedures. This skill set may come from a fellowship training, previous experience with similar techniques, and/or attendance at seminars, conferences, and cadaveric workshops. It is important that interventional pain practitioners understand their abilities and limitations in performing these procedures.
- Practitioners of interventional procedures should understand the potential risks and complications of the procedures they perform and have the knowledge and equipment necessary to resuscitate patients in an emergency.

GENERAL INDICATIONS FOR INTERVENTIONAL PROCEDURES

- Interventional procedures may be diagnostic and/or therapeutic.
- Interventions should be individualized to each patient's condition. It is recognized that many chronic pain conditions do not have precise patho-anatomical diagnoses. While algorithms for interventions prove valuable as a framework in chronic pain, the symptoms, signs, radiological evidence, and response to previous treatments should guide future interventional considerations.
- Interventional procedures are indicated for a variety of acute, chronic, noncancer, and cancer pain patients. Understanding the indications for interventional procedures is essential. Patient selection is pivotal for achieving long-term efficacy and positive outcome measures.
- Although some patients respond to interventional procedures as unimodality therapy, the majority of chronic pain patients respond best when interventions are part of a multidisciplinary approach. Addressing the physical therapy, vocational needs, and psychological issues of the patient along with the indicated procedures enhances the long-term outcome.
- Some patients should have interventions deferred until other serious issues (eg, severe depression, infections) are managed.

USE OF NEW INTERVENTIONAL PROCEDURES

- New interventional procedures are continuously being developed and promoted by specialists in the field and industry.
- Institutional Review Boards (IRB) approval may be necessary before implementing new procedures. Practitioners interested in new procedures are encouraged to consult colleagues and inquire of their IRB before utilizing new procedures that are not FDA approved. Appropriate study protocols remain the hallmark method for evaluating efficacy and risk of new procedures.
- Caution should be used in employing new procedures. Proper indications can take years to completely

understand with some procedures. Potential risks and complications may not be intuitive for a new procedure.

- Formal training may be necessary for some new procedures, while others may require only modification of existing practice.

- Practitioners should understand the differences in benefits and risks between existing and proposed techniques when evaluating new interventional procedures.

GENERAL TECHNIQUES FOR INTERVENTIONAL PROCEDURES

STERILE TECHNIQUE

- Sterile technique should be used for all interventional procedures. The degree of sterility varies from a simple swab with an alcohol-soaked gauze to full operating room sterile procedure. The sterility required depends on several factors, including the likelihood of infection, patient factors (eg, diabetes mellitus), and the severity or difficulty of treating a resultant infection (eg, diskitis from a diskogram).

- Most interventional procedures are elective. Patients with concomitant, systemic infections should generally be rescheduled to a later date for a specific intervention. A risk/benefit analysis is necessary in all cases, such as for a patient with chest wall trauma and developing atelectasis who may benefit greatly from a thoracic epidural.

- Practitioners should understand the concept of preservative-free (often single dose) versus preservative-containing as it pertains to medications used in interventions. There are reasons to use either type of vial in specific situations. Risk/benefit of each should be understood by the interventionalist

- Compounding pharmacies provide medications for some practitioners of interventions. Practitioners should vet or have their institution vet the compounding pharmacy to assure that the pharmacy is compliant with local and national standards for compounders of drugs used by the pain interventionalist.

SEDATION

- The routine use of sedation for interventional procedures is becoming controversial. Under the "Choosing Wisely Campaign" the American Society of Anesthesiologists recommended against the use of intravenous (IV) sedation for diagnostic and therapeutic nerve blocks, or joint injections as a default practice (with the exception of pediatrics).

They further state that IV sedation can be used after evaluation and discussion of risks, including interference with assessing the acute pain relieving effects of the procedure and the potential for false positive responses.

- Most awake patients experience some discomfort during an interventional procedure. Appropriate use of local anesthetics decreases this discomfort to a tolerable level for most patients.

- Judicious amounts of sedation are appropriate by interventionalists who understand how to dose these medications and how to titrate to effect. It should be understand by all that sedation is not an exact science, and each patient reacts differently to the effects of sedation.

- Appropriate resuscitation equipment should be available in all areas where sedation is used for interventional procedures.

- The type of intervention has a significant role in the amount of discomfort the practitioner may expect a patient to experience; for example, a trigger point injection usually has significantly less associated pain than does provocative diskography.

- Some patients tolerate the pain of interventional procedures poorly. The term *needle phobia* is used for patients who experience excessive pain with any type of intervention. A larger percentage of patients cannot tolerate the more invasive procedures. A skilled and experienced clinician can usually determine the amount of pain expected during any given procedure.

- For any specific procedure or patient, the practitioner may decide to employ the use of sedation to help the patient tolerate the associated pain. Use of sedation is appropriate during interventional procedures but is an art that should be practiced carefully.

- Sedation is important, at times, for patient safety. Patients who move or jump during a procedure place themselves at risk of injury from the needle or cannula. This patient movement can be involuntary or reflexive to the needle invasion. Sedation often prevents this movement.

- An awake or semiconscious patient is important in many procedures to inform practitioners if the needle, catheter, and/or cannula are positioned in an unexpected place. Patients under appropriate levels of sedation can still interact with the practitioner and provide valuable feedback. For example, most sedated patients can inform the practitioner when a needle brushes along or contacts a nerve. Avoiding needle penetration of a nerve is often desired. If the patient is too heavily sedated or unconscious, the practitioner loses this important feedback.

- Appropriate levels of sedation often leave the patient amnestic of the procedure. Patients who reliably and routinely provide accurate information during the procedure develop retrograde amnesia. Clinically, this amnesia is acceptable and often beneficial, as patients often need repeat procedures. Unfortunately, in medicolegal cases, this amnesia is often interpreted as unconsciousness; thus documentation of this scenario may be helpful.
- Patients who have undergone sedation for interventions should be discharged in the care of a driver. Exceptions are rare and require sufficient recovery time for the effects of sedation to dissipate.
- Use of sedation always requires a risk/benefit analysis. The standard of care, however, does not require documentation of this risk/benefit analysis. In many cases, the benefits of sedation outweigh the risks.

FLUOROSCOPIC GUIDANCE

- Fluoroscopic guidance has become the standard of care for many interventions performed in pain medicine. This includes procedures such as cervical epidural steroid injections and median nerve blocks. Precise needle location can only be guaranteed for many interventions with fluoroscopic guidance and visualization of appropriate bony landmarks.
- Fluoroscopic guidance provides useful information when nerves, joints, or other intended targets are in proximity to bony landmarks. Many peripheral nerves, such as ilioinguinal/hypogastric nerves, are commonly blocked at a distance from a bony landmark. Use of fluoroscopic guidance in these situations is not as helpful as in other procedures, such as a selective nerve block. The evolving technology of ultrasound is often used for block of peripheral nerves and being touted for other interventional procedures such as stellate ganglion blocks.
- The use of fluoroscopic guidance for all nerve blocks in or around the spine is a subject of debate. The standard of care for access to the lumbar epidural space in perioperative or obstetric anesthesia is without fluoroscopic guidance. Thoracic epidurals are also performed postoperatively without fluoroscopic guidance by anesthesiologists. As many anesthesiology-trained interventionalists learned these techniques safely without fluoroscopy and have practiced them for years in pain clinics without fluoroscopy, it has been difficult for many to see the need for change. Also, any radiation exposure carries some risk, and a substantial cost is associated with the use of fluoroscopy. While cervical procedures were done "blindly" for many years, the presence and size of the

spinal cord and narrowness of the canal in this region makes fluoroscopic guidance necessary for all interlaminar approaches to the epidural space.
- Fluoroscopic guidance has been extremely useful for many interventions. With the injection of appropriate contrast material, information can be gleaned about the characteristic spread of diagnostic and/or therapeutic injectate material.
- Radiation exposure from fluoroscopy can be significant to the patient and/or the practitioner. Judicious use and continuous monitoring of live fluoroscopic times help limit this exposure. Practitioners should protect themselves with leaded gowns, thyroid shields, lined gloves, and protective glasses, when appropriate.

POSTPROCEDURAL MONITORING

- Patients should be monitored following interventions. Patients may require nothing more than observation by office personnel prior to discharge or may require a formal recovery room and continuous vital-sign monitoring.
- The level of monitoring depends on the procedure, the sedation used, and the individual patient. When intravenous sedation is used, heart rate, blood pressure, respiratory rate, and oxygen saturation are commonly monitored noninvasively.

MEDICATIONS

COMMONLY USED MEDICATIONS

- Local anesthetics and corticosteroids are the most frequently used medications in most interventional practices. Other medications, such as hyaluronidase, hypertonic saline, opioids, bretylium, and clonidine, are sometimes used. Many, if not most, of these drugs are used in interventional pain medicine for non-FDA-approved indications. This does not imply that they are not efficacious or that unacceptable risks exist. For a variety of business/legal reasons, many companies choose not to allocate the resources necessary to win FDA approval for a specific indication. The FDA does not limit the use of a drug to approved indications (the agency limits the ability of pharmaceutical companies to market a drug for a nonapproved indication).
- It is essential that interventional practitioners understand which drugs are safe for which procedures. For example, hypertonic saline is an effective drug in the epidural space but is rarely indicated for subarachnoid injection, and care should be taken to avoid intrathecal injection in most cases.

- Occasionally, the indications for certain medications change over time. For example, many practitioners used particulate steroids such as methyl-prednisolone acetate for cervical selective nerve-root injections or cervical transforaminal steroid injections, but it has become clear that there is an intravascular injection risk with a particulate steroid injection in this area. The use of intrathecal corticosteroids is controversial. Although clinical experience and the literature support the use of these agents in select situations, older reports link neurotoxicity with the intrathecal injection of methylprednisolone acetate. Intrathecal corticosteroids should be avoided except in specific situations.
- Interventional practitioners should stay abreast of the literature and alter their practices as findings emerge.
- Unfortunately, when controversy exists, practitioners may have to decide whether or not to use selected drugs based on the local medicolegal environment.

MANAGING ANTICOAGULANTS

- Patients are frequently prescribed intravenous (heparin, streptokinase), subcutaneous (low-molecular-weight heparins [LMWHs]), or oral (warfarin) anticoagulants/thrombolytic drugs for a variety of medical conditions.
- Many anticoagulants pose some undefined but increased risk for patients undergoing interventional procedures.
- Anticoagulants can be classified broadly as drugs that interfere with platelet function and those that interfere with the coagulation cascade as measured by prothrombin time and/or partial thromboplastin time. Many of these drugs have the potential to increase bleeding time and/or produce coagulopathy.
- Some agents, such as the nonsteroidal anti-inflammatory drugs, do not significantly increase the risk of perioperative interventions or of epidural steroid injections and can be continued safely during interventional procedures.
- Drugs such as streptokinase, however, should be avoided in almost all patients scheduled to undergo an interventional procedure.
- LMWHs pose a significant risk in some patients. Practitioners should understand the risks associated with LMWHs and planned interventional procedures.
- Because many interventions are elective, it is desirable and may be possible to stop anticoagulants three to five days beforehand. This may require clearance from the primary or prescribing physician. A bleeding history and/or PT/PTT/INR levels may be necessary in

patients with recent excessive bleeding. Alternatively, the practitioner can hospitalize the patient and initiate intravenous heparin while discontinuing other anticoagulants. Once the effect of oral or subcutaneous drugs has dissipated, the heparin can be reversed with protamine for a short time while the procedure is performed. Anticoagulant therapy can be reinstituted following the procedure.

RISKS AND COMPLICATIONS

- Risks and potential complications should be explained to patients prior to interventional procedures, and alternative treatments should be discussed. This is most commonly done within the context of informed consent when the physician and patient discuss the treatment plan.
- Certain risks, including infection, trauma to a nerve from the needle, medication reaction, and death, are inherent to any procedure. Although death is a highly unexpected outcome of most procedures, its inclusion in a risk discussion or document implies some level of understanding by the patient that potentially serious complications can occur.
- Lack of efficacy is not a risk, but it is helpful to remind patients that no procedure guarantees improvement, and their symptoms could even become worse following the procedure, often for unclear reasons.

EMERGENCIES

- Interventional practitioners must be prepared to handle any potential complication.
- Resuscitative drugs, oxygen, airway management equipment, and suction should be maintained and readily available whenever interventional procedures and sedation are employed.
- The standard of care does not mandate that resuscitative equipment be available in each procedure room; however, transport of such equipment should occur with expediency in case of an emergency.
- Large, busy practices should have adequately trained personnel nearby to help in emergencies. Solo practitioners should know what trained personnel are readily available and how to get their help in case of an emergency.

MEDICOLEGAL RISK MANAGEMENT

- In today's environment, it is impossible to guarantee that anyone can expect immunity or protect himself or herself in all situations. Geography (practice location), type of interventional practice (some procedures carry an inherently greater risk), and good fortune all play a role in avoiding the unpleasant experience of a medical malpractice lawsuit.

- The burden rests on the plaintiff to prove that a physician committed malpractice by breaching the standard of care with resultant damages. To do this, a causal relationship must exist between the alleged breach, the injury, and the alleged damages. A breach in the standard of care that cannot be linked to the injury or damages is not considered malpractice and usually results in a favorable verdict or settlement for the physician.
- Practitioners unfamiliar with the legal environment should obtain the best legal counsel they can afford whenever the possibility of a malpractice suit arises. In some situations, a practitioner may want to hire legal representation soon after an intervention. Other times, one waits until a plaintiff has filed a complaint.

Indications

- Legal cases always involve examination of the indications for any procedure the plaintiffs allege resulted in malpractice.
- If plaintiff's counsel can establish a lack of medical indications for the procedure, standard of care was breached.
- Although this is often not a clearly won point, documentation of indications generally refutes this argument.

Informed Consent

- To perform any procedure without the consent of the patient is considered assault.
- Although informed consent can ethically and legally be obtained orally (by explaining the risks, complications, and alternative treatments, and documenting this explanation in office or progress notes) or be implied (eg, when a patient is undergoing the "nth" injection in a series and willingly lies on the bed in preparation for the injection), a legal debate can ensue whenever written documentation is poor.
- If adequate explanation is given but no documentation exists, the standard has been met, but credibility and the ability to remember the facts years later will be questioned if an unexpected event occurs and legal restitution is sought.
- Documentation of informed consent in writing, therefore, is preferred by legal experts.
- To avoid legal confrontation, therefore, the best informed consent is obtained in writing, is witnessed, and is documented in the patient's chart.

Performance of the Procedure

- Regardless of proper indications or informed consent, if the intervention is carried out in substandard fashion, the practitioner has violated the standard of care.
- Procedures should be carried out in a manner consistent with current textbooks and/or teachings.
- From the legal perspective, the more information documented about the performance of the procedure, the better.
- Many practitioners use legally accepted templates to document their procedures. Practitioners should always have the opportunity to individualize a template, however, when unusual events occur during an intervention.

Complications

- Complications can be expected to occur in any busy interventional practice.
- How the patient is managed following an alleged complication is often critical to the patient's outcome and to avoiding a possible medical malpractice suit or receiving a favorable verdict should one be filed.
- The first step is to listen fully and completely to the patient's complaint. Many physicians become defensive because they fail to realize that the patient is not trying to place blame but, instead, is simply trying to understand the situation.
- The physician should never compromise his or her honesty and integrity. If a complication occurs, it is almost always in the physician's best interest to acknowledge all of the facts and be straightforward and truthful with the patient.
- Patients generally want to know the cause of the complication, and the physician should explain that this is being explored.
- Often the cause of the complication cannot be clearly ascertained, particularly in the immediate postprocedural period.
- Sometimes, there is a causal relationship between the procedure and the event. This does not imply that a breach in the standard of care occurred. If the physician is clear about the cause, he or she should explain it to the patient after careful reflection and assimilation of the facts. It is usually better to wait several days or weeks and deliver accurate information to the patient and/or patient's family than to retract erroneous information given in haste.
- Maintaining a dialogue with the patient and/or patient's family is important as is keeping the patient returning for follow-up, which allows the interventionalist to maintain continuity of care.
- Continuing the doctor/patient relationship can be strained, particularly in the initial months following

an event or if there is a lack of agreement on the facts, but it is often the best way to reach reconciliation and maintain a workable relationship.

- The physician should be very careful in discussions with patients and/or family members after an alleged complication. The relationship of a procedure to a complication may seem intuitive, but a true cause-and-effect relationship may not exist. For example, if a patient dies during a nerve block, the patient's family (and possibly the physician) may assume the procedure caused the death; however, a myocardial infarction, stroke, or malignant ventricular dysrhythmia may have been the actual cause. The physician should avoid accepting blame for an event until all the facts have been accumulated.

BIBLIOGRAPHY

Benzon HT, Gisson AJ, Strichartz GR, et al. The effect of polyethylene glycol on mammalian nerve impulses. *Anesth Analg.* 1987;66:553.

Fishman SM, Smith H, Meleger A, et al. Radiation safety in pain medicine. *Reg Anesth Pain Med.* 2002;27:296.

Horlocker TT, Bajwa ZH, Ashraf Z, et al. Risk assessment of hemorrhagic complications associated with nonsteroidal anti-inflammatory medications in ambulatory pain clinic patients undergoing epidural steroid injection. *Anesth Analg.* 2002;95:1691.

Horlocker TT, Wedel DJ. Neuraxial block and low-molecular-weight heparin: balancing perioperative analgesia and thromboprophylaxis. *Reg Anesth Pain Med.* 1998;23(6, Suppl 2):164.

Horlocker TT, Wedel DJ, Schroeder DR, et al. Preoperative antiplatelet therapy does not increase the risk of spinal hematoma associated with regional anesthesia. *Anesth Analg.* 1995; 80:303.

Johnson SH. Providing relief to those in pain: a retrospective on the scholarship and impact of the Mayday project. *J Law Med Ethics.* 2003;31:15.

Kotani N, Kashikata T, Hashimoto H, et al. Intrathecal methylprednisolone for intractable postherpetic neuralgia. *N Engl J Med.* 2000;343:1514.

Manchikanti L, Staats PS, Singh V, et al. Evidence-based practice guidelines for interventional techniques in the management of chronic spinal pain. *Pain Physician.* 2003;6:3.

Mendelson G, Mendelson D. Legal aspects of the management of chronic pain. *Med J Aus.* 1991;155:640.

Nelson D. Arachnoiditis from intrathecally given corticosteroids in the treatment of multiple sclerosis. *Arch Neurol.* 1976;33:373.

Swerdlow M. Medico-legal aspects of complications following pain relieving blocks. *Pain.* 1982;13:321.

Vincent C, Young M, Phillips A. Why do people sue doctors? A study of patients and relatives taking legal action. *Lancet.* 1994;343:1609.

Wipf JE, Deyo RA. Low back pain. *Med Clin North Am.* 1995;79:231.

55 RADIATION MANAGEMENT FOR PAIN INTERVENTIONS

David M. Schultz, MD

PREREQUISITES

- Before beginning a discussion of radiation safety, it is important to define the terms "X ray" and "x-ray," since the use of these terms is often confusing.
- X rays are produced in an x-ray tube so that we can take an interval "image" of a patient.
- "X ray" refers to a particular particle of energy that constitutes a ray.
  - It is a ray because the particle is energy traveling in a straight line.
  - An X ray is an X particle of energy.
  - In physics, there are many particles of energy, but we are concerned only with the X particle.
  - "X" in this case is an adjective modifying "ray".
- The term "x-ray" can be a verb, noun, or adjective.
  - As a verb, it means to take an image using X rays.
  - As an adjective, it is a descriptor of something that involves X rays, such as an x-ray tube or an x-ray image.
  - As a noun, x-ray refers to the image acquired using X rays as in the sentence, "My x-ray was normal."

WHAT ARE X RAYS?

- For our purposes, X rays should be thought of as very tiny particles of pure energy that travel in a straight line at the speed of light until they collide with electrons associated with atoms or molecules within matter.
- These particles are so tiny that when they enter a human body they do not see the body as organs or tissues, but rather as atoms and molecules.
- These particles can travel between the spaces that separate these atoms and molecules to penetrate deep into the tissue before they encounter an electron orbiting an atom or a molecule.
- Some X rays traverse the entire thickness of a patient's abdomen without colliding with any electron.
  - Those few X rays that happened to traverse the entire anatomy without incident create the radiographic image.
  - In general, fewer than 1% of the X rays that enter an average human abdomen penetrate completely through the abdomen.
- On the other hand, more than 99% of the X rays collide with electrons of atoms and molecules inside the abdomen.
  - These interactions cause many of the X rays to change their direction of travel, lose some of their

energy, and scatter into the room that is occupied by personnel.

- ○ Although the X rays have lost some of their energy, they still travel at the speed of light.
- Therefore, the entire process of X rays entering an abdomen and either traversing it unabated or scattering into the room takes place instantaneously while the X rays are turned on.

HOW ARE X RAYS PRODUCED?

- The production of X rays is a matter of converting electric current into x-ray energy.
- Simply conceived, a beam of electrons is created inside a vacuum tube and accelerated to a high fraction of the speed of light.
- Two properties are used to describe this electron beam: the beam energy, described by the term kV or kilovoltage, and the tube current described by the parameter mA or milliamperes.
  - ○ The kilovoltage determines how fast electrons travel and the milliamperage determines how many of them travel.
- Once the electrons reach their designed speed, they collide with a heavy metal target set within their path and come to an abrupt stop.
  - ○ This abrupt braking of the speed of the electrons results mostly in heat, but a small percentage of the energy results in the production of X rays.
  - ○ X rays produced by the braking action of high-speed electrons are called **bremsstrahlung**.
  - ○ The area on the heavy metal target that produces the X rays is only about 1 mm^2.
- The X rays fan out in all directions from that production point. So, in theory, X rays would travel in all directions throughout the room.
  - ○ However, the vacuum tube in which X rays are produced is housed in a heavy metal shield that blocks X rays that travel in the undesired directions.
  - ○ Only X rays that travel toward the patient are allowed to escape the housing.
  - ○ The escape hatch through which the X rays travel is called the port.
  - ○ Thin sheets of metal, usually copper or aluminum, cover the port itself.
  - ○ These thin sheets of metal are called filters.
  - ○ Their purpose is to block very low-energy nonpenetrating X rays before they have a chance to expose the patient.
  - ○ Such low-energy nonpenetrating x-rays only represent a hazard to the patient and provide no medical-imaging benefit.
  - ○ The operator of the fluoroscope typically has no control over the use of filters because they are

permanently mounted inside the x-ray tube housing and, if any adjustment is available at all, it is performed in the background by the machine to manage radiation production for optimal imaging conditions.

- The x-ray beam that leaves the port of the x-ray tube housing is a diverging beam that originated from the 1-mm^2 area on the metal target.
- As the X rays travel further away from their point of origin, their diverging trajectories result in a continually expanding and widening x-ray beam.
- Billions of X rays constitute the x-ray beam.
- Because all the X rays that are produced originate from a very tiny area and expand into an ever widening area, the intensity of the x-ray beam changes rapidly with increasing distance from the source.
  - ○ It is most intense close to the source and the intensity drops off rapidly with increasing distance from the source.
  - ○ The rate at which the intensity decreases is governed by the inverse square law.
    - ■ This law merely states that when the distance from the source of the x-rays doubles, the intensity of the X rays will drop by a factor of four, since four is the inverse square of two.
    - ■ If the distance from the x-ray source triples, the intensity will drop off by a factor of nine, since the inverse square of three is 1/9.
- It is important that the x-ray beam cover only the area necessary for the medical imaging task. Therefore, the x-ray machine (fluoroscope) has an additional set of restriction devices built into it that may further reduce the area of the x-ray beam. These devices are called collimators.
  - ○ Collimators may be either two sets of blades that can be adjusted in order to create a rectangular field of the desired size or an iris-type device that provides circular collimation.
  - ○ The collimator blades themselves are made of a heavy metal attenuating material so that X rays cannot readily penetrate them.

HOW IS THE IMAGE MADE?

- Once the X rays are properly produced and the x-ray beam area properly collimated, the imaging process can take place efficiently.
- The x-ray beam that is directed into a specified area of the patient is a uniform field of X rays.
- If an image of the raw beam were captured, the image would simply be a neutral gray rectangle representing the entire field.
- As the x-ray beam enters into the patient, the numbers of X rays in the field are reduced by attrition.

○ Within the first thin layer of tissue, many X rays collide with the atoms and molecules of the skin.
○ In the next layer of tissue, there are fewer X rays in the field and some of these X rays will collide with the atoms and molecules of that tissue layer.
- As the X rays continue to penetrate through the patient, more and more X rays are eliminated from the initial field. The X rays either cease to exist because their energy is completely absorbed by the patient or they are degraded in energy and scattered out into the environment.
- The likelihood that X rays will be removed from the initial unattenuated beam will depend upon how much material occupies their path and on the atomic composition of the material that is in the path.
○ For example, X rays that pass through large pockets of air will not likely be attenuated.
○ X rays that pass through bone will more likely be attenuated because of the higher density of bone. Further, bone has a considerable amount of calcium and X rays are more likely to interact with calcium than with elements like carbon, nitrogen, oxygen, and hydrogen.
○ Therefore, as the x-ray beam penetrates deeper and deeper into the patient, an attenuation pattern of the initial beam begins to develop within the field.
○ X rays are more densely populated in areas with pockets of air and less densely concentrated in areas that include the bone.
- When the beam finally emerges from the patient, it will have developed a pattern of relative intensities across the field. This pattern of changing x-ray concentration constitutes the x-ray image.
- As previously stated, more than 99% of the X rays that enter into in a normal adult abdomen are either absorbed by the abdomen or scattered.
- Every time there is an interaction between an X ray and human tissue, energy is exchanged.
○ When an x-ray collides with anatomical structures, they ionize atoms and molecules, producing displaced fast-moving electrons within the tissue.
○ The fast-moving electrons then create a cascade of events that further removes other electrons from other atoms.
○ This entire process takes place within microns of the initial interaction and produces a short path of ionization that changes the biochemistry in the immediate vicinity.
○ This phenomenon cannot be separated from the imaging process and constitutes the first stage of the mechanism by which X rays cause biological effects.
  ■ There is, therefore, always some risk involved with medical x-ray imaging.

HOW IS EXPOSURE TO X-RAYS ASSESSED?

- There are five descriptors relevant to fluoroscopy that are used to describe x-ray quantities. Each of these quantities is designed to help assess the potential risks to one's health from the exposure to the x-rays. These quantities are as follows:
○ Absorbed dose
○ Air kerma
○ Equivalent dose
○ Effective dose
○ Dose area product, a.k.a., air-kerma area product.

ABSORBED DOSE

- The most fundamental quantity for assessing the risk associated with an exposure to x-ray radiation is absorbed dose.
- All other quantities are some adaption or modification of this quantity.
- By definition, absorbed dose is the energy absorbed by tissue per unit mass of tissue.
- Remember that X rays transfer energy to tissues when they collide with electrons of atoms and molecules.
- The amount of energy transferred is related to the amount of ionization produced inside the tissue.
- Therefore, absorbed dose is directly related to the potential for biological effects.
- Absorbed dose can be thought of as a localized concentration of energy deposited in a small mass of tissue.
○ For example, we could consider a small mass of tissue as a cube of about 1-mm dimension. The absorbed dose to neighboring 1-mm cube of tissue could be different than the small volume in which we are measuring dose. In other words, absorbed dose does not generally refer to the energy deposited in a large mass of tissue such as a kidney or liver. In fact, as x-rays penetrate through the patient they are attenuated by attrition and so the absorbed dose also changes with depth in the patient.
- In general, the absorbed dose at the surface of the patient is about 30 to 100 times greater than the absorbed dose when the beam exits the patient.
- The process of x-ray attenuation reduces the absorbed dose by a factor of two for every 4 to 5 cm depth in the patient, depending on beam energy.
○ For a 25-cm thick patient, the exit dose would be about 1%–3% of the entrance skin dose.
- The units of absorbed dose are milligray (mGy).
○ The entrance dose rate to the skin surface of a patient during fluoroscopy might be about 50 mGy per minute, but this varies widely depending on the fluoroscopic conditions.

- Absorbed dose is necessary to assess risk, including risk of radiation-induced cancer or risk of radiation-induced injury. However, absorbed dose might not be sufficient to assess risk. In order to account for the insufficiencies, other dose values are used.

AIR KERMA

- Air kerma is often used to assess the amount of radiation that exists at a point in space and it can easily be converted to the absorbed dose to tissue, should a person occupy that space.
- Air kerma is effectively the absorbed dose to air and is therefore measured in units of milligray (mGy).
- Air kerma is often quoted when one wants to assess the amount of radiation exposing a patient.
- Roughly speaking, the absorbed dose to tissue is about 20%–40% higher than the air kerma, depending on the collimation of the beam.

EQUIVALENT DOSE

- Equivalent dose is only important when reading radiation exposure reports for personnel.
  ○ Many of these reports give the dose in terms of equivalent dose instead of absorbed dose.
- The units of equivalent dose is the millisievert (mSv).
- In some reports, the unit of equivalent dose is the millirem (mrem), which differs from the millisievert by a factor of 100. That is: 1 mSv = 100 mrem.
  ○ The reason this unit is used in personal dosimetry reports is to account for exposures from types of radiation used in industry that are not relevant to medicine.
- Diagnostic and interventional x-ray medicine need not be concerned with equivalent dose.
- Medicine can equate equivalent dose as absorbed dose. That is, one mSv of equivalent dose is the same as 1 mGy of absorbed dose. And 100 mrem of equivalent dose is also the same as 1 mGy of absorbed dose.

EFFECTIVE DOSE

- Effective dose is also measured in millisieverts and should not be confused with the term "equivalent dose."
- Effective dose is a hypothetical dose that would have to be delivered uniformly to the persons' entire body in order to produce the same quantitative risk for stochastic effects as the dose actually delivered. (Stochastic effects include radiation-induced cancer and radiation-induced heritable genetic effects. Effective dose does not relate at all to radiation injury.)

- The reason this is important is that patients and medical workers are exposed nonuniformly to radiation and assessing risk from nonuniform exposures is complex.
  ○ For example, we have already learned that the radiation dose at depth in the patient is quite different than the radiation dose at the surface of the patient but, even more importantly, the physician collimates the field so that many of the organs of the patient are not exposed at all.
- The dose to the patient varies for different organs throughout the body.
  ○ If the exposed organs are not sensitive for radiation-induced cancer, then the risk is very low.
  ○ If the organs exposed are extremely sensitive to radiation, then the risk is higher.
  ○ Furthermore, if we expose less tissue, then the risk is less because less tissue is placed at risk.
- Effective dose is a construct used to remove these factors when comparing doses to individuals who are exposed in entirely different ways.
- Effective dose is calculated from the doses actually delivered to individual tissues and depends on the sensitivities of the tissues exposed.
- Effective dose is also used to calculate personnel exposures.
  ○ For example, if we are exposed during our working hours to radiation while wearing a lead apron, the apron blocks most of the radiation from exposing the sensitive organs of our body. However, other organs are not shielded. To calculate our stochastic risk, we have to know the absorbed dose to the unshielded part of the body, which contains the least sensitive organs and we have to know what penetrated the lead apron to expose the most sensitive organs. This can be a very complex process, which has been addressed for various scenarios.
  ○ Conversion factors have been published that can be used to roughly assess the effective dose from various exposure scenarios.

DOSE-AREA PRODUCT (AKA: AIR-KERMA-AREA PRODUCT)

- Dose-area product is also known as air-kerma-area product.
- It is the multiplicative product of both the air kerma and the area of the x-ray field and is measured in units of Gy cm² or some denomination thereof.
- As the area of the x-ray field gets larger, the patient is exposed to more radiation and thus the risk is increased.
- If the area is decreased, the amount of tissue exposed decreases and thus the risk to the patient also decreases.

- Air-kerma-area product was designed to help assess stochastic risk to the patient from fluoroscopic and radiographic examinations of patients, depending on dose and collimation.
- It was not intended for use in assessing risk for radiation injury.
- Factors used to convert dose-area-product into effective dose have been published.

HOW DO PERSONNEL GET EXPOSED TO RADIATION?

Personnel are exposed to radiation principally from two sources: the patient and the x-ray source. Of these the most important source is the patient.

RADIATION FROM THE PATIENT

- As radiation enters and traverses the tissues of the patient, many x rays collide with electrons that are attached to the atoms and molecules of those tissues.
  - When that happens, x rays lose energy and are redirected away from their initial trajectory.
  - This results in a spray of radiation into the room in all directions.
    - This spray of radiation, called stray or scatter radiation, spreads out in all directions at an intensity that is much reduced from that entering the patient.
    - The stray radiation is most intense on the side of the patient where the beam enters the patient.
    - It is least intense on the other side.
    - Intensity drops off very rapidly with distance from the patient in a fashion that follows the inverse-square law.

RADIATION PENETRATING THE HOUSING

- A second source of radiation exposure, usually of much less concern, is radiation that penetrates through the protective housing of the X-ray source.
- No housing can block 100% of the radiation and a little bit penetrates through the housing.
- As long as the protective housing remains intact and meets regulation requirements, this source of radiation should be relatively minor compared to that emanating from the patient.

A RULE REGARDING RADIATION MANAGEMENT FOR PERSONNEL

- From the previous discussions regarding stray radiation, it is clear that the less radiation used to expose the patient, the less will become stray radiation in the room.

- So, a simple safety rule is to use radiation in a frugal and efficient manner. This will minimize radiation risk both to the patient and to personnel.

THE MOBILE C-ARM FLUOROSCOPE

A typical mobile c-arm fluoroscopy unit is shown in Figure 55-1. The important features that directly affect radiation delivery are:

- Location of the X-ray source
- Location of the image receptor
- Control switches to activate X rays (foot pedal and hand switch)
- Collimator controls
- Magnification controls (field-of-view controls)
- Dose rate controls
- Pulse rate controls
- Information on kVp, mA and fluoroscopy time, air-kerma-area product (KAP), and air kerma (AK) output are provided. Of these, fluoroscopy time, KAP, and AK output are useful tools for monitoring radiation delivery.

WHAT FACTORS DOES THE MACHINE CONTROL?

- In order to maintain image quality at a consistent level during fluoroscopy, fluoroscopes are designed to automatically adjust radiation output. It would, therefore, be a mistake to think that radiation output is the same for all patients, all projections, or all procedures.
- This radiation control mechanism is referred to as the automatic exposure rate control, or the AERC.
- The two principal parameters that are controlled are beam energy and tube current.
  - Beam energy is controlled by varying the kVp in order to achieve an x-ray energy that produces a good compromise between image quality and the ability of the radiation to adequately penetrate the patient.
  - The tube current can be varied in many ways.
    - This includes varying the average mA by varying tube current characteristics such as pulse intensity.
    - If a continuous tube current is employed, the machine varies the magnitude of the mA.
  - The purpose of this control by the machine is to ensure that physician is not distracted by a temporally varying image brightness or by changing noise characteristics of the image.
  - The machine achieves this constant control by examining the signals from the image receptor and

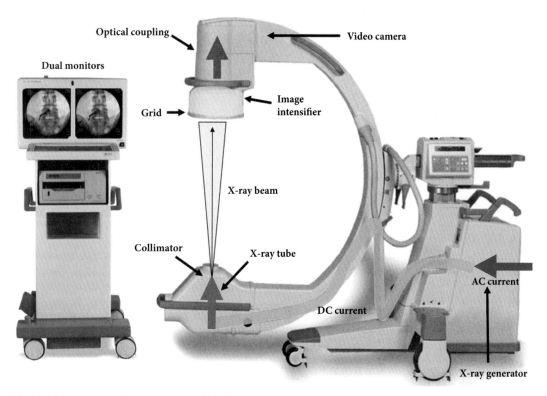

FIG. 55-1. Modern fluoroscope with components labeled.

ensuring that the same average signal is maintained for a large portion of the central area of the image.

- If the signal starts to diminish, the machine will automatically adjust the kVp, the pulse characteristics, or the mA as necessary.
- If the signal from the image starts to increase, the machine will adjust the parameters to decrease the output.
- In some machines, there may be an option for the machine to vary the tube filtration. These functions are typically unnoticed by the operator.
- The FDA puts limits on the amount of radiation output the machine is allowed to produce during standard fluoroscopy and there is, therefore, a maximum kVp and a maximum average tube current at which the machine can operate.
- The FDA does not put limits on the amount of radiation that can be produced in order to perform image acquisition.
- Under normal operation, the fluoroscopic parameters are limited to those combinations that would produce a free-in-air air kerma of 86 mGy per minute at 30 cm from the image receptor.
- Should the occasional situation occur where greater fluoroscopic output is required to improve image quality, the FDA allows manufacturers to design a high level control (HLC) operation into their system.

- Under HLC, the output is allowed to reach 172 mGy per minute at 30 cm from the image receptor.
- The output is still controlled by the machine, but the operator has to select HLC operation.
- The FDA requires that HLC fluoroscopy have a special or different means of activation than that used for standard fluoroscopy.
- Also, during this operation, an audible tone must be present indicating to the operator that they are operating in the HLC mode.
- Not all machines are designed with HLC, as this feature is optional.
- Fluoroscopes use information derived from their AERC to determine the appropriate radiographic techniques required for image acquisition.
- During image acquisition sequences, there is no limit imposed by the FDA as to the radiation output per image.
- Generally, the manufacturer boosts the output rate such that it is significantly higher than the fluoroscopic rate.
- For mobile C-arm devices, the image acquisition rate is generally two to five times greater than that of fluoroscopy. However, this general rule of thumb does not apply to all manufacturers and the actual acquisition rates for any specific unit can be quite different.
- For fixed in-room angiographic machines, the output rates during acquisition can be much higher.

How are AERC and Patient Dose Related?

- The AERC is designed to assure that X-ray output is what it needs to be to penetrate the patient and produce a quality image.
- Radiation does not penetrate large patients very well. Inevitably, image quality will be lower and patient dose higher for larger patients.
- The entrance fluoroscopic skin dose rate can vary by a factor of about 20 or more for a thin, 15-cm thick patient when compared to a large, 30-cm thick patient.

WHAT FEATURES DOES THE OPERATOR CONTROL?

The operator controls the position of the patient relative to the x-ray source, beam orientation, magnification mode, collimation, and dose-rate controls such as pulse rate, noise control, and HLC.

Position of the Patient Relative to the C-arm

- For frontal projections, the X-ray tube is positioned below the patient. This orientation is used for the safety of the operator and personnel since the patient acts as a shield for the upper bodies of personnel.
- Furthermore, if there is a need for the physician to have hands in the beam (not recommended), then the dose rate to the hands will be a great deal less than if the source were above the patient.
- The image receptor must be positioned high enough above the patient to provide clearance for the physician to insert medical devices.
  - But it should be low enough that a significant distance is maintained between the X-ray source and the patient's skin.
  - This will of course depend on patient size.
  - For short procedures that involve only a couple of minutes of fluoroscopy, this is not a critical factor, but it is good practice.
- The FDA requires that the manufacturer provide a separator device for the unit that forces a minimum distance of 38 cm between the 1-mm² port through which X rays exit and the patient's skin.
  - The device is often removed because it can represent a hazard to the patient during surgical interventions. In that case, the forced distance drops to 20 cm.
  - At 20 cm, the intensity of the x-ray beam is over 10 times greater than at the point where regulatory outputs are measured.
  - A suggested distance of the image receptor above the patient might be 30 cm.

- In oblique or lateral orientations, the image receptor should be positioned as close to the patient as possible without interfering with the medical devices.
  - This practice places the X-ray source as far from the patient as possible.
  - Personnel standing on the side of the patient were the x-ray source originates will receive the greatest amount of scatter while those on the image receptor side will receive lower amounts.

The Golden Rule

- The golden rule is to use only the least amount of fluoroscopy necessary to safely and effectively complete the procedure.
- The timer will record the minutes of fluoroscopy used. This should be checked against procedure times typical of that procedure and used as a quality control measure to assure that fluoroscopy is not overused. (Some machines do not record the time of engagement.)
- If the machine does not record true pedal engagement time, then the reading will be of little value.)

Last-Image Hold

- All fluoroscopy units have a feature called "last-image hold."
- After fluoroscopy, the x-ray image most recently displayed during fluoroscopy remains on the screen.
- It is a valuable tool for the physician to use to study the status of the procedure since no radiation is applied during this time.
- If documentation is needed, most units allow the operator to save the image as part of the patient's record, saving the need for additional radiation exposure.

Use of Collimation

- Collimators are used to block off areas of the patient that do not need to be in the image.
- This helps keep the radiation exposure burden to the patient at a minimum and reduces stray radiation.
- Most machines are equipped with virtual collimator tools that allow the operator to manipulate the collimators while watching a virtual indicator showing where the collimator blades are positioned over the last-image display.
- With this tool, the collimator blades are moved into position without the need for a fluoroscopic image.
- When using a lateral beam orientation, collimation can effectively be used to block the beam that would otherwise exist above the posterior skin surface of the patient.
  - This part of the x-ray beam not only exposes the image receptor to unattenuated raw beam, which

reduces image quality, it also presents a radiation hazard if the hands must be manipulating devices at the back of the patient.
- Collimating the field inward to assure all the beam passes internally through the patient markedly reduces the radiation hazard and improves image quality

Use of Magnification

- Electronic magnification of the image is possible by selection of various imaging field sizes.
- Selection of a smaller field size provides a magnified image because the imaged field is expanded across the entire face of the physician's monitor.
- For procedures that use only a few minutes of fluoroscopy, there are no significant radiation management issues regarding the uses of these options.
- For long procedures that use more than 30 minutes of fluoroscopy or require lengthy image acquisition runs, the rule is to use the minimal magnification necessary to complete the procedure safely and effectively. This general rule might or might not have a significant impact on safety, depending on how the machine manages dose rates to the patient as magnification changes. Such management varies greatly among manufacturers.

Dose Rate Controls

- Dose rate controls adjust radiation output rates solely by changing the intensity of the beam.
- Three options are often available: normal mode, low-dose mode, and HLC. Sometimes, more options are available.
- When low dose is used, the machine changes its AERC to work at a low-out level. This saves radiation exposure to everyone and should be used whenever the image quality produced is adequate for the safe and efficient completion of the procedure.
- HLC boosts radiation output for those special situations that require exceptionally good image quality during fluoroscopy. This mode should be used sparingly.

Pulse Rate Controls

- Another way to change radiation output is to use a different pulse frequency for fluoroscopy.
- If kVp, mA, pulse width, and filtration remain the same, but pulse frequency is reduced, then radiation output rate drops.
- If pulse frequency increases, output rate increases. The tradeoff in image quality is in the continuity of motion.
- Lower pulse rates result in jerkier image progression while high pulse rates result in higher fidelity of fluid motion perception. Lower pulse rates also result in

poorer eye integration and a perception of noisier images.
- The lowest pulse rate as is necessary for safe and efficient completion of the procedure should be used.
- An important caveat is that not all manufacturers design fluoroscopic pulse rate options in the same way. The manufacturer might change the pulse intensity or duration when the rate is adjusted. If that happens, then there may not be any dose savings at lower pulse rates. The user must verify with the manufacturer or with a physicist whether or not the lower pulse rate option truly results in a lower dose rate.

Acquisitions

- Typically, the manufacturer uses information on radiation output obtained during fluoroscopy to adjust radiation output for image acquisition runs for improved image quality.
- The user is in control of the rate of acquisition (images per second) and the duration of the acquisition and careful attention should be paid to keeping both to the minimum necessary to safely and efficiently complete the procedure.

RADIATION SAFETY HABITS AND TOOLS

Radiation safety habits and tools should be used in combination to create the safest possible environment for both the patient and the staff. The previous discussions were primarily related to methods to best manage radiation exposures to the patient and, collaterally, to keep stray radiation in the room to a minimum. We will now discuss methods by which the personnel can further protect themselves from radiation exposure.

DISTANCE

- Stray radiation emanating from the patient drops off rapidly as distance from the irradiated area of the patient increases.
- Ancillary personnel should position themselves at the furthest distance from the irradiated site of the patient that is compatible with their ability to effectively and efficiently complete their duties.
- This distance will depend on their responsibilities for care of the patient and will not be the same for all personnel.
- The goal is for each person to minimize their radiation exposure to the least amount necessary to perform their assigned tasks.

- Physicians should learn to maximize their distance by stepping back from the patient when possible before engaging fluoroscopy.
- For serial run acquisitions, the same rule applies but in this case it might be possible to step further back or to step behind a stand-up shield.

SHIELDING

Aprons

- Protective aprons are an essential tool when personnel must freely move about in the room during a procedure.
- Aprons should block a sufficient amount of radiation while not placing too much weight on the shoulders, back, and waist of the individual.
- The National Council on Radiation Protection and Measurements (NCRP) recommends a minimum "lead equivalent" thickness of 0.35 mm. This, combined with other safety measures, should be adequate for pain management personnel.
- The aprons must fit the individual comfortably and protect the front and sides of the body.
- For women, the apron should cover all breast tissue, as the female breast for women under the age of 35 years is the most sensitive organ for radiation-induced cancer.
- It is not necessary to cover the thyroid, but this organ will be discussed later.
- Light-weight aprons are now available and have the advantage that the protective value can be very high. Some physicians have recommended them, but they are not commonly used

Hand Protection

- Radiation-attenuating surgical protective gloves are usually an expensive means to achieve a very minimal benefit.
- Sometimes the gloves are counterproductive to protection.
- Remember, fluoroscopes use an AERC to adjust radiation output to penetrate the patient.
  - If radiation-attenuating gloves are inserted into the fluoroscopy beam, the machine will adjust output to penetrate the gloves.
  - This will result in no protection for the operator and will increase radiation exposure to the patient and increase stray radiation in the room.
  - Physicians should never insert their hands into the radiation field since radiation-attenuating surgical gloves are inadequate for protection and increase radiation dose.

- We have previously discussed the fact that the x-ray tube is positioned below the patient during frontal imaging so that the patient acts as a shield for the physician operator. This is an essential orientation if the hands must be inserted into the field during fluoroscopy, as previously discussed.
- The best method to protect hands is to keep hands out of the fluoroscopy field.
- If hands are visible in the image, they are in the field.
- Physicians should use mechanical aids, such forceps or tongs, to perform tasks that must be completed during active fluoroscopy.
- Using collimation to assist in protection has been discussed previously.

Thyroid Protection

- The thyroid is a hypersensitive organ for children.
- This fact has little relevance to pain management unless the patient is a child.
- For adults, the thyroid loses its sensitivity with increasing age.
- Protection of the thyroid is, therefore, not as essential as it was once thought.
- However, for individuals who work in close proximity to the patient, it is a recommended protective garment

Eye Protection

- The human lens is more sensitive to radiation than previously thought.
- The threshold dose for cataract induction is no more than 0.7 Gy or 700 mGy but may be lower.
  - Although this dose level is relatively high, protection against exposure is recommended for individuals who work in close proximity to the irradiated area of the patient.
- Purchase of personal quality protective eyewear of 0.35-mm lead equivalent is recommended for those individuals but is unnecessary for other personnel.

Leg Protection

- Legs are not radiation sensitive but chronic exposure in close proximity to the patient might result in high doses over many years that theoretically could be consequential.
- Remember, with the x-ray tube under the patient, radiation is most intensely scattered backward off of the patient toward the floor and legs of any worker in close proximity to the patient (ie, the physician).
- Maximizing working distance from the patient effectively avoids undo exposures. Use of stand-alone shields to protect legs can also have great protective value.

Stand Alone or Ceiling Mounted Shields

- Stand-alone or upright radiation shields are a valuable asset to any fluoroscopy suite. Such devices can be used by personnel whose immediate assistance is not required.
- To be effective, the shield must be placed between the protected individual and the source of the radiation, ie, the irradiated anatomy of the patient and/or the x-ray tube.
- Ceiling suspended shields are useful to operators for head and eye protection; however, they may not be practical due to the sterile nature of the procedure.

MONITORING DOSES

The most important radiation safety activity is to assiduously wear and review your radiation exposure monitor(s). This simple device is the best way to assure that your long-term accumulation of radiation exposure never exceeds levels that would be inordinate for your profession.

Whole-Body Exposure Monitoring

- If you wear only one badge, it should be worn outside the protective apron and near the neck and shoulder level.
  - Wearing it attached to a thyroid collar is convenient.
  - If you do not wear a thyroid collar, attaching it to the collar of the protective apron is satisfactory.
- Whether or not a reading is acceptable or unacceptable depends to some extent on what your job duties are.
  - No one should have a reading in excess of 10 mSv (1000 mrem) per month.
  - I recommend physicians remain under 3 mSv (300 mrem) per month, with a target of less than 1 mSv (100 mrem) per month.
  - Ancillary personnel should not exceed 1 mSv per month (100 mrem per month).
- State regulation might require that a worker's effective dose be estimated from this radiation monitor readout. For example, the effective dose might be estimated as one-third of the collar badge reading. This is a crude construct that overestimates the true effective dose, but may be required for regulatory purposes.

Extremity Exposure Monitoring

- Unless the individual is prone to having their hands in the image field during fluoroscopy or acquisition imaging, there should be no need for a hand dosimeter.

- Hand dosimeters are usually rings to be worn on the most exposed finger with the radiation-sensitive detector facing the x-ray source.
- These monitors should never exceed 5 mSv (500 mrem) per month and should be considerably lower than that.
- It is important to remember that these monitors do not necessarily record the exposure to the fingertips, which can be much higher than the sensor reading.
- If an individual is prone to having their hands in the beam and the monitor readings are 500 mrem per month, then the fingertips might still be at risk for long-term radiation damage.
- The best rule is to keep hands out of the live beam unless essential for patient safety.

Under-Apron Monitors (Required by some States and for Pregnancy)

- Sometimes workers wear two monitors, one at the collar and one under the apron at the waist.
- In some States, two monitors are required by regulation.
- For these States, effective dose is calculated using a formula that incorporates the two readings to produce a final official effective dose estimate.
- Pregnant workers may also wear a radiation monitor under their protective apron to determine the potential exposure to the unborn child, and it is recommended that all women of child-bearing potential wear an under-apron monitor before they become pregnant.
  - Monitoring the under-apron exposure before pregnancy provides information about the safety level of the working environment ahead of any pregnancy event and takes the guesswork out of the safety questions that inevitably arise when no precedent under-apron monitoring takes place.
  - Pregnant women may continue to work in an x-ray environment as long as certain regulatory requirements are met, but should discuss risks with their partner before deciding whether to continue to work around radiation.
  - Pregnancy is an important and emotional time for parents and regardless of the level of radiation safety, working around radiation may cause an overriding anxiety for some individuals.
  - While a safe radiation environment can be created for pregnant women to continue working, some pregnant women do not want any radiation exposure.
  - If a woman does wish to continue to working in the x-ray suite while pregnant, she should notify the radiation safety officer who can review her exposure history and provide extra protective measures in order to be extra safe.

○ Extra measures may include a small lap apron to be worn under the lead apron as an extra measure of protection for the conceptus.

○ It might also be worthwhile to have the pregnant woman wear a real-time monitor that can be checked daily to assure that daily exposures do not exceed 3 microSv (0.003mSv or 0.3mrem). This would guarantee the dose to the child over the gestation time would be less than 10% of what is allowed by regulation.

○ A second radiation monitor that records long-term exposure might additionally be required by regulation.

CONCLUSION

• Professionals who work with radiation on a regular basis should be expert in radiation safety so that radiation is managed well and no worker is exposed to unnecessarily high radiation doses that accumulate over time.

• Many professionals have been injured due to lack of knowledge and a cavalier attitude toward radiation. Injuries include radiation-induced cataracts, radiation-induced cancer, and radiation-induced hand injuries.

• Excessive exposure to radiation has been documented or highly suspected to have injured physicians and other personnel in modern times.

• Radiation injury is as relevant today as it has been in the past and will never be entirely vanquished unless professionals understand and abide by radiation safety standards.

56 ULTRASOUND-GUIDED INTERVENTIONAL PAIN PROCEDURES

Dmitri Souzdalnitski, MD, PhD
Imanuel R. Lerman, MD

INTRODUCTION

• *Ultrasound-guided pain management interventions* (UGPMI) has become increasingly popular as evidenced by a dramatic increase in the number of publications and by the growing number of workshops offered at regional, national, and international conferences.

• UGPMI remains essentially an *operator-dependent technique*. Understanding the basic principles of

TABLE 56-1 Principles of Performing Ultrasound-Guided Interventional Procedures

PRINCIPLES OF PERFORMING ULTRASOUND-GUIDED INTERVENTIONAL PROCEDURES

• Maintenance of aseptic technique. Utilize the "Free Hand Technique" to stabilize the ultrasound probe (Figure 56-2).
• A quick scan of the target structures to confirm normal anatomy, recognize common pathology, or anatomic variations is necessary. The landmark structures, target (typically nerves, muscles, tendons, fascia, or bone surface) and structures "to avoid" including blood vessels, pleura, intestine, liver, and other, should be visualized.
• Verification of the target structure on short-axis or long-axis imaging.
• Planning for a safe needle approach to minimize tissue, vascular trauma, or injury to vital structures.
• Visualization of the tip of the needle under real-time ultrasound during its advancement toward the target.
• Injecting an initial small volume of a test solution (hydrolocalization) may help localize the tip of the needle. If the injectate is not visualized during test injection the needle is likely out of the ultrasound beam or the needle tip is intravascular. The visualization of the injectate spread should be observed throughout the injection.
• Trauma to cartilage or tendons, as well as corticosteroid injections in these structures should be avoided during musculoskeletal UGPMI.
• Relevant monitoring and resuscitation equipment should be available in the UGPMI procedural area.

UGPMI, ultrasound-guided pain management interventions.

ultrasound, familiarity with image optimization techniques, a deep knowledge of anatomy, and knowledge of needle visualization techniques are vital for a safe and effective UGPMI. The common principles of performing UGPMI are listed in Table 56-1.

RATIONALE AND ADVANTAGES

• Until recently, interventional pain procedures were being performed with either landmark, neurostimulation, or image-guided techniques. Fluoroscopy is most commonly utilized for pain management interventions, as is computed tomography (CT), though less frequently. UGPMI offers *significant advantages compared to x-ray-based imaging modalities.*

• Ultrasound allows for *soft tissue visualization,* including muscles, tendons, nerves, blood vessels, fluid filled body structures. Ultrasound can distinguish normal and pathological states, and is used to perform a dynamic examination of these structures (Figure 56-1).

○ Ultrasound allows the operator to visualize *real-time needle advancement* and the needle injectate.

○ Ultrasound allows to *avoid ionizing radiation exposure* to both the patient and the healthcare provider.

○ It *does not require iodinated contrast* routinely used with fluoroscopy or CT.

○ Ultrasound machines typically are not expensive, they are portable, require minimal maintenance, and

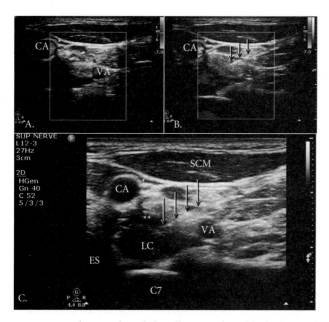

FIG. 56-1. Ultrasound-guided stellate ganglion block (cervical sympathetic block). Stellate ganglion block (SGB) is typically utilized in the diagnosis and treatment of sympathetically medicated pain of the head, neck, and arm. Traditional techniques including landmarks or fluoroscopically guided procedures may result in major complications due to inability to visualize esophagus, vessels, nerves, and other soft tissues during the procedure. Ultrasound-guided SGB allows direct visualization of the relevant anatomical structures. Therefore, risk of nerve, vascular, and soft tissue injury may be decreased. Panels A, B, and C represent a transverse view of the neck at the level of the C7 vertebral body. The compressible jugular vein (*), carotid artery (CA), and vertebral artery (VA) can be viewed under Color Doppler ultrasound (Panels A, B). Color Doppler ultrasound enhances visualization of the moving needle tip as well as during hyrdrolocalization red arrows (Panel B). The esophagus can be easily visualized by asking the patient to swallow, at which time air bubbles will be seen within the lumen. Panel C demonstrates a 2D sonogram of the longus colli (LC) muscle, the needle and needle tip (in an in-plane approach), and the deposition of injectate (**) within the prevertebral fascia. Pre-scan with Color Doppler ultrasound (Panels A, B) can aid in planning for the approach, ie, in-plane or out-of-plane needle advancement.

are *readily available in virtually any clinical setting.* In small practices, the ultrasound unit can be used by multiple specialists (in anesthesiology, cardiology, emergency medicine, gastroenterology, neurology, rheumatology, surgery, and other).

o In many instances UGPMI may result in a *safer procedure* and more reliable and consistent outcomes compared to other imaging modalities.

o UGPMI is potentially very *cost-effective.*

o With relatively basic training followed by hands-on experience, a physician can rapidly become proficient in interventional ultrasound-guided procedures.

o So far, hospitals grant ultrasound privileges based on the scope of practice, and *do not require special certification or board examination.*

DISADVANTAGES

• Ultrasound *images are not always recognizable.* For many current pain physicians imaging under fluoroscopy provides a more recognizable anatomical landmark than with ultrasound.

• *Needle visualization* during its advancement, and following the injectate beyond the immediate needle tip, is sometimes challenging even for an experienced operator. It can be hard to visualize needles in more than one plane, unless 3D ultrasound is employed.

• While bone surfaces are clearly visible with ultrasound, the *images beyond bony structures are lost.*

• USPMI *sometimes require three or more hands at a time.*

• *Deep tissue ultrasound imaging is challenging to use in morbidly obese* patients.

• USPMI is not routinely presented in the residency and fellowship programs; therefore, it *requires additional training.*

BASICS OF THE ULTRASOUND IMAGING

• The ultrasound machine creates sound pulses using the *piezoelectric effect.* The piezoelectric effect is the electromechanical interaction between the mechanical and the electrical state in a crystalline material. When exposed to an electrical field the piezoelectric material can generate a mechanical tension and resultant sound wave. On the other hand, the electromechanical property of quartz crystals and certain ceramics generates an electrical field resulting from sound pressure waves that return to the transducer. Therefore, the ultrasound probe functions as both ultrasound generator and scanner of returning sound waves. The change in the electric field generated from returning sound waves is then relayed to an imaging processing unit and translated into an image representation visualized on the ultrasound machine display screen.

• *Acoustic impedance* is a physical property that describes the portion of sound waves that will reflect off of a material compared to the portion of sound waves that continues to transmit through a material. Acoustic impedance is proportional to the density of the material and the speed of sound waves in the material. Dense objects (such as needles) have larger acoustic impedances compared to less dense objects (such as nerves and muscles). At the interface of two different types of material, a larger difference in acoustic impedance means more sound waves will be reflected rather than transmitted.

- The velocity of the ultrasound sound wave varies. For most tissues, the **acoustic velocity is approximately 1500 m/s to 1600 m/s.**

- Ultrasound waves penetrate depending on frequency, wavelength, and tissue structure. Routine ultrasound *wave frequencies* used in pain management range from 3 to 20 MHz. These frequencies are higher than what a human ear can detect (normally 12 Hz–20 kHz). The acoustic waves generated from the ultrasound transducer probe move through the body, are reflected off of tissues, and are transmitted back to the ultrasound probe. The information is then processed into an image that is exposed on the screen. Higher frequency waves experience more attenuation (loss of intensity) than lower frequency waves. As a result, higher frequency waves are not able to penetrate tissue as deeply as lower frequency waves are. However, higher frequency waves provide better resolution.

- Ultrasound machines often have an assortment of probes. The probes differ in their geometry (linear, curvilinear, footprint). *Linear probes* are typically used for superficial structures, and utilize higher frequencies aimed to improve image resolution. *Curvilinear probes* usually utilize lower frequencies and therefore are routinely applied for procedures aimed at deeper tissue; however, the resolution is proportionally decreased as the depth of the target image is increased.

SONOGRAPHIC ARTIFACTS

- *Artifacts* result from the image procurement and handling. *Anisotropy* is an effect of acoustic beam misalignment causing ultrasound wave degradation. Anisotropy can cause hyperechoic objects to appear hypoechoic and/or anechoic. It can be corrected by probe positioning. *Reverberation* is caused by the reflection of an acoustic beam from multiple surfaces between each surface and the ultrasound transducer. *Duplication* is a mirror image artifact. *Shadowing* is most commonly seen at the edge of fluid containing structures (ie, vessels), when a hypoechoic area is seen seep to an edge of a fluid containing structure (Figure 56-1).

SONOGRAPHIC MODES AND IMAGE OPTIMIZATION TOOLS

- The *A-mode* (A stands for Amplitude) is considered the oldest *ultrasound mode.* The transducer sends a *single pulse* and waits for a return. Echoes are plotted against the depth. Currently, the A-mode is rarely used. *M-mode* (M stands for Motion) detects flow changes; however, this mode is rarely used in interventional pain management. *B-mode* (B stands for Brightness) is the most commonly used mode in pain management. In the the transducer sends a *series of ultrasound pulses* which are separated in time to allow for the probe to detect returning sound waves or *echo pulses.* Some ultrasound machines use complex, internally rotating probes to permit *3D* (three-dimensional) imaging.

- *Color Doppler* is used to identify vascular structures by visualizing flow within them. Usually the movement toward the probe is colored red on the screen, while movement away from the probe is blue. Therefore, either arteries or veins can be presented as red or blue, depending on the position of the probe. *Power Doppler*, also termed Amplitude Doppler, detects the presence of flow, but does not provide velocity or directional information. A single color is used to show flow on the screen. The Power Doppler allows *detection of low flows and smaller vessels.*

- Typical ultrasound machines have an *adjustable depth control.* The target area should be just within the adequate ultrasound depth in order to maximize resolution. Increased depth will reduce resolution and narrow the imaging field. Frequency of the ultrasound transducer will be automatically changed in most ultrasound machines.

- *Auto-focus* features are typically available, but focus can be changed manually, so the target area will be within the focal zone of the beam. Typically there is an indicator on the screen which shows the details of the focal zone set.

- *Time gain compensation* (TGC) allows gain to be adjusted based on depth. Without this correction, target structures will look brighter in the superficial areas and darker in the deep areas. Ultrasound units usually adjust for this automatically by increasing the gain for the more attenuated waves. On the other hand, manual gain compensation helps control the entire image in the way that everything on the screen either looks brighter or darker. Increasing gain reduces resolution, and may increase chances of artifacts. Inadequate gain can make the image too obscure and prevent visualization of important structures.

- *Beam steering* has been more and more used to improve needle visualization during ultrasound-guided interventions. It works by a software-controlled angle optimization of the beam between the probe and the needle. Other technological developments which have improved ultrasound image quality include increased scanner and transducer bandwidth, compound imaging, and other innovative technologies of signal processing.

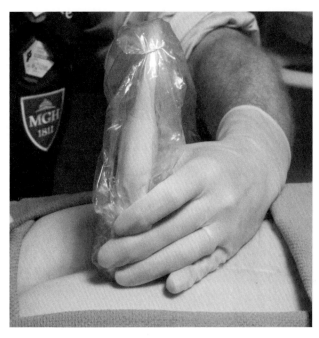

FIG. 56-2. The operator is carrying out a caudal epidural steroid injection under ultrasound guidance. The free-hand technique allows the operator increased stability and control of the ultrasound probe. This technique can dramatically improve needle visibility while undergoing small but accurate movements, including probe (1) sliding, (2) tilting, (3) angulation, and (4) rotation.

- Combinations of ultrasound with fluoroscopy, CT, magnetic resonance imaging, and photoacoustic imaging are under development, and seem very promising in improving the image quality for UGPMI.
- Saving, printing and transferring UGPMI (images and videos) to hospital databases is available in most facilities. The digital image is a widely accepted form of proof of the satisfactorily performed procedure. The targeted anatomical structures, important vital structures, needle advancement, and injectate spread are important to label.

- Use of echogenic needles, needle guides, various advanced needle positioning systems, **hydrolocalization,** and other techniques have been utilized to help *improve needle visualization.* The practicing needle tracking technique is, however, probably most important. One of the most significant adjustments the operator can make while undergoing UGPMI is to utilize the *Free Hand Technique* by placing the operator's little and/or ring finger on the patient while simultaneously holding ultrasound transducer with the index and middle finger (Figure 56-2). In addition, the operator can improve visualization of the needle and target by (1) maintaining adequate probe pressure and alignment, (2) maintaining adequate needle alignment, and (3) gently rotating and tilting of the probe.

INDICATIONS, CONTRAINDICATIONS, AND HEALTH HAZARDS

- Indications to the UGPMI include a variety of musculoskeletal, visceral, vascular, and neurological problems. The level of difficulty of UGPMI performance varies as well. The musculoskeletal procedures seem to be most commonly performed UGPMI, and they are relatively easy to perform. Table 56-2 lists commonly performed UGPMI.
- Contraindications to UGPMI are comparable with other interventional pain management procedures. UGPMI should be avoided in patients with severe infections, infections at the site of the injection, inability to provide consent, or to interact with the patient during the UGPMI procedure or if the patient declines the procedure. Neuraxial procedures are contraindicated in patients with coagulopathy or low platelets.
- There are no known absolute contraindications to the use of ultrasound for the needle guidance. For example, some UGPMI can be safely performed in pregnant patients if supported by patient's obstetrician. However, it is important to remember that ultrasound

TABLE 56-2 Procedures Performed with Ultrasound Guidance

MUSCULOSKELETAL PROCEDURES	PERIPHERAL NERVES PROCEDURES	NEURAXIAL PROCEDURES
• Large Joint Injection	• Greater Occipital Nerve	• Cervical Nerve Root
• Intermediate Joint Injection	• Stellate Ganglion Block	• Third Occipital Nerve Block
• Small Joint Injection	• Intercostal Nerve Block	• Cervical Facet and Medial Branch Block
• Joint Aspiration	• Suprascapular Nerve Block	• Thoracic Paravertebral Block
• Tendons and Ligaments Injections	• Iliohypogastric Nerve Block	• Celiac Plexus Block*
• Peritendonous and Periarticular Injections	• Ilioinguinal Nerve Block	• Lumbar Facet*
• Periarticular Bursae Injections	• Transversus Abdominal Plane (Tap) Block	• Lumbar Nerve Root*
• Sacroiliac Joint Injections	• Lateral Femoral Cutaneous Nerve Block	• Caudal, Sacral Foramina Injections
• Intramuscular Injections	• Genitofemoral Nerve Block	
• Trigger Point Injections	• Pudendal Nerve Block	
• Chemical Denervation with Botulinum Toxin	• Upper and Lower Extremity Peripheral Nerves	

*These procedures are not routinely performed, but still presented in the literature.

energy may have some short-lived biologic effects, for example, local increase in the temperature and cavitation. Therefore, it is suggested that the pain physician should reasonably limit the use of ultrasound to perform UGPMI procedure. The prolonged effects of tissue warming and cavitation in humans are not currently described in the literature.

BIBLIOGRAPHY

Narouze S, Peng PW. Ultrasound-guided interventional procedures in pain medicine: a review of anatomy, sonoanatomy, and procedures. part II: axial structures. *Reg Anesth Pain Med.* 2010;35(4):386–396.

Narouze SN, Provenzano D, Peng P, et al. The American Society of Regional Anesthesia and Pain Medicine, the European Society of Regional Anaesthesia and Pain Therapy, and the Asian Australasian Federation of Pain Societies Joint Committee recommendations for education and training in ultrasound-guided interventional pain procedures. *Reg Anesth Pain Med.* 2012;37(6):657–664.

Peng PW, Narouze S. Ultrasound-guided interventional procedures in pain medicine: a review of anatomy, sonoanatomy, and procedures: part I: nonaxial structures. *Reg Anesth Pain Med.* 2009;34(5):458–474.

57 ACUPUNCTURE—A THERAPEUTIC TOOL FOR PAIN AND PALLIATIVE MEDICINE

Albert Y. Leung, MD

INTRODUCTION

- Acupuncture is an ancient treatment modality used in a variety of illnesses.
- The therapy often consists of stimulating specific points of the body via inserted small needles.
- In addition to the practitioners (over 100,000) certified by the National Certification Commission for Acupuncture and Oriental Medicine, more than 3000 physicians in the United States are currently using acupuncture for treating different symptoms, including chronic pain, nausea, addiction disorders, and cancer-related symptom management.
- Although the empirical principles governing the practice of acupuncture are largely based upon metaphysical doctrines within Traditional Chinese Medicine

(TCM), the latest evidence from basic science research and controlled clinical trials has provided insightful information regarding the clinical indication and neurophysiological mechanisms of acupuncture.

HISTORICAL BACKGROUND

TRADITIONAL CHINESE MEDICINE

- Acupuncture was first used in China approximately 4000 to 5000 years ago. This modality of treatment was considered an integral part of TCM.
- Huangdi Neijiang (Yellow Emperor's Classic text of Internal Medicine), published in 200 BC, was the first textbook that systematically described the concept of TCM and the principles guiding the practice of acupuncture.
- With the advancement of medicinal tools throughout the history of civilization, different materials including stones, bronze, silver, and gold were used in the practice of acupuncture.
- Different methods of needle stimulation including manual manipulation, moxibustion (lighted sticks of a herbal medicine, *artemis vulgaris*), heat, and electroacupuncture (EA) have been applied to this ancient therapeutic technique (Figure 57-1).

MERIDIANS AND QI

- In TCM, the human body is considered a miniature model of the universe. Therefore, the laws governing the universe similarly regulate the human body.
- The main principles forming the foundation of TCM include Yin-Yang and the Five Elements. Yin-Yang emphasizes the balance of a duality of energy, namely Yin and Yang, existing in nature; therefore, an imbalance of the duality was thought to be the cause of illness.

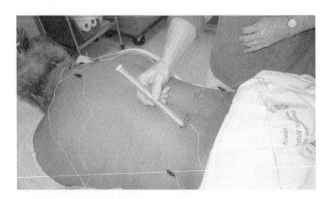

FIG. 57-1. Electroacupuncture with Moxibustion.

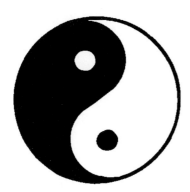

FIG. 57-2. As perceived in Traditional Chinese Medicine, the symbol of Yin-Yang represented the duality that exists in the nature and an imbalance of which will lead to illness.

- The Five Elements Principle embodying the elements of Fire, Earth, Metal, Water, and Wood complements the Yin-Yang Principle.
- Within the Five Elements Principle, each element exerts its unique regulatory effect on the other elements. The energy existing within these systems is called "Qi."
  - The channels conducting the flow of Qi are called the meridians.
  - In TCM, the occurrence of the illness is thought to be due to stagnation or an imbalance of Qi, in either an excess or a deficient state.
  - Manipulating the acupuncture points along the meridians, one can correct the imbalance of Qi,

and thus reestablishing the overall well-being of an individual (Figures 57-2 and 57-3).

ACUPUNCTURE POINTS

- Over 360 classic acupuncture points can be found in a human body. Although it is likely these points have been established over many years of trial and error, they share some common characteristics:
  - Tenderness on palpation
  - High electrical conductance
  - Fibrillation and fasciculation potentials with electromyography
  - Erythema on insertion of a needle
  - Paresthesia in distant parts of the body
- A previous study also found a greater than 70% correlation between myofascial trigger points and acupuncture points.
- In addition, a high correspondence also exists between motor and acupuncture points.
- The pattern of meridians in the extremities highly resembles the distribution of peripheral nerves.
- Practitioners with various training backgrounds in acupuncture also utilize other body systems including the ear, hand, and scalp (Figure 57-4).

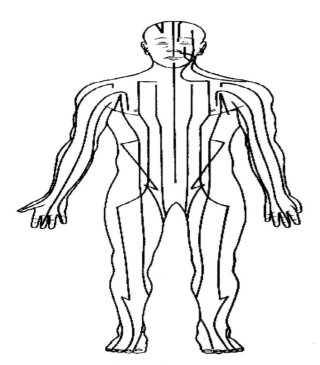

FIG. 57-3. The distribution of classical acupuncture meridians, the channels in which "Qi" flows.

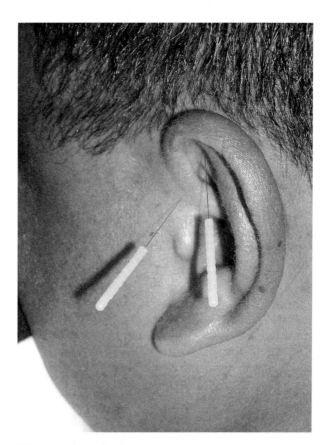

FIG. 57-4. Auricular electroacupuncture.

ACUPUNCTURE IN THE UNITED STATES

- Despite the early acceptance of acupuncture as an alternative therapy in most Asian and European countries, acupuncture did not receive the same degree of attention in the United States until early 1970s.
- Since concluding that acupuncture is "effective" in two conditions (postoperative or postchemotherapy nausea, and dental pain) in 1998, the National Institute of Health (NIH) has funded many projects to assess the efficacy and underlying mechanisms of acupuncture. The investigation leads to an overall better understanding in the underlying mechanisms of acupuncture and more clinical evidence in supporting the use of acupuncture for several chronic pain conditions as discussed in the next two sections of this chapter.

NEUROHUMORAL MECHANISM OF ACUPUNCTURE

PLACEBO OR NOT

- Due to the empirical nature of the principles governing the use of acupuncture, the clinical effect of acupuncture has been doubted by some as a purely placebo response. Several lines of evidence provide strong argument against this notion.
- Acupuncture has been used in Veterinary Medicine in both surgical anesthesia and treating illness in animals.
- Numerous reports regarding the use of acupuncture in pediatric patients can be found in the acupuncture literature.
- Pharmacological evidence suggests that the analgesic effect of acupuncture is partially naloxone reversible in both human and animal studies. This body of published and observational evidence argue against the notion that the observed clinical benefits of acupuncture for the past several thousand years have been a purely placebo effect.
- Evidence supporting the neuromodulatory effect of acupuncture continues to emerge in both animal and human studies.

PERIPHERAL MECHANISM

- The modality-specificity of different peripheral sensory fibers, namely A-β, A-δ, and C-fibers, is well described in literature.
  - Broadly speaking, high-frequency and low-threshold mechano-stimulation is transmitted by the myelinated A-β fibers.
  - Cool and well-localized pain is carried by the less myelinated A-δ fiber, whereas warm, hot, and cold pain sensations are carried by the unmyelinated C-fiber.
- Activation of myelinated primary afferent fibers (A-fibers) will inhibit small unmyelinated primary afferent fibers (c-fibers).
- Acupuncture needles appear to stimulate primarily small myelinated A-δ afferent nerve fibers to achieve its analgesic benefit.

CENTRAL NEUROMODULATORY MECHANISM

In correlation with peripheral neuromodulatory mechanisms, several central mechanisms have been postulated for the clinical benefits observed with acupuncture treatment:

- Endorphinergic system
  - Several lines of evidence strongly support the supraspinal β-endorphin involvement as the main mechanism of acupuncture analgesia.
  - In a cross-perfusion experiment, an acupuncture-induced analgesic effect was transferred from the donor rabbit to the recipient rabbit when the cerebrospinal fluid (CSF) was transferred.
  - The effect of acupuncture analgesia could be reversed with naloxone, and the inhibition of degradation of met-enkephalin by D-phenylalanine or D-leucine enhanced the acupuncture analgesic.
  - Subsequent studies demonstrated that the release of different subtypes of endorphin appeared to be frequency-dependent. For example, antiserum of met-enkephalin, dynorphine A and B reduced 2, 15, and 100 Hz acupuncture effect, respectively, suggesting frequency-dependent endorphin release in response to EA.
  - Other studies also suggest that EA analgesia is mediated through the periadqueductal gray (PAG) and shares the common descending inhibitory mechanisms of the exogenous opioids.
  - The effect of acupuncture in reducing withdrawal symptoms of narcotic addicts further implied the endorphinergic involvement in the acupuncture analgesic mechanisms.
- Nonendorphinergic mechanism
  - The effect of acupuncture on serotonin level has also been implicated in the overall neurohumoral mechanisms of acupuncture as the vasodilatory effect of acupuncture was blocked by the serotonin antagonist (cyproheptadine) but not by naloxone.
  - Inhibition of serotonin inactivation by clomipramine enhanced acupuncture analgesia. Acupuncture could increase plasma cortisol levels in horses and induced the release of both endorphins and adrenocorticotropic hormones. Such an effect appeared to be

bilateral and to had a nonsegmental cranio-caudal gradient, and is not naloxone reversible.

ONGOING RESEARCH IN ACUPUNCTURE

- The neurophysical linkage of acupuncture analgesic related mechanisms at the supraspinal level derived from the latest research using functional imaging in which a supraspinal sedative effect was noted.
- Needle manipulation at the extremities decreased activities in brain regions commonly associated with pain perception. This preliminary evidence suggests that acupuncture may modulate the hypothalamus-limbic system and subcortical gray structures of the human brain.
- Although both sham and real EA activated the reported distributed pain neuromatrix, real EA elicited significantly higher degree of activation than sham EA over the hypothalamus and primary somatosensory-motor cortex and deactivation over the rostral anterior cingulate cortex, suggesting the higher neuromodulatory effect of meridian points over the non-meridian points in the hypothalamus-limbic system.
- In addition, comparing to EA given at minimal intensity, EA provided at optimal intensity induced an overall more robust sedative effect in the supraspinal regions related to pain processing.

CLINICAL APPLICATION

ACUPUNCTURE IN THE TREATMENT OF ACUTE INJURY PAIN

- According to classical acupuncture literature, the anatomy of acupuncture is divided into different channels, so-called meridians, within which lie specific acupuncture points.
- The tendinomuscular meridian subsystem is located on the surface of the body.
- The tendinomuscular meridians can be used for the treatment of pain, swelling, contraction, spasm, and other forms of acute trauma. The best results of this method of acupuncture are obtained when patients are treated within 12 to 24 hours of the injury.

- Twelve tendinomuscular meridians exist in a human body with each one starting at a toe tip or fingertip.
- The tendinomuscular meridians can be activated by
  - stimulating the so-called Ting point(s) of the relevant meridians located at the toe of fingers;
  - stimulating the gathering point(s) of the relevant meridians located in the trunkal areas); and
  - surrounding the lesion with superficially placed needles.

PERIOPERATIVE USAGE OF ACUPUNCTURE

- In addition to alleviating dental pain and postoperative nausea, acupuncture can decrease the postoperative opioid requirement and reduce analgesic-related side effects in low abdominal surgery.
- Anecdotal reports also indicate that acupuncture can be used in other types of surgical procedures such as craniotomy, tonsillectomy, thyroidectomy, and labor-related procedures either as a means of supplemental anesthesia or as a tool for managing postoperative associated side effects.

ACUPUNCTURE IN CHRONIC PAIN MANAGEMENT

- The use of acupuncture in chronic pain management is probably one of the most thoroughly studied areas in medicine.
- Acupuncture has been utilized to treat a variety of chronic pain conditions. Some of these chronic pain conditions have been studied more extensively than others.
- Recent meta-analyses and Cochrane review studies deemed the use of acupuncture in managing several chronic pain conditions efficacious. These conditions include chronic neck and low back pain, and knee osteoarthritis pain (see Table 57-1).
- Acupuncture has also been found to improve physical activity, sense of well-being, and quality of sleep while reducing the need for oral nonopioid analgesic medication.
- On the other hand, similar analyses have not found conclusive or significant benefits for the use of

TABLE 57-1   Summary of Randomized Controlled Trial (RCT) for Pain-Related Acupuncture Studies

PATHOLOGICAL CONDITIONS	NUMBER OF STUDIES	CONCLUSION	AUTHORS	TYPE OF PUBLICATION
Chronic knee pain	13 RCT	Effective	White et al., 2007	Meta-analysis
Fibromyalgia	3 RCT	Inconclusive	Mayhew et al., 2007	Narrative review
Chronic neck pain	10 RCT	Effective	Trinh et al., 2006	Cochrane systemic review
Irritable Bowel syndrome	6 RCT	Inconclusive	Lim et al., 2006	Cochrane systemic review
OA	24 RCT	Effective	Kown et al., 2006	Meta-analysis
Chronic low back pain	33 RCT	Effective	Manheimer et al., 2005	Meta-analysis

TABLE 57-2 **Summary of Randomized Controlled Trial (RCT) for Non-pain-related Acupuncture Studies**

PATHOLOGICAL CONDITIONS	NUMBER OF STUDIES	CONCLUSION	AUTHORS	TYPE OF PUBLICATION
Stroke rehabilitation	5 RCT	Inconclusive	Wu et al., 2006	Cochrane systemic review
Smoking cessation	24 RCT	Not supported	White et al., 2006	Cochrane systemic review
Postoperative nausea and vomiting in adults	24 RCT	Effective	Shiao et al., 2006	Meta-analysis
Postoperative nausea and vomiting in children	12 RCT	Effective	Dune et al., 2006	Meta-analysis
Cocaine dependence	7 RCT	Inconclusive	Gates et al., 2006	Meta-analysis
Depression	7 RCT	Inconclusive	Smith et al., 2006	Meta-analysis
Depression	7 RCT	Inconclusive	Mukaino et al., 2006	Systemic analysis

acupuncture in fibromyalgia, irritable bowel diseases, smoking cessation, depression, stroke rehabilitation, and cocaine dependence (see Table 57-2, Figure 57-5).

ACUPUNCTURE IN PALLIATIVE MEDICINE

- A large body of literature supports the use of acupuncture as a safe and clinically cost-effective palliative modality

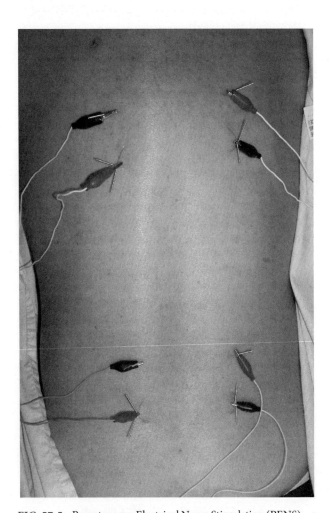

FIG. 57-5. Percutaneous Electrical Nerve Stimulation (PENS)—a form of electroacupuncture for chronic low back pain.

for managing cancer patients with debilitating symptoms such as nausea, xerostomia, pain, and dyspnea.

ADVERSE EVENTS RELATED TO ACUPUNCTURE

- Compared to pharmacological interventions, side effects associated with acupuncture are quite minimal.
- Various adverse events associated with acupuncture have been reported in literature. These adverse events, although rare, include pneumothorax, infection, and spinal lesions.
- If conducted with caution and given by adequately trained practitioners, acupuncture carries minimal risk to the patients.

SUMMARY

- Acupuncture provides a low cost and yet clinically effective treatment option for pain and cancer-related symptom management.
- Ongoing investigation in basic science and clinical trial continues to facilitate the integration of this treatment modality into the main stream medical practice.

BIBLIOGRAPHY

Fei H, Xie GX, Han JS. Differential release of met-enkephalin and dynorphin in spinal cord by electroacupuncture of different frequencies. *Kexue Tongbo*. 1986;31:1512–1515.

Hamza MA, White PF, Craig WF, et al. Percutaneous electrical nerve stimulation: a novel analgesic therapy for diabetic neuropathic pain. *Diabetes Care*. 2000;23(3):365–370.

Helms J. The tendinomuscular meridian subsystem. In: Helms J, ed. *Acupuncture Energetics: A Clinical Approach for Physicians*. Berkeley, CA: Medical Acupuncture Publishers; 1995:103–130.

Hui KK, Liu JJ, Makris N, et al. Acupuncture modulates the limbic system and subcortical gray structures of the human brain: evidence from fMRI studies in normal subjects. *Hum Brain Mapp*. 2000;9(1):13–25.

Kaada B, Eielsen O. In search of mediators of skin vasodilation induced by transcutaneous nerve stimulation: II. Serotonin implicated. *Gen Pharmacol.* 1983;14(6):635–641.

Leung AY, Kim SJ, Schulteis G, et al. The effect of acupuncture duration on analgesia and peripheral sensory thresholds. *BMC Complement Altern Med.* 2008;8:18.

Lim B, et al. Acupuncture for treatment of irritable bowel syndrome. *Cochrane Database Syst Rev.* 2006(4):CD005111.

Liu Y, Varela M, Oswald R. The correspondence between some motor points and acupuncture loci. *Am J Chin Med.* 1975;3(4):347–58.

Manheimer E, White A, Berman B, et al. Meta-analysis: acupuncture for low back pain. *Ann Intern Med.* 2005;142(8):651–663.

Mayhew E, Ernst E. Acupuncture for fibromyalgia—a systematic review of randomized clinical trials. *Rheumatology (Oxford).* 2007;46(5):801–804.

Melzack R, Stillwell DM, Fox EJ. Trigger points and acupuncture points for pain: correlations and implications. *Pain.* 1977;3(1):3–23.

NIH. *NIH Consensus Conference. Acupuncture. J Am Med Assoc.* 1998;280(17):1518–1524.

Shukla S, Torossian A, Duann JR, et al. The analgesic effect of electroacupuncture on acute thermal pain perception—a central neural correlate study with fMRI. *Mol Pain.* 2011;7:45.

Trinh KV, et al. Acupuncture for neck disorders. *Cochrane Database Syst Rev.* 2006(3):CD004870.

White A, Foster NE, Cummings M, et al. Acupuncture treatment for chronic knee pain: a systematic review. *Rheumatology (Oxford).* 2007;46(3):384–390.

White AR, Rampes H, Campbell JL. Acupuncture and related interventions for smoking cessation. *Cochrane Database Syst Rev.* 2006(1):CD000009.

Wu HM, et al. Acupuncture for stroke rehabilitation. *Cochrane Database Syst Rev.* 2006;3:CD004131.

Wu MT, et al. Neuronal specificity of acupuncture response: a fMRI study with electroacupuncture. *Neuroimage.* 2002;16(4):1028–1037.

Yamashita H, Tsukayama H, Hori N, et al. Incidence of adverse reactions associated with acupuncture. *J Altern Complement Med.* 2000;6(4):345–350.

Yarnitsky D, Ochoa JL. Warm and cold specific somatosensory systems. Psychophysical thresholds, reaction times and peripheral conduction velocities. *Brain.* 1991;114(Pt 4):1819–1826.

58 BOTULINUM TOXIN INJECTIONS

Charles E. Argoff, MD

INTRODUCTION

- The botulinum toxins are products of the anaerobic bacterium *Clostridium botulinum.*
- There are seven immunologically distinct serotypes of these extremely potent neurotoxins, types A, B, C1, D, E, F, and G. Only types A and B are available for routine clinical practice.

- Three type A preparations, Botox (onabotulinum toxin A, Allergan, Inc., Irvine, Ca., USA), Dysport (abobotulinum toxin A, Ipsen Ltd., Berkshire, UK), and Xeomin (incobotulinum toxin A, Merz Pharma, Germany), have been developed for commercial use and are currently commercially available in the United States. One type B preparation is currently commercially available as Myobloc in the United States (rimabotulinum toxin B, Solstice Neurosciences).
- These neurotoxins are proteins and vary with respect to molecular weight, mechanism of action, duration of effect, and adverse effects. The bacteria synthesize each toxin initially as a single-chain polypeptide. Bacterial proteases then "nick" both type A and type B proteins, resulting in a dichain structure consisting of one heavy chain and one light chain. Type A is nicked more than type B and there is less than 50% homology between the two toxins.
- Traditionally, most of the known effects of these toxins have been attributed to their ability to inhibit the release of acetylcholine from cholinergic nerve terminals; however, this effect does not appear to explain the apparent analgesic activity of some of these toxins. Inhibition of the release of glutamate, substance P, and calcitonin gene–related peptide reduced afferent input to the central nervous system through effects of the toxins on muscle spindles, and other possible effects on pain transmission independent of the effect on cholinergic transmission of these neurotoxins have been proposed based on the results of laboratory experiments. In particular, Cui and colleagues recently reported in a placebo-controlled study that subcutaneous injections of botulinum toxin type A (onabotulinum toxin A) into the paws of rats before exposure to the formalin model of inflammatory pain induced significant dose-dependent inhibition of both the acute and secondary pain responses. In addition to the demonstration that glutamate release in the periphery is reduced in treated as opposed to control animals, inhibition of the expression of *c-fos* was observed in the dorsal spinal cord in treated animals but not controls. These findings suggest indeed that one of the botulinum toxins (onabotulinum toxin A) very likely operates by noncholinergic mechanisms, which helps explain its analgesic effect.
- The mechanism by which acetylcholine is released by these neurotoxins is a multistep process. It is much better understood at this point than the mechanism by which these neurotoxins may exert their analgesic effects. The toxin must be internalized into the synaptic terminal to exert its anticholinergic effect. The first step in this process is the binding of the toxin to a receptor on the axon terminals of the cholinergic terminals. Each specific botulinum toxin serotype

binds specifically to its own receptor irreversibly, and neither binds nor inhibits the receptor for other serotypes. After the toxin is bound, an endosome is formed that carries the toxin into the axon terminal. The final step involves cleavage of one of the known synaptic proteins that are required for acetylcholine to be released by the axon. Botulinum toxins A, E, and C cleave synaptosome-associated protein 25 (SNAP-25). Botulinum toxins B, D, F, and G cleave synaptobrevin, also known as vesicle-associated membrane protein (VAMP). Botulinum toxin type C also cleaves syntaxin. The specific manner in which each toxin type may cleave the synaptic protein, as well the specific differences in effect on inhibiting acetylcholine release, is beyond the scope of this chapter. It has not yet been conclusively demonstrated how these differences translate into varied clinical responses, including both beneficial and adverse effects.

- Once the toxin is injected into a muscle, weakness occurs within a few days to a week and peaks most often within two weeks, and then gradually muscle weakness resolves with a slow return to baseline. This recovery is associated with sprouting of the affected axon and return of synaptic activity to the original nerve terminals. Regeneration of the cleaved synaptic protein is also required for recovery to occur.
- The duration of the clinical effect of the currently available neurotoxins appears to be approximately three months but may clearly vary from individual to individual. Additionally, the possible differences in duration of action of these toxins for different clinical conditions, for example, cervical dystonia versus migraine headache, have not been well studied to date.

CURRENT FDA-APPROVED USES OF THE BOTULINUM TOXINS

- The first botulinum toxin to be approved by the Food and Drug Administration (FDA) for use in the United States was onabotulinum toxin A (Botox) in 1989. Although originally FDA-approved for the treatment of strabismus, blepharospasm, cervical dystonia, and hemifacial spasm, it is currently also FDA approved for the treatment of overactive bladder in adults who have an inadequate response to or are intolerant of an anticholinergic medication, treatment of urinary incontinence due to detrusor overactivity associated with a neurologic condition, the prophylaxis of headaches in adult patients with chronic migraine (≥15 days per month with headache lasting 4 hours a day or longer, treatment of upper limb spasticity in adult patients, treatment of severe axillary hyperhidrosis that is inadequately managed by topical agents in adult patients,

temporary improvement in the appearance of moderate to severe glabellar lines associated with corrugator and/or procerus muscle activity in adult patients, and the temporary improvement in the appearance of moderate to severe lateral canthal limes associated with orbicularis oculi activity in adult patients.

- The second botulinum toxin to be FDA approved (2009), botulinum toxin type B (rimabotulinum B), is currently approved for cervical dystonia only.
- The second type A botulinum toxin to be FDA approved (2009), abobotulinum toxin A (Dysport), is currently FDA approved for cervical dystonia and the temporary improvement of moderate to severe glabellar lines in adults patients <65 years old. The most recently (2010) introduced and FDA-approved type A botulinum toxin, incobotulinum toxin A (Xeomin), is FDA approved for the treatment of cervical dystonia, treatment of blepharospasm, and the temporary improvement in the appearance of moderate to severe glabellar lines in adult patients.
- Even among initial published studies on the use of either onabotulinum toxin A or rimabotulinum toxin B for cervical dystonia, the analgesic effect of these agents, for example, the ability for these toxins to reduce the pain associated with cervical dystonia, was observed. In fact, the analgesic effect of the neurotoxins appeared to have a greater duration of action than other more direct neuromuscular effects.
- The discussion that follows on the use of either botulinum toxin type A or botulinum toxin type B in the management of painful states other than those noted in the above review of FDA-approved uses involves the off-label uses of these agents.

USE OF THE BOTULINUM TOXINS FOR TREATMENT OF CHRONIC HEADACHE

MIGRAINE HEADACHE

- The botulinum toxins have been used for a number of different headache types with varying responses according to the individual study.
- Initially, Dr. William Binder, a plastic surgeon, rather serendipitously made the observation that many of his patients who had undergone onabotulinum toxin A injections for the treatment of glabellar lines reported notable improvement in their headache control. As a result of this observation, he and his colleagues coordinated a multicenter open-label trial of onabotulinum toxin A in patients with migraine. Thirty-six of seventy-seven (51%) patients with migraine as defined by the International Headache Society (IHS) noted complete relief of their headaches with a mean

duration of effect of 4.1 months. Twenty-seven of seventy-seven (38%) reported a partial response. The site of injection varied from patient to patient but generally included the frontalis, temporalis, corrugator, and procerus muscles, and, in a few patients, suboccipital muscles. The dose of onabotulinum toxin A also varied from patient to patient. Except for brow ptosis, no significant adverse effects were experienced.

- Silberstein et al. reported the results of a multicenter, randomized, controlled study of onabotulinum toxin A involving 123 patients with IHS-defined migraine who experienced between two and eight severe migraine headaches each month. Patients were randomized to one of three groups: placebo, 25 units of onabotulinum toxin A, or 75 units of onabotulinum toxin A. Eleven standard injection sites were used, including the frontalis, temporalis, corrugator, and procerus muscles. Bilateral injections were performed. Compared with placebo, 25 units of onabotulinum toxin A resulted in significantly fewer and less severe migraine headaches each month, a reduction in the amount of acute headache medication used, and a lower incidence of emesis. There was no difference between the group receiving 75 units of onabotulinum toxin A and those receiving placebo. No adverse effects were noted except for 2 cases of diplopia and 13 cases of ptosis.

- In a separate study, Brin and his colleagues presented the results of a randomized, placebo-controlled multicenter study of onabotulinum toxin A in migraine prophylaxis. Patients received injections in either the frontal and temporal regions, frontal region only with placebo injections into the temporal region, temporal region only with placebo injections into the frontal region, or placebo injections into both regions. Only patients who received onabotulinum toxin A injections into both temporal and frontal regions experienced significantly greater pain relief than the placebo group.

- A variety of other studies had been reported primarily, however, as abstracts only. Nevertheless, some interesting observations had been made. In a study of 30 patients with IHS-defined migraine headache experiencing between two and eight attacks each month, patients were randomized to receive either 50 units of onabotulinum toxin A or placebo. Fifteen injection sites were used, including the temporalis, frontalis, corrugator, procerus, trapezius, and splenius capitis muscles bilaterally. Patients were followed for up to 90 days. Compared with placebo-treated patients who did not experience any significant change in headache frequency or severity, those who received onabotulinum toxin A injections had a significant reduction in headache frequency (at 90 days, 2.5 versus 5.8, $P < 0.01$) as well as severity. No significant adverse effects were noted.

- In an open-label study evaluating the effects of onabotulinum toxin A on disability in episodic and chronic migraine, treatment with 25 units of onabotulinum toxin A (frontalis, temporalis, and corrugator muscles) resulted in decreased migraine-associated disability in 58% of the patients.

- Two retrospective studies had emphasized the potential benefit of onabotulinum toxin A as a "disease-modifying" treatment for patients with chronic migraine. Each of these reports suggests (based on nonrandomized data) that increasing benefit might be experienced with repeated treatments with onabotulinum toxin A for patients with chronic migraine. These clinical observations, although not derived from randomized, controlled studies, are important to consider as many injectors do in fact believe that for maximal benefit to be realized from botulinum injections, a patient may indeed have to be treated at least several times. Ultimately, these studies led to the successful completion of the pivotal trials leading to the FDA approval of onabotulinum toxin A for chronic migraine defined as an headache that occurs 15 or more days a month with headache lasting 4 hours or longer for at least 3 consecutive months, with at least one half of the headaches being migraine in people with current or prior diagnosis of migraine.

- One open-label study involving the use of rimabotulinum toxin B for the treatment of chronic migraine headache has been reported. Forty-seven patients with at least four migraine headaches within a four-week period were treated with a total of 5000 units of rimabotulinum toxin B into at least three injection sites. Injection sites were chosen on the basis of pain distribution, "trigger points," and glabellar lines. Thirty patients (64%) reported improvement in headache intensity and severity. One adverse effect experienced with rimabotulinum toxin B treatment in this study that was not experienced by onabotulinum toxin A-treated patients was dry mouth.

TENSION-TYPE HEADACHE

- Several studies involving the use of botulinum toxin for the treatment of IHS-defined tension-type headache have been reported.

- Smuts et al. completed a randomized, controlled study of 37 patients with tension-type headache. Patients received either 100 units of onabotulinum toxin A or placebo into six injection sites: two in the temporalis muscles and four in cervical sites. By the third month postinjection, the treated group experienced a statistically significant reduction in headache severity compared with the placebo-treated group.

- A retrospective study of 21 patients with chronic tension-type headache with concurrent tenderness of the scalp or neck was conducted by Freund and Schwartz. Five injection sites were chosen and the patient received a total of 100 units of onabotulinum toxin A. The injection sites were chosen based on the sites of maximal tenderness as reported by the patient. Eighteen of the twenty-one patients experienced at least a 50% reduction in headache frequency and 20 of the 21 experienced at least a 50% reduction in scalp/neck tenderness to palpation.
- Although several other clinical reports have documented successful treatment of a small number of patients, another small study by Zwart et al. reported on six patients with tension-type headache who were treated with onabotulinum toxin A and failed to show any improvement in pain intensity following injection. One reason for this outcome may have been that in this study, patients received injections only into the temporalis muscle unilaterally.
- In a small randomized controlled study of 10 patients with tension-type headache, onabotulinum toxin A was no more effective than placebo.
- Porta evaluated the difference in response between onabotulinum toxin A and methylprednisolone injections in patients with tension-type headaches. Although both groups improved, patients who had undergone the BTX-A injections experienced improvement for a greater duration (>60 days) compared with the methylprednisolone-treated patients.

CLUSTER HEADACHE

- There have been at least three reports of treatment of cluster headache with botulinum toxin.
- In 1996, a single patient with cluster headache refractory to other treatment was reported by Ginies et al. to respond to the injection of botulinum injection.
- Two patients with intractable cluster headache were reported by Freund and Schwartz to respond to the unilateral injection of 50 units of onabotulinum toxin A into five sites within the temporalis muscle on the affected side. Within 9 days of treatment, the headaches abated for both the patients.
- Robbins reported in an open-label study that for seven patients with chronic cluster headache who were treated with onabotulinum toxin A or rimabotulinum toxin B, treatment was at least moderately effective in four of the seven and not effective in three. He also treated three patients with episodic cluster headache with botulinum toxin and two had at least moderate improvement.

CHRONIC DAILY HEADACHE

- One open-label study, one randomized, controlled study, and one case series have been reported regarding the use of botulinum toxin for the management of chronic daily headache (CDH).
- Four of five treated patients in an open-label study by Klapper and Klapper benefited from injections.
- In a randomized trial of 56 patients with CDH, patients were divided into four groups involving both forehead and suboccipital injections. Only patients who received botulinum toxin injections into each region experienced significant benefit.
- Argoff reported on three patients with CDH who were successfully treated with a total of 5000 units of BTX-B injected into the frontalis, temporalis, corrugator, splenius capitis, splenius cervicis, levator scapular, and trapezius muscles.

USE OF BOTULINUM TOXIN IN THE MANAGEMENT OF MUSCULOSKELETAL PAIN

- Painful musculoskeletal conditions that have been treated with botulinum toxin include chronic temporomandibular joint dysfunction, chronic myofascial pain, chronic cervicothoracic pain, chronic low back pain, plantar fasciitis, and epicondylitis.

TEMPOROMANDIBULAR DISORDERS

- Botulinum toxin type A has been used for a number of the temporomandibular disorders including myofascial dysfunction affecting this joint, bruxism, oromandibular dystonia, and masseter/temporalis hypertrophy.
- In an open-label study of 46 patients with chronic temporomandibular pain, Freund et al. injected onabotulinum toxin A into both masseter muscles (50 units each) and into the temporalis muscles (25 units each) under electromyographic guidance. Outcome measures that showed improvement included pain level as assessed by Visual Analog Scale (VAS) scores, interincisal oral opening, and tenderness to palpation. Approximately 60% of those treated experienced at least 50% improvement in these areas.
- In contrast, Nixdorf et al. completed a double-blind, placebo-controlled crossover trial evaluating the use of onabotulinum toxin A in the management of chronic moderate to severe orofacial pain of myogenic origin. Similar to Freund and colleagues' open-label study, 25 units of toxin was injected into each temporalis

muscle and 50 units was injected into each masseter muscle. Crossover occurred at 16 weeks. Pain intensity and unpleasantness were the primary outcome variables used. No significant difference was determined between placebo and active treatment in this study; however, only 15 patients entered the study and only 10 patients completed it, and these small numbers may have made it difficult to see a statistical difference between the two groups.

- The dose of botulinum toxin used for treatment of the temporomandibular disorders depends on the size(s) of the muscle(s) involved as well as the type of toxin used. For the temporalis and medial pterygoid muscles, the recommended doses of onabotulinum toxin A are between 5 and 25 units in multiple injection sites. For the masseter muscle, the recommended dose of onabotulinum toxin A is 25–50 units, also in multiple injection sites. For the lateral pterygoid muscle, the recommended dose of type A toxin is between 5 and 10 units. For each of these muscles, the recommended doses of type B toxin are between 1000 and 3000 units, again with multiple injection sites within each muscle.

CERVICOTHORACIC DISORDERS

- A number of studies have examined the role of botulinum toxin in the treatment of chronic cervical or thoracic pain most often associated with myofascial dysfunction.
- In their study of the use of onabotulinum toxin A injections into cervical paraspinal, trapezius, and thoracic paraspinal muscles, Wheeler et al. were not able to detect any significant differences in pain reduction between treated and placebo patients.
- Freund and Schwartz, in their randomized controlled study of 26 patients with chronic neck pain following "whiplash" injuries, demonstrated a statistically significant reduction in pain for the patients treated with onabotulinum toxin A compared with placebo. One hundred units of toxin were injected into five "tender" sites and these were compared with a similar number of saline injections. Improvement was noted after four weeks.
- Cheshire et al. injected myofascial trigger points in the cervical paraspinal or shoulder girdle area in six patients with either onabotulinum toxin A (50 units spread out over two to three areas) or saline. In this randomized, controlled, crossover study, crossover occurred at eight weeks. Four of the six patients experienced at least 30% pain reduction in response to toxin but not saline injections.

- In a prior study by Wheeler et al., 33 patients with cervical myofascial pain were injected with either 50 or 100 units of onabotulinum toxin A or placebo. No significant differences were observed between the two groups.
- Using a novel injection technique, injecting the whole muscle in a grid-like pattern instead of the areas of tenderness only, and using doses of onabotulinum toxin A ranging from 20 to 600 units, Lang, in an open-label study of the use of type A toxin in the treatment of myofascial pain, noted that 60% of patients experienced good to excellent results 22–60 days following injection.
- In a 12-week randomized, double-blind, placebo-controlled study, 132 patients with cervicothoracic myofascial pain were treated with onabotulinum toxin A or saline by Ferrante et al. No significant differences in outcome were seen between the groups. Patients receiving onabotulinum toxin A were treated with 50–250 units of toxin total divided among five injection sites.
- Porta, in a single-blinded study, evaluated the difference between lidocaine/methylprednisolone injections and onabotulinum toxin A injections in affected myofascial trigger points within the psoas, piriformis, and scalenus anterior muscles. Doses of 80–150 units of toxin were used. Each group received benefit, but the toxin-treated patients experienced a greater duration of relief.
- Opida has presented 31 patients with posttraumatic neck pain who he has treated with rimabotulinum toxin B injections in an open-label study. Seventy-one percent of his patients noted significant reductions in pain and headache frequency and severity.
- Taqi et al. have shown in two separate open-label studies that either type of botulinum toxin may be effective in the treatment of myofascial pain.
- Several case reports on the use of rimabotulinum toxin B injections in the management of chronic myofascial pain have suggested generally good results.

CHRONIC LOW BACK PAIN

- Use of botulinum toxin in the management of chronic low back pain has also been explored.
- Foster et al., in a randomized controlled study involving 31 patients with chronic low back pain, studied the effect of 200 units of onabotulinum toxin A (five sites at paravertebral levels L1 to L5 or L2 to S1, 40 units/site) compared with placebo injections. Pain and extent of disability were noted at baseline as well as at three and eight weeks using the VAS scale as well as

the Owestry Low Back Pain Questionnaire. At both three and eight weeks, more patients who had received botulinum toxin injections (73.3%/60%) experienced 50% or greater pain relief than the placebo-treated group (25%/12.5%). At eight weeks, there was less disability in the botulinum toxin-treated group than in the placebo-treated group.

- Knusel et al. treated patients with low back pain associated with painful muscle spasm with different doses of onabotulinum toxin A and noted that only those treated with the highest doses (240 units) experienced greater relief than placebo-treated patients.

PIRIFORMIS SYNDROME

- There have been reports of the use of botulinum toxin for the treatment of piriformis muscle syndrome as well.
- Childers et al. concluded, following completion of a randomized, controlled, crossover study of nine patients with piriformis muscle syndrome who were treated with both onabotulinum toxin A (100 units) and placebo, that there was a trend toward greater pain relief for patients receiving toxin as opposed to placebo. Electromyographic and fluoroscopic guidance were used for the injections.
- Fannucci et al. reported that 26 of 30 patients with piriformis syndrome who were injected with onabotulinum toxin A under CT guidance obtained relief of their symptoms within five to seven days.
- Fishman performed a dose ranging study with rimabotulin toxin B in the management of piriformis syndrome using electromyographic guidance and observed notable symptom improvement as well.

OTHER MUSCULOSKELETAL CONDITIONS

Abobotulinum toxin A (Dysport) has been studied as a treatment for patients with chronic plantar fasciitis. In a short-term, randomized, multicenter, double-blind, placebo-controlled study, 40 patients were randomized to receive 200 units of abobotulinum toxin A or saline injections given directly at the calcaneal origin of the plantar fascia. More patients in the active treatment group achieved a response at week 6 (25% vs. 5% for placebo; at study endpoint (week 18), 63.1% of the active treatment group reported improvement versus 55% of the placebo group). More than one randomized controlled study has documented the potential benefit of the use of one of the botulinum toxin preparations for the treatment of otherwise refractory chronic lateral epicondylitis. Several less well-controlled studies have suggested a possible role for the use of onabotulinum toxin A in the management of osteoarthritis of the knee.

USE OF BOTULINUM TOXIN IN THE MANAGEMENT OF NEUROPATHIC PAIN AND OTHER PAINFUL CONDITIONS

- The use of botulinum toxin for the treatment of neuropathic pain remains novel and there are only a few reports describing initial results in the management of postherpetic neuralgia, complex regional pain syndrome, trigeminal neuralgia, and spinal cord injury pain.
- Although reduction of pain is not the usual primary outcome measurement used in studies of botulinum toxin and spasticity, a study of patients treated with onabotulinum toxin A for spasticity by Wissel et al. noted the analgesic benefit of this treatment for 54 of 60 patients treated.

GENERAL CONSIDERATIONS FOR TREATMENT

- Currently, none of the available botulinum toxins is FDA approved for a specific painful state other than chronic migraine; therefore, use in pain management other than for chronic migraine (not including cervical dystonia) is in an off-label manner. Patients should be informed of such prior to treatment.
- Significant side effects are uncommon. Increased pain, muscle weakness, and a flu-like syndrome have been reported. Spread of toxin has been noted, with weakness sometimes involving muscles that were not directly injected. Autonomic side effects appear to be more commonly seen with type B toxin.
- Contraindications to treatment with botulinum toxin include pregnancy (category C), concurrent use of aminoglycoside antibiotics, myasthenia gravis, Eaton–Lambert syndrome, or known sensitivity to the toxins.
- Treating more frequently than the recommended interval of 12 weeks may lead to the development of antibodies to the toxin, which may also be associated with the development of clinical resistance.
- There is no valid way to reliably and consistently convert doses of type A toxin to doses of type B toxin at present.
- The use of botulinum toxin for pain management is as part of a comprehensive treatment program that has been developed based on an accurate diagnosis.
- Current storage/handling recommendations for each of the toxins should be followed.
- Whenever possible, an injection technique including needle size that is the least likely to cause additional pain should be used.
- Guidance techniques such as electromyography, ultrasound, CT, or fluoroscopy should be used at the discretion of the injector.

- Prolonged observation following the injections is generally not warranted.
- Follow-up should be arranged for four to six weeks following injections.
- More than one series of injections may be required to achieve maximal analgesic response.

BIBLIOGRAPHY

Argoff C. Successful treatment of chronic daily headache with Myobloc (abstract). *J Pain.* 2002;3(Suppl 1):10.

Argoff CE. A focused review on the use of botulinum toxins for neuropathic pain. *Clin J Pain.* 2002;18:S177–S181.

Aurora SK, Dodick DW, Turkel CC, et al. Onabotulinum toxin A for treatment of chronic migraine: results from the double-blind, randomized, placebo-controlled phase of the PREEMPT 1 trial. *Cephalagia.* 2010;30(7):793–803.

Barrientos N, Chana P. Efficacy and safety of botulinum toxin type A (Botox®) in the prophylactic treatment of migraine. Paper presented at: American Headache Society 44th Annual Scientific Meeting; 2002; Seattle, Wa.

Binder WJ, Brin MF, Blitzer A, et al. Botulinum toxin type A (BOTOX®) for treatment of migraine headaches: an open-label study. *Otolgolaryngol Head Neck Surg.* 2000;123:669–676.

Botox prescribing information. Available at: www.allergan.com/assets/pdf/botox_pi.pdf. Accessed April 20, 2014.

Brin MF, Swope DM, O'Brien C, et al. Botox® for migraine: double blind, placebo-controlled, region-specific evaluation (abstract). *Cephalalgia.* 2000;20:421.

Cheshire WP, Abashian SW, Mann JD. Botulinum toxin in the treatment of myofascial pain syndrome. *Pain.* 1994;59:65–69.

Childers MK, Wilson DJ, Gnatz SM, et al. Botulinum toxin type A use in piriformis muscle syndrome: a pilot study. *Am J Phys Med Rehabil.* 2002;81:751–759.

Cui M, Li Z, You S, et al. Mechanisms of the antinociceptive effect of subcutaneous Botox®: inhibition of peripheral and central nociceptive processing. *Arch Pharmacol.* 2002;365:33.

Diener HC, Dodick DW, Aurora SK, et al. Onabotulinum toxin A for treatment of chronic migraine: results from the double-blind, randomized, placebo-controlled phase of the PREEMPT 2 trial. *Cephalagia.* 2010;30(7):804–814.

Dubin A, Smith H, Tang J. Evaluation of botulinum toxin type B (Myobloc™) injections in a patient with painful muscle spasms (abstract). *Pain.* 2002;3(Suppl a):11.

Dysport prescribing information. Available at: www.dysport.com/pdfs/Dysport_Patients_PI_Sept2013.pdf. Accessed April 20, 2014.

Eross EG, Dodick DW. The effects of botulinum toxin type A on disability in episodic and chronic migraine. Paper presented at: American Headache Society 44th Annual Scientific Meeting; 2002; Seattle, Wa.

Fannucci E, Masala S, Sodani G, et al. CT-guided injection of botulinum toxin for percutaneous therapy of piriformis muscle syndrome with preliminary MRI results about denervation process. *Eur Radiol.* 2001;11:2543–2548.

Ferrante M, Bearn L, Rothrock R, et al. Botulinum toxin type A in the treatment of myofascial pain. Presented at: Annual meeting of the American Society of Anesthesiologists; 2002.

Fishman LM. Myobloc™ in the treatment of piriformis syndrome: a dose finding study. Paper presented at: American Academy of Pain Medicine's Annual Scientific Meeting; 2002; San Francisco, Ca.

Foster L, Clapp L, Erickson M, et al. Botulinum toxin A and chronic low back pain: A randomized, double blind study. *Neurology.* 2001;56:1290–1293.

Freund B, Schwartz M. Treatment of whiplash-associated neck pain with botulinum toxin A: a pilot study. *Headache.* 2000;40:231–236.

Freund B, Schwartz M, Symington J. Botulinum toxin: new treatment for temporomandibular disorders. *Br J Oral Maxillofac Surg.* 2000;38:466–471.

Freund BJ, Schwartz M. A focal dystonia model for subsets of chronic tension headache (abstract). *Cephalalgia.* 2000;20:433.

Freund BJ, Schwartz M. The use of botulinum toxin A in the treatment of refractory cluster headache: Case reports. *Cephalalgia.* 2000;20:329–330.

Ginies PR, Fraimout JL, Kong A, et al. Treatment of cluster headache with subcutaneous injection of botulinum toxin. Paper presented at: 8th World Congress on Pain; 1996; Vancouver.

Gobel H, Lindner V, Krack PK, et al. Treatment of chronic tension-type headache with botulinum toxin (abstract). *Cephalagia.* 1999;19:455.

Guyer BM. Mechanism of botulinum toxin in the relief of chronic pain. *Curr Rev Pain.* 1999;3:427–431.

Jabbari B, Machado D. Treatment of refractory pain with botulinum toxins—an evidence-based review. *Pain Med.* 2011, November;12(11):1594–1606.

Klapper JA, Klapper A. Use of botulinum toxin in chronic daily headaches associated with migraine. *Headache Q.* 1999;10:141–143.

Klapper JA, Mathew NT, Klapper A, et al. Botulinum toxin type A (BTX-A) for the prophylaxis of chronic daily headache (abstract). *Cephalalgia.* 2000;20:292–293.

Knusel B, DeGryse R, Grant M, et al. Intramuscular injection of botulinum toxin type A (Botox®) in chronic low back pain associated with muscle spasm. Paper presented at: American Pain Society Annual Scientific Meeting; 1998; San Diego, Ca.

Lang A. A pilot study of botulinum toxin type A (BOTOX®), administered using a novel injection technique, for the treatment of myofascial pain. *Am J Pain Manage.* 2000;10:108–112.

Lew MF. Review of the FDA-approved uses of botulinum toxins, including data suggesting efficacy in pain reduction. *Clin J Pain.* 2002;18:S142–S146.

Mathew NT, Kallasam J, Kaupp A, et al. "Disease modification" in chronic migraine with botulinum toxin type A: long-term experience. Paper presented at: American Headache Society 44th Annual Scientific Meeting; 2002; Seattle, Wa.

Mauskop A. Long-term use of botulinum toxin type A (Botox®) in the treatment of episodic and chronic migraine headaches. Paper presented at: American Headache Society 44th Annual Scientific Meeting; 2002; Seattle, Wa.

Meunier FA, Schiavo G, Molgo J. Botulinum neurotoxins: from paralysis to recovery of functional neuromuscular transmission. *J Physiol.* 2002;96:105–113.

Myobloc prescribing information. Available at: www.myobloc .com/hp_about/PI_5-19-10.pdf. Accessed April 20, 2014.

Nalamachu S. Treatment with botulinum toxin type B (Myobloc™) injections in three patients with myofascial pain. Paper presented at: American Academy of Pain Medicine's Annual Scientific Meeting; 2002; San Francisco, Ca.

Nixdorf DR, Heo G, Major PW. Randomized controlled trial of botulinum toxin A for chronic myogenous orofacial pain. *Pain*. 2002;99:465–473.

Opida C. Open-label study of Myobloc (botulinum toxin type B) in the treatment of patients with transformed migraine headaches (abstract). *J Pain*. 2002;3(Suppl 1):10.

Opida CL. Evaluation of Myobloc™ (botulinum toxin type B) in patients with post-whiplash headaches. Paper presented at: American Academy of Pain Medicine's 18th annual meeting; 2002; San Francisco, Ca.

Peterlein CD, Funk JF, Hölscher A, et al. Is botulinum toxin A effective for the treatment of plantar fasciitis? *J Pain*. 2012, July;28(6):527–533.

Porta M. A comparative trial of botulinum toxin A and methylprednisolone for the treatment of tension-type headache. *Curr Rev Pain*. 2000;4:31–35.

Porta M. A comparative trial of botulinum toxin type A and methylprednisolone for the treatment of myofascial pain syndrome and pain from chronic muscle spasm. *Pain*. 2000;85:101–105.

Robbins L. Botulinum toxin for cluster headache. Presented at: 10th Congress of the International Headache Society; New York; 2001.

Schwartz M, Freund B. Treatment of temporomandibular disorders with botulinum toxin. *Clin J Pain*. 2002;18:S198–S203.

Settler PE. Therapeutic use of botulinum toxins: background and history. *Clin J Pain*. 2002;18:S19–S24.

Silberstein S, Mathew N, Saper J, et al. Botulinum toxin type A as a migraine preventive treatment. *Headache*. 2000;40:445–450.

Simpson LL. Identification of the characteristics that underlie botulinum toxin potency: implications for designing novel drugs. *Biochemie*. 2000;82:943–953.

Simpson LL. Kinetic studies on the interaction between botulinum toxin type A and the cholinergic neuromuscular junction. *J Pharmacol Exp Ther*. 1980;212:16–21.

Smith H, Audette J, Dey R, et al. Botulinum toxin type B for a patient with myofascial pain. Paper presented at: American Academy of Pain Medicine's Annual Scientific Meeting; 2002; San Francisco, Ca.

Smuts JA, Baker MK, Wieser T, et al. Treatment of tension-type headache using botulinum toxin type A. *Eur J Neurol*. 1999;6(Suppl 4):S99-S102.

Taqi D, Gunyea I, Bhakta B, et al. Botulinum toxin type A (Botox®) in the treatment of refractory cervicothoracic myofascial pain (abstract). *Pain*. 2002;3(Suppl 1):16.

Taqi D, Royal M, Gunyea I, et al. Botulinum toxin type B (Myobloc™) in the treatment of refractory myofascial pain (abstract). *Pain*. 2002;3(Suppl 1):16.

Tsui JKC. Botulinum toxin as a therapeutic agent. *Pharmacol Ther*. 1996;72:13–24.

WE MOVE. Practical considerations for the clinical use of botulinum toxin type B: a self-study continuing medical education activity. February 2002.

Wheeler A, Goolkasian P, Gretz S. Botulinum toxin A for the treatment of chronic neck pain. *Pain*. 2001;94:255–260.

Wheeler AH, Goolkasian P, Gretz SS. A randomized, double blind, prospective pilot study of botulinum toxin injection for refractory, unilateral, cervicothoracic, paraspinal, myofascial pain syndrome. *Spine*. 1998;23:1662–1666;1667.

Wissel J, Muller J, Dressnandt J, et al. Management of spasticity associated pain with botulinum toxin A. *J Pain Symptom Manage*. 2000;20:44–49.

Xeomin prescribing information. Available at: www.xeomin.com/ files/Xeomin_PI.pdf. Accessed April 20, 2014.

Zwart JA, Bovim G, Sand T, et al. Tension headache: botulinum toxin paralysis of temporal muscles. *Headache*. 1994;34:458–462.

59 CHRONIC OPIOID THERAPY FOR NONCANCER PAIN

Sean Li, MD

BACKGROUND

- The earliest recorded use of opiates in the human civilization was described by Homer in 300 BC when it was given to Helen, the daughter of Zeus, to treat her grief over the absence of Odysseus.

- The general consensus today is that the Sumerians, who inhabited what is now known as Iraq, cultivated the poppy plant for the opium containing seeds in 3000 BC. They called this plant "hul gil" or joy plant. Chronic pain is defined as "pain that persists 6 months after an injury and beyond the usual course of an acute disease or a reasonable time for a comparable injury to heal, that is associated with chronic pathologic processes that cause continuous or intermittent pain for months or years that may continue in the presence or absence of demonstrable pathology; may not be amenable to routine pain control methods; and healing may never occur."

- Prevalence of chronic pain has dramatically increased, fueling the exploding healthcare costs and the consequence of the opioid abuse epidemic.

- Opioids have become the most commonly prescribed class of medications in the United States.

- Awareness for right to pain relief by patient advocate groups in the early 1990s, followed by new pain management guidelines set by the Joint Commission on the Accreditation of Health Care Organizations (JACHO) in 2000, along with aggressive marketing strategies by opioid manufacturers, has cultivated a culture of opioid overutilization.

- Recent report by the Institute of Medicine (IOM) recognizes that there are more than 116 million Americans suffering from chronic pain. The IOM concluded that opioids are a safe and effective class of medications for acute postoperative pain, procedural pain, and end-of-life pain. In treating chronic pain, the IOM does include opioids among other treatment modalities; they acknowledge a serious crisis in opioid abuse but also recognized the lack of clinical evidence in their long-term efficacy. Opioid therapy should be reserved for patients with moderate to severe persistent chronic pain refractory to nonopioid and intervention pain management modalities to improve functioning and quality of life.
- Opioids should be started only after careful assessment of the risks and benefits of opioid therapy for the individual patient.
- The initiation, titration, monitoring, and maintenance of opioid medications should only be carried out under the care of an adequately trained healthcare provider.

EVIDENCE

- Much of what is practiced in the prescribing of opioids for chronic pain has been adapted from experiences with treating cancer pain. The "analgesic ladder" was first introduced by the World Health Organization (WHO) in the 1980s
- The short-term (less than 6 months) use of opioids for the treatment of noncancer chronic pain has been shown to be effective in several systematic reviews.
- Furlan et al. reviewed 41 randomized trials in 6019 patients suffering from nociceptive, neuropathic, mixed, and fibromyalgia pain and concluded that opioid use over 5 to 16 weeks was more effective than placebo despite a 33% dropout rate.
- Chou and Huffman found opioids to be moderately effective in the treatment of chronic noncancer pain compared to placebo based on study periods less than 12 weeks.
- Interestingly, tramadol was the only pain medication to show fair evidence in the treatment of chronic osteoarthritis pain in the systematic review by Manchikanti et al. In this comprehensive systematic review of 111 trials, only 4 studies evaluated the effectiveness of opioid use beyond 6 months.
- Furthermore, Trescot et al. reviewed the efficacy of chronic opioid therapy in terms of functional improvement among chronic pain patients in addition to their pain relief. For treatment of chronic noncancer pain beyond six months, there is weak evidence supporting morphine and transdermal fentanyl; there is limited evidence for other more commonly used opioids, including hydrocodone and oxycodone.

SIDE EFFECTS AND COMPLICATIONS

- Chronic opioid administration is associated with side effects that may lead into serious complications.
- Common side effects include nausea, vomiting, pruritus, delayed gastric emptying, sedation, sexual dysfunction, muscle rigidity, myoclonus, sleep disturbance, and constipation.
- Serious life-threatening side effects are associated with high-dose opioid use (above 100 mg daily morphine equivalent) and long-term administration beyond six months. Serious side effects of opioid use include respiratory depression, cardiovascular collapse from histamine release, cardiac arrhythmia, endocrine system dysfunction leading to adrenal suppression, reduced libido, testicular atrophy in males, and menstrual dysfunction in females.
- Chronic high-dose opioids will eventually lead to tolerance and physical dependence, which is a physiological phenomenon. This should be distinguished from addiction and abuse that are pathologic diagnoses associated with psychosocial dimensions resulting in overuse and/or misuse of opioids despite harm.
- Opioid-induced hyperalgesia (OIH) is another important concept associated with increased pain after chronic high-dose opioid administration that may limit its usefulness.

OPIOID-INDUCED HYPERALGESIA

- Opioid induced hyperalgesia (OIH) is another potential complication of opioid therapy resulting from a pronociceptive process related but different from tolerance.
- The phenomenon of pain sensitization from the chronic administration of opioids was first observed in 1870 by Albutt in patients receiving morphine for pain.
- OIH was observed by Mao in animal models and later observed in the clinical setting in patients who received remifentanil infusions in the operating room.
- OIH and tolerance may present as uncontrolled pain. The two concepts are not interchangeable.
- Tolerance is a physiologic response to opioid molecules in the body that occur with prolonged use. This can be overcome by increasing the dose.
- OIH occurs both peripherally and centrally where pain is worsened with increased doses and improved with reducing or stopping opioids.

EQUIANALGESIA

- Currently, there are numerous forms of weak and strong opioids available for human use in the United States.
- The common target of all opioids is the mu receptor.
- The most common routes of administration for chronic pain in an outpatient setting are oral and transdermal.
- Table 59-1 is a sample of common opioids and their route of administration, duration of action, suggested initial dose, and morphine equivalent.
- When selecting an opioid, the clinician must take into account the severity of pain complaint, duration of action, and the best route of administration.
- For opioid-naive patients, slow and careful titration of the opioid dose is necessary to achieve adequate analgesia while minimizing side effects and the chance of overdose.
- Patients must be thoroughly consulted on the potential side effects and complications of the opioids used.

METHADONE

- The unique pharmacokinetics and molecular properties of methadone allow it to be very effective as an analgesic in treating chronic pain, but also potentially dangerous if abused or inappropriately prescribed.
- Once regarded as a common treatment for opioid addiction maintenance because of its extremely long five-day half-life, the use of methadone in the treatment of chronic pain has increased, but has been followed by a disproportionately large spike in related deaths.
- Due to its long pharmacokinetic half-life, active metabolites of methadone may build up to toxic levels before the patient reports pain relief. The accumulation of these metabolites may result in lethal respiratory arrest after the patient has taken additional doses when pain relief is not obtained.
- There is incomplete cross-tolerance of methadone and other opioids.
- Although the potency of methadone and morphine is similar, one must not convert from high morphine equivalent doses (1:1) directly based upon this conversion scheme.
- A safer alternative is to wean a patient's opioid dosing to less than 60 mg/d of morphine equivalent prior to converting to methadone.
- At higher doses above 100 mg/d, methadone is associated with QTc prolongation and we recommend obtaining a baseline electrocardiogram before initiating methadone therapy.
- Patients should be monitored closely when initiating methadone therapy.
- If in doubt, consult a pain management physician who is experienced with prescribing methadone.

TITRATION

- Dosing of opioids should be targeted to both pain relief and functional improvement while keeping patient safety above all other treatment goals.

TABLE 59-1   Common Opioids Used in Clinical Practice

DRUG	AVAILABLE ROUTE OF ADMINISTRATION	DURATION OF ANALGESIA (h)	EXTENDED RELEASE OPTION	SUGGESTED INITIAL DOSE FOR OPIOID NAIVE	MORPHINE EQUIVALENT (per mg of opioid)
Morphine	IV/SQ/IM/PO/PR/IT	3–4	Kadian® MS Contin®	10–30 mg/6 h	1.0
Hydrocodone	PO	4–8	N/A	5–10 mg/6 h	1.0
Oxycodone	PO	3–6	Oxycontin®	5–10 mg/6 h	1.0–1.5
Hydromorphone	IV/SQ/IM/PO/IT	3–4	Exalgo®	2–4 mg/4 h	0.2
Oxymorphone	IV/SQ/IM/PO	3–6	Opana ER®	5–10 mg/6 h	0.2–0.3
Fentanyl	IV/SQ/IM/TD/TM	1–2 (TM) 48–72 (TD)	Duragesic®	12–25 mcg/72 h	30 mg/d Morphine PO ~12 mcg/h fentanyl TD
Methadone	IV/SQ/IM/PO	6–8*	N/A	2.5–5 mg/8 h	1.0*
Tramadol	PO	4–6	Ultram ER®	50 mg/4–6 h	0.1
Tapentadol	PO	6–8	Nucynta ER®	50–75 mg/8 h	0.15
Buprenorphine patch	TD	24	Butrans Patch®	5–10 mcg/7 d	30 mg/d Morphine PO ~5 mcg/h TD

*Starting dose of methadone should be reduced 25%–50% due to incomplete cross-tolerance. Conversion ratio also varies based on initial daily morphine requirements. Due to its long half-life (five days) there is potential for drug accumulation prior to dose efficacy. Extreme caution and close monitoring are required when starting methadone. Only for use by or in consultation with physicians experienced with methadone prescribing.

IV, intravenous; SQ, subcutaneous; IM, intramuscular; PO, oral; PR, rectal; IT, intrathecal; TD, transdermal; TM, transmucosal; mg, milligrams; mcg, micrograms; h, hour.

- Clinicians must adopt a healthy respect for the potential side effects and complications associated with chronic opioid use.
- Dosing should be tailored to the individual patient.
- Equianalgesic tables and dosing charts are only be used as rough estimates and regarded with extreme caution.
- The best practice is to "start low and go slow."
- When there is doubt, one should consult with a trained pain management specialist experienced with opioid dosing.

OPIOID ROTATION

- To ensure goal-oriented and safe prescribing of opioids, one may decide to switch from one formulation to another or the route of administration instead of dose escalation.
- The indications to "rotate" opioids may include poor analgesic efficacy, intolerable side effects, ineffective administration route, drug interactions, developing tolerance, and financial constraints.
- The rationale for opioid rotation is based on the pharmacogenetic variability of individual response to opioids and their incomplete cross-reactivity. For example, 9% of Caucasians are unable to metabolize codeine phosphate to the active metabolite morphine in the liver.
- To initiate an opioid rotation, the clinician should convert daily dose of existing opioid(s) to morphine equivalent dose and end up with a reduced target dose of the new opioid to account for the incomplete cross-tolerance between the formulations. This incomplete cross-tolerance can be variable and unpredictable; an initial reduction of 50%–75% with a supplement as needed with breakthrough or immediate release medications is recommended.
- Methadone conversion should be regarded with additional care because of its unique pharmacokinetic profile (see section on methadone).
- Occasionally, patients may benefit from an "opioid holiday" when tolerance and pain relief are clinically plateaued.
- The physician may choose to administer a complete holiday where opioids are withheld versus a limited holiday where long-acting opioids are held while intermittent dosing is maintained.

MONITORING

- The decision to start chronic opioid therapy should be made with the patient's interest and safety in mind.
- Patients need to be screened for depression, potential abuse. This can be carried out with a multidisciplinary approach and mental health or addiction specialists in high-risk patients or the use of standardized questionnaires for assumed low-risk patients.
- One should set realistic functional goals and assess functional status, pain relief, side effects, and abuse risk at each follow-up visit.
- Applying the 4 A's (Analgesia, Activity, Aberrant behavior, and Adverse side effects), one can quickly assess the appropriateness of continuing opioid treatment.
- Opioid agreements, urine drug testing, and pill counts are essential tools to build provider-patient trust, ensure proper administration of medication, and preventing abuse.
- Regular follow-up evaluations are essential to maintain a motto of "trust but verify".
- On a regular interval, the provider must outline and document treatment goals and end-points.
- Society guidelines for chronic opioid management are available. (American Pain Society, American Society of Interventional Pain Physicians).

SUMMARY

- Opioids are an important class of analgesics that have been used throughout civilization for thousands of years to treat pain.
- Recent increase in chronic pain and public awareness has put the use of opioids under increased scrutiny.
- The pendulum has swung away from generous prescribing of opioids due to the real public health crisis of opioid abuse.
- Concurrently, the evidence is lacking for the use of opioids in the treatment of chronic noncancer pain.
- Therefore, opioids must be prescribed with restraint and caution with careful clinical judgment, clear end-points, judicious monitoring, and cotreatment with mental health/addiction specialists.

BIBLIOGRAPHY

Albutt C. On the abuse of hypodermic injections of morphia. *Practitioner.* 1870; 5:327–331.

Bajwa AH, Smith HS. Overview of the treatment of chronic pain. 2013. Available at: www.uptodate.com.

Benzon HT, Raja, S, Cohen SP, et al. *Essentials of Pain Medicine,* 3rd ed. Philadelphia, Pa.: Elsevier; 2011:85–100.

Brownstein MJ. A brief history of opiates, opioid peptide, and opioid receptors. *Proc Natl Acad Sci.* 1993;90:5391–5393.

Centers for Disease Control and Prevention (CDC). Vital signs: risk for overdose from methadone used for pain relief—United States, 1999–2011. *MMWR Morb Mortal Wkly Rep.* 2012;61:493.

Chou R, Fanciullo GJ, Fine PG, et al. Clinical guidelines for the use of chronic opioid therapy in chronic non-cancer pain. *J Pain.* 2009;10:113.

Chou R, Huffman L. Use of chronic opioid therapy in chronic non-cancer pain: a systematic review. *American Pain Society.* 2009.

Furlan AD, Sandoval JA, Mailis-Gagnon A, et al. Opioids for chronic non-cancer pain: a meta-analysis of effectiveness and side effects. *Can Med Assoc J.* 2006;174:1589–1594.

Gupta S, Atcheson R. Opioid and chronic non-cancer pain. *J Anaesthesiol Clin Pharmacol.* 2013;29:6–12.

Guignar B, Bossard AE, Sessler DI, et al. Acute opioid tolerance: intraoperative pain and morphine requirement. *Anesthesiology.* 2000;93:409–417.

Institute of Medicine (IOM). *Relieving Pain in America: A Blueprint for Transforming Prevention, Care, Education, and Research.* Washington, DC: The National Academies Press; 2011.

Kuehn BM. Prescription drug abuse rises globally. *J Am Med Assoc.* 2007;297–1306.

Manchikanti L, Helm S, Fellows B, et al. Opioid epidemic in the United States. *Pain Physician.* 2012;15:ES9–ES38.

Manchikanti L, Koyyalagunta L, Datta S, et al. A systematic review of randomized trials of long-term opioid management for chronic non-cancer pain. *Pain Physician.* 2011;14:91–121.

Manchikanti L, Singh V, Datta S, et al. Comprehensive review of epidemiology, scope, and impact of spinal pain. *Pain Physician.* 2009;12:E35–E70.

Mao J. Opioid-induced abnormal pain sensitivity: implications in clinical opioid therapy. *Pain.* 2009;100:213–217.

Silverman SM. Opioid induced hyperalgesia: clinical implications for the pain practitioner. *Pain Physician.* 2009;12:679–684.

Trescot AM, Helm S, Benyamin R, et al. Opioids in the management of chronic non-cancer pain: an update of the American Society of Interventional Pain Physicians (ASIPP) guidelines. *Pain Physician.* 2008;11:S5–S62.

World Health Organization. *Cancer Pain Relief.* Geneva: World Health Organization; 1990.

Yue QY, Hasselstrom J, Svenssson JO. Pharmacokinetics of codeine and its metabolites in Caucasian healthy volunteers; comparisons between extensive and poor hydroxylators of debrisoquine. *Br J Clin Pharmacol.* 1991;31:635–642.

60 NEUROLYSIS

Raimy R. Amasha, MD
Michael A. Erdek, MD

BACKGROUND

- Neurolytic (neuorablative) techniques confer analgesia through the intentional injury of a nerve(s) by chemical, thermal, cryogenic, or surgical means.
- This technique may be indicated for patients suffering from intractable pain after failure of more conservative management.

- Chemical neurolysis is not without risk and thus infrequently used in the treatment of nonmalignant, or nonterminal origin unless benefits clearly outweigh the inherent risks.
- Aside from the analgesic effect of neurolysis, it may also provide prolonged relief of muscle spasticity in conditions such as paraplegia, poststroke hemiparesis, or multiple sclerosis.
- The efficacy of neurolysis, if successful, is often measured in weeks to months. The risk of serious life-altering complications must be weighed against this anticipated benefit of pain reduction.
- In the context of terminal cancer pain, quality of life may often be more important than longitudinal functional status.
- Risks of neurolysis include neuritis and deafferentiation pain, motor deficit, and potential unintentional damage to nontargeted tissue.
- One of the most important factors that determine the success of neurolysis is patient education. Neurolysis is not a panacea for the patient's condition, but rather one component to their treatment.
- Often employed in refractory pain conditions, neurolysis offers potentially optimal results as part of a multidisciplinary approach to pain.
- Neurolysis confers the opportunity to improve pain control, help reduce opioid requirements, and thus limit drug side effects.
- In combination with neurolytic techniques, disease-modifying therapies, pharmacologic medications, neurosurgical procedures, and behavioral and psychiatric therapies are often utilized in refractory chronic pain.
- Generally provided by anesthesiologists and neurosurgeons, neurolytic therapy is most commonly considered after a diagnosis of advanced, irreversible disease has been established.

NEUROABLATIVE MODALITIES

- In actual practice, the modalities used to produce neurolysis are chemical, thermal, cryogenic, and surgical, with thermal being the most commonly used to treat neck and back pain in nonmalignant pain.
- Chemical neurolysis is generally performed with either ethyl alcohol or phenol.
- Ethyl alcohol is the classic neurolytic agent, first reported for subarachnoid injection by Dogliotti in 1931.
- Ethyl alcohol is commercially available as undiluted (absolute or 100%) vials, is hypobaric relative to cerebrospinal fluid, may cause pain with injection, and systemic toxicity may present as mild alcohol intoxication.

- Concentrations of ethyl alcohol between 50% and 100% are typically used for neurolytic blocks.
- Alcohol destroys nerve fibers and subsequent wallerian degeneration of axonal fibers and Schwann cells. The basal lamina of the Schwann cell sheath may remain intact allowing for new Schwann cell proliferation and nerve regeneration.
- In comparison, phenol may be compounded with contrast medium, saline, or, for intrathecal use, glycerine can be used. Phenol is hyperbaric relative to cerebrospinal fluid, painless on injection, and systemic toxicity may manifest as cardiovascular collapse or convulsions. Concentrations between 4% and 10% typically are used to obtain a neurolytic block.
- Chemical neurolysis is less commonly performed with glycerol. Gasserian ganglion block is performed using 100% glycerol. Essentially, this use is confined almost exclusively to treatment of trigeminal neuralgia.
- Thermocoagulation has been touted as efficacious as glycerol neurolysis in trigeminal neuralgia according to recent report.
- Radiofrequency thermocoagulation is performed by creating a high-frequency current produced by a generator connected to an electrode.
- The electromagnetic field around the tip of the electrode rapidly vibrates the tissue, which causes the tissues to heat up. A thermo couple at the tip of the electrode monitors the temperature and a lesion is formed if the temperature within the neuronal tissues exceeds 40°C.
- The lesion size correlates with the electrode size, temperature generated, duration of radiofrequency application, and local tissue characteristics.
- Radiofrequency ablation offers the advantage of being precise, reproducible, and effective. It also has the ability to stimulate before ablation to avoid ablating wrong nerve elements, which adds a considerable margin of safety.
- Lumbar facet nerve (medial branch) ablation is perhaps the most common application of radiofrequency ablation. It may also be used in cervical facet nerve ablation and sacroiliac joint nerve ablation.
- Additional applications of radiofrequency ablation have included biacuplasty for intradiscal pain, aimed at neuroablation of nerve fibers of the posterior annulus.
- Chemical neurolysis remains the preferred intervention over radiofrequency for disrupting a more diffuse neural network, such as with pancreatic cancer supplied by the celiac plexus or cervical cancer supplied by the superior hypogastric plexus.
- The use of extreme cold (cryoablation) is less commonly employed. This technique represents an alternative approach to the repetitive use of chemical neurolysis or radiofrequency ablation.
- Cryoablation uses a cryoprobe often with N_2O to cool the probe tip (to approximately −60°C) (see Chapter 62).
- Axonal and neuronal disruptions occur as a consequence of cooling, with the amount of destruction depending on the size of the cryoprobe, freezing time, tissue permeability to water, and presence of vascular structures.
- Cryoablation has a lower incidence of neuritis and neuroma formation compared with chemical neurolysis.
- Surgical neurolysis has also been described as a means for pain control in a subset of patient.

RISKS AND LIMITATIONS

- The risks and limitations of neuroablation include temporary analgesia (weeks to months), postablative neuritis, neurologic deficit, damage to adjacent structures (neural and non-neural tissue), and failure to achieve desired effect due to overlapping nerve supply.
- The quality of analgesia may be less than after a local anesthetic block and there is a potential for long-term complications.
- Long-term complications include weakness interfering with function and ambulation, numbness, secondary traumatic injury, neuropathic pain, and dysesthesias.
- Careful judgment and scrupulous technique must be employed to relieve pain without producing untoward effects.
- The mechanism of neurolysis, whether chemical, thermal, or cryoablative, has the potential to damage tissue relatively indiscriminately, thus requiring a trained physician.
- Verifying needle placement with fluoroscopic or CT-guided imaging technology, serial aspiration, electrical stimulation, and/or test doses of local anesthetic are all methods of reducing extraneous tissue injury.
- Damage to non-nerve tissue may occur, such as skin slough after peripheral neurolysis, aortic dissection or spinal infarction during celiac plexus neurolysis, or renal infarct during lumbar sympathectomy.
- Incomplete pain relief may occur for several reasons, including the sheltering of neural targets by tumor and scarring, failure to address overlapping sensory fields, and inadequate neurolysis.
- To this end, durability of neurolysis may be maximized by targeting alternate sites unencumbered by tumor burden (ie, retrocrural vs. antecrural celiac plexus neurolysis) and by maximizing lesion size by increasing the concentration of the injectate and/or ensuring adequate exposure time.

NEUROLYSIS ADVANTAGES

- Treatment with a single (or repeated) intervention targeting a painful lesion via neurolysis potentially reduces:
  - The need for multiple drugs to control pain symptoms.
  - High-dose requirements of pain medications.
  - Opioid-mediated side effects.
  - Collateral effects of drugs on unrelated organ systems (ie, opioid-related respiratory depression).
- Moreover, neurolysis provides an effective means to improve quality of life and decrease healthcare costs, hospital admissions, and outpatient visits.
- Neuroablative techniques may have a niche in rural areas, developing nations, and any setting where health care is limited as overall consumption of healthcare resources is lessened and the effect of analgesia may be prolonged.

NEUROLYSIS VS. SYSTEMIC PHARMACOTHERAPY

- Many of the purported benefits of pharmacotherapy (opioids and adjuncts) relate to the dynamic nature of cancer characterized by unpredictably variable patterns of progression, regression, and recurrence.
- Indications where pharmacotherapy may provide benefit over neurolytic modalities include pain arising from varied etiologies (ie, widespread tumor invasion, postradiation necrosis, chemotherapy-induced pain) or pain maintained by a multiple mechanisms (ie, nociceptive, visceral, and neuropathic).
- However, opioids, a mainstay in cancer treatment, are not without serious side effects, including somnolence, decreased bowel motility, nausea and vomiting, pruritis, and respiratory depression.
- Literature supports that timely neurolytic therapies in the management of amenable cancers reduce high-dose opioid therapy and its associated toxicity.
- Thus it is not unreasonable to consider neurolysis an effective adjunct, when appropriate, to allow for reduced dosage of opioids.

NEUROLYSIS VS. INTRASPINAL PHARMACOTHERAPY

- Spinal opioid therapy and systemic pharmacotherapy are more similar to each other than to those of neuroablative approaches.
- The effects of spinal and systemic analgesics are reversible, titratable, and applicable to a wide variety of pain in diverse populations, and do not involve local tissue destruction.

- In contrast to neurolysis, intraspinal opioid therapy more often provides effective relief of generalized pain, widely disseminated or multifocal pain, and pain that cannot be accurately targeted.
- Although both neuroablation and spinal opioid therapy are interventional and associated with greater initial cost, technical expertise, sophisticated equipment, and risk versus noninterventional therapy, patients status postneurolysis may require less frequent follow-up. In contrast, spinal drug delivery requires a commitment on the part of the clinical team, patient, family, and institution. This includes the hospital, home care nursing, and pharmacies, and requires careful attention to titration of medication over time.
- On this basis, neuroablation may be more practical than continuous spinal opioid administration in rural areas, developing nations, and hospices that emphasize effective, resource-conscious care.

NEUROLYSIS VS. LOCAL ANESTHETIC BLOCKADE

- Local anesthetic blockade is often utilized, in the setting of cancer pain, as a diagnostic, prognostic, and therapeutic nerve block. As such, these blocks may provide relief (albeit temporary) from chronic pain, muscle spasm, sympathetically maintained pain, urgent relief in pain crisis, and chronic catheter-based infusion.
- Although the utility of local anesthetic blockade can be extended by relying on continuous infusion, such therapies are limited by many of the same factors that limit the utility of spinal administration, most notably, risk of local anesthetic toxicity or motor weakness.
- There is recent evidence that regional anesthesia with local anesthetic may reduce the risk of tumor metastasis and recurrence. This benefit may be due to the attenuation of immunosuppression by regional anesthesia. A variety of malignancies exhibit increased activity of voltage-gated sodium channels. Blockade of these channels by local anesthetics may help inhibit tumor progression.
- Furthermore, opioids promote angiogenesis, cancer cell proliferation, and metastasis. With this recent literature, it may further guide interventional techniques utilized and the medications provided to cancer patients. They may benefit from use of local anesthetics, perhaps not as a sole analgesic, but in addition to other potential therapies.

LIFE EXPECTANCY

- Disease stage (especially metastatic status), treatability, baseline functional status, and clinician experience help predict probable survival, although life expectancy can only be approximated at best even by experts.

- The effects of neuroablation may endure an average of three to six months, with a wide therapeutic range.
- Duration of relief may be influenced by incomplete neurolysis, new pain due to disease progression, and/or iatrogenic postdenervation neuropathic pain (neuralgia).
- Consideration of neurolysis must be carefully individualized based on the nature and severity of pain, functional status, the likelihood of efficacy relative to more conservative measures, and the goals and expectations of the patient and his/her family.
- An equally important determinant of whether a patient may undergo neurolysis is the extent to which their disease has affected liver and bone marrow function, coagulation status, and whether their chemotherapy or radiotherapy has adversely affected their platelets. A patient with an inability to clot could suffer from untoward complications secondary to needle manipulation.
- Treatment with a significant degree of inherent risk may be more liberally considered when conservative measures have proven unsuccessful; however, the physician's guiding principle always remains, "*primum non nocere.*"

PAIN CHARACTERISTICS

- Neurolytic procedures are most appropriate and effective for well-localized pain in a single area that the patient can be identified.
- Neuropathic pain responds poorly to neurolysis.
- When extended to provide coverage for pain that is distributed more extensively or that is present in multiple areas, treatment is more prone to fail and may be associated with increased risk for undesired neurologic deficit.
- The exception is visceral pain, which, although it is often vague and broadly based, is generally amenable to neurolysis. Although diffuse, visceral pain is typically well circumscribed and elicits a reliable, consistent report.
- Patients with vague pain ("I can't describe it; it just hurts" or "It feels bad all over") or whose complaints are inconsistent or change over time are poor candidates for neurolysis. Such a patient presentation confounds selection of the optimal intervention and may be compounded by extraneous components including social or psychological factors.
  - Other indications that expressions of pain may reflect global malaise include selection of all the descriptors offered by assessment tools like the McGill Pain Questionnaire or Brief Pain Inventory or selection of predominantly affective (emotionally laden) descriptors (eg, wretched, cruel, agonizing, miserable).
  - Nevertheless, psychological disturbances commonly accompany established painful disorders and are not specifically contraindications, but when these disturbances are prominent and pharmacologic control is feasible, it is preferred over neurolysis.
- Neurolysis is best reserved for pain that is limited to a single site.
- Cancer pain is, however, often multifocal, especially with progressive disease.
  - Even with multifocal pain, treatment can be considered if a single source of pain is dominant, anticipating that reducing the foremost pain complaint may facilitate control of secondary pain with conservative treatment.
  - Despite the presence of multiple lesions, many patients appreciate pain in only a single site, especially in the case of bone metastases.
  - The clinician should be aware, especially in this setting, that despite a single apparent site of pain, neurolytic procedures are associated with the risk that "new" pain will be unmasked once the primary complaint is eliminated, perhaps partially as a consequence of spinal gating mechanisms. When feasible, a preliminary local anesthetic block may help exclude this possibility.
- The customary biologic behavior of the underlying malignancy and the growth pattern of a tumor in a given patient are other factors to consider before proceeding with neurolysis:
  - With rapid progression, pain may exceed the topographic boundaries of what would otherwise have been a successful procedure. Alternatively, rapid systemic progression, organ failure, and metabolic abnormalities (eg, hypercalcemia, anemia) may render the urgent need for an aggressive procedure of little utility.
- Despite an absence of controlled trials, clinicians agree that somatic or visceral pain appears to respond more favorably to neurolytic blockade than neuropathic pain. Although often relieved by local anesthetic blockade, neuropathic pain responds less frequently to the additional nerve injury that occurs with neurolysis.
- Recent literature has described novel uses for neurolysis. Such reports describe intraoperative radiofrequency nerve ablation as a useful modality when the lesion (tumor) is near vital structures (ie, great vessels, hilum, or heart). This use may also be beneficial if resectability can only be determined at the time of operation, or in patients with secondary tumors of the

viscera (ie, lung) combined with limited resection to preserve tissue parenchyma.

- Absolute contraindications to neurolysis, other than inadequate informed consent, are few, and even relative contraindications are not etched in stone in the context of palliative care.
  - In addition to those discussed above, relative contraindications include local infection, bleeding diathesis, spinal cord compression, and the extensive spread of solid tumor at or along the site of the injection.

SPECIFIC NEUROLYTIC PROCEDURES

PERIPHERAL NERVES

- With a few exceptions, neurolysis of peripheral mixed motor and sensory nerves is generally avoided.
- Neurolytic blocks of peripheral nerves in the extremities may produce analgesia, but also extremity weakness or even paralysis due to the predominance of mixed (sensorimotor) nerves.
- Additional risks include new/worsened pain secondary to higher incidence of neuritis (more common with alcohol than phenol) and risk of procedural failure secondary to overlapping sensory innervations.
- With intercostal neurolysis the risks include pneumothorax and the need for associated lesions above and below the peripheral sites to account for overlapping innervation.
- Subarachnoid neurolysis is an alternative to intercostal neurolysis in experienced hands and may produce a predominantly sensory lesion with reduced risk of neuralgia.
- For cranial nerves alcohol, phenol, or radiofrequency ablation of the fifth cranial nerve or its branches and, occasionally, of the ninth and tenth cranial nerves is employed. This technique is used for orofacial pain that is unresponsive to radiotherapy and often employed by neurosurgeons and pain physicians.
- Although its availability is limited, gamma knife has specific usages as in trigeminal neuralgia and is predominantly utilized by neurosurgeons and radiation therapists.

SYMPATHETIC NERVES

- Neurolysis of sympathetic nerves is used to treat refractory visceral pain, sympathetically maintained pain, hyperhidrosis, and peripheral ischemia. Successful treatment is associated with a very low incidence of neuralgia and no numbness or motor weakness.
- Celiac plexus or splanchnic nerve block is often considered in the course of treatment for abdominal and back pain secondary to visceral or retroperitoneal malignancy and can be accomplished by a variety of approaches.
  - Although usually performed percutaneously by an anesthesiologist or endoscopically by a gastroenterologist, injections can be performed at the time of surgery, and splanchnic nerves can be lesioned via thoracoscopy.
- As recent research suggests, neurolysis of the celiac plexus in patients with nonmetastatic pancreatic cancer may demonstrate some advantage over only pharmacotherapy with regard to reported pain score. However, the efficacy of the procedure becomes readily apparent when comparing postprocedure functional status and side-effect burden of medications between the two groups.
- Superior hypogastric plexus neurolysis targets the sympathetic nervous system near the sacral promontory bilaterally and is effective for visceral pelvic pain (ie, gynecologic cancers).

CENTRAL NERVOUS SYSTEM/AXIAL

- Although of historical significance, subarachnoid neurolytic blocks are rarely performed for patients with cancer pain. Complications of intrathecal neurolytic blocks include bowel and bladder dysfunction, dysesthesia, aseptic meningitis, and muscle weakness.
- Implanted intrathecal pumps have largely supplanted these blocks and can be used to manage recurrent pain when the disease progresses, including painful metastases at distant sites.

VASCULAR EFFECTS OF NEUROLYTIC AGENTS

- Vasospasm of segmental lumbar arteries may have catastrophic consequences and may be induced with either alcohol or phenol. The fact remains that phenol and alcohol will destroy all types of tissue and may cause a contractile response in blood vessels, which may lead to loss of neural function.
- Therefore, the risk of paraplegia after neurolysis of the celiac plexus and other ganglia must be discussed during informed consent.

CONCLUSION

- Neurolytic techniques include surgical, cryogenic, thermal, or chemical injury to nerves.
- The indications for neurolysis extend beyond its analgesic effect, but also to relieve muscle spasticity, and to curtail escalating pharmacotherapy and its associated drug side effects.

- Neurolytic procedures are most appropriate and effective for discrete, well-localized pain in a single area that can be reliably identified.
- Visceral pain, although often vague and broadly based, is generally amenable to neurolysis.
- Cancer pain is often multifocal, especially with progressive disease. Prior to undertaking any invasive procedure, the interventionalist must weight the probable benefits vs. the potential risks and act under the auspices of sound judgment.

BIBLIOGRAPHY

Amasha RR, Christo PJ. *Cancer Pain: Etiology, Barriers, Assessment, and Treatment.* Pain Report 14, Dannemiller Foundation; 2013. Available at: http://cme.dannemiller.com

Arcidiacono PG, Calori G, Carrara S, et al. Celiac plexus block for pancreatic cancer pain in adults. *Cochrane Database Syst Rev.* 2011, March 16;(3).

Bender MT, Pradilla G, Batra S, et al. Glycerol rhizotomy and radiofrequency thermocoagulation for trigeminal neuralgia in multiple sclerosis. *J Neurosurg.* 2013, February;118(2):329–336.

Bonica JJ, Buckley FP, Moricca G, et al. Neurolytic blockade and hypophysectomy. In: Bonica JJ, Chapman CR, et al. eds. *The Management of Pain.* 2nd ed. Philadelphia, Pa.: Lea and Febiger; 1990: 1980–2039.

Brogan S, Junkins S. Interventional therapies for the management of cancer pain. *J Support Oncol.* 2010, March–April;8(2):52–59.

Candido K, Stevens RA. Intrathecal neurolytic blocks for the relief of cancer pain. *Best Pract Res Clin Anaesthesiol.* 2003, September;17(3):407–428.

Cohen S, Hurley R, Buckenmaier CC, et al. Randomized placebo-controlled study evaluating lateral branch radiofrequency denervation for sacroiliac joint pain. *Anesthesiology.* 2008;109:279–288.

Erdek MA, Halpert DE, Gonzalez FM, et al. Assessment of celiac plexus block and neurolysis outcomes and technique in the management of refractory visceral cancer pain. *Pain Med.* 2010, January;11(1):92–100.

Kambadakone A, Thabet A, Gervais DA, et al. CT-guided celiac plexus neurolysis: a review of anatomy, indications, technique, and tips for successful treatment. *Radiographics.* 2011, October;31:1599–1621.

Kapural L, Mekhail N. Radiofrequency ablation for chronic pain control. *Curr Pain Headache Rep.* 2001;5(6):517–525.

Kyriacou S, Pastides PS, Singh VK, et al. Exploration and neurolysis for the treatment of neuropathic pain in patients with a sciatic nerve palsy after total hip replacement. *Bone Joint J.* 2013, January;95-B(1):20–22.

Lee DG, Jang SH. Ultrasound guided alcohol neurolysis of musculocutaneous nerve to relieve elbow spasticity in hemiparetic stroke patients. *NeuroRehabilitation.* 2012;31(4):373–377.

Linden PA, Wee JO, Jaklitsch MT, et al. Extending indications for radiofrequency ablation of lung tumors through an intraoperative approach. *Ann Thorac Surg.* 2008, February;85(2):420–423.

Lloyd JW, Barnard JDW, Glynn CJ. Cryoanalgesia: a new approach to pain relief. *Lancet.* 1976;2(7992):932–934.

Loev M, Varklet VL, Wilsey BL, et al. Cryoablation: a novel approach to neurolysis of the ganglion impar. *Anesthesiology.* 1998;88:1391–1393.

Mao L, Lin S, Lin J. The effects of anesthetic on tumor progression. *Int J Physiol Phathophysiol Pharmacol.* 2013;5(1):1–10. Epub 2013.

Mazza E, Carmignani L, Stecco A, et al. Interventional radiology in the palliative treatment of pancreatic cancer. *Tumori.* 1999, January–February;85(1 Suppl 1):S54–S59.

Mercadante S, Intravaia G, Villari P, et al. Intrathecal treatment in cancer patients unresponsive to multiple trials of systemic opioids. *Clin J Pain.* 2007;23(9):793–798.

Molley RE, Benzon HT. Neurolytic blocking agents: uses and complications. In: Benzon HT, Rathmell JP, Wu CL, et al. eds. *Raj's Practical Management of Pain.* 4th ed. Philadelphia, Pa.: Elsevier; 2008:839–850.

Penman ID. Coeliac plexus neurolysis. *Best Pract Res Clin Gastroenterol.* 2009;23(5):761–766

Rohof OJ. Radiofrequency treatment of peripheral nerves. *Pain Pract.* 2002, September;2(3):257–260.

Soloman M, Mekhail M, Mekahil N. Radiofrequency treatment in chronic pain. *Expert Rev. Neurother.* 2010;10(3):469–474.

Straube, S, Derry S, Moore RA, et al. Cervico-thoracic or lumbar sympathectomy for neuropathic pain and complex regional pain syndrome. *Cochrane Database Syst Rev.* 2010, July 7;(7)

Yang FR, Wu BS, Lai GH, et al. Assessment of consecutive neurolytic celiac plexus block (NCPB) technique outcomes in the management of refractory visceral cancer pain. *Pain Med.* 2012, April;13(4):518–521.

61 COMPLEMENTARY AND ALTERNATIVE MEDICINE

Michael Kurisu, DO

INITIAL APPROACH

Complementary and alternative medicine (CAM) offers numerous approaches to treat pain.

- These therapies are being increasingly used by the public, and many are now subject to the same rigorous trials as allopathic treatments.
- Evidence indicates that the number of patients visiting alternative medicine practitioners increases each year.
- Educated patients and patients with severe pain conditions are most likely to use CAM.
- This increased prevalence of CAM behooves us to learn about these therapies and, at the very least, "integrate" them into our clinical thought processes, if not into our practices.

- *Integrative medicine* is the term used to describe combined allopathic and complementary modalities for treatment of pain and disease.
- Integrative therapies can be safely integrated with ongoing treatments. Just like other treatments, use of Integrative therapies requires attention to drug interactions, cross-reactivity, and side effects.
- Always ask patients about their use of Integrative medicine and stop all supplements before initiating invasive or surgical procedures.

DIETARY THERAPY

- Diet modulation can alter pain by mechanisms involving oxidant production and cytokine biology.

WEIGHT LOSS

- Evidence indicates that body weight increases with chronic pain and that early weight gain may increase the incidence of chronic pain later in life.
- Unhealthy weight gain early in life may increase the incidence of chronic pain later in life.
- Excess body weight is a multifactorial problem that has reached epidemic proportions in the Western world. Thus, weight control must be part of any pain treatment plan.

RAW VEGETARIAN DIET

- Increases fiber and antioxidant intake.
- May help reduce symptoms of fibromyalgia.

OMEGA-3 FATTY ACIDS

- *Source*: flax seeds, walnuts, and fish.
- *Active ingredient*: α-linoleic acid (ALA).
- *Mechanism of action*: decrease prostaglandin E2 (PGE2) and leukotriene B4 (LTB4) inflammation; increase prostaglandin inhibitor (PGI2) and PGI3; cause vasodilation, platelet inhibition, and blunt inflammatory response.
- *Indications*: studied extensively in rheumatoid arthritis, in which they reduce morning stiffness and number of tender joints.
- *Risks*: increased bleeding time, decreased thrombus formation.

SOY

- *Source*: soybeans.
- *Active ingredient*: soy is the only dietary source of isoflavones (phytochemicals similar in structure to mammalian estrogen).

- *Mechanism of action*: metabolized to its biologically active forms (genistein and daidzein) by intestinal bacteria. Approximately 30%–50% of the ingested isoflavone is absorbed, and serum levels increase in a dose-dependent manner.
- *Indications*: can be used as a primary source of protein because it meets human protein requirements. Soy enhances pain suppression by reducing inflammation and decreasing production of tumor necrosis factor α (TNFα) in macrophages.
- Soy is an antimutagenic, antioxidant agent with anti-inflammatory and cardioprotective effects.
- *Contraindications*: soy allergies or hypersensitivities, pregnancy, lactation, presence of estrogen receptor-positive tumors.

SOY OIL

- *Active ingredient*: polyunsaturated fatty acids.
- *Mechanism of action*: decreases pain by reducing pro-inflammatory eicosanoids and cytokines and reducing TNFα.
- *Indications*: analgesia supported by findings of increased paw-lick latency in rats fed soy oil.

ANTHOCYANINS

- *Source*: bright pigments found in plants and fruits, such as tart cherries, blueberries, bilberries, cranberries, elderberries, and grapes.
- *Active ingredient*: anthocyanin.
- *Mechanism of action*: inhibits prostaglandin synthesis with anti-inflammatory and antioxidant properties.
- *Indications*: Growing evidence indicates that fruits and vegetables help reduce the incidence of chronic pain, cancer, and cardiovascular disease. Studies show anthocyanin extracts to be better anti-inflammatory agents than aspirin, better antioxidants than vitamin E, and better inhibitors of cyclooxygenases 1 and 2 than ibuprofen. Anthocyanins may be effective for treatment of chronic pain, such as arthritis pain.
- *Contraindications*: none known.

SUCROSE

- *Source*: carbohydrates, principally from cane sugar and cane beet.
- *Active ingredients*: glucose and fructose.
- *Mechanism of action*: decreases nociceptive transmission in the central nervous system, enhances levels of opioid-induced antinociception, and reduces tolerance to morphine.

- *Indications*: analgesia. sucrose use significantly reduced the crying induced during infant heel lancing for blood collection. Rat studies also show a decrease in paw withdrawal from a hot plate.
- *Risks*: dental caries, diabetes, coronary artery disease, obesity.

HERBAL THERAPY

ST JOHN'S WORT

- *Source*: a flower containing flavonoids, naphthodian-thrones, and glucinols.
- *Active ingredient*: hypericin, available as 0.3% hypericin (ie, LI 160).
- *Mechanism of action*: inhibits reuptake of norepineph-rine, serotonin, and dopamine.
- *Indications*: superior to tricyclic antidepressants with fewer side effects for depression and dysphoria; minor wounds; AIDS.
- *Risks*: decreases concentration of protease inhibitors in HIV patients; may potentiate monoamine oxidase inhibitors; photosensitization.
- *Contraindications*: pregnancy, excessive exposure to sunlight.

GINSENG

- Source: Panax quinquefolius.
- Active ingredients: the saponin glycosides known as ginsenosides and panaxosides, steroidal compounds, and coumarin.
- Mechanism of action: Ginsenosides stimulate and inhibit the central nervous system and stimulate TNFα production by alveolar macrophages.
- Indications: cancer prevention and treatment, diabetes treatment, stimulation of immune system, to increase stamina.
- Risks: may cause adverse drug interactions with monoamine oxidase inhibitors; increase effect of insulin and sulfonylureas, causing hypoglycemia; inhibit analgesic action of opioids; antagonize effect of anticoagulants.

BLACK CURRANT, EVENING PRIMROSE, AND BORAGE SEED OIL

- *Active ingredient*: γ-linolenic acid (GLA).
- *Indications*: GLA (1–3 g/d) has some efficacy in patients with rheumatoid arthritis and breast pain.
- *Mechanism of action*: astringent, sequestering, and anti-inflammation properties.

- *Risks*: may exacerbate temporal lobe epilepsy and manic–depressive disorder.

MYROBALAN

- *Source*: bark extract of the plant *Terminalia arjuna* native to India.
- *Active ingredients*: tannins, triterpenoid saponins (including arjunic and terminic acid).
- *Mechanism of action*: reduces triglycerides and choles-terol; may enhance elimination of cholesterol.
- *Indications*: beneficial to patients with ischemic heart disease and chest pain; some evidence to support its use as a treatment of heart failure. A randomized, controlled, clinical trial indicated that it is better than placebo and similar to isosorbide mononi-trate in preventing provocable ischemia on the treadmill test.
- *Dose*: 500 mg tid.
- *Risks*: no contraindications or interactions. Related *Terminalia oblongata*, at high doses, is linked to dyspnea. Hepatic necrosis may occur at high doses.
- *Contraindications*: none recorded.

KAVA KAVA

- *Source*: plant (*Piper methysticum*) cultivated in the Pacific islands.
- *Active ingredient*: kava lactones (pyrones 5%–12%), chalcones. The extract used in studies, WS 1490, contains 70% kava pyrones.
- *Mechanism of action*: acts in the limbic system; binds to GABA receptors and increases GABA binding sites; also inhibits norepinephrine uptake, antagonizes dopa-mine, inhibits monoamine oxidase B, and decreases glutamate release. Kava kava has anticonvulsant, anti-inflammatory, and antiplatelet properties.
- *Indications*: treatment of anxiety (70 mg tid), sleep-lessness (210 mg qhs), and menopausal symptoms.
- *Risks*: oculomotor disturbance; may potentiate alco-hol and psychotherapeutic agents; and, rarely, liver damage.
- *Contraindications*: liver disease, pregnancy.

CAPSAICIN

- *Source*: pepper plant.
- *Active ingredient*: capsaicin.
- *Mechanism of action*: inhibits substance P.
- *Indications*: topical treatment of postherpetic neuralgia, inflammation, diabetic neuropathy.
- *Risks*: skin rash.

DEVIL'S CLAW

- *Source*: roots, stems, leaves of South African plants in the sesame family (*Harpagophytum radix, Harpagophytum procumbens, Harpagophytum zeyheri*).
- *Active ingredient*: harpagosidelts such as harpagoside are metabolized into harpagogenin, which may be responsible for decreasing inflammation.
- *Mechanism of action*: not clear.
- *Indications*: inflammation, rheumatism (50–100 mg harpagoside/d), pain, and appetite, bile, and gastric stimulation.
- *Risks*: may cause miscarriage.
- *Contraindications*: duodenal or gastric ulcers, gallstones, heart disease, pregnancy, use of warfarin.

WILLOW BARK EXTRACT

- *Source*: bark from branches of willow tree, *Salicis alba*.
- *Active ingredient*: phenolic glycosides (salicin, salicortin, piecin, fragilin, tremulacin, triandrin) and tannins.
- *Mechanism of action*: similar to aspirin but slower to take effect than aspirin.
- *Indications*: rheumatoid arthritis, inflammation, fever, headaches, influenza, myofascial pain.
- *Risks*: gastrointestinal irritation and bleeding; interaction with anticoagulants.

ASPEN OR GOLDENROD (PHYTODOLOR)

- *Source*: Phytodolor is 3:1:1 preparation of *Populus tremula, Fraxinus excelsior*, and *Solidago virgaurea* derived from common ash, aspen, and goldenrod.
- *Active ingredient*: salicylic acid derivatives, phenolic acid, flavonoids, and triterpene saponins.
- *Mechanism of action*: thought to suppress inflammation by inhibiting arachidonic acid metabolism via the cyclooxygenase and lipoxygenase pathways.
- *Indications*: musculoskeletal pain, inflammation, rheumatoid arthritis, optimization of muscle and joint function.
- *Contraindications*: Some people experience gastrointestinal upset, allergic reactions, and other less common adverse effects.

MARIJUANA

- *Source*: cannabis plant, *Cannabis sativa*.
- *Active ingredient*: Δ9-tetrahydrocannabinol (THC).
- *Mechanism of action*: agonist to CB1 receptors (ie, arachidonyl cyclopropylamide).

- *Indications*: used to manage allodynia and chronic hyperalgesia associated with cancer pain; may improve pain, mood, and sleep.
- *Risks*: hallucinations at high doses.
- Further research on THC and marijuana use is needed.

TURMERIC

- *Source*: perennial plant of the ginger family, *Curcuma longa*.
- *Active ingredient*: curcumin or diferuloylmethane.
- *Mechanism of action*: thought to suppress inflammation by inhibiting the cyclooxygenase and lipoxygenase pathways. Also support for antioxidant pathways by alteration of serum lipids.
- *Indications*: skin, pulmonary, GI, musculoskeletal, liver, rheumatologic.
- *Contraindications*: patients with gallstones, stomach ulcers, and bile duct obstructions should not eat large amounts of turmeric.

SUPPLEMENTS

GLUCOSAMINE

- *Source*: Glucosamine is an amino sugar produced from shells of shellfish and is a key component of cartilage.
- *Active ingredient*: glucosamine, a constituent of proteoglycans in cartilage.
- *Mechanism of action*: stimulates chondrocytes to produce cartilage.
- *Indications*: osteoarthritis, inflammation, progressive joint space loss.
- *Risks*: may increase insulin resistance.
- *Contraindications*: pregnancy, shellfish allergy

VITAMIN D

- *Source*: cholecalciferol.
- *Active ingredient*: 25-hydroxy vitamin D.
- *Mechanism of action*: produced phytochemically in the skin from 7-dehydrocholesterol, which then reacts with ultraviolet UVB light to produce vitamin D3 in skin. Binds to Vit D receptor in cells in most organs.
- *Indications*: osteoporosis, osteoarthritis, inflammation, depression.
- *Risks*: renal stones, diarrhea, hypercalcemia.

COENZYME Q10

- *Source*: component of the electron transport chain.
- *Active ingredient*: ubiquinone or ubiquinol.

- *Mechanism of action*: inhibition of both the initiation and propagation of lipid and protein oxidation.
- *Indications*: migraines, cancer, blood pressure.

OTHER MODALITIES

OSTEOPATHIC MEDICINE

- Holistic philosophy of health care practiced by Osteopathic physicians.
- Use of hands-on Osteopathic Manual Treatments (OMT) to treat somatic dysfunction within the body.
- OMT has been shown to be effective for treating a variety of issues such as back pain, headache, and otitis media.

MASSAGE

- *Mechanism of action*: relaxation and release of tense and taut muscle fibers; activates large afferent fibers, releasing endorphins.
- *Indications*: myofascial pain and muscle fatigue.
- One study found a significant difference between visual analog scale pain scores during rest and massage, but no difference was observed on electromyogram.

TRANSCUTANEOUS ELECTRICAL NERVE STIMULATION (TENS)

- *Mechanism*: pulsed electrical activity over the skin on a painful area activates large afferent fibers stimulating inhibitory dorsal horn neurons and releasing endorphins.
- *Indications*: TENS is a useful adjunctive treatment modality that helps many with chronic pain. It reduces scores on scales measuring anxiety and improves sleep.

ACUPUNCTURE

- *Mechanism of action*: Neurohumoral hypothesis suggests that pain relief is partly mediated by stimulating Aδ afferents and initiating a cascade of endorphins and monoamines activated by stimulating *de qi* (a sensation of numbness and fullness). Only limited evidence supports acupuncture as better than no treatment or placebo.
- Injection of bee venom into an acupoint may cause an anti-inflammatory and antinociceptive effect by stimulating a dormant immune reaction.
- *Indications*: chronic pain.
- *Risks*: relatively safe. Serious adverse events are rare.
- *Contraindications to bee venom*: allergy.

YOGA

- Increases strength, flexibility, feelings of well-being, and vitality.
- Significantly reduces pain intensity, functional disability, and pain medication usage in one study with two-month follow-up.

EXERCISE

- Strength training, stretching, endurance training, isometric strengthening, and aerobic exercises.
- Meta-analysis demonstrated that exercise therapy is beneficial for chronic low back pain.

BIBLIOGRAPHY

Anderson JW, Johnstone BM, Cook-Newell ME. Meta-analysis of the effects of soy protein intake on serum lipids. *N Engl J Med.* 1995;333:276–282.

Andersson, Lucente T, Davis AM, et al. A comparison of osteopathic spinal manipulation with standard care for patients with low back pain. *N Engl J Med.* 1999;341:1426–1431.

Anderson, Seniscal C, et al. A comparison of selected osteopathic treatment and relaxation for tension-type headaches. *Headache.* 2006;46:1273–1280.

Bharani A, Ganguli A, et al. Efficacy of terminalia arjuna in chronic stable angina: a double-blind, placebo-controlled, crossover study comparing terminal arjuna with isosorbide mononitrate. *Indian Heart J.* 2002;54:1705.

Deal CL. Neutraceuticals as therapeutic agents in osteoarthritis. *Rheum Dis Clin North Am.* 1999;25:379–395.

Dwivedi S, Jauhari R. Beneficial effects of terminalia arjuna in coronary artery disease. *Indian Heart J.* 1997;49:507.

Eisenberg DM, Davis RB, Ettner SL, et al. Trends in alternative medicine use in the United States, 1990–1997: Results of a follow-up national survey. *J Am Med Assoc.* 1998;280:1569.

Ernest E, White AR. Prospective studies of the safety of acupuncture: a systematic review. *Am J Med.* 2001;110:481.

Ezzo J, Berman B. Is acupuncture effective for the treatment of chronic pain? A systematic review. *Pain.* 2000;86:217.

FAO/WHO/UNU Expert Consultation. *Energy and Protein Requirements.* Geneva: World Health Organization; 1985: series 724.

Fraser J. Psychophysiological effects of back massage on elderly institutionalized patients. *J Adv Nurs.* 1993;18:238.

Hayden, van Tulder MW, Tomlinson G, et al. Strategies for using exercise therapy to improve outcomes in chronic low back pain. *Ann Intern Med.* 2005;142:776–785.

Iversen L, Chapman V. Cannabinoids: a real prospect for pain relief? *Curr Opin Pharmacol.* 2002;2:50.

Jamison RN, Stetson B, Sbrocco T. Effects of significant weight gain on chronic pain patients. *Clin J Pain.* 1990;6:47.

Jha HC, von Recklinghausen G, Zilliken F. Inhibition of *in vitro* microsomal lipid peroxidation by isoflavonoids. *Biochem Pharmacol*. 1985;34:1367.

Katzung BG, ed. *Basic and Clinical Pharmacology*. 8th ed. New York: Lange; 2001.

Kremer JM, Lawrence DL. Dietary fish oil and olive oil supplementation in patients with rheumatoid arthritis: clinical and immunological effects. *Arthritis Rheum*. 1990;33:810.

Kwon Y, Lee J. Bee venom injection into an acupuncture point reduces arthritis associated edema and nociceptive responses. *Pain*. 2001;90:271.

Lake JK, Power C, Cole TJ. Back pain and obesity in the 1958 British birth cohort: cause or effect? *J Clin Epidemiol*. 2000;53:245.

Lee J, Kwon Y. Bee venom pretreatment has both an antinociceptive and antiinflammatory effect on carrageenan-induced inflammation. *J Vet Med Sci*. 2001;63:251.

Linde K, Mulrow CD. *St John's Wort for Depression*. Oxford: Cochrane Collaboration, Cochrane Library; 2000; Issue 2.

Little C, Parsons T. Herbal therapy for treating rheumatoid arthritis. *Cochrane Database Syst Rev*. 2001;1:CD002948.

Mills, Henley CE, Barnes LL, et al. The use of osteopathic manipulative treatment as adjuvant therapy in children with recurrent acute otitis media. *Arch Pediatr Adolesc Med*. 2003;157:861–866.

Pisticelli SC, Burstein AH, Chaitt D. Indinavir concentrations and St John's wort. *Lancet*. 2000;355:547.

Pittler MH, Ernest E. Efficacy of kava extract for treating anxiety: systematic review and meta-analysis. *J Clin Pharmacol*. 2000;20:84.

Rao JK, Mihaliak K, Kroenke K, et al. Use of complementary therapies for arthritis among patients of rheumatologists. *Ann Intern Med*. 1999;131:409.

Reginster JY, Deroisy R, Rovati LC. Long-term effects of glucosamine sulphate on osteoarthritis progression: a randomized, placebo controlled clinical trial. *Lancet*. 2001;357:251.

Richards KC. Effect of back massage and relaxation intervention on sleep in critically ill patients. *J Adv Nurs*. 1998;7:288.

Rossi AL, Blostein-Fujii A, DiSilvestro RA. Soy beverage consumption by young men: increased plasma total antioxidant status and decreased acute, exercise-induced muscle damage. *J Nutraceuticals Functional Med Foods*. 2000;3:33.

Schenk RC. New approaches to the treatment of osteoarthritis: oral glucosamine and chondroitin sulfate. *AAOS Instruct Course Lect*. 2000;49:491.

Schofield D, Braganza JM. Shortcomings of an automated assay for total antioxidant status in biological fluids. *Clin Chem*. 1996;42:1712.

Seltzer Z, Dubner R, Shir Y. A novel behavioral model of neuropathic pain disorders produced in rats by partial sciatic nerve injury. *Pain*. 1990;43:245.

Shir Y, Ratner A, Raja SN, et al. Neuropathic pain following partial nerve injury in rats is suppressed by dietary soy. *Neurosci Lett*. 1998;240:73.

Simopoulos AP. Omega-3 fatty acids in health and disease and in growth and development. *Am J Nutr*. 1991;54:438.

Sims J. The mechanism of acupuncture analgesia: a review. *Complement Ther Med*. 1997;5:102.

Tanaka T, Leisman G. The effect of massage on localized muscle fatigue. *BMC Complementary Alternative Med*. 2002;2:9.

Ward RC. *Foundations for Osteopathic Medicine*. Baltimore, Md: Williams & Wilkins; 1997:3–14.

Ware MA, Gamsa A, Persson J. Cannabis for chronic pain: case series and implications for clinicians. *Pain Res Manag*. 2002;7:95–99.

Williams K, Petronis J, Smith D, et al. Effect of Iyenagar yoga therapy for chronic low back pain. *Pain*. 2005;115:107–117.

Wood C. Mood change and perceptions of vitality: a comparison of the effects of relaxation, visualization and yoga. *J R Soc Med*. 1993;86:254.

Wu ES, Loch JT 3rd, Toder BH, et al. Flavones. 3. Synthesis, biological activities, and conformational analysis of isoflavone derivatives and related compounds. *J Med Chem*. 1992;18:3519.

Yagasaki K, Kaneko M, Miura Y. Effect of soy protein isolate on cytokine productivity and abnormal lipid metabolism in rats with carrageenan-induced inflammation. *Soy Protein Res (Japan)*. 2001;4:65.

62 CRYONEUROLYSIS

Lloyd Saberski, MD

INTRODUCTION

- Cryoneurolysis temporarily destroys a nerve through the application of extreme cold.
- When a cryoprobe touches a nerve, the extreme cold degenerates the nerve axons without damaging surrounding connective tissue.

PHYSICS

- The cryoprobe consists of an outer tube and a smaller inner tube that terminates in a fine nozzle.
- The working principle of a cryoprobe is based on the expansion of compressed gas (nitrous oxide or carbon dioxide).
- High-pressure gas (650–800 psi) is passed between the tubes and released via a small orifice into a chamber at the tip of the probe. Expansion of the gas within the chamber causes a substantial reduction in pressure (80–100 psi) and a rapid decrease in temperature that cools the probe tip surface to approximately −70°C. This causes an ice ball to form around the exterior of the probe tip.
- The low-pressure gas flows back through the center of the inner tube to the console where it is vented.
- The sealed construction of the cryoprobe ensures that no gas escapes from the probe tip, handle, or hose.

Larger myelinated fibers cease conduction at 10°C, which is before unmyelinated fibers cease conduction, but at 0°C, all nerve fibers entrapped in the ice ball stop conduction. The clinical difference is moot as long as the temperature is below −20°C for 1 minute.

HISTOLOGY

- Histologically, the axons and myelin sheaths of the neurons degenerate after cryoneurolysis (wallerian degeneration), but the epineurium and perineurium remain intact, thus allowing subsequent nerve regeneration.
- The duration of the block depends on the rate of axonal regeneration after cryolesion, which is reported to be between 1 and 3 mm/d.
- Since axonal regrowth is constant, the return of sensory and motor activity is a function of distance between the cryolesion and the end organ.
- The absence of external damage to the nerve and the minimal inflammatory reaction following freezing ensure that regeneration is exact. Thus, the regenerating axons are less likely to form painful neuromas.

INDICATIONS

- Cryoneurolysis is best suited for clinical situations in which analgesia is required for weeks to months.
- The median duration of pain relief ranges from two weeks to five months.
- Cryoanalgesia is suitable for painful conditions that originate from small, well-localized lesions of peripheral nerves, such as neuromas, entrapment neuropathies, and axonal injury or severance from a surgical incision.
- The longer-than-expected periods of analgesia that have been reported may arise from the patient's enhanced ability to participate in physical therapy or from effect of prolonged analgesia on the central processing of pain (preemptive analgesic effect).
- Sustained blockade of afferent impulses with cryoanalgesia may reduce plasticity (windup) in the central nervous system and decrease pain permanently.

TECHNIQUE

- Cryoablative procedures can be performed open or closed (percutaneous), depending on the clinical setting. For management of chronic pain, however, open cryoneurolysis should be avoided if the procedure can be performed percutaneously.

OPEN CRYONEUROLYSIS FOR POSTOPERATIVE CRYOANALGESIA

- Most frequently, open procedures are performed to contribute to postoperative analgesia.
- Under direct visualization, the operator identifies the neural structure of concern and applies the cryoprobe for 1–4 minutes. (The time required is determined by tissue heat, blood supply, and the distance of the probe from the nerve.)
- Care is taken not to freeze adjacent vascular structures.
- The cryoprobe is withdrawn only after thawing, as removal with an intact ice ball can tear tissue.

Postthoracotomy Pain

- Intraoperative intercostal cryoneurolysis is an easily performed open procedure on intercostal nerves just lateral to the transverse process, before branching of the collateral intercostal nerve. (A closed intercostal cryoneurolysis is much more difficult to perform and carries the risk of pneumothorax.)
- Postthoracotomy cryoanalgesia is an effective means of treating incisional pain but is not effective for pain from visceral pleura supplied by autonomic fibers or for ligamentous pain of the chest secondary to intraoperative rib retraction.

Post-Herniorrhaphy Pain

- Cryolesioning of the ilioinguinal nerve will decrease analgesic requirements during the postoperative period.
- After repair of the internal ring, the posterior wall of the inguinal canal, and the internal oblique muscle, the ilioinguinal nerve on the surface of the muscle is identified and elevated above the muscle for cryoablation.

PERCUTANEOUS CRYONEUROLYSIS FOR CHRONIC PAIN

- Percutaneous (closed) cryoablation is the technique of choice for outpatient chronic pain management. It has the advantage of easy application with few complications.

Test Blocks

- Cryoanalgesia for chronic pain syndromes should always be preceded by diagnostic/prognostic local anesthetic test blocks.
- A favorable result occurs when the local anesthetic injection decreases pain and the patient can tolerate the numbness that replaces the pain.
- Care must always be taken regarding correct anatomic placement of the needles. When necessary, fluoroscopic guidance should be used.

- The smallest amount of local anesthetic required to achieve blockade must be used.
- A tuberculin syringe injecting tenths of a millimeter at a time ensures that the local anesthetic does not contaminate other structures, which would obfuscate interpretation of the block.

Percutaneous Cryoablation

- To perform a successful percutaneous cryoablation, it is essential to achieve proper placement of the cryoprobe.
- The preferred introducers are large-bore (12-, 14-, and 16-gauge) intravenous catheters, with the size based on the size of the cryoprobe.
- The nerve stimulator located at the tip of the cryoprobe can be used to determine if the cryoprobe is near a motor nerve.
- The operator freezes the nerve for 2–3 minutes.
- Often, patients feel an initial discomfort as the cooling begins, but this should quickly dissipate.
- Prior to removal of the probe, the tip should be thawed to prevent tissue damage from an ice ball sticking to the tissues.
- In general, with closed procedures, two freeze cycles, each 2 minutes in duration, followed by their respective thaw cycles, are sufficient.

INDICATIONS FOR CRYONEUROLYSIS IN CHRONIC PAIN

Intercostal Neuralgia

- Percutaneous cryoneurolysis of the intercostal nerves can be used to treat a variety of pain syndromes, including postthoracotomy pain, traumatic intercostal neuralgia, rib fracture pain, and, occasionally, postherpetic neuropathy.

Painful Neuroma

- Painful neuromas are typically associated with lancinating, shooting pain and are exacerbated by movement or deformation of nearby soft tissues.
- A cryoneurolysis is considered after careful mapping has isolated a discrete pain generator (neuroma).
- In these cases, cryoneurolysis is most effective when the volume of local anesthetic necessary for analgesia during the test block was 1 mL or less.

Pain Associated with Harvest of Iliac Crest Bone for Fusion

- This pain is often responsive to cryoablation in cases where more conservative therapies have failed.

Cervical and Lumbar Facet and INTERSPINOUS Ligament Pain

- Because this pain is typically exacerbated with movement, physiotherapy programs frequently fail.
- Fluoroscopically guided cryoneurolysis can improve analgesia, range of motion, and rehabilitation.

Coccydynia

- The test injection should be performed bilaterally and should provide short-term analgesia.
- To perform cryoneurolysis of the coccygeal nerve, the probe must be inserted into the canal and contact the nerve.
- Accurate placement of the ice ball is facilitated by using the 100-Hz stimulator and by gauging patient response.
- Care should be taken to prevent bending the relatively large cryoprobe when inserting it in the canal.

Perineal Pain

- Pain over the dorsal surface of the scrotum, perineum, and anus that has not been responsive to conservative management can at times be effectively managed with cryoneurolysis from inside the sacral canal with bilateral S4 lesions.
- Insertion of the cryoprobe through the sacral hiatus up to the level of the fourth sacral foramen for placement of a series of cryolesions can provide good analgesia for six to eight weeks.
- Bladder dysfunction only rarely results from this procedure.

Ilioinguinal, Iliohypogastric, and Genitofemoral Neuropathies

- These conditions often complicate herniorrhaphy, general abdominal surgery, or cesarean sections.
- Patients present with a sharp/lancinating or dull pain radiating into the lower abdomen or groin. The pain is exacerbated by lifting and defecation.
- Significant care and time must be spent in localizing the nerve, and use of the sensory nerve stimulator is required.
- The difficulty with localization has led to frequent misdiagnoses of the pain generator. In an effort to improve the accuracy of diagnosis, Rosser et al. developed a "conscious pain mapping technique." In a lightly sedated patient, a general surgeon working with a pain management specialist performs a laparoscopic evaluation of the abdomen in an operating suite. This allows easy visualization of the genitofemoral nerve, lateral femoral cutaneous nerve, and other structures.

Neuralgia Due to Irritation of the Infrapatellar Branch of the Saphenous Nerve

- This condition occurs weeks to years after blunt injury to the tibial plateau or following knee replacement.
- The nerve is vulnerable as it passes superficial to the tibial collateral ligament, piercing the sartorius tendon and fascia lata, inferior and medial to the tibial condyle.

Peroneal Neuralgias

- Neuralgia due to irritation of the deep peroneal, superficial peroneal and intermediate dorsal cutaneous nerves can occur weeks to years after injury to the foot and ankle.
- These superficial sensory nerves pass through strong ligamentous structures and are vulnerable to stretch injury with inversion of the ankle, compression injury due to edema, and sharp trauma from bone fragments.

Superior Gluteal Nerve Neuralgia

- This condition arises from irritation of the superior gluteal nerve which arises from the lumbosacral plexus proximal to where the sciatic nerve is usually located and is commonly seen following injury sustained while lifting.
- The superior gluteal nerve is vulnerable as it passes in the fascial plane between the gluteus medius and gluteus minimus musculature and can be injured by shearing between the gluteal musculature with forced external rotation of the leg and by extension of the hip under mechanical load.
- The clinical presentation consists of sharp pain in the lower back, dull pain in the buttock, and vague pain to the popliteal fossa.

Cranial Neuralgia

- Facial nerves can be cryolesioned.
- As these areas are relatively vascular, it is wise to inject a few milliliters of saline containing 1:100,000 epinephrine prior to insertion of the cryoprobe introducer cannula and to apply a postprocedural ice pack for 30 minutes to reduce pain and swelling.

Supraorbital Nerve Neuralgia

- This condition often occurs at the supraorbital notch.
- Vulnerable to blunt trauma, this nerve is often injured by deceleration against an automobile windshield (seen when there is an airbag failure).
- The pain of supraorbital neuralgia often manifests as a throbbing frontal headache. It is commonly confused with migraine and frontal sinusitis.

Infraorbital Neuropathy

- The infraorbital nerve is the termination of the second division of the trigeminal nerve.
- An irritative neuropathy can occur at the infraorbital foramen secondary to blunt trauma or fracture of the zygoma with entrapment of the nerve in the bony callus.
- Commonly confused with maxillary sinusitis, the pain of infraorbital neuralgia usually manifests as pain exacerbated with smiling and laughter.
- A referred pain to teeth is common, and a history of dental pain and dental procedures is typical.

Mandibular Neuropathy

- The mandibular nerve can be irritated at many locations along its path.
- Commonly injured as the result of hypertrophy of the pterygoids after chronic bruxism, it can also be irritated by loss of oral cavity vertical dimension from tooth loss and altered dentition.
- It is often associated with a referred pain to the lower teeth.

Injury to the Mental Nerve

- The mental nerve is the terminal portion of the mandibular nerve.
- Injury to this nerve frequently occurs in edentulous patients.
- This pain can be reproduced easily with palpation.

Auriculotemporal Neuropathy

- The auriculotemporal nerve can be irritated at a number of different sites, such as immediately proximal to the parietal ridge at the attachment of the temporalis muscle and, less commonly, at the ramus of the mandible.
- Patients often present with temporal pain associated with retroorbital pain.
- Pain is often referred to the teeth.
- Patients frequently awaken at night with temporal headache.

FUTURE DIRECTIONS

- Cryotechnology offers promise for a wide variety of pain management needs.
- Its unparalleled track record for safety is remarkable.
- Its effective and safe use on sensory and mixed nerves contrasts with the radiofrequency technology that potentially produces deafferentation.

- The preemptive anesthetic effect may make this a technique of choice for "wind-down" (calming the central nervous system during neuropathic pain states).
- Lack of controlled studies, lack of uniform training, and poor communication among providers have impeded widespread adoption of the technology.
- Currently there are no commercial units for nerve cryolesioning; the used market may be only choice for now.

BIBLIOGRAPHY

Evans P. Cryo-analgesia: the application of low temperatures to nerves to produce anesthesia or analgesia. *Anaesthesia*. 1981;36:1003.

Moesker AA, Karl HW, Trescot AM. Treatment of phantom limb pain by cryoneurolysis of the amputated nerve. *Pain Pract*. 2014;14(1):52–56.

Raj P. Cryoanalgesia. In: *Practical Management of Pain*. Chicago, Il.: Year Book Medical; 1986:779.

Rosser J, Goodwin M, Gabriel N, et al. Patient-guided mini-laparoscopy. *Pain Clin*. 2001;3(6):11.

Ryan AT, Grechushkin V, Durkin B, et al. Prospective evaluation of cryoneurolysis for refractory neuralgia. *J Vasc Interven Radiol*. April 2013;24(4 Suppl):S22. [Note: This is the publication of abstract only in proceedings of a conference.]

Sidebottom AJ, Carey EC, Madahar AK. Cryoanalgesia in the management of intractable pain in the temporomandibular joint: a five-year retrospective review. *Br J Oral Maxillofacial Surg*. 2011, December;49(8):653–656.

Wolter T, Deininger M, Hubbe U, et al. Cryoneurolysis for zygapophyseal joint pain: a retrospective analysis of 117 interventions. *Acta Neurochirurgica*. 2011, May;153(5):1011–1019.

63 SPINAL CORD STIMULATION

Richard B. North, MD

INTRODUCTION

- The clinical goal of spinal cord stimulation (SCS) for pain relief is to achieve a 50% or more reduction in pain.
- This generally involves overlapping the area of pain with stimulation-induced paresthesia.
- The technical goal of SCS for pain relief is to apply sufficient electrical stimulation to cause paresthesia overlap of the pain without causing discomfort or motor effects.
- SCS does not affect acute pain or predispose to injury, by making one insensate to pain.

MECHANISM OF ACTION

- The "gate control theory of pain," published in 1965, provided a scientific basis for the use of electrical stimulation to treat pain by proposing that a "gate" regulates transmission of pain sensations from the dorsal horn in the spinal cord to the brain. According to the theory, this gate opens when small fiber afferents are unusually active and closes when large fiber activity is dominant. By selectively depolarizing large fiber afferents in the dorsal columns, SCS can close this gate without causing motor effects. The gate control theory, however, fails to explain the fact that in some abnormal pain states large fibers themselves can signal hyperalgesia.
- A frequency-related conduction block might interfere with signals at the point where dorsal column fibers split from dorsal horn collaterals. This would explain why patients with pain who have a SCS prefer a minimum stimulation rate of 25 pulses per second.
- Animal studies using clinical range parameters indicate that the sympathetic nervous system and GABAergic interneurons might play a role when stimulation relieves ischemic or neuropathic pain.
- Validated computer-generated models that predict the distribution of SCS current flow and voltage gradients in the spinal canal and cord have revealed the potential recruitment of the pathways adjacent to the dorsal columns and of the dorsal roots.
- SCS changes the neurotransmitter and neurotransmitter metabolite concentrations in cerebrospinal fluid (CSF), including glutamate glycine and serotonin.
- Administration of the opioid antagonist naloxone has no effect on SCS efficacy, indicating that SCS is not mediated by opioid systems.

ELECTRICAL STIMULATION BASICS

- Stimulation Pulse
  - Contains the energy applied to the nerve
  - Characterized by strength (amplitude) and duration (pulse width)
  - Total charge per phase is measured in coulombs
  - Net charge is zero (avoiding electrochemical effects).
- Four parameters are used in SCS
  - Electrode Polarity
  - Amplitude
  - Pulse Width
  - Frequency (pulse repetition rate, the reciprocal of interpulse interval).
- Electrode polarity
  - For current to flow and thus for stimulation to occur, there must be at least one negative electrode (cathode) and one positive electrode (anode)

- Depolarization occurs under the cathode at a lower threshold than under the anode
  - To increase the charge density on cathode, increase the number of anodes
  - Controls the shape and density of the electrical field, which in turn will determine the nerve fibers that are activated
  - Multiple electrodes placed cephalad/caudad and medial/lateral over the spinal cord can be used to steer the current.
- Amplitude
  - Measured in volts or milliamps
  - Primary control over intensity of stimulus sensation
  - Higher the amplitude, the greater the size of the electrical field
  - Larger electrical fields depolarize nerves over a larger area
  - High amplitudes can cause uncomfortable side effects.
- Pulse width
  - Duration of stimulation pulse, typically measured in microseconds
  - Greater pulse width will depolarize fibers with higher threshold (sequential recruitment)
  - Adjustment in pulse width can activate fibers that normally would require higher amplitudes, resulting in uncomfortable side effects
  - Can be used to control the intensity of the stimulation pulse, in conjunction with amplitude adjustments.
- Frequency (pulse repetition rate)
  - Higher frequency increases the number of action potentials delivered by the nerve—up to the point at which conduction block can occur
  - Change in frequency results in changes in sensation
    - Low frequency = pulsing sensation
    - High frequency = flutter sensation, up to the point at which "flicker fusion" occurs
  - Higher frequency increases battery depletion.
- Electrical Basics
  - Ohm's law: Voltage (V) = Current (I) × Resistance (R)
  - We can control V and I but not R
  - Patient factors that affect R
    - Cerebrospinal fluid (CSF) depth
    - Fluids: CSF, blood, injectates
    - Dural thickness
    - Epidural fat
    - Scar tissue
  - CSF depth can change with posture, and scar tissue can build around the contacts over time.
- SCS system types
  - No controlled studies have been conducted to compare the efficacy of the different technologies
  - Voltage controlled

- Since voltage remains constant, current will change depending on the resistance (see Ohm's law)
  - Current controlled
    - Adjusts voltage depending on changes in resistance to maintain a constant current
  - Single source current control
    - One power source supplies all contacts
    - More current flows through electrodes with less resistance
  - Multiple independent current control (true "multichannel")
    - Each electrode has own independent power source

PATIENT SELECTION

GENERAL INDICATIONS

- An established and specific diagnosis should exist for the pain.
- All acceptable, less invasive treatment options should be exhausted.
- Psychiatric comorbidities, significant drug habituation, and issues of secondary gain should be addressed.
- Test stimulation with temporary electrode placement should relieve the pain.

SPECIFIC INDICATIONS

- The most common indication for SCS in the United States is "failed back surgery syndrome" with lumbar radiculopathy. Use of complex electrode arrays and careful psychophysical tests might help achieve coverage of associated axial low back pain. Nociceptive or mechanical axial low back pain might be harder to treat than neuropathic or deafferentation pain.
- In Europe, SCS is also used to treat ischemic pain arising from peripheral vascular disease in the lower extremities. In these patients, SCS can improve red blood cell flow velocity, capillary density, and perfusion pressures and might enhance limb salvage.
- SCS provides pain relief and anti-ischemic effects when used to treat intractable angina pectoris. Fortunately, SCS does not mask the pain of myocardial infarction.
- SCS might relieve segmental pain from spinal cord injury, postcordotomy dysesthesias, and other spinal cord lesions (such as multiple sclerosis).
- Pain from peripheral nerve injury or neuralgia, causalgia, and "reflex sympathetic dystrophy" (complex regional pain syndrome) responds to SCS.
- SCS is efficacious in cases of postamputation pain syndrome, including phantom limb and stump pain.

- Other applications of SCS include the management of intractable pain associated with lower extremity spasticity, evoked potential monitoring, cerebral blood flow, autonomic hyperreflexia, and motor disorders.

CONTRAIN-DICATIONS

- Coagulopathy
- Sepsis
- Untreated, major comorbidity (eg, depression)
- Serious drug behavior problems
- Inability to cooperate or to control the device
- Secondary gain
- Demand cardiac pacemaker (without ECG monitoring or changing the pacemaker mode to a fixed rate)
- MRI needs (for most systems).

SYSTEM DESIGN AND USE

- Modeling studies show that:
  - The longitudinal position of an electrode dictates whether it achieves paresthesia at any given segmental level.
  - Bipolar stimulation is most effective on longitudinal midline fibers.
  - The optimal contact separation is 1.4 times the thickness of the meninges and CSF (6–8 mm).
- Anatomic factors determine the appropriate position and spacing of spinal cord electrodes for the treatment of low back and leg pain. Although advancing electrodes cephalad would seemingly broaden the area of paresthesia, the decreasing thickness of ascending fibers in the dorsal column and the varying thickness of CSF might elicit excessive local segmental effects.
- **Test stimulation to define electrode position, if not to optimize results, should begin with closely spaced** bipoles, cathode cephalad to anode; an anode(s) may be added cephalad to create a longitudinal tripole. Creating a transverse tripole by adding lateral anodes should mitigate recruitment of lateral structures.
- In patients with failed back surgery syndrome who have low back and lower extremity pain, low thoracic electrode placement is most effective.

IMPLANTABLE DEVICES

Electrodes

- SCS electrodes are available as multicontact catheters (arrays of electrodes on a single carrier) inserted through a Tuohy needle or as insulated "paddles" or "plates" the width of which usually requires laminectomy or laminotomy (Figure 63-1).
- No single approach is the best for all patients. Percutaneous leads can be implanted with minimal tissue disruption, while laminotomy leads require surgical removal of ligament and/or bone for implantation. Some patients, eg those who have had prior surgery at the level of electrode implantation,

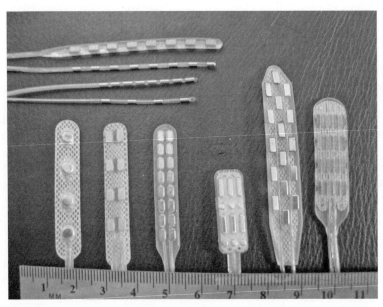

FIG. 63-1. Some multicontact SCS electrode arrays are placed through a Tuohy needle; others require laminectomy.

require surgical electrode placement even for an SCS trial.

- The percutaneous method offers longitudinal access to multiple levels of the spinal canal and, with fluoroscopy, allows the clinician to position the electrode optimally in a conscious patient.
- Insulated electrodes (requiring a small laminectomy) compare favorably with percutaneous electrodes for low back and lower extremity pain and require half the battery power. Clinical outcome has been reported to be significantly better with insulated than percutaneous electrodes at 1–2 years but not at 3 years.
- Posteriorly insulated "paddle" leads mitigate painful stimulation of the ligamentum flavum.
- In a single-center study, dual percutaneous electrodes, placed side by side bracketing the midline, were found to be inferior to a single electrode placed in the midline for the treatment of axial low back pain. However, many physicians find that two or more leads are advantageous.
- Intractable low back pain has been effectively treated with insulated arrays of two or three parallel columns of multiple contacts.
- Manufacturers are producing new electrodes with new contact configurations and an increased number of contacts.

Pulse Generators

- Implanted pulse generators can be programmed postoperatively with the patient in the appropriate position to determine which contacts should be active and which should be configured as anodes or cathodes.
- "Multichannel" systems (or single-channel generators gated to multiple outputs) are technically and clinically more reliable than single-channel systems.
- Radiofrequency-coupled passive implants used to deliver energy are not encumbered by components with a limited life, but the external antenna that accompanied the first generation of these systems was inconvenient, could irritate the skin, and could cause fluctuations in stimulation amplitude. Newer systems are being developed to overcome these difficulties.
- The convenience of primary cell battery-operated "implanted pulse generators" (IPGs) might improve patient compliance unless patients compromise usage to maximize battery life (dictated by the amount of power required for a given amplitude, width, repetition rate, and time in use).
- Patients control IPGs with an external magnet (on–off and some adjustment in stimulation parameters) and/or remote transmitter (for more complicated adjustments).

COMPUTERIZED STIMULATOR ADJUSTMENT

- The number of possible cathode and anode combinations increases proportionately with the number of contacts (eg, 50 for an array of four, 6050 for an array of eight).
- Further adjustments must be made to pulse parameters (width, rate, and amplitude).
- Each combination must be considered for amplitudes ranging from perception to discomfort.
- Computer analysis of these data for several populations of patients has resulted in the ability to make technical comparisons and in the development of rules and expert systems.
- A patient can make computerized adjustments directly using a graphic input device to control stimulus amplitude, draw areas of pain and stimulation paresthesias, and rate pain on a visual analog scale.
- The benefits of computerized adjustment include improved efficacy, battery life, and cost-effectiveness.

TRIAL PROTOCOLS

- A temporary epidural electrode may be placed percutaneously for a trial of SCS.
- The level of pain relief obtained and patient performance during a trial demonstrate the feasibility of long-term treatment by implanting a device.
- During a trial, longitudinal mapping of the epidural space indicates the optimal placement of an eventual chronic implant and provides information that helps in the choice of which electrode and generator to use.
- An SCS trial is a third-party-payer prerequisite for long-term SCS treatment in the United States. This requirement may be met by test stimulation immediately before implantation. Most SCS trials in the United States, however, last between three days and one week.
- Percutaneous trial electrode placement allows:
  - The efficacy to be assessed during the procedure in a fluoroscopy room (less expensive than an operating room).
  - The incremental withdrawal of the electrode at the bedside for assessment of a greater number of anode and cathode positions and pulse parameters.
  - Assessment under everyday conditions of activity and posture and with the patient's pain medications reduced.

○ The patient and the physician to gain information that will assist with implantation of a system for chronic use (specific array location, type of array (percutaneous vs. paddle, number of columns), power requirements, programming specifics).

- Because a prolonged trial might increase the risk of infection and of epidural scarring that might compromise implantation, it is wise to limit a trial to approximately one week, extending it on an individual basis.
- A percutaneous extension cable, intended for later removal, allows an implanter to adapt a temporary electrode for chronic use.
  ○ This option saves the expense of a second electrode but, unlike a simple percutaneous lead that can be removed at the bedside, requires one trip to the operating room for placement and another for internalization or removal.
  ○ Because percutaneous lead extensions increase the risk of infection, urgency to end the trial might lead to inappropriate implantation.
  ○ Increased incisional pain might confound trial results.
- Surgical electrode placement is sometimes required (eg, if prior spinal surgery precludes percutaneous access).
  ○ Surgical placement allows use of the insulated electrodes that prolong battery life and mitigate side effects, such as pain caused by the unwanted recruitment of small fibers in the ligamentum flavum.
- After a screening trial, clinicians should offer implantation for chronic use to patients who report at least 50% pain relief, have improved or stable analgesic requirements and activity levels, and wish to proceed with the therapy.
- Other outcome measures are difficult to assess on the basis of a trial.

OUTCOMES

- Reported "success" rates (generally defined as a minimum of 50% pain relief) vary from 12% to 88% at follow-ups of 0.5–8 years.
- More than two decades of data address additional outcome measures of patient satisfaction with treatment, activities of daily living, work status, medication requirements, and changes in neurologic function.
- Outcome results must be adjusted when the rate of permanent implantation is low (approximately 40%). This adjustment is less crucial when the implantation rate exceeds 75%.

POTENTIAL COMPLICATIONS AND ADVERSE EFFECTS

- Generator failure
- Electrode fatigue fracture
- Electrode migration/malposition
- Unpleasant sensations or damage to the implanted system from exposure to electromagnetic fields (eg, diathermy, security systems)
- Spinal cord or nerve injury
- CSF leak
- Infection
- Bleeding (eg, epidural hematoma in the worst case scenario leading to paralysis).

COST-EFFECTIVENESS

- In 1993, the World Health Organization (WHO) reported that "SCS appears to be cost-effective versus alternative therapies."
- Since that time, the cost-effectiveness of SCS versus reoperation and SCS versus conventional medical management for failed back surgery syndrome has been shown using data from randomized, controlled trials.
- Several modeling studies also support these conclusions.
- The cost effectiveness of SCS increases as the number of adverse events requiring expensive revisions decreases.

FUTURE DEVELOPME'NTS

- Multicontact, multichannel stimulation devices that are functionally equivalent to multiple stimulators
- Automated, enhanced, patient-interactive adjustment methods
- Improved electrode and system designs
- Improved (viz, rechargeable) power sources.

BIBLIOGRAPHY

Barolat G, Massaro F, He J. Mapping of sensory responses to epidural stimulation of the intraspinal neural structures in man. *J Neurosurg.* 1993;78:233.

Barolat G, Oakley JC, Law JD. Epidural spinal cord stimulation with multiple electrode paddle leads is effective in treating intractable low back pain. *Neuromodulation.* 2001;4:59.

ECRI. *Spinal Cord (Dorsal Column) Stimulation for Chronic Intractable Pain.* Health Technology Assessment Information Service, Plymouth Meeting, Pa.: ECRI; 1993.

Hautvast RWM, DeJongste MJL, Staal MJ, et al. Spinal cord stimulation in chronic intractable angina pectoris: a randomized, controlled efficacy study. *Am Heart J.* 1998;136:1114.

Holsheimer J. Effectiveness of spinal cord stimulation in the management of chronic pain: analysis of technical drawbacks and solutions. *Neurosurgery*. 1997;40:990.

Holsheimer J, Nuttin B, King GW. Clinical evaluation of paresthesia steering with a new system for spinal cord stimulation. *Neurosurgery*. 1998;42:541.

Holsheimer J, Struijk JJ. How do geometric factors influence epidural spinal cord stimulation? A quantitative analysis by computer modeling. *Stereotact Funct Neurosurg*. 1991;56:234.

Jacobs MJ, Jorning PJ, Beckers RC, et al. Foot salvage and improvement of microvascular blood flow as a result of epidural spinal cord electrical stimulation. *J Vasc Surg*. 1990;12:354.

Kemler MA, Barendse GAM, van Kleef M, et al. Spinal cord stimulation in patients with chronic reflex sympathetic dystrophy. *N Engl J Med*. 2000;343:618.

Kumar K, Taylor RS, Jacques L, et al. Spinal cord stimulation versus conventional medical management for neuropathic pain: a multicentre randomised controlled trial in patients with failed back surgery syndrome. *Pain*. 2007;132:179.

Linderoth B, Meyerson BA. Spinal cord stimulation, I. Mechanisms of action. In: Burchiel K, ed. *Pain Surgery*. New York: Thieme; 1999.

Melzack R, Wall PD. Pain mechanisms: a new theory. *Science*. 1965;150:971.

National Institute for Health and Clinical Excellence. Spinal cord stimulation for chronic pain of neuropathic or ischaemic origin: NICE technology appraisal guidance 159. Available at: http://www.nice.org.uk/nicemedia/live/12082/42367/42367.pdf.

North RB. Spinal cord stimulation for axial low back pain: single versus dual percutaneous electrodes. In: *International Neuromodulation Society Abstracts*. Lucerne; 1998:212.

North RB, Calkins SK, Campbell DS, et al. Automated, patient-interactive, spinal cord stimulator adjustment: a randomized controlled trial. *Neurosurgery*. 2003;52:572.

North RB, Ewend MG, Lawton MT, et al. Spinal cord stimulation for chronic, intractable pain: superiority of "multichannel" devices. *Pain*. 1991;44:119.

North RB, Kidd D, Shipley J, et al. Spinal cord stimulation versus reoperation for failed back surgery syndrome: a cost effectiveness and cost utility analysis based on a randomized, controlled trial. *Neurosurgery*. 2007;61:361.

North RB, Kidd DH, Olin JC, et al. Spinal cord stimulation electrode design: prospective, randomized, controlled trial comparing percutaneous and laminectomy electrodes, Part I: Technical outcomes. *Neurosurgery*. 2002;51:381.

North RB, Kidd DH, Zahurak M, et al. Spinal cord stimulation for chronic, intractable pain: two decades' experience. *Neurosurgery*. 1993;32:384.

North RB, Olin JC, Kidd DH. Spinal cord stimulation electrode design: a prospective, randomized controlled trial comparing percutaneous and laminectomy electrodes. *Stereotactic Funct Neurosurg*. 1999;73:134.

North RB, Sieracki JM, Fowler KR, et al. Patient-interactive, microprocessor-controlled neurological stimulation system. *Neuromodulation*. 1998;1:185.

Rigoard P, Delmotte A, D'Houtaud S, et al. Back pain: a real target for spinal cord stimulation? *Neurosurgery*. 2012;70:574.

64 EPIDURAL STEROID INJECTIONS

Anita Gupta, DO, PharmD
Steven P. Cohen, MD

BACKGROUND

- Back pain is a common complaint for which patients are seen.
- Most episodes of acute back pain resolve on their own within 12 weeks and extensive therapeutic intervention is not necessary.
- Among chronic low back pain cases, epidemiological studies using validated instruments suggest that around 40% are neuropathic in nature.

The process of selecting patients for specific therapies is particularly important in the potential application of interventional therapies such as nerve blocks.

- Deyo and Weinstein suggest that workup screening must answer three questions:
  ○ Is there systemic disease causing the pain?
  ○ Is there social or psychological distress that is amplifying or prolonging the pain?
  ○ Is there nerve compromise that might dictate surgical evaluation?
- One bases the recommended therapy on the most likely of the differential diagnoses, which are vast for complaints of back pain.
- Not all patients referred or selected for epidural steroid injections (ESIs) manifest the classic symptoms of radiculopathy (Table 64–1) or spinal stenosis, or are considered appropriate candidates.
- The correlation between diagnostic imaging and the effectiveness of ESIs is weak, so clinical judgment must be an additional and compelling component in the decision to perform ESI.
- Approximately two-thirds of patients with an acute herniated disc will experience resolution or remission of their pain within six months.
- A similar percentage will experience resorption of their herniated disc(s).

TABLE 64-1 **Classic Signs of Radiculopathy**

- Sharp, sudden, shooting pain
- Low back source: pain into the extremity below the knee
- Cervical spine source: pain into the upper extremity
- Increased pain with coughing, sneezing, or straining
- Onset often associated with lifting a heavy load while in an awkward position
- Repetitive spinal motions can be causative in fatigued, anxious, poorly conditioned individuals

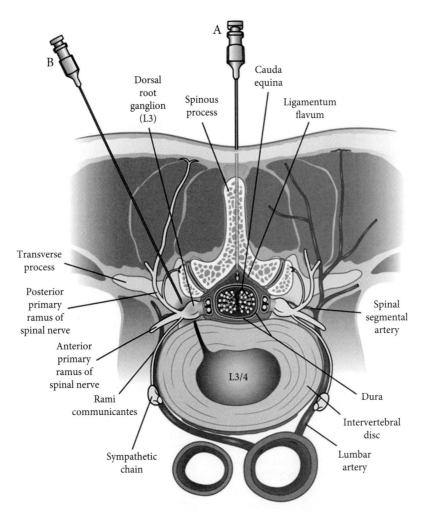

FIG. 64-1. Schematic drawing illustrating L3/4 interlaminar (A) and transforaminal (B) epidural needle placement in relation to anatomical structures in a patient with an L3/4 herniated disc. Adapted from Rathmell J. Atlas of Image-Guided Intervention in Regional Anesthesia and Pain Medicine, 2nd ed. Philadelphia, Pa.: Lippincott Williams & Wilkins; 2012.

- Epidural steroid injections (ESIs) are the most widely utilized pain management procedure in the world and despite the extensive literature on the subject, there continues to be considerable controversy surrounding their safety and efficacy.

- The results of clinical trials and review articles are heavily influenced by specialty, with those done by interventional pain physicians more likely to yield positive findings.

- Overall, more than half of controlled studies have demonstrated positive findings, suggesting a modest effect size lasting less than three months in well-selected individuals.

- Transforaminal injections may be more likely to yield positive results than interlaminar or caudal injections, and subgroup analyses indicate a slightly greater likelihood for a positive response for lumbar herniated disc, compared to spinal stenosis or axial spinal pain (Figure 64–1).

- Serious complications are rare following epidural steroid injections, provided proper precautions are taken.

- Although there are no clinical trials comparing different numbers of injections, guidelines suggest that the number of injections should be tailored to individual response, rather than a set series.

- Most subgroup analyses of controlled studies show no difference in surgical rates between ESIs and control patients; however, randomized studies conducted by spine surgeons, in surgically amenable patients with standardized operative criteria, indicate that in some patients the strategic use of ESI may prevent surgery.

- As with all treatments for chronic pain, the goals of treatment with epidural steroid injections include decreasing the frequency and/or the intensity of the pain, improving the patient's functional capacity, and enhancing the patient's ability to cope with residual pain.

RATIONALE FOR EPIDURAL STEROID INJECTIONS

- It is well established that radiculopathy may represent pathoanatomical changes resulting from a toxic spill of inflammatory mediators from the disc in addition to the primary problem of mechanical compression of nerve roots by herniated discs. Neuromuscular coordination defects are thought to cause inadequate distribution of physical forces that create pressures that exceed the viscoelastic characteristics of the annulus.
- The posterior longitudinal ligament is thinner in the lumbosacral spine area, and the shift of weight-bearing during aging from the anterior elements of the spine to the more delicate posterior elements of the spinal arch, including the pedicles, lamina, and facet joints, leads to either frank herniation of the disc or leakage of the contents of the nucleus pulposus.
- The disc contains phospholipase A-2 (PLA-2), interleukins, and proteoglycans.
- These are spilled into the epidural space, and are potent instigators of inflammation.
- Ingrowth of new nerves into the healing annulus may result in subsequent discogenic pain.
- Saal et al. showed that PLA-2 from the disc was one of the offending agents in creating nerve root swelling after McCarron et al. demonstrated that only small amounts of nucleus pulposus content were necessary to precipitate an inflammatory response.
- Corticosteroids inhibit PLA-2. Since the effect of PLA-2 is to release arachidonic acid from cell membranes, inhibiting this enzyme (which can be achieved with epidural steroids) decreases the release of inflammatory mediators.
- Chen et al. demonstrated in an animal model that PLA-2 can "cause nerve root and corresponding behavioral and electrophysiologic changes consistent with sciatica."
- Cytosolic glucocorticoid receptors are present in all cells and when activated by corticosteroids, they are transported to the nucleus where many changes in gene expression occur, resulting in changes in levels of different mediators. This may explain the prolonged effects on nociception.
- The traditional concept behind the injection of depo-steroids into the epidural space is that localized

placement maximizes the anti-inflammatory and antinociceptive effects and decreases the physical size of the nerve root, thereby decreasing the patient's symptoms.
- Once this result is achieved, resumption of normal activity and participation in focused physical therapy and rehabilitation are expected.
- There have also been suggestions that steroids have nonreceptor effects that include moderate blockade of nociceptive C fibers, membrane stabilization, reduction in ectopic discharges from inflamed tissue, and perhaps a reduction in CNS sensitization associated with acute and chronic pain.
- Finally, the anti-inflammatory actions of the local anesthetic frequently used has not been fully characterized, but likely includes the suppression of ectopic discharges from injured neurons, enhancing blood flow to ischemic nerve roots, and the washout of inflammatory mediators.

INDICATIONS AND POTENTIAL COMPLICATIONS

- The two most common steroid preparations used are triamcinolone and methylprednisolone.
- With recent reports of CNS toxicity with intra-arterial particulate steroids, there is a trend toward using dexamethasone. However, these toxicities have only been demonstrated with transforaminal injection.
- These are chemically altered such that their solubility is diminished, resulting in an estimated dwell time of two to three weeks.
- The drugs exert systemic effects so caution is advised with their use in patients with congestive heart failure, renal insufficiency, and diabetes secondary to the fluid retention and metabolic effects.
- Concern about the intrathecal placement of these compounds is based on historical and scientific data suggesting it may result in arachnoiditis.
- The potential for inducing adhesive arachnoiditis is low and any such symptoms are generally less of a concern than the potential for procedure-related side effects such as backache, postdural puncture headache, paresthesias, bleeding, and infection, or even anxiety-related symptoms such as lightheadedness and nausea.
- Patients with back pain are often treating the musculoskeletal component of their pain with nonsteroidal anti-inflammatory drugs (NSAIDs). A common question is, "Can patients on such medications safely receive an epidural injection with a 17-gauge needle?"
- Horlocker et al. examined at the incidence of hemorrhagic complications related to NSAID use in patients receiving epidural steroid injections.

- ○ One thousand thirty-five patients underwent 1214 injections, the majority of them in the midline and at lumbosacral spine levels.
- ○ Thirty-two percent had used NSAIDs within one week.
- ○ Five and two-tenths percent of patients had a minor, hemorrhagic complication defined as blood appearing in the needle or catheter.
- ○ No spinal hematomas were detected. Four percent of patients experienced worsening of their primary symptoms or a new neurologic deficit.
- ○ Significant risk factors identified included increased patient age, needle gauge, the procedural approach used, attempts at multiple levels, the number of needle passes, the volume of the injectate, and accidental dural puncture.
- ○ The authors conclude that epidural steroid injections are safe in patients taking NSAIDs.
- ○ There are also concerns about the potential increase in the intensity of symptoms if NSAIDs are withheld.
- Liu et al. reported on the benefit of using 20-gauge Tuohy needles. Although effective in increasing patient comfort and lessening the risk of postdural puncture headache, because of the higher incidence of false-positive loss of resistance their use might also require confirmation of correct placement using fluoroscopy, adding expense and logistical issues to the equation. The loss of resistance technique with these smaller needles was most inaccurate in males and patients older than 70.
- A contemporary point of view holds that clinicians must establish a differential diagnosis for the patient's complaints through the distillation of data from history taking, physical examination, and laboratory tests.
- Distinguishing internal disc disruption, which may result in referred pain to the thigh(s) and leg(s) in the absence of neuropathology, from radiculopathy, which is generally associated with dermatomal pain and nerve root sensory and/or motor changes, is important.
- Epidural steroid injections are of questionable benefit in mechanical pain secondary to internal disc disruption. There is sound evidence that they provide relief in radiculopathy. Studies are mixed as to whether patients with neurogenic claudication receive somewhat less, or comparable benefit to those presenting with radiculopathy.
- Fanciullo et al. surveyed 25,479 patients referred to 23 specialty spine care centers with spinal and radicular pain regarding the application of published guidelines that qualify patients for (mostly lumbar) epidural steroid injections.
  - ○ Whereas it is felt that younger patients with a recent onset of radicular pain and no history of back surgery represent the best candidates, the authors reported that epidural steroid injections were recommended for only 7.9% of the studied patients.
- ○ These patients were characterized by complaints of radiating pain in a dermatomal distribution, and neurologic signs on examination.
- ○ Patients who received epidural steroid injections had a higher incidence of comorbid conditions such as congestive heart failure, hypertension, peripheral vascular disease, and diabetes mellitus.
- ○ This is significant since most reported cases of epidural abscess related to epidural steroid injections have occurred in diabetics.
- ○ In his editorial on this study, Abram notes that the diagnosis of radiculopathy is the most consistent predictor of outcome with epidural steroid treatment, including patients with the provisional diagnosis of spinal stenosis.
- ○ The application of guidelines as documented by Fanciullo et al. resulted in a relatively small proportion of patients being referred for epidural steroid injections, many of whom had protracted symptoms and/or previous surgical treatment—groups less likely to respond to epidural steroid injections.
- A short-term response would generate frequent requests for repeated treatment, leading to risks of steroid-related and/or procedure-related complications in groups of patients perhaps already at risk.

INTERVENTIONAL TECHNIQUE

- Many, many studies have been published, but the lack of consistency of research design, type(s) of patients included, therapeutic protocol, and quality and duration of follow-up have been a significant problem in comparing the results and unifying the therapeutic approach based on randomized controlled trials (Figure 64-2).
- The addition of fluoroscopy to the armamentarium theoretically limits the complications of this procedure by allowing confirmation of correct needle placement and demonstrating the clinically relevant spread of the injectate, but its ability to improve outcomes has yet to be evaluated in clinical trials.
- The widespread availability of fluoroscopy has allowed for the growth of the transforaminal/selective nerve root block (SNRB) technique.
- This places the corticosteroid at a site in which the drug is more likely to reach the anterior epidural space, the most common site of pathology.
- Lutz et al. advocated the (anatomically) "safe triangle" approach for transforaminal blocks to enhance the accuracy of drug deposition, and provide a relatively high steroid concentration at the chosen site.

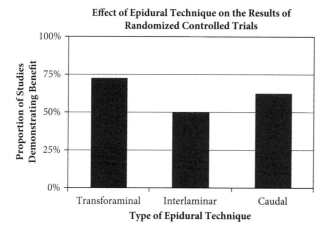

Effect of Epidural Technique on the Results of Randomized Controlled Trials

FIG. 64-2. Effect of epidural technique on the results of randomized controlled trials. Notes: (1) Based on all randomized, placebo-controlled studies performed since 1970, as cited in PubMed and EMBASE. (2) Benefit tabulated at initial visit for primary outcome measure. Adapted from Cohen SP, Bicket, MC, Jamison D, et al. A comprehensive, evidence-based review. *Reg Anesth Pain Med.* 2013;38:175–200.

However, the use of a "safe triangle" has been called into question.
- After 60 years of clinical use, there still is no consensus as to what the best technique is for delivering steroids to the affected nerve root or epidural space.
- The majority of practitioners use the loss of resistance technique to identify the epidural space, with patients in the prone position. Fluoroscopy is used more in nonacademic than academic venues.
- The most frequent injectate includes a combination of local anesthetic and corticosteroid.
- A recent meta-analysis and systematic review suggests that even without steroids, epidural injections themselves may provide some benefit.
- A cautionary tone is not unreasonable considering that closed claim data are beginning to indicate that ESIs – especially in the cervical region – are a major source of claims, leading some insurance companies to apply a surcharge for malpractice coverage for pain management physicians (personal communication).
- Clinical trials are mixed regarding whether epidural steroid injections provide long-term relief, reduce the need for surgery, or decrease healthcare utilization.
- A thorough review comparing the transforaminal to interlaminar and caudal techniques suggests that the transforaminal approach may provide superior benefit.
- Although deductive reasoning suggests that the use of fluoroscopy may improve outcomes, there is no difference in the results of clinical trials between those that used fluoroscopy and those that did not, and one cost minimization analysis suggested that epidural steroids performed under fluoroscopy are not cost-effective.

- Epidural steroid injections are inherently nondiagnostic. Selective nerve root blocks, in which the local anesthetic injectate is limited to a single nerve root, are diagnostic but have limited specificity. If the targeted nerve root is a source of pain, the addition of steroids can improve the therapeutic value.
- Studies are decidedly mixed regarding whether or not epidural steroid injections are cost-effective and whether or not they have a surgery-sparing effect.
- Despite media-hyped reports of serious complications following ESI, the procedures are very safe.
- Elevated glucose levels may occur for several days after epidural steroid injections, but there are no long-term adverse effects on glycemic control.
- Death and spinal cord infarction have been reported following transforaminal epidural steroid injections, and are postulated to result from a direct toxicity of the steroids to the blood brain barrier ("chemical burn") with a resultant breakdown in the barrier. This may occur in any spinal region, but is more common in the cervical and thoracic regions. This has not been demonstrated with dexamethasone in animal studies. In addition, there are no reports of death and spinal cord infarct with the use of dexamethasone. The use of heavy sedation for cervical epidural steroid injections may increase the risk of complications.
- It has been suggested that inadvertent intrathecal injection of depo-steroids may result in arachnoiditis; however, this complication is exceedingly rare.

EVIDENCE AND OUTCOMES

- A recent comprehensive review of epidural steroid injections was completed by Cohen et al. (Tables 64-2 to 64-4).
- Published success rates for ESIs vary widely between 18% and 90%.
- Patients with less disease burden (ie, shorter duration, lower baseline disability and pain scores, no opioid use) with a herniated disc are more likely to benefit from ESIs. Whereas some studies have demonstrated a better response in patients with herniated disc than spinal stenosis, an equal number have not.
- Patients with less disease burden (eg, short duration of pain, not on opioids or disability, good function, intermittent rather than constant pain, lower pain scores, shorter duration, no previous surgery) generally respond better to epidural steroid injections than those with a higher disease burden. However, in clinical trials a high proportion of these patients who receive a "control" injection will also improve.
- The presence of psychopathology and adverse social factors (eg, secondary gain, low job satisfaction)

TABLE 64-2 Studies Comparing TF, IL, and Caudal ESI

STUDY	DESIGN	SUBJECTS	INTERVENTIONS	RESULTS	COMMENTS
Ackerman and Ahmad (2007)	Randomized evaluator blinded	90 patients with S1 radiculopathy from HNP	TF: 40 mg triamcinolone + 4 mL NS IL: 40 mg triamcinolone + 4 mL NS C: 40 mg triamcinolone + 19 mL NS	TFESI > ILESI or caudal ESI at 24 weeks	Patients with ventral epidural spread, more common in TFESI group, had better outcomes
Candido et al. (2008)	Randomized	60 patients with unilateral radiculopathy from HNP and DDD	TF and IL: 80 mg methylprednisolone + 1 mL NS + 1 mL 1% lidocaine	No difference between TFESI and ILESI up to 6 months	Study underpowered.
Gharibo et al. (2011)	Randomized	42 patients with unilateral radiculopathy from disc disease <1 year	TF: 40 mg triamcinolone + 1 mL 0.25% bupivacaine IL: 80 mg triamcinolone + 2 mL 0.25% bupivacaine	TFESI > ILESI at 2 weeks follow-up	Short follow-up period
Kolsi et al. (2000)	Randomized	30 patients with sciatic or femoral neuralgia	TF and IL: 3.75 mg cortivazol + 2 mL 0.5% lidocaine	No difference between TFESI and ILESI up to 4 weeks	TFESI > ILESI for initial mean pain score decrease
Kraemer et al. (1997)	Randomized	182 patients with LBP	TF, IL, and paravertebral injections not described	TFESI > ILESI > paravertebral local anesthetic up to 3 months	IM steroid injection added in saline group
Lee et al. (2009)	Randomized evaluator blinded	192 patients with axial LBP due to HNP or SS	TF: 20 mg triamcinolone + 4 mL 0.5% lidocaine IL: 40 mg triamcinolone + 8 mL 0.5% lidocaine	TFESI > ILESI up to 4 months	TF injections received half ILESI dose on each side. Differences between groups greater for SS patients
Rados et al. (2011)	Randomized	64 patients with chronic unilateral lumbar radiculopathy	TF: 40 mg methylprednisolone + 3 mL 0.5% lidocaine IL: 80 mg methylprednisolone + 8 mL 0.5% lidocaine	No difference between TFESI and ILESI through 6 months	TFESI contained half the steroid dose and >50% less LA
Thomas et al. (2003)	Randomized	31 patients with lumbosacral radiculopathy from HNP <3 months	TF and IL: 5 mg dexamethasone in 2 mL solution	TFESI > ILESI up to 6 months	Fluoroscopy used for TFESI, while ILESI done blindly
Lee et al. (2009)	Retrospective	233 patients with lumbosacral radiculopathy from SS or HNP	TF small volume: 40 mg triamcinolone + 2 mL 0.5% lidocaine TF large volume: 40 mg triamcinolone + 8 mL 0.5% lidocaine IL: 40 mg triamcinolone + 8 mL 0.5% lidocaine C: 40 mg triamcinolone + 15 mL 0.5% lidocaine	Satisfaction and pain scores: TFESI and ILESI > caudal ESI up to 2 months Function: TFESI > ILESI > caudal ESI	Functional benefits of TFESI more pronounced at 2 weeks. Injectate volumes not standardized

Study	Type	Population	Intervention	Results	Comments
Manchikanti et al. (1999)	Retrospective case control	225 patients with low back and leg pain	TF: 1.5–3 mg betamethasone + 1 mL 1% lidocaine IL: 120 mg depo-methylprednisolone + 10 mL 0.5% lidocaine, with 80 mg methylprednisolone on subsequent injections C: 80 mg depo-methylprednisolone + 1-mL 0.5% lidocaine	TFESI and caudal ESI > ILESI at 1–3 months follow-up, but no difference between groups at 3–6 and 6–12 months follow-up	Longer pain duration in caudal ESI group. Variable steroid dose in TFESI and variable follow-up period
Schaufele et al. (2006)	Retrospective case control	40 patients with lumbosacral radiculopathy from single-level HNP	TF: 80 mg methylprednisolone + 1–2 mL 2% lidocaine IL: 80 mg methylprednisolone + 2–3 mL 1% lidocaine	TFESI > ILESI; variable follow-up period averaging 3 weeks	Higher baseline pain scores in ILESI group. Short follow-up period
Smith et al. (2010)	Retrospective case control	38 patients with lumbosacral radiculopathy from SS	TF: 80 mg methylprednisolone + 1–2 mL 2% lidocaine IL: 80 mg methylprednisolone + 2–3 mL 2% lidocaine	No difference between TFESI and ILESI; variable follow-up averaging 4–6 weeks	Study underpowered.
Mendoza-Lattes et al. (2009)	Retrospective case-control	93 patients with mostly lower lumbar radiculopathy	Caudal: Up to 3 injections of 2 mL of 40 mg/mL depo-methylprednisolone or 3 mL of 6 mg/mL betamethasone Transforaminal: Up to 3 injections of a 1:1 solution containing 1.5–2 mL of bupivacaine 0.25% mixed with depomethylprednisolone or betamethasone	C = TF through 2-years follow-up	16 pts lost to follow-up. Equivalent rates of surgery between groups. Low volumes used for caudal injections. Included some pts with stenosis and spondylolisthesis

TF, transforaminal; IL, interlaminar; C, caudal; ESI, epidural steroid injection; LBP, low back pain; LA, local anesthetic; SS, spinal stenosis; HNP, herniated nucleus propulsus; DDD, degenerative disc disease.

Adapted from Cohen SP, Bicket, MC, Jamison D, et al. A comprehensive, evidence-based review. *Reg Anesth Pain Med.* 2013;38:175–200.

TABLE 64-3 Randomized Studies Comparing Different Steroid Mixtures and Approaches for ESI

STUDY	DESIGN	SUBJECTS	INTERVENTIONS	RESULTS
Studies Comparing Different Doses of Steroids				
Owlia et al. (2007)	Randomized case-matched for age/gender	84 patients with lumbar radiculopathy from HNP	ILESI with methylprednisolone 40 mg or 80 mg + 2–4 mL 2% lidocaine	No significant difference between groups for VAS improvement. Fewer complications in low-dose group
Kang et al. (2011)	Randomized double blind	160 patients with lumbar radiculopathy from HNP	2 TFESI at 1 week intervals of triamcinolone 5 mg, 10 mg, 20 mg, or 40 mg	Significant pain reduction in all groups except 5 mg after first injection. Nonsignificant trend of better pain reduction with increasing dose after second injection
Revel et al. (1996)	Randomized	60 patients with lumbosacral pain from failed back surgery syndrome	Caudal ESI with either: A: Prednisolone 125 mg in 5 mL alone B: Prednisolone 125 mg in 5 mL + 40 mL NS	High volume injection > low volume for VAS reduction at 18 months
Studies Comparing Different Types of Steroids				
Dreyfuss et al. (2006)	Randomized	30 patients with unilateral cervical radiculopathy	TFESI with 0.75–1 mL 4% lidocaine + either: A: Dexamethasone 12.5 mg B: Triamcinolone 60 mg	Nonsignificant trend favoring particulate steroid
Lee et al. (2009)	Retrospective	159 patients with cervical radiculopathy who failed IL ESI or had previous surgery	TFESI with either: A: Dexamethasone 10 mg B: Triamcinolone 40 mg	Nonsignificant trend favoring particulate steroid
Kim and Brown (2011)	Randomized single blinded	60 patients with lumbar radiculopathy ≥ 6 months	ILESI with 10 mL consisting of 2 mL 0.25% bupivacaine + NS + either: A: Dexamethasone 15 mg B: Methylprednisolone 80 mg	Nonsignificant trend favoring particulate steroid
Park et al. (2010)	Randomized	106 patients with lumbar radiculopathy	TFESI with 1 mL 1% lidocaine + either: A: Dexamethasone 7.5 mg B: Triamcinolone 40 mg	Particulate > nonparticulate steroid for pain reduction
Noe and Haynsworth (2003)	Retrospective	52 patients with low back pain referred for ESI	ILESI with either: A: Betamethasone 15 mg B: Methylprednisolone 80 mg	Particulate > nonparticulate steroid for pain reduction, improvement in disability
Shakir et al. (2013)	Retrospective	441 patients with cervical radiculopathy	TFESI with 1 mL of 1% lidocaine + either: A: Dexamethasone 15 mg B: Triamcinolone 40 mg	No difference in pain score reduction between groups
Studies Comparing Different Injection Levels				
Jeong et al. (2007)	Randomized single blinded	239 patients with lumbosacral radiculopathy from HNP or SS scheduled for one level TFESI from L1 to S1	TFESI with 40 mg triamcinolone + 0.5% 0.5 mL bupivacaine, of either location: A: Ganglionic—at location of exiting nerve root B: Preganglionic—at supra-adjacent intervertebral disk	Nonsignificant trend favoring preganglionic > ganglionic at one month, but no differences at 6 months follow-up
Lee et al. (2006)	Retrospective	33 patients with lumbar radiculopathy receiving on level TFESI from L1 to S1	TFESI with triamcinolone 40 mg + 0.5 mL 0.5% bupivacaine at either A. Conventional approach B. Preganglionic approach (one level above conventional approach)	Preganglionic TFESI trends toward but is not significantly better than conventional approach at 2 weeks follow-up

TF, transforaminal; IL, interlaminar; ESI, epidural steroid injection; SS, spinal stenosis; HNP, herniated nucleus propulsus.

Adapted from Cohen SP, Bicket, MC, Jamison D, et al. A comprehensive, evidence-based review. *Reg Anesth Pain Med.* 2013;38:175–200.

TABLE 64-4 Review Articles Evaluating Epidural Steroid Injections Stratified by Specialty

STUDY, YEAR	TYPE OF REVIEW	TYPE OF EPIDURAL	PRIMARY AUTHOR SPECIALTY	CONCLUSIONS
Staal et al. (2009)	Systematic	Lumbar	Epidemiology	There is limited to moderate evidence that ESIs are not better than placebo or other treatments for pain relief or disability.
Ranquis et al. (2010)	Systematic	Perioperative Lumbar	Neurosurgery	ESIs reduce postoperative pain and analgesic consumption, and risk of not returning to work, but do not affect quality of life.
Armon et al. (2007)[1]	Systematic	Lumbar	Neurology	Does not impact function, decrease rate of surgery, or provide pain relief for >3 months.
Carragee et al. (2008)	Systematic	Cervical	Orthopedic Surgery	There is support for short-term, but not long-term symptomatic improvement of radicular symptoms with epidural corticosteroids.
Karnezis (2008)	Evidence-based	Lumbar	Orthopedic Surgery	Epidural steroid injections may provide only short-term relief from pain in lumbar radiculopathy but have no long-term effect.
Deyo et al. (2009)	Narrative	Lumbar	Internal Medicine	Increases in expenditures for ESIs are not accompanied by improvements in patient outcomes.
Roberts et al. (2009)	Systematic	Lumbar	Physical Medicine	Fair evidence-supporting TFESIs for treatment of radicular symptoms, good evidence for surgery sparing. TFESIs are superior to ILESI for radicular pain.
Benny and Azari (2011)	Systematic	Lumbar Transforaminal	Physical Medicine	There is strong evidence for TFESI for both short-term and long-term relief.
Balague et al. (2012)	Narrative	Lumbar	Rheumatology	Although there is some biological and animal data in favor of corticosteroids for LBP and sciatica, clinical evidence remains scarce. However, ESI can have some short-term benefit.
Rho and Tang (2011)	Narrative	Lumbar	Physical Medicine	There is strong evidence to support the use of TFESI for radicular pain caused by HNP or spinal stenosis. There is evidence for IL and caudal ESI, but less than for TFESI.
Quraishi (2012)	Systematic and Meta-Analysis	Systematic	Surgery	Appropriately performed TFESI should result in short-term improvement in pain, but not disability. The addition of steroids provides no additional benefit to local anesthetic.
Eckel and Bartynski (2009)	Narrative	Lumbar and Cervical	Interventional Radiology	Epidural steroid injections are highly effective in a large proportion of patients, including patients with axial pain (neck or low back pain), radiculopathy, or spinal stenosis with neurogenic claudication.
Diwan et al. (2012)	Systematic	Cervical	Anesthesiology	The evidence is good for cervical ESI for HNP with radiculitis.
Manchikanti et al. (2012)	Systematic	Lumbar TFESI	Anesthesiology	The evidence is good for TFESI for HNP with radiculitis and fair for spinal stenosis.
Benyamin et al. (2012)	Systematic	Lumbar Interlaminar	Anesthesiology	The evidence is good for lumbar ILESI for HNP with radiculitis and fair for spinal stenosis.
Parr et al. (2012)	Systematic	Caudal	Anesthesiology	Good evidence for short- and long-term relief for HNP with radiculitis, and fair evidence for spinal stenosis, failed back surgery syndrome or axial pain.
MacVicar et al. (2013)	Comprehensive	Lumbar TFESI	Physical Medicine/ International Spinal Intervention Society	In a substantial proportion of patients with lumbar radicular pain caused by contained disc herniations, lumbar TF injection of corticosteroids is effective in reducing pain, restoring function, reducing the need for other health care, and avoiding surgery.

Adapted from Cohen SP, Bicket, MC, Jamison D, et al. A comprehensive, evidence-based review. *Reg Anesth Pain Med.* 2013;38:175–200.

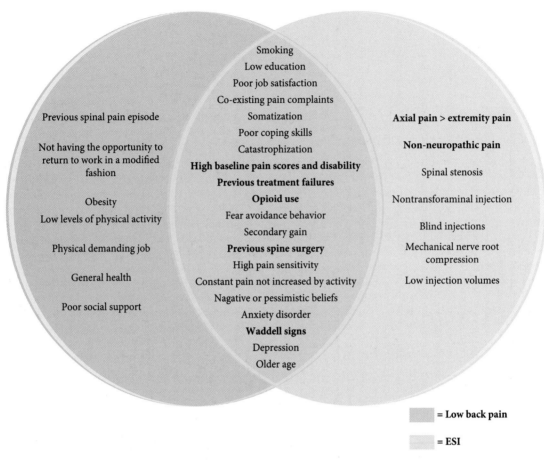

FIG. 64-3. Venn diagram depicting predictors of a poor outcome for low back and epidural steroid injections. Characteristics in bold denote major risk factors for negative outcome. Adapted from Cohen SP, Bicket, MC, Jamison D, et al. A comprehensive, evidence-based review. *Reg Anesth Pain Med.* 2013;38:175–200.

are associated with a poorer treatment outcome (Figure 64-3).

- Randomized trials suggest that doses of depomethyl prednisolone or triamcinolone greater than 40 mg do not increase effectiveness, and that even lower dosages may be just as effective.
- When performing a transforaminal epidural steroid injection for a paracentral disc herniation, it may be better to inject at the level of pathology (ie, L4-5 for an L4-5 herniated disc affecting the L5 nerve root) than at the level of symptoms.
- Patients with cancer-related pain who are thought to have tumor invasion of nerve roots (which causes an inflammatory pathology), and those with acute herpes zoster, may benefit from ESIs.

CONCLUSION

- Back pain is a common, pervasive, and expensive problem.

- Neuropathic pain comprises a much higher percentage of patients with chronic low back pain (approximately 40%) than has previously been appreciated.
- Patients with neuropathic pain respond better to epidural steroids than those with mechanical back pain.
- Treating the cause of the pain is more likely to be successful than merely treating the symptom of pain.
- Patients should be actively evaluated for all the procedures including ESIs, each time they present for treatment.
- There is little basis for performing a routine series of epidural steroid injections. Instead, the number of injections should be determined based on patient response.
- The clinical decision as to what type of procedure to perform should be symptoms, imaging, and physical exam findings.
- ESIs are not to be viewed as generic treatment for all patients with back pain complaints.
- ESIs should be but one component of a coordinated multidisciplinary treatment program that balances the continuation of effective therapy with the cessation

of any therapy that is not working or is causing side effects.
- ESIs can help patients achieve the goals of acute and chronic pain management.

BIBLIOGRAPHY

Abram SE. Treatment of lumbosacral radiculopathy with epidural steroids. *Anesthesiology*. 1999;91:1937–1941.

Abram SE. Factors that influence the decision to treat pain of spinal origin with epidural steroid injections. *Reg Anesth Pain Med*. 2001;26:2–4.

Benoist M. The natural history of lumbar disc herniation and radiculopathy. *Joint Bone Spine*. 2002;69:155–160

Bicket M, Gupta A, Brown C, et al. Epidural injections for spinal pain: what constitutes a treatment versus a control. A systematic review and meta-analysis. *Anesthesiology*. 2013;9(4),907–931. In press.

Cannon DT, Aprill CN. Lumbosacral epidural steroid injections. *Arch Phys Med Rehabil*. 2000;81:S-87–S-98.

Chen C, Cavanaugh JM, Ozaktay AC, et al. Effects of phospholipase A2 on lumbar nerve root structure and function. *Spine*. 1997;22:1057–1064.

Cluff R, Mehio A-K, Cohen SP, et al. The technical aspects of epidural steroid injections: a national survey. *Anesth Analg*. 2002;95:403–408.

Cohen SP, Bicket, MC, Jamison D, et al. Epidural steroids: a comprehensive, evidence-based review. *Reg Anesth Pain Med*. 2013;38:175–200.

Cribb G, Jaffray D, Cassar-Pullicino V. Observations on the natural history of massive disc herniation. *J Bone Joint Surg (Br)*. 2007;89:782–784.

Dawley JD, Moeller-Bertram T, Wallace MS, et al. Intra-arterial injection in the rat brain: evaluation of steroids used for transforaminal epidurals. *Spine*. 2009;34(16):1638–1643.

Deyo RA, Weinstein JN. Primary care: low back pain. *N Engl J Med*. 2001;344:363–370.

Even J, Crosby C, Song Y, et al. Effects of epidural steroid injections on blood glucose levels in patients with diabetes mellitus. *Spine*. 2012;37:E46–E50.

Fanciullo GJ, Hanscom B, Seville J, et al. An observational study of the frequency and pattern of use of epidural steroid injection in 25,479 patients with spinal and radicular pain. *Reg Anesth Pain Med*. 2001;26:5–11.

Henschke N, Maher C, Refshauge K, et al. Prognosis in patients with recent onset low back pain in Australian primary care: inception cohort study. *Br Med J*. 2008;337:a171.

Hollmann MW, Durieux ME. Local anesthetics and the inflammatory response. *Anesthesiology*. 2000;93:858–875.

Hopwood MB, Manning DC. Lumbar epidural steroid injections: is a clinical trial necessary or appropriate? *Reg Anesth Pain Med*. 1999;24:5–7.

Horlocker TT, Bajwa ZH, Ashraf Z, et al. Risk assessment of hemorrhagic complications associated with nonsteroidal antiinflammatory medications in ambulatory pain clinic patients undergoing epidural steroid injection. *Anesth Analg*. 2002;95:1691–1697.

Jeong H, Lee J, Kim S, et al. Effectiveness of transforaminal epidural steroid injection by using a preganglionic approach: a prospective randomized controlled study. *Radiology*. 2007;245:584–590.

Kainer M, Reagan D, Nguyen D, et al. Fungal infections associated with contaminated methylprednisolone in Tennessee. *N Engl J Med*. 2012;367:2194–2203.

Kang S, Hwang B, Son H, et al. The dosages of corticosteroid in transforaminal epidural steroid injections for lumbar radicular pain due to a herniated disc. *Pain Physician*. 2011;14:361–370.

Klein GR, Vaccaro AR, Cwik J, et al. Efficacy of cervical epidural steroids in the treatment of cervical spine disorders. *Am J Anesthesiol*. 2000;9:547–550.

Liu SS, Melmed AP, Klos JW, et al. Prospective experience with a 20-gauge Tuohy needle for lumbar epidural steroid injections: is confirmation with fluoroscopy necessary? *Reg Anesth Pain Med*. 2001;26:143–146.

Lutz GE, Vad VB, Wisneski RJ. Fluoroscopic transforaminal lumbar epidural steroids: an outcome study. *Arch Phys Med Rehabil*. 1998;79:1362–1366.

McCarron RF, Wimpee MW, Hudkins PG, et al. The inflammatory effect of nucleus pulposus: a possible element in the pathogenesis of low-back pain. *Spine*. 1987;12:760–764.

Mulligan KA, Rowlingson JC. Epidural steroids. *Curr Pain Headache Rep*. 2001;5:495–502.

Owlia M, Salimzadeh A, Alishiri G, et al. Comparison of two doses of corticosteroid in epidural steroid injection for lumbar radicular pain. *Singapore Med J*. 2007;48(3):241–245.

Pinto RZ, Maher CG, Ferreira ML, et al. Epidural corticosteroid injections in the management of sciatica: a systematic review and meta-analysis. *Ann Intern Med*. 2012;157:865–877.

Rathmell J, Aprill C, Bogduk N. Cervical transforaminal injection of steroids. *Anesthesiology*. 2004;100:1595–1600.

Rathmell J, Michna E, Fitzgibbon D, et al. Injury and liability associated with cervical procedures for chronic pain. *Anesthesiology*. 2011;114:918–926.

Riew K, Park J, Cho Y, et al. Nerve root blocks in the treatment of lumbar radicular pain: a minimum five-year follow-up. *J Bone Joint Surg Am*. 2006;88(8):1722–1725.

Rowlingson JC. Epidural steroids: do they have a place in pain management? *Am Pain Soc J*. 1994;3:20–27.

Ryan M, Taylor T. Management of lumbar nerve root pain by intrathecal and epidural injection of depot methylprednisolone acetate. *Med J Aust*. 1981;2:532–534.

Saal JS, Franson R, Dobrow E, et al. High levels of inflammatory phospholipase A2 activity in lumbar disc herniation. *Spine*. 1990;15:674–678.

Slipman CW, Lipetz JS, Jackson HB, et al. Therapeutic selective nerve root block in the nonsurgical treatment of atraumatic cervical spondylotic radicular pain: a retrospective analysis with independent clinical review. *Arch Phys Med Rehabil*. 2000;81:741–746.

Southern D, Lutz GE, Cooper G, et al. Are fluoroscopic caudal epidural steroid injections effective for managing chronic low back pain? *Pain Physician*. 2003;6:167–172.

Straus B. Chronic pain of spinal origin: the costs of intervention. *Spine*. 2002;27:2614–2619.

Tonkovich-Quaranta LA, Winkler SR. Use of epidural corticosteroids in low back pain. *Ann Pharmacother*. 2000;34:1165–1172.

Whynes DK, McCahon RA, Ravenscroft A, et al. Cost effectiveness of epidural steroid injections to manage chronic lower back pain. *BMC Anesthesiology*. 2012;12:26.

Wilkinson H. Intrathecal depomedrol: a literature review. *Clin J Pain*. 1992;8:49–56.

Wilkinson I, Cohen S. Epidural steroid injections. *Curr Pain Headache Rep*. 2012;16:50–59.

Wilkinson I, Cohen SP. Epidural steroids for spinal pain and radiculopathy: a narrative, evidence-based review. *Curr Opin Anaesthesiol*. 2013. In press.

65 FACET JOINT BLOCKS

Maxim S. Eckmann, MD
Somayaji Ramamurthy, MD

INTRODUCTION

- Back pain and neck pain are the most common causes of chronic pain and disability.
- Although radicular pain secondary to herniated disc is most commonly suspected, pain originating from facet joints is likely to be the etiology of 15%–40% of nonradicular low back pain and 40%–60% of nonradicular neck pain.
- These joints, also known as the zygapophyseal joints, are formed by the articulation of the articular processes of the adjacent vertebrae.
- These sinuarthrodial joints are subject to degenerative arthritis, thus becoming one of the factors contributing to nonradicular back and neck pain.
- Pain originating from facet joints can coexist with other causes of multifactorial back and neck pain, including radicular, myofascial, sacroiliac, and intradiscal pathology.

DIAGNOSIS

- History and clinical examination findings have been shown unable to predict whether or not pain is originating from the facet joints. However, paraspinal tenderness has been associated with increased rate of successful treatment with lumbar facet denervation.
- Imaging studies including MRI have not been useful in pinpointing facet joints as the cause of pain, although Single Photon Emission Computed Tomography (SPECT) scan findings have been reported to have a high correlation with the pain relief following joint injection with corticosteroids.

- At present, state-of-the-art diagnosis can be established only by local anesthetic injections. Injection of local anesthetic and/or steroid either into the joint or blocking the nerve supply of the joint is used in establishing the diagnosis.

CONSERVATIVE THERAPY

- Nonradicular low back pain or neck pain is managed in our clinic using manual methods consisting of mobilization, physical therapy, and home exercises with significant success.
- In patients who have significant pain and restriction of motion it may be necessary to inject the facet joint or block the medial branches to provide analgesia for physical therapy and mobilization.

FACET JOINT INJECTION

- These injections are performed under fluoroscopic guidance using nonionic radiocontrast material.
- Greater than 50% pain relief with the injection of local anesthetic into the joint is considered diagnostic.
- Steroids such as methylprednisolone acetate (Depo-Medrol), triamcinolone, and betamethasone are commonly mixed with the local anesthetic for therapeutic purposes.
- The role of the joint injections is controversial and the present trend is to use medial branch blocks for diagnostic and therapeutic purposes.

MEDIAL BRANCH BLOCKS

- Each lumbar facet joint is supplied by a branch of the posterior ramus from the nerve root at the corresponding level and the branches from the nerve root one level above (Figure 65-1).
- For example, the L4–5 facet joint receives a medial branch from the L5 posterior primary ramus and a branch from the medial branch of the L4 nerve root.
- The cervical facet joint receives innervation from the same level and one level above and below.
- To significantly denervate each joint, the medial branches of all the nerves supplying the joint have to be blocked.
- In the lumbar region, the medial branches are blocked under fluoroscopic guidance at the junction of the transverse process and the superior articular process.
- In the cervical region, the nerve is blocked at the waist of the articular process.
- In the thoracic region, the nerve is blocked superior to the tip of the transverse process or more proximally as the nerve courses over the pedicle and lamina toward the joint capsule.

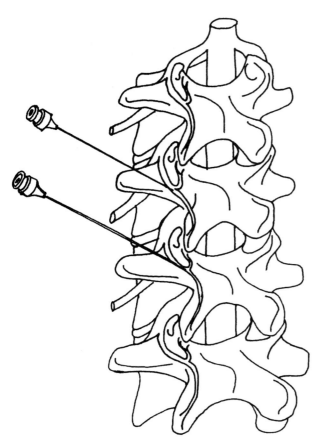

FIG. 65-1. Medial branch blocks.

INTERPRETATION AND CONFIRMATION

- A single injection with the local anesthetic can produce false-positive results in 40% of patients.
- The most accurate technique consists of using double-blind, randomized injections of placebo, a short-acting local anesthetic such as lidocaine, and a longer-acting local anesthetic such as bupivacaine.
- In most clinical situations, it is more practical to use short- and long-acting local anesthetic agents to assess whether the duration of pain relief corresponds to that of the local anesthetic agent.
- Some clinicians use corticosteroids such as methylprednisolone acetate (Depo-Medrol) and Sarapin (pitcher plant) to provide long-term pain relief.
- Longer duration of pain relief has been achieved by using neurolytic techniques with 4% phenol, cryogenic nerve block, or most commonly radiofrequency lesions.
- Well-controlled studies indicate that radiofrequency lesion provides predictable long-term pain relief in patients with cervical facet joint pain secondary to trauma.
- While evidence for the long-term efficacy of lumbar medial branch nerve radiofrequency lesions is

increasing, precise anatomic lesion placement and careful patient selection are considered important in achieving significant outcomes.

COMPLICATIONS

- The incidence of serious complications following injections into the facet joint is very low, although there are reports of infection and subarachnoid injection following facet joint injections.

BIBLIOGRAPHY

Cohen SP, Hurley RW, Christo PJ, et al. Clinical predictors of success and failure for lumbar facet radiofrequency denervation. *Clin J Pain.* 2007, January;23(1):45–52.

Cohen SP, Raja SN. Pathogenesis, diagnosis, and treatment of lumbar zygapophysial (facet) joint pain. *Anesthesiology.* 2007, March;106(3):591–614.

Dolan AL, Ryan PJ, Arden NK, et al. The value of SPECT scans in identifying back pain likely to benefit from facet joint injection. *Br J Rheumatol.* 1996;35:1269.

Lord S, Barnsley L, Walis B, et al. Percutaneous radiofrequency neurotomy for chronic cervical zygapophyseal joint pain. *N Engl J Med.* 1996;335:1721.

Manchikanti L, Pampati V, Fellows B, et al. The diagnostic validity and therapeutic value of lumbar facet joint nerve blocks with or without adjuvant agents. *Curr Rev Pain.* 2000;4:337.

Saal JS. General principles of diagnostic testing as related to painful lumbar spine disorders: a critical appraisal of current diagnostic techniques. *Spine.* 2002;27:2538.

66 NEUROSURGICAL TECHNIQUES
Kenneth A. Follett, MD, PhD

INTRODUCTION

- Neurosurgical techniques include "anatomic" (eg, spinal reconstruction, microvascular decompression), augmentative ("neuromodulation"), and ablative procedures.
- Neuroaugmentative therapies have largely replaced neuroablative therapies as treatments of choice for intractable pain, but ablative therapies may be appropriate for certain patients.
- Expertise overlaps among medical specialties involved in pain care. Some techniques reviewed in this chapter

(eg, spinal cord stimulation and intrathecal analgesic administration) are provided by pain physicians trained in specialties other than neurosurgery as well as by neurosurgeons.

- Pain medicine practitioners should be familiar with the indications for common neurosurgical techniques and refer patients for such procedures when appropriate.

PATIENT SELECTION FOR SURGICAL PAIN THERAPIES

- A surgical procedure is not usually the first treatment option for intractable pain.
- Treatment of intractable pain should follow a rational process with the simplest, safest methods used first and interventional treatments reserved for later in the course. The approach to patients with pain should be flexible, however, and treatment should be tailored to meet individual needs. For some individuals, this means that a surgical procedure may be appropriate earlier rather than later in the course of treatment.
- In general, surgical treatment of intractable pain is appropriate for individuals in whom:
  - Conservative therapies have not provided adequate pain relief.
  - Other treatments are associated with unacceptable side effects (eg, medication side effects).
  - Further direct treatment of the underlying cause of pain is not possible, practical, or appropriate.

  - There are no contraindications to surgery (eg, infection, coagulopathy).
  - The pain has a definable organic cause.
- Surgical treatment is not appropriate in patients with significant or untreated psychological or psychiatric disorders or overt dysfunction. Thus, formal psychological evaluation is appropriate for many individuals being considered for surgical treatment of intractable pain. Patients with psychological risk factors are not necessarily precluded from surgical treatment, but the treatment program should address the psychological issues to facilitate good outcomes.

NEUROSURGICAL TECHNIQUES FOR INTRACTABLE PAIN

- Indications for anatomic (eg, spinal reconstruction, microvascular decompression), augmentative (neuromodulation), and ablative procedures overlap in many instances (Table 66-1). If anatomic procedures are not indicated, augmentative therapies are generally preferred as initial surgical treatments for pain management because of their relative safety and reversibility; however, ablative therapies have an early role in the treatment of certain pain syndromes.
- Factors that must be considered when selecting a therapy include pain etiology (cancer-related vs. nonmalignant); pain location; pain characteristics (nociceptive vs. neuropathic); patient life expectancy; and

TABLE 66-1   **Neurosurgical Pain Therapies**

PAIN THERAPY	HEAD/NECK	UPPER TRUNK, SHOULDER, ARM	LOWER TRUNK, LEG	DIFFUSE
Anatomic	X	X	X	X
Augmentative				
Peripheral nerve stimulation	X	X	X	
Spinal cord stimulation		X	X	X
Thalamus (PVG-PAG) stimulation	X	X	X	
Motor cortex/deep brain stimulation	X	X	X	
Intrathecal/epidural drug infusion		X	X	X
Intraventricular drug infusion	X	X	X	X
Ablative				
Neurectomy	X	X	X	
Sympathectomy	X	X	X	
Ganglionectomy	X	X	X	
Rhizotomy	X	X	X	
Spinal DREZ lesioning		X	X	
Cordotomy			X	
Myelotomy			X	
Nucleus caudalis DREZ lesioning	X			
Trigeminal tractotomy	X			
Mesencephalotomy	X	X		
Thalamotomy	X	X	X	X
Cingulotomy	X	X	X	X
Hypophysectomy		X	X	X

PVG, periventricular gray matter; PAG, periaqueductal gray matter.

psychological, social, and economic issues relevant to the pain complaint. The advantages and disadvantages of anatomic, augmentative, and ablative therapies should be weighed according to these factors and a specific intervention can then be selected from within one of these general approaches.

- Specific interventions vary in their appropriateness as treatments for pain in specific body regions (Table 66-1).

ANATOMIC TECHNIQUES

- Anatomic techniques, such as spinal decompressive (eg, laminectomy, discectomy) and reconstructive procedures may be performed to treat pain, neurologic deficits, or orthopedic abnormalities.
- "Microvascular decompression" is useful for treatment of the paroxysmal, lancinating pain of trigeminal neuralgia, glossopharyngeal neuralgia, and nervus intermedius neuralgia that is refractory to pharmacologic treatment.
- Microvascular decompression is a major surgery and is most appropriate for healthy patients, generally under the age of 65.
  - The rationale of this surgery is to eliminate compression of the affected cranial nerve by a blood vessel (usually a small artery) that generally occurs near the entry of the nerve into the brainstem.
  - The advantage of microvascular decompression compared with percutaneous (eg, radiofrequency rhizotomy for trigeminal neuralgia) or open ablative procedures for cranial neuralgias is the absence of postoperative sensory deficit, which is an obligate outcome of most ablative procedures.
- Pain may recur over months or years in some patients but relief is maintained in most patients.

AUGMENTATIVE TECHNIQUES

- Augmentative therapies involve either stimulation or neuraxial drug infusion.
- Compared with ablative therapies, augmentative therapies are:
  - Relatively safe, reversible, and "adjustable"
  - Cost more (initial device costs and upkeep)
  - Require maintenance (eg, refilling of infusion pumps, replacement of stimulation system battery packs)
  - Have the potential for device-related complications
- General indications for augmentative therapies are similar to those for other neurosurgical pain treatments with the additional criterion that estimated patient life expectancy should be sufficient to warrant implantation of a neuroaugmentative device.

STIMULATION THERAPIES

- The Food and Drug Administration (FDA) has approved spinal cord stimulation (SCS) and peripheral nerve stimulation (PNS) therapies for pain management.
- Other stimulation therapies in clinical use include deep brain stimulation and motor cortex stimulation, but these are not FDA approved therapies.

Spinal Cord Stimulation

- SCS is appropriate for treatment of neuropathic pain that is relatively focal, especially in the arm or leg, and static in nature.
- Common applications include radicular pain associated with failed back surgery syndrome, complex regional pain syndrome, and extremity pain related to peripheral neuropathy or root injury. SCS may be useful for neuropathic pain affecting the trunk (eg, postherpetic neuralgia, postthoracotomy pain) and phantom limb pain (postamputation stump pain does not improve consistently with SCS).
- SCS has been used as a treatment for refractory angina pectoris and for interstitial cystitis, but it is not approved by the FDA for these indications.
- Stimulation leads may be implanted percutaneously or surgically. Surgical ("laminotomy," "plate," or "paddle") leads offer the advantages of a lower incidence of dislodgement ("migration"), lower stimulation amplitude requirements, longer pulse generator battery life, and broader distribution of stimulation contacts, providing more programming options.
- The success rate of SCS (more than 50% reduction in pain) in the failed back surgery syndrome and complex regional pain syndrome populations is reported generally as approximately 50%–65%, but critical reviews indicate long-term success rates are lower.
- SCS is less consistently successful in the treatment of other pain syndromes, for example, phantom limb pain and postherpetic neuralgia, but warrants a trial because of its relative ease and safety.

Peripheral Nerve Stimulation

- The indications for PNS are similar to those for SCS except that the distribution of pain should be limited to the territory of a single peripheral nerve.
- Extremity pain that might be appropriately treated with PNS can sometimes be treated equally well with SCS, and many physicians find it easier to implant a percutaneous SCS lead than a PNS lead (which may require an open procedure).
- The outcomes of PNS are generally similar to those of SCS, and PNS can be very effective for the treatment of occipital neuralgia.

Intracranial Stimulation

- Intracranial stimulation therapies include deep brain stimulation (DBS) of the somatosensory thalamus and periventricular–periaqueductal gray matter and motor cortex stimulation.
- These therapies are used primarily for treating pain of nonmalignant origin, such as pain associated with failed back surgery syndrome, neuropathic pain following central or peripheral nervous system injury, or trigeminal pain.
- Neither DBS nor motor cortex stimulation has the approval of the FDA for the treatment of pain, although DBS has been used clinically for more than two decades.

Deep Brain Stimulation

- The targets for focal electrical stimulation of the brain include the ventrocaudal nucleus (ventroposterolateral and ventroposteromedial nucleus) and periventricular–periaqueductal gray matter (PVG–PAG).
- The DBS sites are chosen generally on the basis of the pain characteristics. Nociceptive pain and paroxysmal, lancinating, or evoked neuropathic pain (eg, allodynia, hyperpathia) tend to respond best to PVG–PAG stimulation, which may activate endogenous opioid systems. Continuous neuropathic pain responds most consistently to DBS of the sensory thalamus (ventrocaudal nucleus).
- Success rates of DBS for the treatment of intractable pain are difficult to determine from the literature because patient selection, techniques, and outcome assessments vary among studies. Although 60%–80% of patients undergoing a screening trial with DBS have sufficient pain relief to warrant implantation of a permanent stimulation system, 25%–35% of patients undergoing a DBS trial have good long-term pain relief, but some investigators have reported 80% success rates.
- DBS results are better in patients with pain related to failed back surgery syndrome and peripheral neuropathic pain (e.g., complex regional pain syndrome) than in patients with central pain syndromes (eg, thalamic pain, spinal cord injury pain, anesthesia dolorosa, postherpetic neuralgia, phantom limb pain).

Motor Cortex Stimulation

- Motor cortex stimulation (MCS) has received attention as an alternative to thalamic and PVG–PAG stimulation. Overlap exists between indications for DBS and MCS, but MCS is thought to have a lower risk of serious complication because the electrode is placed epidurally rather than within the brain parenchyma.
- The primary indication for MCS is treatment of localized neuropathic pain. Because of technical issues related to electrode placement, the face is the easiest region of the body to treat, and MCS may be particularly effective for the treatment of trigeminal neuropathic pain. Treatment of pain affecting the trunk or, in particular, the legs is difficult because of technical difficulties in positioning the stimulation electrode over the appropriate region of motor cortex.
- Approximately 50%–70% of patients undergoing MCS are reported to have good long-term pain relief, but controlled clinical trials of efficacy are needed. As with DBS, MCS seems to be most effective for patients with no anesthesia in the distribution of the pain being treated.

NEURAXIAL DRUG INFUSION

- Neuraxial analgesic administration is indicated primarily for the treatment of pain syndromes with a significant nociceptive/somatic component (eg, cancer-related pain) because nociceptive/somatic pain typically responds to opioid therapy. Neuropathic pain may improve with intrathecal analgesic administration, but some evidence suggests this may require nonopioid analgesics and polyanalgesia.
- The most common application of intrathecal analgesic is management of pain related to failed back surgery syndrome, which typically includes both nociceptive (low back) and neuropathic (extremity) components.
- Use of intrathecal analgesics for the treatment of cancer-related pain is well-accepted. The use of this therapy for chronic nonmalignant pain remains controversial, in part due to concern that patients with noncancer pain will require long-term therapy resulting in tolerance, that neuropathic pain (common in chronic nonmalignant pain syndromes) does not respond adequately to opioids, and the efficacy and cost-effectiveness of the therapy have not been determined in controlled trials.
- The key advantage of neuraxial analgesic administration compared with other pain therapy is its versatility:
  ○ It has a wide range of indications, including nociceptive and mixed nociceptive/neuropathic pain syndromes.
  ○ It can be used to treat focal or diffuse pain as well as axial and/or extremity pain. It is used commonly to treat pain below cervical levels but can be effective for head and neck pain, especially if analgesic agents are delivered intraventricularly.
  ○ It can be used in the setting of changing pain (eg, in a patient with progressive cancer).

- Significant disadvantages include device costs, medication costs, and need for maintenance (eg, pump refills and battery replacement).
- Most patients achieve good long-term relief of pain (degree of pain relief, patient satisfaction, and dose requirements).
- Serious complications of the therapy are uncommon.

ABLATIVE TECHNIQUES

- Ablative neurosurgical therapies are often considered the last resort for pain treatment, but in some instances they are procedures of choice and should be considered earlier rather than later. Thus, phantom-limb pain in the setting of spinal nerve root avulsion or "end zone" pain arising from spinal cord injury can be treated effectively by dorsal root entry zone (DREZ) lesioning, and cordotomy might be more appropriate than intrathecal analgesia for the treatment of cancer-related pain in a patient with a short life expectancy.
- Ablative therapies target almost every level of the peripheral and central nervous systems:
  ○ Peripheral techniques interrupt nociceptive input into the spinal cord (eg, neurectomy, ganglionectomy, rhizotomy).
  ○ Spinal interventions alter afferent input, dorsal horn neuronal activity, or rostral transmission of nociceptive information (eg, DREZ lesioning, cordotomy, myelotomy).
  ○ Supraspinal intracranial procedures may interrupt rostral transmission of nociceptive information (eg, mesencephalotomy, thalamotomy) or influence perception of painful stimuli (eg, cingulotomy).
- Ablative therapies are most appropriate for the treatment of nociceptive pain rather than neuropathic pain. Neuropathic pain that is intermittent, paroxysmal, or evoked (eg, allodynia, hyperpathia) may improve after an ablative procedure, but continuous, dysesthetic neuropathic pain does not typically improve.

PERIPHERAL TECHNIQUES

Sympathectomy

- Sympathectomy is indicated primarily for the treatment of sympathetically maintained pain and vasospastic disorders.
- Although sympathectomy can be effective when sympathetic blocks reliably relieve the pain, the procedure has fallen into disfavor as a treatment for intractable nonmalignant pain because of inconsistent results.
- SCS may provide better long-term outcomes with lower morbidity than sympathectomy, so SCS may be the treatment of choice for sympathetically maintained noncancer pain.

Neurectomy

- Neurectomy may be useful in individuals who develop pain following peripheral nerve injury, including that associated with limb amputation, when an identifiable neuroma is the cause of pain.
  ○ As an exception to this rule, however, sectioning the lateral femoral cutaneous nerve may provide good long-lasting relief of meralgia paresthetica.
- Neurectomy is not useful for treatment of nonspecific stump pain after amputation or for other nonmalignant peripheral pain syndromes.
- The utility of neurectomy is limited because pain arising from a pure sensory nerve is not common, and mixed sensory–motor nerves cannot be sectioned without risk of functional impairment.

Dorsal Rhizotomy/Ganglionectomy

- Dorsal rhizotomy and ganglionectomy serve similar purposes in denervating somatic and/or visceral tissues. Ganglionectomy produces more complete denervation than dorsal rhizotomy because some afferent fibers enter the spinal cord through the ventral root and are not affected by dorsal rhizotomy. Ganglionectomy effectively eliminates input from dorsal and ventral root afferent fibers by removing their cell bodies, which are located within the dorsal root ganglion.
- Both rhizotomy and ganglionectomy can be used to treat pain in the trunk or abdomen, but neither procedure is useful for treatment of pain in the extremities unless function of the extremity is already lost, because denervation removes proprioceptive as well as nociceptive input and produces a functionless limb.
- To be successful, denervation must extend over several adjacent levels. Limited denervation does not provide adequate pain relief, probably because of overlap of segmental innervation of dermatomes.
- These procedures are most appropriate for the treatment of cancer-related pain; noncancer pain does not improve consistently.
- When these procedures are used to treat neuropathic pain (eg, postherpetic neuralgia of the trunk), lancinating, paroxysmal, or evoked pain may improve, but continuous dysesthetic pain does not typically improve.
- In the setting of cancer, rhizotomy and ganglionectomy can be useful for thoracic or abdominal wall pain; for perineal pain in patients with impaired bladder, bowel, and sex function; and for pain in a functionless extremity. Multiple sacral rhizotomies

can be performed (eg, to treat pelvic pain from cancer) by passing a ligature around the thecal sac below S1.

Cranial Nerve Rhizotomy

- Rhizotomy is especially useful in treating the paroxysmal, lancinating pain of classical trigeminal and glossopharyngeal neuralgia. In contrast, atypical facial pain syndromes (constant, burning pain) do not improve with ablative techniques and may intensify following rhizotomy.
- Percutaneous trigeminal rhizotomy can be accomplished with radiofrequency, glycerol injection, or balloon compression. These techniques are performed on an outpatient basis, are well tolerated, and have high success rates in relieving paroxysmal pain of cranial neuralgias.
- Open rhizotomy (ie, via craniotomy or craniectomy) is usually performed for treatment of glossopharyngeal and nervus intermedius neuralgia and may be required for treatment of some trigeminal neuralgias.
- Early pain relief is achieved in more than 95% of patients undergoing percutaneous or open rhizotomy. Pain may recur after months or years.
- Stereotactic radiosurgery rhizotomy for the treatment of trigeminal neuralgia is an alternative to percutaneous or open rhizotomy or microvascular decompression.
  - Unlike other surgical treatments for trigeminal neuralgia, pain relief does not occur for several weeks following radiosurgical treatment. Radiosurgery is, therefore, not appropriate for patients with severe acute exacerbation of pain that cannot be controlled adequately with medications because it does not afford prompt pain relief.

C2 Ganglionectomy

- C2 ganglionectomy is indicated for the treatment of occipital neuralgia.
- It is especially effective for patients with posttraumatic occipital neuralgia who have no migraine component to their headache.
- Long-term pain relief may be comparable to that achieved with occipital nerve stimulation without the need for implanted devices and long-term follow-up.

SPINAL TECHNIQUES

Dorsal Root Entry Zone Lesioning

- DREZ lesioning of the spinal cord can relieve neuropathic trunk or extremity pain. DREZ lesioning of the nucleus caudalis has been used to treat neuropathic facial pain.

- DREZ lesioning disrupts input and outflow in the superficial layers of the spinal cord dorsal horn where afferent nociceptive fibers terminate and some of the ascending nociceptive fibers originate. DREZ lesioning also disrupts the spontaneous abnormal activity and hyperactivity that develops in spinal cord dorsal horn neurons in the setting of neuropathic pain.
- DREZ lesioning is best reserved for localized neuropathic pain. The most successful applications are related to treatment of neuropathic pain arising from spinal nerve root avulsion (cervical or lumbosacral) and "end zone" or "boundary" pain following spinal cord injury.
- As with other ablative procedures, DREZ lesioning is most effective for relieving paroxysmal or evoked neuropathic pain rather than continuous neuropathic pain.

Cordotomy

- Cordotomy can be an effective method of pain control, especially for cancer-related pain in individuals with short life expectancies for whom it is difficult to justify the costs of implanted drug infusion systems.
- Cordotomy disrupts nociceptive afferent fibers ascending in the spinothalamic tract in the anterolateral quadrant of the spinal cord.
- Cordotomy is a one-time procedure with no required long-term follow-up or maintenance, which can be important for individuals who may find it difficult to return to a medical facility for refilling of an infusion system or for whom costs of ongoing medical care become burdensome.
- Cordotomy is used most commonly to treat cancer-related pain below the mid- to low-cervical dermatomes. It is not generally used to treat noncancer pain due to risk of post-cordotomy dysesthesias or neurologic complication.
- Cordotomy can be performed as an open or percutaneous procedure. Percutaneous techniques are less invasive, but some surgeons lack the required expertise and equipment.
  - Lancinating, paroxysmal, and evoked (allodynic or hyperpathic) pain that sometimes follows spinal cord injury or occurs as part of peripheral neuropathic pain syndromes can improve following cordotomy, but continuous neuropathic pain does not improve. Laterally located pain responds better than midline or axial pain (eg, visceral pain). Midline and axial pain may require bilateral procedures to achieve pain relief.
- The risk of complications, including weakness; bladder, bowel, and sexual dysfunction; and respiratory depression (if the procedure is performed bilaterally at cervical levels), is significantly greater with bilateral

procedures. The risk of respiratory depression subsequent to a unilateral high cervical procedure mandates that pulmonary function be acceptable on the contralateral side. Cordotomy provides good pain relief in 60%–80% of patients, but pain tends to recur over time. Approximately one-third of patients have recurrent pain in three months, half at one year, and two-thirds at longer follow-up intervals.

Myelotomy

- Myelotomy can provide significant pain relief in properly selected individuals, including some who fail treatment with intrathecal analgesics.
- Commissural myelotomy was developed to provide the benefits of bilateral cordotomy without the inherent risk of lesioning both anterior quadrants of the spinal cord. This is accomplished by sectioning spinothalamic tract fibers from both sides of the body with one lesion as they decussate in the anterior commissure. Identification of a dorsal column visceral pain pathway has led to the development of punctate midline myelotomy to treat abdominal and pelvic pain. Compared with cordotomy, bilateral and midline pain can be treated with a single procedure with lower morbidity and mortality.
- Myelotomy is indicated primarily for cancer-related pain, generally in the abdomen, pelvis, perineum, and legs, and is most effective for nociceptive rather than neuropathic pain. Early, complete pain relief is achieved in most patients, but pain tends to recur, so only 50%–60% of patients achieve good long-term pain relief.
- The risk of bladder or bowel complications or sexual dysfunction is less than that associated with bilateral cordotomy, but remains sufficiently high so this procedure is restricted in most instances to patients with cancer-related pain who have preexisting dysfunction.

SUPRASPINAL CRANIAL TECHNIQUES

- Ablative neurosurgical procedures directed at the brainstem are not common, in part because relatively few patients require such interventions and because relatively few neurosurgeons have the expertise to perform them.

Mesencephalotomy

- Mesencephalotomy is indicated for intractable pain involving the head, neck, shoulder, and arm. Most commonly, the procedure is used to treat cancer pain.
- Mesencephalotomy disrupts nociceptive fibers ascending in the brainstem and can be viewed as a supraspinal version of cordotomy.

- Pain relief is achieved in many patients, but mesencephalotomy does not provide consistent long-term relief of central neuropathic pain.
- Side effects and complications, especially oculomotor dysfunction, are common.
- The utility of mesencephalotomy has diminished subsequent to the advent of neuraxial analgesic administration. Intraventricular morphine infusion can provide good relief of head, neck, shoulder, and arm pain with a lower incidence of complications.

Thalamotomy

- Thalamotomy has been used to treat cancer-related and noncancer pain. In the setting of cancer, thalamotomy is most appropriate for patients who have widespread pain (eg, from diffuse metastatic disease) or who have midline, bilateral, or head/neck pain that other procedures are not likely to relieve.
- The incidence of complications of thalamotomy is lower than for mesencephalotomy, so thalamotomy may be preferable for the treatment of head, neck, shoulder, and arm pain in patients who are not candidates for neuraxial analgesia.
- Thalamotomy can also be useful for patients who are not candidates for cordotomy, for example, those with pain above the C5 dermatome or with pulmonary dysfunction.
- The procedure can be accomplished via stereotactic radiofrequency or radiosurgical techniques.
- Medial thalamotomy appears to be most effective for treating nociceptive pain (eg, cancer pain), with acceptable long-term pain relief obtained in 30%–50% of patients. Neuropathic pain syndromes respond less consistently to thalamotomy.
- As with other ablative procedures, paroxysmal, lancinating neuropathic pain or neuropathic pain with elements of allodynia and hyperpathia (ie, evoked pain) may improve following thalamotomy, whereas continuous neuropathic pain tends not to improve.

Cingulotomy

- Cingulotomy is used rarely to treat intractable pain. When used, it is most often for treatment of cancer pain, but it has been used for noncancer pain as well.
- Approximately 50%–75% of treated patients benefit from the procedure, at least short-term. In the cancer population, pain relief generally is maintained at least three months.
- The utility of cingulotomy for chronic noncancer pain is less certain; some studies indicate relatively good long-lasting pain relief and others only 20% long-term success.

- Because cingulotomy is performed to treat psychiatric disease and carries the stigma of "psychosurgery," formal review by an institutional ethics committee may be warranted before using this procedure to treat intractable pain.

Hypophysectomy

- Hypophysectomy (surgical, chemical, or radiosurgical) is used rarely but is reported to provide good relief of cancer-related pain.
- It is typically thought to be most effective for hormonally responsive cancers (eg, prostate, breast cancer), but may relieve pain associated with other tumors as well. It is indicated primarily for the treatment of diffuse pain associated with widespread disease.
- Hypophysectomy alleviates pain in 45%-95% of treated patients. Pain relief occurs independent of tumor regression; the specific mechanism of pain relief is unknown.

SUMMARY

- In general, augmentative neuromodulation techniques have supplanted ablative procedures as treatments of choice for intractable pain due to generally good outcomes and the low risk of serious or permanent complication.
- Augmentative techniques are superior to ablative techniques for the treatment of neuropathic pain that has a continuous, dysesthetic component. Ablative procedures can be effective for treatment of paroxysmal, lancinating neuropathic pain, especially that of trigeminal or glossopharyngeal neuralgia.
- Pain management physicians should be familiar with the variety of neurosurgical techniques available to treat pain, their indications, and general outcomes and should incorporate these treatments into the care of their patients when appropriate. Otherwise, with the increasing amount of attention paid to augmentative therapies to treat intractable pain, ablative therapies that might be appropriate for some patients may be overlooked as treatment options.

BIBLIOGRAPHY

Coffey RJ, Lozano AM. Neurostimulation for chronic non-cancer pain: an evaluation of the clinical evidence and recommendations for future trial designs. *J Neurosurg.* 2006;105(2):174–189.

Cohen SP, Dragovich A. Intrathecal analgesia. *Anesthesiol Clin.* 2007;25(4):863–882.

Deer T. Current and future trends in spinal cord stimulation for chronic pain. *Current Pain Headache Reports.* 2001; 5(6):503–509.

Doleys DM, Olson K. *Psychological Assessment and Intervention in Implantable Pain Therapies.* Minneapolis, Mn: Medtronic Inc; 1997.

Dougherty PM, Lee J-I, Dimitriou T, et al. Medial thalamotomy. In: Burchiel KJ, ed. *Surgical Management of Pain.* New York: Thieme; 2002:795–802.

Gildenberg P. Mesencephalotomy. In: Burchiel KJ, ed. *Surgical Management of Pain.* New York: Thieme; 2002:786–793.

Hodge CJ, Christensen M. Anterolateral cordotomy. In: Burchiel KJ, ed. *Surgical Management of Pain.* New York: Thieme; 2002;732–742.

Jasper JF, Hayek SM. Implanted occipital nerve stimulators. *Pain Physician.* 2008;11(2):187–200.

Karavelis A, Foroglou G, Selviaridis P, et al. Intraventricular administration of morphine for control of intractable cancer pain in 90 patients. *Neurosurgery.* 1996;39(1):39–57.

Lozano AM, Vanderlinden G, Bachoo R, et al. Microsurgical C-2 ganglionectomy for chronic intractable occipital pain. *J Neurosurg.* 1998;89(3):359–365.

Maesawa S, Salame C, Flickinger JC, et al. Clinical outcomes after stereotactic radiosurgery for idiopathic trigeminal neuralgia. *J Neurosurg.* 2001;94(1):14–20.

Nauta HJW, Westlund KN, Willis WD. Midline myelotomy. In: Burchiel KJ, ed. *Surgical Management of Pain.* New York: Thieme; 2002:714–731.

Ramirez LF, Levin AB. Pain relief after hypophysectomy. *Neurosurgery.* 1984;14(4):499–504.

Rasche D, Rinaldi PC, Young RF, et al. Deep brain stimulation for the treatment of various chronic pain syndromes. *Neurosurg Focus.* 2006;21(6):1–8.

Sindou MP, Mertens P. Surgery in the dorsal root entry zone for pain. *Seminars in Neurosurgery.* 2004;15:221–232.

Taha JM, Tew JM Jr. Comparison of surgical treatments for trigeminal neuralgia: Reevaluation of radiofrequency rhizotomy. *Neurosurgery.* 1997;38(5):865–871.

Velasco F, Arguelles C, Carrillo-Ruiz JD, et al. Efficacy of motor cortex stimulation in the treatment of neuropathic pain: a randomized double-blind trial. *J Neurosurg.* 2008;108(4):698–706.

Yen CP, Kung SS, Su YF, et al. Stereotactic bilateral anterior cingulotomy for intractable pain. *J Clin Neurosci.* 2005;12(8):886–890.

67 RADIOFREQUENCY ABLATION

Sunil J. Panchal, MD

HISTORY

- Radiofrequency (RF) lesioning or ablation was first used in the treatment of pain to improve the predictability of the size of lesions created during percutaneous lateral cordotomy for unilateral malignant pain.

- RF lesioning is now used to treat a variety of pain disorders, including joint disease and disk-related pain.
- The rationale for the use of RF in pain is straightforward: the destruction of the nerves that signal pain should relieve pain.
- This oversimplistic view of neural activity has led to less than satisfactory results with neuroablation and restriction of its use to certain conditions.

PRINCIPLES

- RF lesioning involves inserting a small insulated electrode with an uninsulated (active) tip through soft tissue toward a site.
- The tissue impedes the flow of current through the needle, causing the current to be dissipated as heat (Joule heating).
- Heat is not generated in the electrode tip because the electrode offers minimal resistance to flow. The tip absorbs heat from the surrounding tissue, however, eventually achieving thermal equilibrium with the entire system.
- The greatest density of current occurs adjacent to the tip of the electrode; as a result, the adjacent tissue becomes the hottest part of the lesion.
- The amount of heat generated controls the quality of the lesion; temperature control determines the size of the lesion.
- The lesion is spherical around the active tip and progresses only a very small distance beyond the cannula tip.
- Unlike direct current techniques, RF uses continuous high-frequency waves of about 1 MHz.
  - Direct current generates lesions by dielectric mechanisms similar to electrolysis; RF generates lesions by ionic means. Thus, compared with direct current lesions, RF lesions are more uniform in size, more predictable, and do not form gas as a byproduct of electrolysis.
  - RF generators have automatic temperature controls that allow precise control over tissue temperature and the extent of the lesion.
  - Sensory and motor electrical stimulation can be used to locate a specific nerve and prevent unwanted collateral nerve damage.
  - Tissue resistance (impedance) can be measured: High impedance (>2000 ohms) suggests electrical disconnection and low impedance (<200 ohms) implies a short circuit.
- The most common reason for failure to generate a lesion is a poor electrical connection, usually related to cable damage.

CIRCUIT PRINCIPLES

- The circuit consists of a RF generator, which initiates the current; an active electrode, which delivers the current; a thermistor or thermocouple, which monitors the temperature; and a passive electrode with a large surface area, which returns the current.
- Current in the region of the active electrode generates heat, which in turn heats the electrode tip solely as a result of local tissue warming.
- The heat generated is a function of the amount of current that flows in the region of the electrode and the resistance of the surrounding tissue.
- Current flows from the active to the passive electrode, however, because, compared with the active electrode, the passive electrode has much greater surface area and less current density; thus, heating and tissue damage do not usually occur at the passive electrode.
- Tissue damage is related to the temperature generated; therefore, heating of the active electrode is an important safety feature that allows control of lesion size. Five factors affect the size of a lesion:
  - *Temperature*: At higher temperatures, the size of the lesion increases.
  - *Thermal equilibrium*: the more rapid the tissue equilibrium, the more uniform the lesion. Lesion size initially rises exponentially with time but becomes independent of time after approximately 30 seconds.
  - *Electrode size*: Larger electrodes generate larger lesions.
  - *Duration of treatment*: It has been demonstrated that lesion size can be increased with longer treatment time to a limited degree.
  - *Local tissue characteristics*: Lesions in tissues in contact with tissue of low electrical resistance, such as blood and cerebrospinal fluid, may be small or irregular in shape because the current was siphoned through paths with relatively little impedance. Similarly, lesions created next to heat-absorbing bone may suffer from irregular heating. Circulation of blood also provides a heat sink.
- Thus, choosing a proper electrode, achieving quick thermal equilibrium to a controlled temperature near nonconductive tissues, helps ensure optimal results.
- To ensure refinement of technique, it is essential that the following parameters be recorded for every lesion: type of electrode, temperature, time, voltage, and current.
- The actual tip may not even be incorporated into the lesion, so nerves in contact with the tip may be only partially blocked; furthermore, electrodes placed tangential to the nerve often generate a more effective lesion.
- The effect of RF on tissue depends on the temperature generated: >45°C, irreversible tissue injury occurs;

between 42°C and 45°C, temporary neural blockade occurs.

- The larger the lesion, the larger the zone of irreversibility. Early in its use, clinicians believed that heat was selective for small-diameter neural fibers, but this has not borne out by histologic analysis.

EQUIPMENT

- Cannulas used for RF lesioning come in various lengths and diameters and may be straight or curved.
- Reusable and disposable needles are available.
- Selection depends on the depth of the intended target, the desired size of the lesion, and operator experience and comfort level with cannula placement.
- Cannula systems are available in 50-, 100-, and 150-mm lengths with 5-, 10-, and 15-mm active tips.
- When performing RF ablation, it is critical to have additional cannulas for backup, as well as backup connector cables to be prepared for possible defects/malfunctions.

ADVANTAGES

- With a typical temperature gradient of 10°C/mm, the lesion size can be effectively controlled and predicted by selecting the appropriate target temperature.
- Lesion temperature can be monitored with a thermocouple electrode, allowing for adjustment of energy output to maintain the target temperature.
- Appropriate placement of the electrode is facilitated with electrical stimulation and impedance monitoring.
- The stimulation feature allows the operator to determine if the active tip is too close to a neural target that is undesirable for lesioning, such as a nerve root.
- Conventional stimulation testing consists of sensory testing at 50 Hz up to 1.0 V and motor testing at 2 Hz up to 2.5 V. This range stimulates structures in a 1-cm radius of the active tip.
- Impedance monitoring provides additional information about the type of tissue in which the active tip is located (bone differs from muscle, etc.) and assists in confirming appropriate location.
- The discomfort associated with this minimally invasive technique is of limited duration, and most RF lesions can be performed with mild sedation.
- It is very important to maintain the patient's ability to report his or her experience during sensory and motor testing to maintain safety.
- The incidence of morbidity and mortality is low when performed by a skilled operator.
- The procedure can be repeated if necessary.

GENERAL INDICATIONS, PROGNOSTIC TESTS, AND COMPLICATIONS

- RF ablation is a useful tool in the treatment of pain that occurs in a well-defined and fairly limited anatomic location where we have a clear understanding of the neuroanatomy involved for nociception.
- Appropriate patients are those in whom reasonable conservative treatment failed to provide adequate analgesia or was limited by side effects.
- Possible associated motor or sensory deficits must be discussed with the patient as part of the informed consent process prior to embarking on RF ablation.
- Psychological assessment helps eliminate patients who may not respond in a reliable manner to any intervention.
- A prognostic block is advised to assess possible magnitude of response to neuroablation.
- Some practitioners routinely perform a series of prognostic blocks using local anesthetics of different durations as well as a placebo injection to determine if the patient exhibits a consistent response.
- Complications associated with RF ablation include neurologic deficits from the intended target or nearby neural structures, deafferentation pain, neuritis, burn injury at breaks in the needle insulation, hematoma, and infection.
- All RF procedures are performed under sterile conditions with fluoroscopic guidance.

HEAD AND NECK PAIN

TRIGEMINAL NEURALGIA

- Idiopathic (typical) trigeminal neuralgia (ITN) is the most common form of cranial neuralgia, occurring with a mean annual incidence of 4 or 5 patients per 100,000 population.
- Unilateral sharp, lancinating pain limited to the somatosensory territory of one or more divisions of the trigeminal nerve with short attacks and associated trigger points is characteristic of ITN. Other features include absence of pain between attacks; frequent remissions, especially early in the course of the disease; normal neurologic examination; and high degree of pain relief in response to oral carbamazepine.
- The cause of ITN is unknown; however, in most patients, the trigeminal nerve root is compressed by adjacent vessels, most commonly the superior cerebellar and anterior inferior cerebellar arteries.
- Patients with ITN who no longer experience pain relief with medications or develop side effects can be treated effectively by percutaneous RF trigeminal rhizotomy, glycerol rhizotomy, or balloon compression.

Each procedure has advantages and disadvantages; however, RF trigeminal rhizotomy has the highest selectivity.

ANATOMY

- The trigeminal nerve originates in the brainstem and synapses in the gasserian ganglion before dividing into the ophthalmic, maxillary, and mandibular nerves, which pass through the foramen ovale.

TRIGEMINAL RHIZOTOMY TECHNIQUE

- Trigeminal rhizotomy, used to treat ITN, can also effectively treat facial pain associated with tumors, multiple sclerosis, and cluster headaches.
- Oral intake is restricted 6 hours prior to the procedure, and atropine (0.4 mg intramuscularly) is administered 30 minutes before the procedure to reduce oral secretions and prevent bradycardia during sedation.
- Short-acting sedatives can be administered during the procedure.
- The patient lies supine with the head in neutral position.
- The patient's blood pressure, heart rate, and oxygen saturation are monitored continuously during the procedure.
- Three anatomic landmarks are marked on the face: 3 cm anterior to the external auditory meatus, beneath the medial aspect of the pupil, and 2.5 cm lateral to the oral commissure. The first two delineate the site of the foramen ovale, and the third delineates the site of needle entry.
- The needle is placed into the foramen ovale anteriorly. Positioning and adequate fluoroscopy are critical. The fluoroscope is positioned to obtain both submentovertex and lateral views.
- A standard 100-mm-long, 20-gauge cannula with a stylet penetrates the skin 2.5 cm lateral to the oral commissure.
- The surgeon's finger prevents the cannula from penetrating the oral mucosa and guides it into the medial portion of the foramen ovale.
- The needle is advanced toward the intersection of a coronal plane passing through a point 3 cm anterior to the tragus and a sagittal plane passing through the medial aspect of the pupil.
- Using lateral fluoroscopy, the cannula should be directed 5–10 mm below the sella floor along the clivus, toward the angle formed by the shadows of the petrous bone and the clivus.
- A needle depth of about 6–8 cm is enough to achieve entrance into the foramen ovale and is signaled by a wince and a brief contraction of the masseter muscle.

- Proper positioning of the cannula within the trigeminal cistern allows free flow of cerebrospinal fluid (CSF) once the stylet is removed; however, CSF may not be obtained in patients who have had a previous percutaneous ablative procedure.
- Paresthesia after stimulation at 50 Hz should be evident in the affected division at less than 1 V, and motor stimulation at 2 Hz should be minimal. Ideally, the threshold for motor stimulation should be at least twice the sensory stimulation threshold.
- Three sequential low-temperature burns are used, starting at 60°C for 1 minute, then increasing to 63°C and 65°C.
- The disappearance of the trigger zones and the development of the patient's inability to differentiate between sharp and dull stimulation are considered safe endpoints for the coagulation.
- Hypalgesia of 75% or more is a good endpoint.
- After RF ablation, patients should receive half of the daily dose of anticonvulsant medications, which thereafter is slowly tapered and eventually discontinued.
- After RF ablation, mild facial numbness occurs in 98%, major dysesthesias in 10%, and anesthesia dolorosa (deafferentation pain) in up to 1.5%.
- Other complications include carotid artery puncture; injury to abducens, trochlear, or oculomotor nerves; epilepsy; infection; and alteration of salivation.

TRIGEMINAL RHIZOTOMY OUTCOMES

- Pain is immediately relieved in 99% of patients.
- The rate of pain recurrence is similar to that of microvascular decompression: approximately 15%–20% in 10–15 years.
- Kanpolat et al. performed a 25-year follow-up in 1600 patients whose ITN was treated with RF and found that 97.6% had acute pain relief. Pain relief was reported in 92% of patients with single or multiple procedures at 5 years; 94.2% of the patients who underwent multiple procedures had pain relief; and at 20-year follow-up, 41% of single procedure and 100% of multiple procedure patients experienced pain relief.

SPINE PAIN

OVERVIEW OF FACET ARTHROPATHY

- The pathophysiology of back pain is a complex issue, and the etiology of the pain is even more complex.
- The facet joint has a significant role in back pain, and the history and physical examination form the basis for the diagnosis of pain due to facet arthropathy.

Unfortunately, neither is specific enough to make a decision leading to definitive therapy.

- Physical examination reveals tenderness over the facet joints and associated muscle spasm. The pain is exacerbated by extension or lateral bending, and the range of motion is limited in all directions.
- A sequence (usually two sets) of diagnostic injections of the medial branches is performed under fluoroscopy to help secure a more definitive diagnosis.
- The lack of a corresponding cutaneous innervation to the facet joint makes it impossible to determine when complete blockade has occurred; however, when the patient can extend the spine without reproducing the preblock pain, we can assume that the block has worked. The specificity of the test is also limited because the medial branch nerve innervates muscles, ligaments, and periosteum in addition to the facet joints.

Anatomy

- The facet joints are paired diarthrodial synovial joints formed by the inferior articular process of one vertebra and the superior articular process of the vertebra below.
- The facet joints are present from the C1–2 junction to the L5–S1 junction.
- Each facet joint has a dual innervation supply: The medial branch, from the posterior ramus of a spinal nerve root, divides into two branches that supply the facet joint at the same level and the joint at the level below. There is also some evidence of joint innervation from a third ascending branch, which originates directly from the mixed spinal nerve.
- In the cervical facet region, the medial branch predominately supplies the facet joints, with minimal innervation of the posterior neck muscles.
- The C3 dorsal ramus is the only cervical dorsal ramus below C2 that regularly has a cutaneous distribution.
- The C3–4 to C7–T1 facet joints are supplied by the medial branches from the same level and the level above.
- The medial branches of the C3 ramus differ anatomically from those of lower cervical levels: The posterior rami nerve divides early in its course into deep and superficial (third occipital nerve) branches. The deep C3 medial branch descends to innervate the C3–4 facet joint, and the superficial medial branch traverses the C2–3 facet joint before entering the joint capsule.
- In the lumbar region, the medial branch is located in a groove at the base of the superior articular facet, and it sends a branch medially and to the inferior pole of the joint at the same level and a descending branch to the superior pole of the joint below.

- The thoracic facet joint innervation is similar to the lumbar region, except for the T5 to T8 levels, where the medial branches travel laterally from the foramen, cross the superior lateral border of the transverse process, and course medially to innervate the corresponding facet joint and the level below.

CERVICAL FACET DENERVATION

- Chronic cervical pain is one of the most difficult syndromes to treat.
- Percutaneous RF neurotomy has been increasingly used in the treatment of chronic cervical pain, especially pain originating from the cervical zygapophyseal joints. Few definitive data exist, however, on the efficacy of such procedures for several reasons: inadequate patient selection; inaccurate surgical anatomy; lack of controls; no controlled diagnostic blocks prior to RF ablation; and possible inaccurate placement of electrodes on the target nerve.
- In a controlled trial of the procedure, the outcomes were favorable for patients with chronic cervical zygapophyseal joint pain after percutaneous RF neurotomy with multiple lesions of target nerves. The median time that elapsed before the pain returned to at least 50% of the preoperative level was 263 days in the active treatment group compared with 8 days for the placebo group.

Technique

- In the traditional prone position, a 22-gauge, 5-cm needle with a 4-mm exposed tip is introduced 1–2 cm lateral to the waist of the articular pillar, guided by posterior–anterior and lateral views on fluoroscopy. This approach allows the practitioner to reach the desired target without encountering the vertebral artery.
- In the supine position, the head is rotated to the opposite side, and the fluoroscope is positioned approximately 10° obliquely. The needle is inserted into the posterior triangle and passed anteriorly under intermittent fluoroscopy until the transverse process is reached. Compared with the prone position, the supine approach positions the needle more tangential to the nerve and should give better results.
- Stimulation should be performed at 50 and 2 Hz and should cause few radicular symptoms and no motor stimulation.
- Lesioning is up to 80°C for 90 seconds.

THORACIC FACET DENERVATION

- The indication is thoracic facet joint syndrome; however, few data are available regarding the outcome measures of thoracic facet denervation. One report indicated that after a mean follow-up period of 31 months, 44% of patients were pain-free and another 39% of patients had greater than 50% pain relief.

Technique

- The patient is positioned prone with an abdominal cushion.
- The transverse process for each branch is identified using fluoroscopy, and the medial branch passes over the junction of the superior articular process and the transverse process.
- Stimulation should be at 50 Hz and less than 1 V, and motor stimulation should not be seen when 2 Hz is used at 2 V.
- Lesioning is up to 80°C for 90 seconds.

LUMBAR FACET DENERVATION

- The indication for denervation is persistent facet-mediated low back pain with a good response to diagnostic blocks.
- The lumbar facet is innervated by the medial branch of the posterior ramus of the corresponding nerve root and also the nerve root cephalad to it. The nerve loops over the junction of the transverse process and superior articular process.
- Reported long-term success rates include approximately 45% of patients achieving 50% relief at mean follow-ups of 2 years in one study and 3.2 years in another.

Technique

- The patient is positioned prone with an abdominal cushion to reduce lumbar lordosis.
- The patient's back is prepared in a sterile fashion, and the C-arm fluoroscopic device is used to identify the junction of the sacral ala with the superior articulating process of S1; the second and third targets are the superior and medial aspects of the transverse processes at L5 and L4.
- After the skin and subcutaneous tissues are anesthetized, the first cannula is placed so that it touches the groove between the sacral ala and superior articulating process of S1 (L5 dorsal ramus); the remaining cannulas are placed superomedial of the transverse processes of L5 and L4.
- At the level of the sacral ala and the transverse processes, the cannula is slipped over the leading edge of the periosteum.
- The RF cannulas should lie parallel to the nerve to be lesioned.

- The next step is checking the impedance and stimulation.
- Then lesioning is performed up to 80°C for 90 seconds.

SACROILIAC JOINT DENERVATION

- The sacroiliac joint is a source of low back pain, with a referral pattern similar to that for pain originating in the lumbar facet joints.
- RF denervation to provide long-term analgesia for patients with sacroiliac pain was first described in 2001. Ferrante et al. described a bipolar technique in which two needles are positioned approximately 1-cm apart, with multiple lesions performed along the length of the posterior surface of the joint. Over a 6-month follow-up period, 36.4% of patients achieved at least 50% pain relief. Following this, several retrospective studies targeted the lateral branches as they exit the sacral neuroforamina with success rates from 52% to 64% of patients achieving >50% pain relief.
- A randomized, placebo-controlled study of treatment of the lateral branches had a 57% success rate at six months.
- An in vitro study suggests that more complete lesions would be created with cannulae spacing of 4–6 mm, and leads to the possibility of improving results from strip lesions.

KNEE JOINT DENERVATION

- A double-blind, randomized controlled study of RF denervation of the knee articular nerve branches in chronic osteoarthritis patients had a 59% success rate of >50% relief at 12 weeks, which was statistically significant.

NEUROPATHIC PAIN

- Fourouzanfar et al. described the use of RF for ablation of the stellate ganglion, with 40% of patients achieving greater than 50% pain relief at a mean follow-up of 52 weeks.
- RF lesioning of the dorsal root ganglion has been reported to treat neuropathic pain, but prospective controlled trials are lacking.
- In general, neuroablative therapies are rarely used to treat neuropathic pain since an additional insult/injury to the nervous system carries a risk of increasing the pain from a preexisting nervous system injury. An exception to this rule is in the treatment of terminal cancer pain as the pain relief of the neurolytic

procedure will outlast the life of the patient. In other words, the time it takes for the additional injury from the neurolytic to cause pain is longer than the life of the patient.

PULSED RADIOFREQUENCY

- Observations of pain relief in patients who did not have evidence of complete nerve ablation led to theories that other mechanisms of pain relief may be associated with RF. In vitro studies suggest that changes in mitochondria morphology and axonal structures may explain reduced pain behavior in animal neuropathic pain models.
- Thus, investigators attempted to apply an RF field without increasing temperature (thereby avoiding tissue destruction).
- Pulsed RF achieves this goal by periodically interrupting the energy output, allowing time for heat to dissipate and avoiding a significant rise in temperature.
- Pulsed RF delivers energy from 1 to 10 Hz, with each cycle lasting 5–50 milliseconds. The most common setting reported is 2 Hz and 20 ms.
- The optimal parameters for pulsed RF are unknown. Sluijter, who first described this technique, advocated using 45 V for 120 seconds, which is thought to be the highest setting that will not increase temperature.
- Pulsed RF is used by clinicians in a variety of targets formerly treated with conventional RF with the hope of achieving analgesia while avoiding the complications associated with ablation.

FUTURE NEEDS

- Even though RF has been available for several decades, only a few controlled trials provide information on long-term outcomes for its use in a myriad of pain syndromes.
- Enough data exist to support the use of RF in trigeminal neuralgia, facet arthropathy, and sacroiliac pain, but there clearly is a need for further detailed investigation.
- Studies are also needed to determine the mechanism of action of pulsed RF.

BIBLIOGRAPHY

Choi WJ, Hwang SJ, Song JG, et al. Radiofrequency treatment relieves chronic knee osteoarthritis pain: a double-blind randomized controlled trial. *Pain*. 2011;152:481–487.

Cohen SP, Abdi S. Lateral branch blocks as a treatment for sacroiliac joint pain: a pilot study. *Reg Anesth Pain Med*. 2003;28:113.

Cohen SP, Hurley RW, Buckenmaier CC, et al. Randomized placebo-controlled study evaluating lateral branch radiofrequency denervation for sacroiliac joint pain. *Anesthesiology*. 2008;109: 279–288.

Ferrante FM, King LF, Roche EA, et al. Radiofrequency sacroiliac joint denervation for sacroiliac syndrome. *Reg Anesth Pain Med*. 2001;26:137.

Goupille P, Cotty P, Fouquet B, et al. Denervation of the posterior lumbar vertebral apophyses by thermocoagulation in chronic low back pain: results of the treatment of 103 patients. *Rev Rhum Ed Fr*. 1993;60:791.

Kanpolat Y, Sauas A, Bekar A, et al. Percutaneous controlled radiofrequency trigeminal rhizotomy for the treatment of idiopathic trigeminal neuralgia: 25-year experience with 1600 patients. *Neurosurgery*. 2001;48:524–534.

Kline MT, Yin W. Radiofrequency techniques in clinical practice. In: Waldman, ed. *Interventional Pain Management*. Philadelphia, Pa.: WB Saunders; 2001:243.

Lord SM, Barnsley L, Wallis B, et al. Percutaneous radiofrequency neurotomy for chronic cervical zygapophyseal-joint pain. *N Engl J Med*. 1996;335:1721.

Maxwell RE. Clinical diagnosis of trigeminal neuralgia and differential diagnosis of facial pain. In: Rovit RL, Murali R, Jannetta PJ, eds. *Trigeminal Neuralgia*. Baltimore, Md.: Williams & Wilkins; 1990:53.

North RB, Han M, Zahurak M, et al. Radiofrequency lumbar facet denervation: analysis of prognostic factors. *Pain*. 1994;57:77.

Panchal SJ, Belzberg AJ. Facet blocks and denervations. In: Burchiel KJ, ed. *Surgical Management of Pain*. New York: Thieme; 2002:666.

Saberski L, Fitzgerald J, Ahmad M. Cryoneurolysis and radiofrequency lesioning. In: Raj PP, ed. *Practical Management of Pain*. St. Louis, Mo: Mosby; 2000:759.

Slavin KV, Burchiel KJ. Surgical options for facial pain. In: Burchiel KJ, ed. *Surgical Management of Pain*. New York: Thieme; 2002:855.

Sluijter M, Cosman E, Rittman W, et al. The effect of pulsed radiofrequency fields applied to the dorsal root ganglion: a preliminary report. *Pain Clin*. 1998;11:109–117.

Stolker RJ, Vervest AC, Groen GJ. Percutaneous facet denervation in chronic thoracic spinal pain. *Acta Neurochir (Wien)*. 1993;122:82.

Sweet WH. The pathophysiology of trigeminal neuralgia. In: Gildenberg P, Tasker R, eds. *Textbook of Stereotactic and Functional Neurosurgery*. New York: McGraw–Hill; 1998:1667.

Taha JM. Percutaneous radiofrequency trigeminal gangliolysis. In: Burchiel KJ, ed. *Surgical Management of Pain*. New York: Thieme; 2002:841.

Taha JM, Tew JM Jr. A prospective 15-year follow up of 154 consecutive patients with trigeminal neuralgia treated by percutaneous stereotactic radiofrequency thermal rhizotomy. *J Neurosurg*. 1995;83:989.

Taha JM, Tew JM Jr. Surgical management of vagoglossopharyngeal neuralgia and other uncommon facial neuralgia. In: Tindall G, ed. *The Practice of Neurosurgery*. Baltimore, Md.: Williams & Wilkins; 1996:3065.

68 PERIPHERAL NERVE STIMULATION

Timothy R. Deer, MD
Richard G. Bowman, MD
Jason E. Pope, MD

INTRODUCTION

The positioning of a lead to conduct electrical current on or about a named peripheral nerve is called Peripheral Nerve stimulation (PNS). It is a therapy done to treat neuropathic pain of the trunk, limb or, cranium, based on a working diagnosis of a peripheral nerve causing pain in the proper distribution.

PNS can be used as a solo therapy, as a hybrid approach with Spinal Cord Stimulation (SCS), field stimulation, or Dorsal Root Ganglion Spinal Cord Stimulation (DRGSCS). It can also be used in combination with physical medicine, oral medications, and injections.

PNS has been utilized in clinical practice since its first use in clinical practice over forty years ago. The initial procedure involved an invasive cut-down, fascial graft, and suturing of a paddle type lead around or on the nerve. This invasive approach fell out of favor because of trauma, scarring, and poor results. The recent advent of the use of a percutaneous approach has led to new enthusiasm for the procedure.

THEORY

The use of PNS is growing in clinical practice, but the majority of physicians do not understand the mechanism of action. Even scientists who spend their careers on this issue are uncertain, but have postulated theories to support its use in chronic pain patients.

The majority of scientific analysis suggests that PNS works by changing the milieu in the peripheral nerve including a change in the fibers carrying the chronic pain signal. Some models suggest this may change the neural discharge and create a longer lasting change in the pathways that impact the pain message.

Some theories suggest the impact on the peripheral nerve creates an activation of the large diameter fibers in the spinal cord changing pain signals. Evidence suggests this may be mediated by the Dorsal Root Ganglion (DRG), or may also impact the dorsal column transmission.

INDICATIONS FOR PNS AND PNfS

PNS is indicated for patients having pain in the distribution of a named nerve based on anatomical knowledge. The pain ideally is of a neuropathic nature with characterization of burning, shooting, or lancinating. The response to a local anesthetic block is not predictive of a positive outcome, but may be helpful in establishing a diagnosis.

Peripheral Nerve Field Stimulation (PNfS) is indicated when pain of neuropathic character is located outside of the distribution of a named peripheral or spinal nerve. The use of a lead in the subcutaneous tissue is placed to impact the nerve fibers branching from a nerve. PNfS is an option as a monotherapy or as a combination with SCS in the axial back often called hybrid stimulation.

This chapter will focus on proper treatment using PNS.

DIAGNOSTIC EVALUATION: PNS

A history of pain of neuropathic character should be elicited from the patient. The pain should match the nerve distribution. Initial attempts at treatment should include physiotherapy, oral and transdermal medications, and peripheral nerve blocks if appropriate.

History and Physical examination is important to determine comorbidities and additional physical limitations or issues.

EMG/NCS should be considered if the diagnosis is unclear. These diagnostic tests are helpful in identifying large fiber injury, but may be less sensitive in identifying small nerve fiber injury.

Diagnostic injection of local anesthetic may be helpful in diagnostic evaluation, but is not predictive of a successful outcome based on current published information.

TENS units have been used to help predict ability to tolerate electrical current topically, but have not been shown to be predictive of positive outcomes. In some new novel devices, the use of adhesive is required. In these situations a history of adhesive or tape allergy is very important.

Prior to implant the physician should evaluate the skin to assure there is no local infection or other skin issues that may impact implantation.

Psychological evaluation has been shown to be an important screening tool prior to implant of a SCS device. In PNS, many physicians prefer to continue this policy of working in collaboration with a psychologist and psychiatrist in obtaining clearance for the implant.

PNS IN THE PAIN TREATMENT ALGORITHM

In many situations the patient has neuropathic pain in a distribution that could be successfully impacted by SCS or PNS. In that setting the physician must decide where to place each therapy in the algorithm. We should consider the advantages and disadvantages of each.

TARGETS FOR PNS

The use of PNS has been helpful to many patient groups in the past two decades. These therapies are commonly positioned in areas where named nerves are easily accessible and where a power sources can potentially be accommodated.

Targets that are commonly a focus of this surgery include:

- supraorbital nerve
- infraorbital nerve
- greater occipital nerve
- ulnar nerve
- median nerve,
- suprascapular nerve
- intercostal nerves
- ilioinguinal nerve
- iliohypogastric nerve
- genitofemoral nerve
- lateral femoral cutaneous nerve
- saphenous nerve
- sciatic nerve
- posterior tibial nerve
- superficial peroneal nerve
- sural nerve

ADVANTAGES OF PNS

The risks of each procedure should be considered against the benefit. PNS has a major advantage in that it has diminished risks since there is no spinal invasion required. The major risk of PNS is local infection.

PNS is focal in its impact. This can be ideal when extraneous stimulation or paresthesias are not desired.

PNS can be helpful in patients who have severe spinal abnormalities from previous spinal surgery, congenital deformity, or degenerative disease.

DISADVANTAGES OF PNS

PNS is limited in its scope and may not be helpful in conditions where the pain is outside of the area or distribution of the potential targets for stimulation.

However, PNS may induce local scarring and increase the impedance around the lead. This can lead to failure of the therapy.

Unpleasant paresthesias can occur if the lead is placed too superficial. These complaints normally center around "burning pain" while the device is activated. In cases where the device is too deep the patient may experience unwanted motor recruitment.

In cases where the device is placed in areas of anatomical bony prominences or in regions which hardware crosses joints, the patient may experience pain or device migration.

The tools utilized for PNS techniques were developed for dorsal column stimulation and then adopted for the periphery. This creates a barrier for more peripheral nerve targets.

TECHNIQUES FOR IMPLANT

PREOPERATIVE TESTING

If local anesthetic with mild sedation is planned; the patient should be evaluated by the anesthesiologist prior to surgery for preoperative evaluation and assessment of risks.

In most cases an array of lab testing is done before surgery including assessment of bleeding parameters, electrolytes, and cell counts. Urinalysis is appropriate if at risk for chronic infection. In diabetics, an evaluation of glucose control is indicated and a consultation with the managing physician is in order if abnormalities exist. Chest films and electrocardiogram are often obtained preoperatively by the Anesthesia team. Pregnancy testing should be done if appropriate.

ANESTHESIA FOR LEAD PLACEMENT

The method of needle and lead placement determines the options for anesthesia. In cases where the lead is placed based on landmarks, the patient may be moderately sedated and local anesthetic may be used abundantly. In cases where the lead placement is determined by placement by ultrasound or nerve stimulation the patient is often only mildly sedated and the use of local anesthetic is limited to the skin wheel for initial cut or needle placement.

In some settings, placement involves a surgical dissection to the nerve, exposure of the nerve and placement of a cuff type lead around the nerve. In these settings the anesthetic balance can be much more difficult.

PREOPERATIVE ANTIBIOTIC

The choice of antibiotic for preoperative prophylaxis should be based on history of patient allergy, history of recent infections, and most importantly local pathogens specific to the geographic area of implant. In many settings the staphylococcus bacteria are resistant to both methicillin and to cephalosporins. In these instances the use of vancomycin alone or in combination with gentamycin is often considered.

The antibiotic should be infused with proper timing to allow for proper serum levels prior to surgical incision, commonly within 30 minutes in incision, as recommended by the CDC.

The use of postoperative antibiotics is controversial, but many implanters choose to use them for the duration of the trial, or in the first seven days post permanent implant.

POSITIONING AND SURGICAL SITE PREPARATION

When positioning the patient careful attention should be placed on allowing proper exposure of the planned surgical area for both the lead and the IPG if needed. Also the team should use caution in positioning the limbs in areas that induces pressure on other peripheral nerves around joints. In the patient undergoing little or no sedation the second consideration is often moot.

The choice of prep solution for the skin should be based on patient allergies and local bacterial pathogens.

Draping should be widely outside the planned surgical field. Exposure should include the planned lead location, any areas of potential tunneling and the IPG site if indicated. The C-arm should be wrapped in a sterile fashion and room traffic should be held to a minimum.

Recently Deer and Provenzano outlined proper strategy for wound infection mitigation the placement of implantable devices.

IDENTIFYING THE NERVE

There are different methods to identify the nerve. They are outlined in this section.

LANDMARKS

Some implanters prefer to implant the lead at a desired depth in the tissues adjacent to the nerve. Parameters used in this setting include tissue plane, bony landmarks, and theorized nerve branch location.

ULTRASOUND

Ultrasound is a relatively new addition to lead placement. After proper training, a physician can use ultrasound to identify tissue structures. The needle can be seen as well as the nerve, vascular structures, adipose planes, and muscle planes. The goal is to place the lead adjacent to the nerve with the least possible tissue trauma. Ultrasound has been used in occipital nerve placement for occipital nerve stimulation (ONS), ilioinguinal nerve stimulation, and stimulation of multiple nerves of the trunk and extremities.

FLUOROSCOPY

Fluoroscopy is used to facilitate placement by landmarks. The picture from the C-arm is used to document general position and to compare the trial position with the permanent implant lead position. Because of the change in body position impacting x-ray view and parallax error impacting angles the fluoroscopic view is not always accurate.

NERVE STIMULATION

Recent developments in devices have led to the use of nerve stimulation to place a sheath through which a PNS device can be placed. In order to do this technique it is helpful to use as little anesthetic as possible, to use fluoroscopic guidance for landmarks or ultrasound guidance for nerve location assistance, and to have a conversant and responsive patient.

NEEDLE AND LEAD PLACEMENT

The needle is placed after a small skin incision to assist entry. Most physicians prefer a needle with a plastic stylet to allow bending the needle. Once the needle is placed into the proper location as noted about, the lead is engaged. As the lead is advanced to the needle bevel, the needle is pulled back to deploy the lead. In trialing the lead is then tested for location and secured with a suture or tape. In permanent lead placement a cut down is made and the lead is sewn to the fascia. Many physicians use an anchor, but the alternative technique is to use a nonabsorbable suture to sew the electrode array directly to the fascia.

INTRAOPERATIVE AND POSTOPERATIVE PROGRAMMING

Once the lead is in place and confirmed to be in good position the physician or technical assistant must program the lead. In current systems this involves hooking a cable to the lead and activating contacts on the system. There is an ability to use a cathode, and anode, or keep the lead neutral. Increasing the number of cathodes spreads the focus of the current. Increasing the number of anodes focuses the current toward any existing cathode. If more than one lead is placed in close proximity it is possible to program between the two or three leads to spread the field. This is called "cross talking."

PERMANENT WITH AN INTERNAL PROGRAMMABLE GENERATOR (IPG)

In currently available devices the lead is connected to an IPG. This involves making a pocket in the subcutaneous tissue at a size compatible with the IPG and then connecting the lead to the device. A tunneling tool is often used to pass the lead from the site of the original needle placement to the pocket.

PERMANENT WITHOUT AN IPG

In the United States the development of a device that can be placed without the need for an internalized generator has been used in patients. This device is currently in a pivotal United States trial seeking FDA approval. The procedure involves placement of a lead via a sheath after nerve stimulation, and then tunneling a tiny receiver to a location a few centimeters away. The power source and programming are worn on the skin and no IPG is required.

Recent presentations have shown the possibility of placing a lead that can communicate with an external programming source and microwave technology that can lead to the elimination of an IPG, and the possibility that a smart phone app can be used to interface with the device.

HYBRID SYSTEMS

The use of a Spinal Cord Stimulator (SCS) with a PNS or PNfS in combination is called hybrid stimulation. The possibility of using more than one target for Neuromodulation in the same patient is intriguing and may lead to better outcomes.

POSTOPERATIVE CARE

The risks of PNS are quite low compared to alternative procedures, but the surveillance of the patient post operatively can be very helpful in reducing complications. The patient should be seen in follow-up for wound evaluation and check. Observation for skin color, fever, and erythema are important. The patient may also need reprogramming in the immediate postoperative period. This is particularly common after the lead scars in to the surrounding tissue.

The other risk to consider in the postoperative period is lead movement. In the first six weeks the lead is often in the process of stabilizing with a fibrous sheath around the materials. Once this occurs movement is rare. Methods of securing the leads in the first six weeks include anchoring, tines on the end of the lead to promote scarring, and placing a strain relief at the pocket to relieve pressure on the wiring.

LONG TERM OUTCOMES

In a prospective study of acute nerve stimulation Deer, Levy, and Rosenfeld published a study showing relief in the use of a device that did not require an IPG. This study has been followed up by a multicenter randomized trial that is currently in progress.

Almost twenty years ago Hassenbusch and Stanton Hicks published results on a large prospective trial treating Complex Regional Pain Syndrome (CRPS) The success rate in this study was greater than sixty percent even with what would currently be considered antiquated devices.

Recent studies have been performed showing the use of PNS to treat migraine, facial pain, and pain of the axial spine. The results have been favorable in reducing illness behavior, pain levels, and functional activity.

CONCLUSION

The use of PNS and PNfS are helpful in many patients who suffer from chronic pain. Current devices were designed to treat the spine and are used in the periphery as indicated. New work on product development will lead to more custom treatment based on the involved nerve. PNS as a solo therapy will become more commonly applied to patients in the future, but the possibility of using it as a series of therapy targets in the same patient is intriguing and may represent an ideal situation.

BIBLIOGRAPHY

Chung JM, Lee KH, Hori Y, et al. Factors influencing peripheral nerve stimulation produced inhibition of primate spinothalamic tract cells. *Pain.* 1984;19:277–293.

Deer TR, Levy RM, Rosenfeld EL. Prospective clinical study of a new implantable peripheral nerve stimulation device to treat chronic pain. *Clin J Pain.* 2010;26(5):359–372.

Deer TR, Pope JE, Kaplan M. A novel method of neurostimulation for the nervous system: The StimRouter Implantable Device.

Techniques in Regional Anesthesia and Pain Management. 2012; 16(2):113–117.

Deer TR, Provenzano DA. Recommendations for reducing Infection in the practice of implanting spinal cord stimulation and intrathecal drug delivery devices: A physician's playbook. *Pain Physician.* 2013; 16(3):E125–E128.

Gybels J, Kupers R. Central and peripheral electrical stimulation of the nervous system in the treatment of chronic pain. *Acta Neurochir Suppl (Wien).* 1987;38:64–75.

Hassenbusch SJ, Stanton-Hicks M, Schoppa D, et al. Long-term results of peripheral nerve stimulation for reflex sympathetic dystrophy. *J Neurosurg.* 1996;84:415–423.

Huntoon MA, Hoelzer BC, Burgher AH, Hurdle MF, Huntoon EA. Feasibility of ultrasound-guided percutaneous placement of peripheral nerve stimulation electrodes and anchoring during simulated movement: Part two, upper extremity. *Reg Anesth Pain Med.* 2008;33(6):558–565.

Huntoon MA, Huntoon EA, Obray JB, Lamer TJ. Feasibility of ultrasound-guided percutaneous placement of peripheral nerve stimulation electrodes in a cadaver model: Part one, lower extremity. *Reg Anesth Pain Med.* 2008;33(6):551–557.

Law JD, Swett J, Kirsch WM. Retrospective analysis of 22 patients with chronic pain treated by peripheral nerve stimulation. *J Neurosurg.* 1980;52:482–485.

Levy RM. Algorithms for treatment of neuropathic pain syndromes. In: North RB, Levy RM, eds. *Neurosurgical Management of Pain.* New York: Springer-Verlag; 1997:337–339.

Long DM, Erickson D, Campbell J, et al. Electrical stimulation of the spinal cord and peripheral nerves for pain control: A 10-year experience. *Appl Neurophysiol.* 1981;44:207–217.

Mangram AJ, Horan TC, Pearson ML, Silver LC. Guideline for Prevention of Surgical Site Infection, 1999. *Infection Control and Hospital Epidemiology, CDC.* April 1999; 20(4):250–280.

McRoberts WP, Cairns KD, Deer T. Stimulation of the peripheral nervous system for the painful extremity. In: Slavin KV, ed., *Peripheral Nerve Stimulation.* Basel: Karger, 2011;156–170.

Melzack R, Wall PD. Pain mechanisms: A new theory. *Science.* 1965;150:971–979.

Mironer YE, Hutcheson JK, Satterhwaite JR, LaTourette PC. Prospective, two part study of the interaction between spinal cord stimulation and peripheral nerve field stimulation in patients with low back pain: Development of a new spinal-peripheral neurostimulation method. *Neuromodulation.* 2011;(14):151–155.

Nashold BS Jr, Goldner JL, Mullen JB, et al. Long-term pain control by direct peripheral-nerve stimulation. *J Bone Joint Surg Am.* 1982;64:1–10.

Perryman L. Peripheral Nerve Stimulation (PNS) For Chronic Craniofacial Neuropathic Pain With A Novel Wirelessly Powered Miniature Implantable Neurostimulator Electrode Array. INS Meeting; Berlin, Germany; 2013.

Reverberi C, Dario A, Barolat G. Spinal cord stimulation (SCS) in conjunction with peripheral nerve field stimulation (PNfS) for the treatment of complex pain in failed back surgery syndrome (FBSS). *Neuromodulation.* 2013;16(1):78–82; discussion 83.

Schon LC, Kleeman TJ, Chiodo CP, et al. A prospective analysis of peripheral nerve stimulation for intractable lower extremity nerve pain. Paper presented at: 16th Annual Summer Meeting of the American Foot and Ankle Society; July 13–15, 2000; Vail (Colorado).

Shetter AG, Racz GB, Lewis R, et al. Peripheral nerve stimulation. In: North RB, Levy RM, eds. *Neurosurgical Management of Pain.* New York: Springer-Verlag; 1997; 261–270.

Silberstein SD, Dodick DW, Saper J, et al. Safety and efficacy of peripheral nerve stimulation of the occipital nerves for the management of chronic migraine: Results from a randomized, multicenter, double-blinded, controlled study. *Cephalalgia.* 2012;32(16):1165–1179.

Waisbrod H, Panhans C, Hansen D, et al. Direct nerve stimulation for painful peripheral neuropathies. *J Bone Joint Surg Br.* 1985;67:470–472.

Wall PD, Gutnick M. Properties of afferent nerve impulses originating from a neuroma. *Nature.* 1974;248:740–743.

Wall PD, Sweet WH. Temporary abolition of pain in man. *Science.* 1967;155:108–109.

69 | PERIPHERAL NERVE FIELD STIMULATION

Eric Grigsby, MD, MBA
Devon Schmidt, BA

INTRODUCTION

DEFINITION

- Peripheral nerve field stimulation, Subcutaneous peripheral nerve stimulation, Percutaneous electrical nerve stimulation, Subcutaneous electrical nerve stimulation, and Subcutaneous target stimulation are a few of the many terms used to describe the singular technique discussed in this chapter. For our purposes, the technique will be called Peripheral Nerve Field Stimulation (PNFS).
- PNFS directly targets regions of pain. In contrast to traditional neurostimulation, where well-defined, major neural structures receive electrical stimulation, this technique is used to alter the function of small, highly arborized nerves immediately at the site of pain. A named nerve is not frequently identified

USE: PAST AND PRESENT

- Historically, spinal cord stimulation has delivered poor results in treatment of nociceptive, axial back pain.
- Descriptions of electrical stimulation targeting the area under the skin of painful locations, such as the low back, began to appear in the literature in the late 1990s.
- Targeting regions of pain by stimulating the adjacent subcutaneous tissue is useful in situations where pain

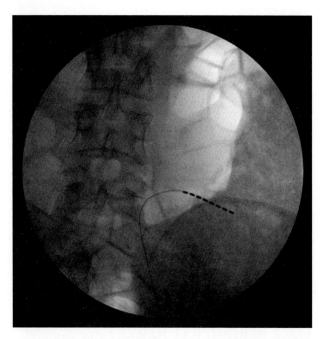

FIG. 69-1. Lower lumbar PNFS with a single eight-contact lead.

relief is difficult to obtain with conventional neuro-stimulation methods that target the spinal cord (SCS) or well-defined peripheral nerves (PNS).

• Because certain painful regions and pain types, including head pain, axial back pain (Figure 69-1), abdominal pain, groin pain, posthernia repair pain (Figure 69-2), and scar pain, have been notoriously difficult to manage with SCS and PNS, PNFS is often

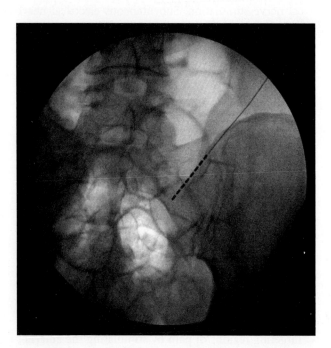

FIG. 69-2. Inguinal PNFS with a single eight-contact lead.

applied prior to or in combination with traditional neurostimulation techniques.

SCIENTIFIC FOUNDATION

• The mechanism of action for PNFS is not well defined. Several theories have been developed to explain the physiological effect produced by this technique; however, no studies have been published to directly address the mechanism of action. Some postulate that pain relief derived by targeting the subcutaneous tissue in a painful region is obtained through a mechanism similar to that provided by SCS, a mechanism built on the foundation of Melzack and Wall's "gate control" theory of pain.

• According to Ehrlich and Lamp, electrical stimulation induces paresthesia through the modulation of large fiber activity combined with the subsequent influence on afferent information from smaller fibers.

• Essentially, PNFS maintains its therapeutic function by modulating the information received at the spinal cord.

• PNFS may also modulate how pain is perceived through one or more of the following manners:
  ○ Stimulation changes the immediate dermal dynamics, thereby altering the effects of local blood flow
  ○ Stimulation has a direct local effect modulating anti-inflammatory membrane depolarization characteristics
  ○ Stimulation provides sensitivity to neurotransmitters.

• While clinical evidence does not favor one mechanism over another, it does indicate that the mechanism of PNFS does not act in a fashion similar to transdermal electrical neurostimulation (TENS).

• PNFS has shown effect at both low frequencies (2–10 Hz) and high frequencies (<50 Hz) unlike conventional TENS therapies which use produce effect through high-frequency stimulation.

• There have been reports of success with PNFS in patients that did not respond to TENS.

SYSTEM

ELECTRODES

• PNFS is a relatively new technique; therefore, equipment designed specifically for subcutaneous use is just beginning to enter the market.

• SCS leads have often been implanted in the subcutaneous tissue for pain relief.

• Both eight and four contact electrodes have been used depending on the stimulation strength and programming capabilities required.

- Paddle type leads or cylindrical leads may be used in PNFS.
- When deciding what type of lead to use, it is important to keep in mind the difference in the electrical field produced by each type of lead, with respect to the therapeutic stimulation necessary.
  - Paddle leads produce a unidirectional, linear electrical field.
  - Cylindrical leads cause an electrical field to radiate from the source.
  - While there is no evidence to support use of one over the other, the electric field produced by cylindrical electrodes may provide a benefit for PNFS, as the lead is usually implanted in the epicenter of pain.
- Electrodes used for the trial are not identical to the leads used for permanent implant; however, they often mimic an identical configuration.
- Many practitioners use the same number of contacts, as they would anticipate using for permanent implant.
- Some practitioners advocate the use of monoelectrodes for the purposes of the trial.

GENERATOR

- Both types of implantable pulse generators, constant voltage and constant current generators, have been manufactured for the purpose of neurostimulation.
- No studies have been published to evaluate the effectiveness of one type of generator over another for PNFS.
- Burgher and associates postulated that different effects may occur when constant current generators are used rather than constant voltage generators. Further analysis of this concept is needed.
- There have been no published studies designed to compare the use of two implantable generators versus one. However, case reports indicate that the use of a single generator has led to better results than when a patient has multiple implanted generators.
- The decision regarding the use of a rechargeable battery when compared to a nonrechargeable system can be made based on the types of leads implanted, the number of leads used, and the stimulation settings required by the patient during the trial.
- The decision on type of IPG is analogous to SCS.
- The lead array, stimulation parameters, and expected IPG replacement interval will drive the decision in the absence of other scientific guidance.

CONFIGURATION

- A variety of configurations can be used with PNFS.
- Case reports have had successful results with 1×8, 2×8, 1×4, 2×4, and 4×4 configurations.

- The type and number of leads depend on the location of pain and the size of the region.
- "Bracketing" or "cross-talk" are terms describing a configuration that attempts to produce paresthesia in the region between leads. This technique is often used when targeting a large area of pain.
- Falco and associates have described a situation where they were able to produce pain relief with an interlead distance of 34 cm and coverage of 377 cm^2.

TRIAL

- Trial length can vary from three days to two weeks.
- Measures taken to prevent infection often include procedural intravenous antibiotics and thorough cleansing of the incision site.
- The procedure can be performed with local anesthestic alone or local anesthetic plus conscious sedation.
- The target site is marked with permanent ink and landmarks can be used to guide the implanter.
- Some implanters advocate the use of an external nerve-mapping probe to identify the proper site and lateral fluoroscopic guidance is often used to confirm lead location.
- If the patient has a large body mass index it may also be advisable to utilize ultrasound while implanting the lead to ensure optimal positioning.
- A 14G needle is commonly used to advance the lead into the proper position (Table 69-1).
- Needle length and shape can be adjusted to conform to the shape of the target anatomy, for example, the head or face.
- Once the lead is placed, leads are secured to the skin with steri-strips.

TABLE 69-1   Subcutaneous Lead Insertion

LOCATION	DEPTH
Preprocedure techniques	**Optimal**
1. Define target area with patient 2. Mark areas to avoid 3. Outline target site	1. Needle produces "tenting" 2. Loss of resistance during needle insertion (indicating dermal layer penetration)
Procedure techniques	**Suboptimal**
1. Ultrasound guidance 2. External nerve stimulation 3. Fluoroscopic guidance 4. Patient guidance	1. Skin indentation—needle is too shallow 2. Discomfort in response to stimulation—lead is too shallow 3. Indifference to stimulation—lead is too deep 4. Muscle twitching—lead is too deep

- An external generator is then attached to the temporarily implanted leads and the patient experiences stimulation for the duration of the trial.
- Programming can occur immediately after the trial or can be initiated in the days immediately following procedure.

PERMANENT IMPLANT

- To produce optimal outcomes and minimize risk, system implant should include a vigilant preoperative routine including preoperative showering with antiseptic soap, and a multiday antibiotic regimen.
- Leads are implanted with the meticulous planning and guidance techniques similar to those used for the trial.
- Upon implant, the incision used to permanently implant the leads is lengthened to accommodate anchors and necessary connections.
- Leads are often anchored to the fascia immediately adjacent to the lead.
- In addition to the anchor, some authors advocate the use of a nondissolvable suture to further secure the leads.
- It is recommended that the electrodes be secured near the contact array because this location represents the sturdiest portion of the lead providing maximum anchor support.
- Generator placement is determined by lead implantation site. Common sites include the abdominal wall, lateral thigh, gluteal, or infraclavicular region.
- Upon deciding the optimal generator location, strategic placement of connections and anchors is crucial in producing the best outcomes with this therapy and preventing future complications.
- The implant surgery is the foundation for PNFS therapy. Integrating lead placement, extension connection, and IPG implant into a seamless rational procedure is essential to produce an effective treatment strategy (Table 69-2).

TABLE 69-2   **Surgical Plan**

DEPENDENT VARIABLES	CONSIDERATIONS
Lead location(s)	1. Pain type and location addressed with PNFS 2. Lead type (Paddle, Cylindrical) 3. Lead array (Octrode, Quatrode) 4. Configuration (Single Lead, Dual Leads, Bracket)
Anchor/connection locations	1. Lead location and configuration 2. Generator location 3. Tunneling route
Generator location	1. Patient preference 2. Lead location

PATIENT ASSESSMENT AND CANDIDACY

- To date, there are poorly defined indications associated with PNFS.
- Pain syndromes reported in the literature include:
  - Axial back pain
  - Cervical pain
  - Abdominal pain
  - Groin pain
  - Postsurgery pain
  - Headache
  - Angina
  - Atypical facial pain.
- Patients who receive PNFS have often previously failed treatments, including medical management, physical therapy, TENS, local injections, and nerve blocks.
- The appropriate patient for PNFS should have previously reported a successful trial, defined by greater than 50% improvement in pain.
- The above description illustrates the patient population that commonly receives PNFS. This portrait is based on case studies and clinical anecdotes.
- Prospective case controlled studies are needed to better define the appropriate patient population for neurostimulation in the subcutaneous tissue underlying the location of pain.

LIMITATIONS AND FUTURE DIRECTIONS

- PNFS is limited by a lack of high-level data regarding its use.
- There are no professional guidelines for use of PNFS and there are inconsistencies surrounding appropriate indications for use.
- While clinical experience and case reports have begun to elicit interest in the use of the technique, controlled clinical trials are needed to develop standards of care for this therapy and to define the patient population with the greatest change for success.
- At the time of this writing, such clinical trials are under way in the United States, Europe, and Australia.

BIBLIOGRAPHY

Abejón D, Deer T, Verrills P. Subcutaneous stimulation: how to assess optimal implantation depth. *Neuromodulation.* 2011;14:343–434.

Aberjon D, Krames E. Peripheral nerve stimulation or is it peripheral subcutaneous field stimulation; what is in a Moniker? *Neuromodulation.* 2009;12(1):1–3.

Burgher AH, Huntoon MA, Turley TW, Doust MW, Stearns Lj. Subcutaneous peripheral nerve stimulation with inter-lead stimulation for axial neck and low back pain: case series and review of the literature. *Neuromodulation.* 2012;15:100–107.

Ellrich J, Lamp S. Peripheral nerve stimulation inhibits nociceptive processing: an electrophysiological study in healthy volunteers. *Neuromodulation.* 2005;8:225.

Falco FJE, Berger J, Vrable A, et al. Cross talk: a new method for peripheral nerve stimulation. An observational report with cadaveric verification. *Pain Physician.* 2009;12:965–983.

Ghoname EA, Craig WF, White PF, et al. Percutaneous electrical nerve stimulation for low back pain: a randomized crossover study. *J Am Med Assoc.* 1999;282:941–942.

Goroszeniuk T, Kothari S, Hamann W. Subcutaneous neuromodulating implant targeted at the site of pain. *Regional Anesthesia and Pain Medicine.* 2006;31(2):168–171.

Goroszeniuk T, Pang D, Al-Kaisy A, Sanderson K. Subcutaneous target stimulation—peripheral subcutaneous field stimulation in the treatment of refractory angina: preliminary case reports. *Pain Practice.* 2012;12(1):71–79.

Ignelzi RJ, Nyquist JK. Direct effect of electrical stimulation on peripheral nerve evoked activity: implications in pain relief. *Journal of Neurosurgery.* 1976;45(2):159–165.

Krutsch JP, McCeney MH, Barolat G, et al. A case report of subcutaneous peripheral nerve stimulation for the treatment of axial back pain associated with postlaminectomy syndrome. *Neuromodulation.* 2008;12:112–115.

Melzack R, Wall PD. Pain mechanisms: a new theory. *Science.* 1965;150:971–979.

Mironer YE, Hutcheson JK, Satterthwaite JR, Latourette PC. Prospective, two-part study of the interaction between spinal cord stimulation and peripheral nerve field stimulation in patients with low back pain: development of a new spinal peripheral neurostimulation method. *Neuromodulation.* 2010;14(1):151–155.

Paicius RM, Bernstein CA, Lemper-Cohen C. Peripheral nerve field stimulation for the treatment of chronic low back pain: preliminary results of long-term follow up: a case series. *Neuromodulation.* 2007;10:279–290.

Reverberi C., Dario A., Barolat G. Spinal cord stimulation (SCS) in conjunction with peripheral nerve field stimulation (PNFS) for the treatment of complex pain in failed back surgery syndrome (FBSS). *Neuromodulation.* 2012;16:78–83.

Sator-Katzenschlager S, Fiala K, Kress H., et al. Subcutaneous target stimulation (STS) in chronic noncancer pain: a nationwide retrospective study". *Pain Practice.* 2010;10(4):279–286.

Shealy CN, Mortimer JT, Reswick JB. Electrical inhibition of pain by stimulation of the dorsal columns: preliminary clinical report. *Anesth Analg.* 1967;46:489–491.

Stanton-Hicks M, Salamon, J. Stimulation of the central and peripheral nervous system for the control of pain. *J Clin Neurophysiol.* 1997;14(1):46–62.

Verills P, et al. Peripheral nerve stimulation: a treatment for chronic low back pain and failed back surgery syndrome? *Neuromodulation.* 2009;12:68–75.

Wall PD, Sweet WH. Temporary abolition of pain in man. *Science.* 1967;6:155(3758):108–109.

Yakovlev A, Resch B. Treatment of chronic intractable atypical facial pain using peripheral subcutaneous field stimulation. *Neuromodulation.* 2010;13:137–140.

70 PALLIATIVE CARE

Kristin D. Forner, MD
Eric Roeland, MD

PALLIATIVE CARE VS. HOSPICE

- Many medical providers believe that Palliative care is same as Hospice care. Palliative care is not synonymous with hospice care, as palliative care is not constrained to any time limit in the course of illness. All patients with poorly controlled symptoms, regardless of life expectancy or disease trajectory, are eligible for palliative care. Hospice care on the other hand is relegated for those at the end of life.

- "Palliative" is derived from the French word *palliatif* or the Latin word *palliativus*, meaning "under cloak or cover," as in to "cloak or cover" one's symptoms. Palliative care includes symptom management and begins early in the course of illness.

- In addition, palliative care also provides a whole-person assessment through a transdisciplinary approach, and can engage patients and families in assessing the patients and family goals of care. *Goals of care* refers to a patient-specific plan that honors the patient's wishes when addressing future medical care.

- Early integration of palliative care to standard cancer care has been demonstrated to improve survival and quality of life. As such, national guidelines recommend that palliative care be integrated into standard oncologic care at the time of diagnosis.

- Hospice care is end-of-life care. Based upon the 1982 Medicare hospice benefit, patients must have a prognosis of six months or less to qualify for hospice care, which consists of symptom management and end-of-life care (Table 70-1).

PALLIATIVE CARE TEAM

- "Palliative care" is the preferred term to "palliative medicine" as nonmedical members are a part of the *palliative care* team.

- A palliative care team is an interdisciplinary team comprised of physicians, nurse practitioners, nurses, social workers, chaplains, pharmacists, nutritionists, and physical therapists, all working together to care for the whole patient.

- The International Association for the Study of Pain defines pain as "an unpleasant sensory and emotional experience associated with actual or potential tissue damage, or described in terms of such damage." Pain is not just a physical experience, but can affect the whole patient as well.

TABLE 70-1 Common Misperceptions of Hospice and Palliative Care

MISPERCEPTION	TRUE/FALSE	FACT
Palliative care is the same as hospice care.	False	Palliative care can be provided at any point in the course of illness. Hospice care is reserved for the end-of-life when a patient has an expected prognosis of six months or less.
Hospice patients must die within six months or they are kicked off hospice.	False	Physicians are not perfect prognosticators. Hospice appropriateness is determined at 90 and then 60-day intervals. At these intervals, the hospice physician determines if the patient is appropriate for hospice. If the hospice physician believes the patient is likely to die in the next six months if the disease runs its expected course, and can describe his/her medical reasoning, patients can continue to remain on hospice.
A patient must be DNR to enroll in hospice.	False	DNR is not a federal mandate to enroll in hospice. Some hospice programs will allow patients to be full code, but this is specific to each hospice program.
Patients cannot receive life-prolonging therapies once on hospice.	False	Antibiotics, blood transfusions, radiation, and chemotherapy are not recognized federal exclusions to receive hospice care. However, many hospice programs will not cover these services because they are more expensive than what the Medicare benefit will cover.
Once a patient has signed onto hospice, they have to stay on hospice.	False	Patients and/or healthcare proxies can choose to sign off hospice services at any time.
Hospice means the patient has "given up" or there is "nothing left to do."	False	Hospice is actually about what *can be done* at the end-of-life, with an emphasis on quality of life and dignity.

- In line with this definition, a palliative care team brings together multiple areas of expertise to address a patient's "total suffering": the physical, emotional, psychological, spiritual, and social concerns that can arise with advanced illness.

WHO CAN RECEIVE PALLIATIVE CARE?

- According to the National Hospice and Palliative Care Organization data from 2012, patients who are appropriate to receive palliative care include those with cancer, and those with noncancer diagnoses such as dementia, failure to thrive (or debility), heart disease, HIV, neurologic diseases including amyotrophic lateral sclerosis, liver disease, pulmonary disease, renal disease, stroke, traumatic brain injury, or coma. Any patient, at any stage in the course of these illnesses, is a candidate for palliative care.

WHY IS PALLIATIVE CARE BENEFICIAL?

- Palliative care teams treat a variety of symptoms. The most common symptoms they evaluate and treat include pain, delirium, constipation, nausea and vomiting, and dyspnea. Palliative care teams diagnose and treat symptoms more accurately and effectively than the primary providing teams.
- In a seminal study published in the *New England Journal of Medicine*, nonsmall cell lung cancer (NSCLC) patients who received early palliative care in comparison to patients who did not, had an improved quality of life at 12 weeks. Patients assigned to early palliative care had a 2.7-month survival benefit. This finding rivals the survival benefits that come with standard first-line metastatic NSCLC chemotherapy regimens.

Palliative care teams help patients determine their goals of care, and then helps develop plans for patients to achieve these goals. Evidence has proven that the earlier palliative care teams are involved in patients' hospitalizations, the more likely patients are to die outside of a hospital (largely either at home with hospice or in an inpatient hospice or palliative medicine facility).

- Cost savings is an unintended consequence of providing evidence-based, patient-centered care. Per admission, palliative care consultations save hospitals approximately $2000 for patients who are discharged alive, and almost $5000 for patients who die in the hospital. Per day, the cost savings are $174 for patients who are discharged alive, and $374 for patients who die in the hospital.

WHY REFER?

- A referral to a palliative care team is appropriate when symptoms are out of control, a transdisciplinary evaluation may be beneficial, a patient has concerns beyond the physical domain and these concerns are contributing to suffering (Figure 70-1), medication management is complicated due to comorbid psychosocial issues or maladaptive coping, or procedural pain management interventions are not appropriate or effective.

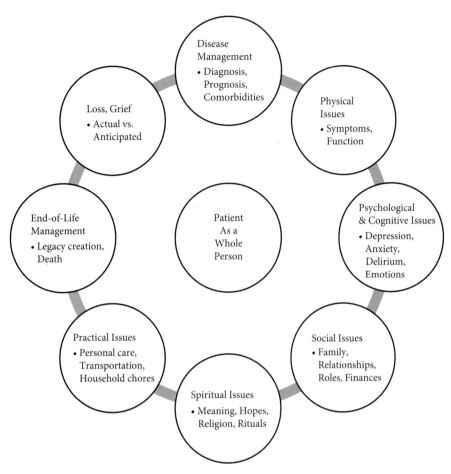

FIG. 70-1. Domains of the whole person in advanced illness.

MOST COMMON SYMPTOMS AND THERAPIES

- Dyspnea
  - Nonpharmacologic methods: positioning, mindfulness, and breathing training
  - Oxygen
  - Opiates
  - Anxiolytics
  - Neuroleptics
  - Steroids
  - Bronchodilators
- Nausea and vomiting
  - Dopamine antagonists
  - Histamine antagonists
  - Acetylcholine antagonists
  - Serotonin antagonists
  - Neurokinin antagonists
  - Prokinetic agents
  - Antacids
- Constipation
  - Stool softeners
  - Fiber
  - Stimulant laxatives
  - Osmotic laxatives
  - Lubricants
  - Enemas
  - Opiate antagonists
  - Prokinetic agents
- Insomnia
  - Sleep hygiene
  - Sleep hormone Melatonin
  - Antidepressant Trazodone
  - Anxiolytics
  - Histamine antagonists
  - Neuroleptic Chlorpromazine
- Anorexia and cachexia
  - Corticosteroids
  - Megestrol
  - Cannabinoids
  - Antidepressant Mirtazapine
  - Exercise
  - Nutritional support

- Fatigue
  - Stimulant Methylphenidate
  - Corticosteroids
- Diarrhea
  - Nutritional support, including fluid and electrolyte replacement
  - Opiates
  - Anticholinergics
  - Bulk-forming agents
  - Octreotide
- Mucositis
  - Topical oral formulations (lidocaine, diphenhydramine, ketamine)
- Malignant bowel obstruction
  - Corticosteroids
  - Antiemetics
  - Histamine antagonists
  - Acetylcholine antagonists
  - Octreotide

WHEN REFER?

- To date, no data suggests that early palliative care causes harm. In fact, early palliative care integration leads to improved symptom management, higher likelihood of patient goal-directed care, and higher the cost savings.
- Ideally, palliative care teams work collaboratively with pain specialists to assist one another with patients in need of both services. Effective palliation requires appropriate referrals and collaboration among palliative care and pain anesthesia teams.

UNIQUE MEDICAL SCENARIOS CHARACTERISTIC OF HOSPICE AND PALLIATIVE CARE

TERMINAL DELIRIUM

- Delirium is characterized by an acute onset, inattention, an altered level of consciousness, and cognitive impairment. Terminal delirium is delirium in the setting of physical signs of the dying process (hypotension, low urine output, or mottling of the skin of the extremities).
- Terminal delirium occurs in up to 83% of patients at the end of life, and it can be highly distressing for patients and family members.
- Unlike typical delirium where neuroleptics are considered first-line therapy, terminal delirium is best treated with benzodiazepines.
- Up to 26% of patients with terminal delirium require palliative sedation. When palliative sedation is

required, benzodiazepines and barbiturates are most commonly used.

UNIQUE DRUG DELIVERY

- Many patients at the end of life are unable to swallow. As such, patients often receive medications by buccal, rectal, or parenteral routes.
- Intravenous administration of drugs in the hospice setting may be limited if registered nurses are not available. As a result, the subcutaneous route is frequently used and can be utilized safely by vocational nurses. Data regarding the routine subcutaneous administration of drugs is lacking.
- The transdermal route is also empirically used without any evidence to support its use.

WEIGHING THE RISKS AND BENEFITS OF THERAPIES

- A hospice patient's goals of care may conflict with life-prolonging therapies. In these situations, the palliative care physician balances the patient's choice, safety, and quality of life when making decisions. Examples include oral gratification in a patient with dysphagia or refusing antibiotics for treatable infections.
- Palliative care teams may have to balance the risks and benefits of a therapy, even when palliative treatments may risk significant side effects, or even death. For example, effective palliation of delirium with neuroleptics may result in a prolonged QTc interval or effective palliation of pain may result in somnolence.
- Palliative care teams are responsible for educating patients, family members, and colleagues about the risks and benefits of treatments they prescribe, and communicating with them about how these treatments correspond with their goals of care.

WHY SHOULD ANESTHESIOLOGISTS CHOOSE PALLIATIVE CARE TRAINING?

- There exists a paucity of Hospice and Palliative Medicine–trained anesthesiologists. However, this training combination makes sense as anesthesiologists receive unparalleled education and training in analgesic, sedative, and infusion pharmacology and titration, and this experience and knowledge is often necessary in palliative care. In addition, anesthesiologists use medications such as propofol, ketamine, lidocaine, dexmedetomidine, and methadone regularly, all of which may be used with the patient who has palliative care needs.

- Anesthesiologists are skilled and comfortable caring for critically ill patients, as palliative patients often are.
- Anesthesiologists are also experts in procedural interventions for pain management, often overlooked by their family medicine and internal medicine colleagues. For those who do not complete a pain medicine fellowship, procedures such as epidural infusions of local anesthetics, intrathecal catheters utilizing a variety of agents, and visceral and peripheral nerve blocks and catheters can benefit select palliative care patients. For those dual trained in palliative care and pain anesthesia, the range of effective palliative procedures is even greater.
- Palliative care teams are consulted to assist with time-limited trials of respite and palliative sedation. Sedation may be utilized to provide relief from severely distressing symptoms, either until a new treatment plan can be started or titrated appropriately (respite sedation), or until the end of life (palliative sedation). In these situations, anesthesiologists with their expertise in sedation pharmacology, especially in relation to the use of propofol, dexmedetomidine, ketamine, and midazolam infusions, are particularly skilled.
- Palliative care teams are regularly called to assist with compassionate extubations. Facilitating communication between these patients, their family members, and the medical teams is a common task for palliative care providers. Ensuring that compassionate extubations are executed in a dignified and peaceful way is critically important. Based on their experience with airway management, anesthesiologists are ideally suited to manage compassionate extubations.

HOSPICE AND PALLIATIVE MEDICINE TRAINING

- In 2006, Hospice and Palliative Medicine was officially recognized by the American Board of Medical Specialties as a subspecialty. In 2012, there were 78 ACGME-recognized Hospice and Palliative Medicine one-year fellowship programs in the United States, from which approximately 140 fellows graduate each year.
- The American Board of Anesthesiology cosponsored fellowship training in Hospice and Palliative Medicine in 2006. The first examination was offered in 2008, and "grandfathering" into the subspecialty, without taking the board examination, ended in 2012. As of March 2013, there were 111 certified Hospice and Palliative Medicine trained Anesthesiologists in the United States.
- Currently, Hospice and Palliative Medicine certification is the only subspecialty approved by 10 accreditation boards: the American Board of Anesthesiology, the American Board of Internal Medicine, the American

Board of Emergency Medicine, the American Board of Family Medicine, the American Board of Obstetrics and Gynecology, the American Board of Pediatrics, the American Board of Physical Medicine and Rehabilitation, the American Board of Psychiatry and Neurology, the American Board of Radiology, and the American Board of Surgery (Table 70-2; Figure 70-2).

TABLE 70-2 Starting Doses of Commonly Used Palliative Medicine Drugs

CATEGORY	DRUG NAME	RECOMMENDED STARTING DOSE
Opioids	Fentanyl	25–75 mcg q 15 min IV PRN, 25 mcg TD q 72 h, or lozenge 200 mcg q 1 h
	Hydrocodone	1–2 tabs q 4 h PO PRN
	Hydromorphone	1–4 mg q 1 h PO PRN, 0.5-1 mg q 15 min IV PRN
	Loperamide	4 mg PO, then 2 mg PO after each loose stool
	Methadone	5 mg PO q 8 h
	Morphine	2.5–10 mg q 1 h PO PRN, 4–10 mg q 15 min IV PRN
	Oxycodone	IR: 5 mg q 1 h PO PRN
	Tramadol	50–100 mg q 6 h PO PRN
Anxiolytics	Alprazolam	0.25 mg PO BID
	Clonazepam	0.25 mg PO q 8–12 h
	Diazepam	2–10 mg PO q 6–8 h
	Lorazepam	0.5–1 mg PO or IV q 6–8 h
	Midazolam	0.2 mg/kg loading dose, divided into 2 doses given q 30 min PRN, continuous infusion is 25% of required loading dose per hour
Neuroleptics	Chlorpromazine	25–100 mg q 6–12 h PO or IV
	Haloperidol	0.5–5 mg q 4–6 h PO or IV
	Olanzapine	2.5 mg daily PO
	Quetiapine	25 mg BID PO
	Risperidone	0.5 mg BID PO
Steroids	Dexamethasone	1–20 mg daily PO or IV
	Prednisone	5–80 mg daily PO
Dopamine antagonists	Metaclopramide	10–20 mg q 6 h PO or IV
	Prochlorperazine	10–20 mg q 6 h PO
	Promethazine	25 mg q 6 h PO
Acetylcholine antagonists	Atropine	0.4–0.6 mg q 3–4 h IV
	Diphenoxylate/ Atropine	2 tabs q 6 h PO
	Glycopyrrolate	0.1–0.4 mg q 4–6 h IV
	Scopolamine patch	1–3 patches q 72 h
	Scopolamine	0.1–0.4 mg q 4 h IV
Histamine antagonists	Diphenhydramine	25–50 mg daily PO

(Continued)

TABLE 70-2   Starting Doses of Commonly Used Palliative Medicine Drugs *(Continued)*

CATEGORY	DRUG NAME	RECOMMENDED STARTING DOSE
	Meclizine	25--50 mg q 6 h PO
	Hydroxyzine	25–50 mg q 6 h PO
Serotonin antagonists	Ondansetron	4–8 mg q 8 h PO or IV
	Granisetron	1 mg daily or BID PO
Somatostatin analogue	Octreotide	100–400 mcg q 8 h SC
Antacids	Cimetidine	300 mg daily or QAC or 400–600 mg q 12 h PO
	Famotidine	20–40 mg daily PO or IV
	Lansoprazole	15–30 mg daily PO
	Omeprazole	20–40 mg daily PO
	Ranitidine	150–300 mg daily PO
	Sucralfate	1 g QAC and QHS PO
Stool softeners	Sodium docusate	250 mg daily PO
Fiber	Psyllium	1 tsp TID PO
	Methylcellulose	1 Tbp TID PO
Stimulant laxatives	Senna	1 tab daily PO
	Bisacodyl	1 tab daily PO or 10 mg daily PR
Osmotic laxatives	Lactulose	15–60 mL BID to TID PO
	Polyethylene glycol	17 g daily PO
	Magnesium hydroxide	15–30 mL daily to TID PO
Enema	Sodium phosphate	120 mL PR
	Tap water or saline	500–1000 mL PR
	Mineral oil	30–60 mL PR
Opioid antagonist	Methylnaltrexone	8 mg QOD SC if < 136 lbs, 12 mg QOD SC if > 136 lbs
Prokinetic agent	Erythromycin	150 mg q 6 h PO
Antidepressants	Amitriptyline	10–25 mg QHS PO
	Bupropion	100 mg BID PO
	Citalopram	20 mg daily PO
	Desipramine	10–25 mg daily PO
	Escitalopram	10 mg daily PO
	Fluoxetine	20 mg Qam PO
	Ketamine	0.5 mg/kg QHS PO
	Mirtazapine	15 mg QHS PO
	Nortriptyline	10–25 mg QHS PO
	Paroxetine	20 mg Qam PO
	Sertraline	50 mg QHS PO
	Trazodone	50 mg QHS PO
	Venlafaxine	37.5 mg BID PO
Sleep agent	Melatonin	1–10 mg 45–60 min before sleep PO
Appetite stimulants	Megestrol acetate	400 mg daily PO
	Dronabinol	2.5 mg BID PO
Stimulant	Methylphenidate	5 mg at 0800 and noon PO
Mucositis mixes	Ketamine	20 mg in 2–3 mL cherry syrup, swish and spit q 3 h PRN
	Morphine	0.2% solution, swish and spit q 3 h PRN
	Diphenhydramine/ 2% viscous xylocaine/Maalox	1:1:1, swish and spit q 3 h PRN

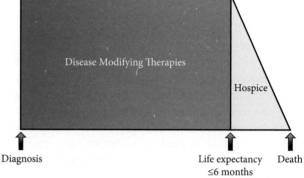

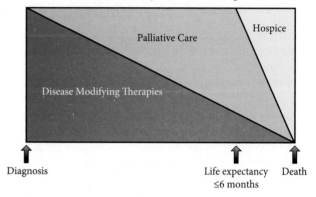

FIG. 70-2. The old and new models of palliative care and hospice integration in illness.

BIBLIOGRAPHY

Braiteh F, El Osta B, Palmer L, et al. Characteristics, findings, and outcomes of palliative care consultations at a comprehensive cancer center. *J Pall Med.* 2007;10:948–955.

Bruera E, Hui D. Palliative care research: lessons learned by our team over the last 25 years. *Pall Med J.* 2013;0:1–13.

Casarett DJ, Inouye SK. Diagnosis and management of delirium near the end of life. *Ann Intern Med.* 2001;135:32–40.

Fine PG. The evolving and important role of anesthesiology in palliative care. *Anesth Analg.* 2005;100:183–188.

Merskey H, Bogduk N. "Part III: Pain Terms, A Current List with Definitions and Notes on Usage". *Classification of Chronic Pain.* 2nd ed. Seattle, Wa: IASP Task Force on Taxonomy, IASP Press; 1994:209–214.

Morrison RS, Penrod JD, Cassel B, et al. Cost savings associated with US hospital palliative care consultation programs. *Arch Intern Med.* 2008;168(16):1783–1790.

Poulose JV, Do YK, Neo PS. Association between referral-to-death interval and location of death of patients referred to a hospital-based specialist palliative care service. *J Pain Symptom Manage.* 2012.

Roeland E, Mitchell W, Elia G, et al. Symptom control in stem cell transplantation: a multidisciplinary palliative care team approach. Part 1: physical symptoms. *J Supp Onc.* 2010;8:100–116.

Smith TJ, Temin S, Alesi ER, et al. American Society of Clinical Oncology Provisional Clinical Opinion: the integration of palliative care into standard oncology care. *J Clin Oncol.* 2012;30(8):880–887.

Temel JS, Greer JA, Muzikansky A, et al. Early palliative care for patients with metastatic non-small-cell lung cancer. *N Engl J Med.* 2010;363(8):733–742.

Wu P. *Palliative Medicine Pocket Companion.* 2nd ed. The Institute for Palliative Medicine at San Diego Hospice, 2012.

71 REGENERATIVE INJECTION THERAPY aka PROLOTHERAPY

Felix Linetsky, MD

Michael Stanton-Hicks, MB, BS

Lloyd Saberski, MD

INTRODUCTION

- Regenerative injection therapy (RIT), also known as prolotherapy or sclerotherapy, is an interventional technique for the treatment of chronic musculoskeletal pain caused by connective tissue diathesis.
- This technique originated in the United States in the mid-1840s for the treatment of hernias.
- RIT became popular in the treatment of musculoskeletal pathology in the 1930s.
- Since then, the scope of applications has expanded gradually.
- It has been proposed recently that pain reduction after RIT is due to chemomodulation or temporary neurolytic action of the injectate. The literature suggests that dextrose/lidocaine or dextrose/glycerin/phenol/lidocaine solutions have a more prolonged pain-relieving action compared with that of lidocaine alone. More so, an injection of sclerosing polidocanol reverses neurovascular ingrowth in painful tendinosis.

CLINICAL ANATOMY

- According to Willard, the connective tissue complex in the cervical, thoracic, and lumbar areas incorporates various ligaments and paravertebral fasciae to form a continuous connective tissue stocking surrounding, interconnecting, and supporting various soft tissue, vertebral, neurovascular, and osseous structures. This arrangement provides bracing and

hydraulic amplification effect to the musculature, enhancing its strength by up to 30%.
- The anterior compartment contains the paravertebral fascia muscles, vertebral bodies, intervertebral disc, and anterior and posterior longitudinal ligaments. The middle compartment includes the contents of the spinal canal. The posterior compartment begins medially at the ventral aspect of z-joint capsules and laterally at the posterolateral aspects of the transverse processes and converges at the apices of the spinous processes.
- Movements of the cranium and spine are accomplished through various types of joints. These include:
  - *Syndesmoses*, that is, anterior longitudinal ligament, posterior longitudinal ligament, transverse apical and alar ligaments, anterior atlanto-occipital membrane, posterior atlanto-occipital membrane, ligamentum flavum, interspinous ligaments, and supraspinous ligaments.
  - *Synovial*, that is, atlanto-axial, atlanto-occipital, zygapophyseal, costotransverse, and costovertebral joints.
  - *Symphysis*, for example, intervertebral discs.
  - *Combined*, for example, sacroiliac joint, which is a synovial/syndesmotic articulation.
- Connective tissues receive segmental innervation from the respective ventral and dorsal rami.
  - Dorsal rami usually divide into medial and lateral branches (except the first cervical, fifth lumbar, fourth and fifth sacral, and coccygeal that form only a medial branch).
  - Medial branches of the dorsal rami (MBDR) innervate z-joints, multifidus muscles, interspinous muscles and ligaments, and supraspinous ligaments.
  - Free nerve endings and Pacini and Ruffini corpuscles have been identified in superficial layers of all ligaments, including supraspinous and interspinous, with a sharp increase in their quantity at the attachment to the spinous processes (enthesis), rendering them a source of nociception equal to that of z-joint capsules.
  - In comparison, the vascular supply is much less abundant in normal connective tissue this is essential for proper homeostasis. Conversely in the internal disc disruptions, tendinosis, and osteoarthritis, the neurovascular ingrowth is well documented.
- Pain arising from affected connective tissue such as ligaments and tendons may mimic any referral pain patterns known.
  - Original patterns of referral pain from interspinous syndesmotic joints, that is, interspinous ligaments, were published by Kellgren in 1939 and were subsequently confirmed in the 1950s by Feinstein and Hackett.

○ Pain patterns from cervical synovial articulations were brought to light by Aprill, Dwyer, and Bogduk in 1990; these were expanded to include upper cervical and thoracic articulations by Dreyfus in 1994.

○ Also in 1994, Dussault described z-joint pain patterns in the cervical and lumbar areas, and Fortin described pain patterns from the sacroiliac joints.

○ The size of this chapter precludes reproduction and comparison of these pain maps, which was published recently. There is a significant overlap between pain patterns from the synovial, syndesmotic, and symphysial joints, which is due to a common segmental innervation.

PATHOPHYSIOLOGY

- Connective tissues are bradytrophic; their regenerative capabilities are much slower than those of any other tissue.
- The natural healing process consists of three overlapping phases: inflammation, granulation with fibroplasia, followed by contraction with remodeling.
- Connective tissue response to trauma varies with the degree of injury.
  ○ In the presence of cellular damage, regenerative response takes place.
  ○ In the presence of damage to the extracellular matrix, a combined regenerative, reparative response takes place.
- Cell replication in combined regenerative, reparative processes is controlled by chemical and growth factors.
- Natural healing, in the best circumstances, may restore connective tissue to its preinjury length but only to 50%–75% preinjury tensile strength.
- The most frequent degenerative changes in ligaments and tendons are hypoxic, followed by lipoid, mucoid, and calcific degeneration. A combination of all of these has been observed.
- Modulation of regenerative and degenerative pathways remains a therapeutic challenge, and application of nonsteroidal anti-inflammatory drugs (NSAIDs) and steroids is of limited value.
- Experimental studies have demonstrated that repeated injections of 5% sodium morrhuate at the fibroosseous attachments (entheses) increased strength of the bone ligament junction by 28%, ligament mass by 44%, and thickness by 27% in comparison to saline controls.
- More recent studies proved reduction of pain hyperplasia and hypertrophy in tendinosis after sclerosing injections of neovessels.

INDICATIONS FOR RIT

- Discogenic low back pain.
- Enthesopathy: a painful degenerative pathologic process that results in deposition of poorly organized tissue, degeneration, and tendinosis at the fibroosseous interface, and transition toward loss of function. (*Note*: Enthesis is the zone of insertion of ligament, tendon, or articular capsule to bone. The outer layers of the annulus represent a typical enthesis.)
- Tendinosis/ligamentosis: a focal area of degenerative changes due to failure of the cell matrix adaptation to excessive load and tissue hypoxia often accompanied with a neurovascular ingrowth and thickening of the tendons with a strong tendency toward chronic pain and dysfunction.
- Pathologic ligament laxity: a posttraumatic or congenital condition leading to painful hypermobility of the axial and peripheral joints.
- Chronic pain from ligaments or tendons secondary to repetitive or occupational sprains or strains, such as "repetitive motion disorder."
- Chronic postural cervical, thoracic, lumbar, and lumbosacral pain.
- Lumbar and thoracic vertebral compression fractures with a wedge deformity that exert additional stress on the posterior ligamento tendinous complex.
- Recurrent painful subluxations of the ribs at costotransverse, costovertebral, and/or costosternal articulations.
- Osteoarthritis, spondylosis, spondylolysis, and spondylolisthesis.
- Painful cervical, thoracic, lumbar, lumbosacral, and sacroiliac instability.

SYNDROMES AND DIAGNOSTIC ENTITIES TREATED WITH RIT

- Cervicocranial syndrome: cervicogenic headaches, secondary to ligament sprain and laxity, atlanto-axial and atlanto-occipital joint sprains, and midcervical zygapophyseal joint sprains
- Temporomandibular pain and muscle dysfunction syndrome
- Barre–Lieou syndrome
- Torticollis
- Cervical disc syndrome without myelopathy
- Cervicobrachial syndrome (shoulder/neck pain)
- Hyperextension/hyperflexion injury syndromes
- Cervical, thoracic, and lumbar zygapophyseal syndromes
- Cervical, thoracic, and lumbar sprain/strain syndrome
- Costotransverse joint pain

- Costovertebral arthrosis/dysfunction
- Slipping rib syndrome
- Sternoclavicular arthrosis and repetitive sprain
- Tietze's syndrome/costochondritis/chondrosis
- Costosternal arthrosis
- Xiphoidalgia syndrome
- Acromioclavicular sprain/arthrosis
- Scapulothoracic crepitus
- Iliocostal friction syndrome
- Iliac crest syndrome
- Iliolumbar syndrome
- Painful lumbar disc syndrome
- Interspinous pseudoarthrosis (Baastrup's disease)
- Lumbar instability
- Lumbar ligament sprain
- Spondylolysis
- Sacroiliac joint pain, subluxation, instability, and arthrosis
- Sacrococcygeal joint pain; coccydynia
- Gluteal tendinosis with or without concomitant bursitis
- Myofascial pain syndromes
- Ehlers–Danlos syndrome
- Ankylosing spondylitis (Marie–Strümpell disease)
- Failed back syndrome
- Fibromyalgia syndrome
- Laxity of ligaments
- Patellar, Achilles, trochanteric, rotator cuff, and elbow tendinosis

CONTRAINDICATIONS TO RIT

- Allergy to proliferant or anesthetic solutions or their components, for example, phenol, dextrose, or sodium morrhuate.
- Acute nonreduced subluxations or dislocations, arthritis, bursitis, or tendinitis (septic, gouty, rheumatoid, or posttraumatic).
- Recent onset of a progressive neurologic deficit involving the segment to be injected, including but not limited to severe intractable cephalgia, unilaterally dilated pupil, bladder dysfunction, and bowel incontinence.
- Request for a large quantity of narcotics before and after treatment.
- Neoplastic or septic inflammatory lesions involving osseous structures.
- Lack of improvement after infiltration of the putative nociceptive structure with a local anesthetic or severe exacerbation of pain.
- Febrile disorder or acute medical/surgical conditions that render a patient's status unstable.

COMMONLY USED SOLUTIONS

Five types of injectates are currently used for RIT and they are:

- Osmotic shock agents such as hypertonic dextrose, glycerin, or distilled water.
  - The most common solution is commercially available lidocaine and 50% dextrose. For example, 3 mL of 1% lidocaine mixed with 3 mL of 50% produces a hyperosmolar lidocaine solution with 25% dextrose (Table 71-1).
- Chemotactic sclerosing agents such as sodium morrhuate, Sotradecol, or polidocanol.
- Chemical irritants such as phenol, Sarapin, 5% Tetra-cycline.
  - A diluted 1:4, 6% phenol in 50% glycerin solution was used at donor harvest sites at the iliac crest for neurolytic and pain controlling responses.
- Dextrose/phenol/glycerin (DPG or P2G) solution consists of 25% dextrose, 2.5% phenol, and 25% glycerin. Dilutions with a local anesthetic are presented in Table 71-1.
- Particulates such as pumice suspension.

BIOLOGIC AGENTS

- Whole blood, Platelet Rich (PRP), and Poor Plasma (PPP), Autologous Conditioned Serum (ACS), Adipose and Bone Marrow Aspirates Mesenchymal Stem Cells (MSC), fresh harvested and culture expanded.
- Human Growth Hormone (HGH), Testosterone (water soluble).

TABLE 71-1 Dilutions of Injectates with Neurolytic Properties and their Osmolarities

50% dextrose diluted with local anesthetic makes the following "PROLIFERATING" CONCENTRATIONS:
1:4 proportion 10% dextrose = 555 mOsm/L.
1:3 proportion 12.5% dextrose = 694 mOsm/L.
2:1 proportion 16.5% dextrose = 916 mOsm/L.

NEUROLYTIC CONCERNTRATIONS:
3:2 proportion 20% dextrose = 1110 mOsm/L.
1:1 proportion 25% dextrose = 1388 mOsm/L.
Dextrose / phenol / glycerin (DPG):
25% dextrose, 25% glycerin, 2.5% phenol.

ALL DILUTIONS NEUROLYTIC:
1:3 proportion = 1026 mOsm/L; phenol 0.62%
1:2 proportion = 1368 mOsm/L; phenol 0.83%
2:3 proportion = 1641 mOsm/L; phenol 0.5%
1:1 proportion = 2052 mOsm/L; phenol 1.25%

Almost all of the injectates produce irritation and an inflammatory stage after injection. Any solution with osmolality greater than a 1000 mOsm/L is potentially neurolytic (see Table 71-1).

MECHANISM OF ACTION

- The RIT mechanism of action is complex and multifaceted. The three most important components are:
  - Chemomodulation of collagen through inflammatory proliferative, regenerative/reparative responses is induced by the chemical and biologic properties of the injectates and mediated by cytokines and multiple growth factors.
  - Chemoneuromodulation of peripheral nociceptors provides stabilization of antidromic, orthodromic, sympathetic, and axon reflex transmissions. The literature suggests that a dextrose/lidocaine or glycerin/phenol/lidocaine combination has a much more prolonged action than lidocaine alone.
  - Modulation of local peritendinous hemodynamics with sclerosants changes the intratendinous blood flow, reverses neurovascular ingrowth, pain, and tendinosis with return of tendons to normal size and loading activity.

TECHNICAL CONSIDERATIONS

- Any innervated tissue or structure may contain nociceptors. To confirm nociceptive involvement, the structure proper or its nerve supply is injected with a local anesthetic and an analgesic response is assessed.
- For RIT purposes, tissue pain generators are identified by local tenderness and are confirmed by needling and local anesthetic blocks of the tissue bed, taking its nerve supply into account.
- In experienced hands, using palpable landmarks for guidance, the following posterior column elements innervated by the dorsal rami may be safely injected without fluoroscopic guidance: spinous process, supraspinous and interspinous ligaments, lamina, posterior zygapophyseal joint capsule, transverse process, and cervicodorsal fascia, as well as posterior sacroiliac, sacrotuberous, and sacrospinous ligaments and posterior sacrococcygeal ligaments.
- The dextrose/lidocaine solution is an effective diagnostic and therapeutic tool for pain arising from posterior column elements when used in increments of 0.5–1.0 mL injected at each bone contact in the following sequence:

- In the presence of midline pain and tenderness, the interspinous ligaments are blocked initially in the midline.
- If tenderness remains at the lateral aspects of the spinous processes, injections are carried out to the lateral aspects of the apices of the spinous processes, thus blocking off the terminal filaments of the MBDR of the dorsal rami.
- Persistence of paramedial pain dictates blocks of the facet joint capsules, costotransverse joints, sacroiliac ligaments, and apices of transverse processes in the lumbar region and the posterior tubercle of the transverse processes in the cervical region with their respective tendon insertions.
- Perseverance of lateral tenderness dictates investigation of the structures innervated by the lateral branches of the dorsal rami, that is, iliocostalis tendon insertions to the ribs.
- In this fashion, all potential nociceptors on the course of MBDR are investigated from the periphery to the center. Using the above-described sequence, the practitioner is able to make a differential diagnosis of pain arising from vertebral and paravertebral structures innervated by MBDR and lateral branches of the dorsal rami. (See Figures 71-1 and 71-2.)
- Pain from pathology of the upper cervical synovial joints presents a diagnostic and, more so, a therapeutic challenge. Because of the previously mentioned overlaps of pain patterns, it is usually a diagnosis of exclusion.
- Regarding therapeutic intervention, radiofrequency (RF) lesions and corticosteroid injections do not always produce the desired therapeutic value in upper cervical synovial joint pain.
  - Intra-articular atlanto-axial and atlanto-occipital joint injections of 6% phenol have secured a long-lasting therapeutic effect in selected patients.
  - Intra-articular injections of 25% dextrose into the above-mentioned joints, as well as into midcervical synovial joints, were reported to relieve persistent pain after RF and capsular injection failure.
- Painful lumbar disc syndrome also remains a therapeutic challenge.
  - Original studies in the 1950s advocated injection of irritating solutions into the lumbar intervertebral disc. Chemonucleoannuloplasty was revisited in the last decade by the enthusiastic work of Klein et al.
  - They reported significant pain improvement and return-to-work ratio after intradiscal injections of 25% dextrose mixed with chondroitin sulfate and glucosamine. The pilot group consisted of 30 patients with up to 2 years' follow-up. These patients have

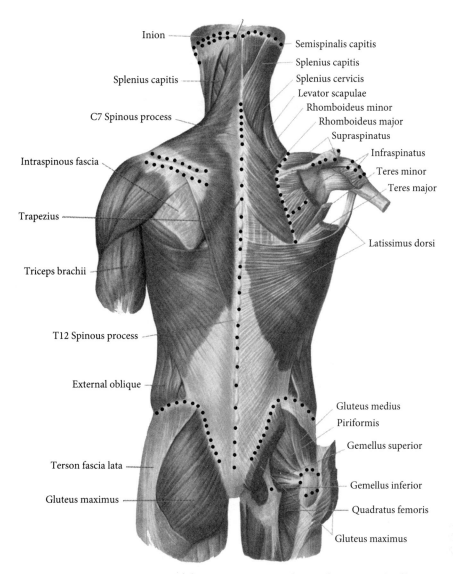

FIG. 71-1. Dots represent some of the most common enthesopathy areas at the fibroosseous insertions (enthesis) in the occiput, humerus, trochanter, iliac crest, and spinous processes. Dots also represent the most common location of needle insertions during RIT. (Please note: not all of the locations must be treated in each patient.) Dotted vertebral and paravertebral structures are innervated by their respective medial and lateral branches of the dorsal rami. From Sinelnicov. *Atlas of Anatomy*. Vol. 1. Meditsina, Moskow; 1972. Modified and prepared for publication by Tracey James.

failed previous conservative care, laminectomies, fusions at adjacent levels, or intradiscal electrothermal annuloplasty (IDET).

○ Thirty patients were reported to have a significant pain improvement and return-to-work ratio after lumbar intradiscal injection of a mixed solution containing dextrose, chondroitin sulfate, and glucosamine chloride. These patients had failed previous conservative care, laminectomies, fusions at adjacent levels, or IDET.

• Pennsylvania researchers received and reported good results with lumbar intradiscal injections of 25% dextrose for treatment of painful mechanical and chemical discopathy, suggesting that 25% dextrose may provide an immediate and long-lasting neurolytic action.

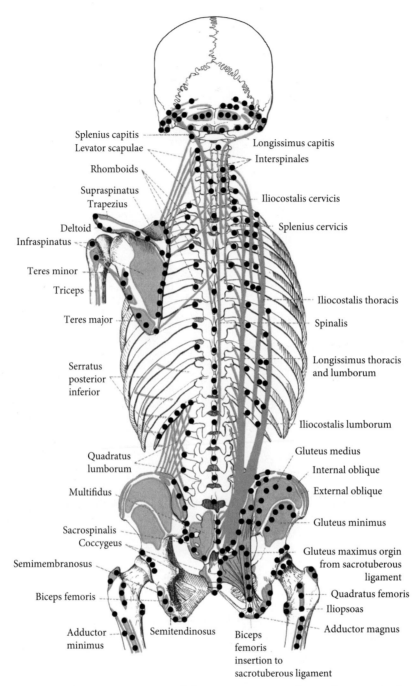

FIG. 71-2. Dots represent some of the most common enthesopathy areas in the fibroosseous insertions of ligaments and tendons (enthesis) at the occiput, humerus, trochanter, iliac crest, and spine, ichial tuberosity, sacrum, and spinous processes. Dots also represent the most common location of needle insertions and infiltrations during RIT. (Please note: not all of the locations must be treated in each patient.) Dotted vertebral and paravertebral structures are innervated by their respective medial and lateral branches of the dorsal rami. From Sinelnicov. *Atlas of Anatomy*. Vol. 1, Meditsina, Moskow; 1972. Modified and prepared for publication by Tracey James.

CONCLUSION

- RIT/prolotherapy is a valuable method of treatment for correctly diagnosed chronic painful conditions of the musculoskeletal systems.

- Thorough familiarity of the physician with clinical anatomy and pathophysiology, as well as anatomic variations, is necessary to use this technique effectively.
- Manipulation under local joint anesthesia and a series of local anesthetic blocks for diagnosis of somatic

pain are other commonly used options in conjunction with RIT.

- RIT in an ambulatory setting is an acceptable standard of care in the community.
- Recent literature reports that NSAIDs and steroid preparations have limited usage in degenerative painful conditions of ligaments and tendons or chronic painful overuse injuries. Regenerative injections and proper rehabilitation up to six months or a year supported with acetaminophen and opioid analgesics may be more appropriate.
- Preceptorships are available through the American Academy of Regenerative Orthopedic Medicine (AAROM), www.AAROM.org, Tel: (727) 787 5555.

BIBLIOGRAPHY

Aprill C, Dwyer A, Bogduk N. Cervical zygapophyseal joint pain patterns II: a clinical evaluation. *Spine.* 1990;15(6):458–461.

Ashton I, Ashton A, Gibson S, et al. Morphological basis for back pain: the demonstration of nerve fibers and neuropeptides in the lumbar facet joint capsule but not in ligamentum flavum. *J Orthop Res.* 1992;10:72–78.

Best T. Basic science of soft tissue. In: Delee J, Drez D, eds. *Orthopedic Sports Medicine Principles and Practice.* Vol 1. Philadelphia, Pa.: WB Saunders; 1994:7–53.

Bogduk N. *Clinical Anatomy of the Lumbar Spine and Sacrum.* 3rd ed. London: Churchill Livingstone; 1997.

Dreyfuss P, Tibiletti C, Dreyer SJ. Thoracic zygapophyseal joint pain pattern: a study in normal volunteers. *Spine.* 1994;19:807–811.

Dussault R, Kaplan PA, Reeves KD. Facet joint injection: diagnosis and therapy. *Appl. Radiol.* 1994;35–39.

Gray's Anatomy. 38th British ed. Edinburgh: Churchill Livingstone, Pearson Professional Limited; 1995.

Gedney EH. Use of sclerosing solution may change therapy in vertebral disk problem. *The Osteopathic Profession.* 1952, April;34(38, 39):1113.

Hackett G, Hemwall GA, Montgomery GA. *Ligament and Tendon Relaxation—Treated by Prolotherapy.* 5th ed. Springfield, Il.: Charles C Thomas; 1991.

Jozsa L, Kannus P. Human tendons, anatomy, physiology and pathology. In: *Human Kinetics.* Champaign, Il.: 1997.

Klein RG, Derby R, O'Neill C, et al. Biochemical injection treatment for discogenic low back pain: a pilot study. *Spine.* 2003;3:220–226.

Klein R, Dorman TA, Johnson CE. Proliferant injections for low back pain: histologic changes of injected ligaments & objective measurements of lumbar spine mobility before and after treatment. *J Neurol Orthop Med Surg.* 1989;10:2.

Kon E, Filardo G, Delcogliano M, et al. Platelet-rich plasma: new clinical application: a pilot study for treatment of jumper's knee. *Injury.* 2009, June;40(6):598–603. Epub 2009 Apr 19.

Leadbetter WB. Cell-matrix response in tendon injury. *Clin Sports Med.* 1992;11:533–578.

Linetsky FS, Botwin K, Gorfine L, et al. Position paper of the Florida Academy of Pain Medicine on regenerative injection therapy: effectiveness and appropriate usage. *Pain Clin.* 2002; 4(3):38–45.

Linetsky F, Alfredson H, Crane D, et al. Treatment of chronic painful musculoskeletal injuries and disease with regenerative injection therapy (RIT): regenerative injection therapy principles and practice (Chapter 81). In: Deer TR, editor-in-chief. *Comprehensive Treatment of Chronic Pain by Medical Intervention, and Integrative Approaches; The Textbook on Patient Management.* American Academy of Pain Medicine/Springer Science + Business Media (www.springer.com); 2013:889–913.

Linetskyx F, Derbyx R., Miguelx R, Saberskix L, Stanton-Hicksx M. Pain management with regenerative injection therapy (RIT) (Chapter 62). In: Boswell M, Eliot Cole B, eds. *Weiner's Pain Management: A Practical Guide for Clinicians.* 7th ed. Boca Raton, Fl.: CRC Press; 2006:939–966.

Linetsky F, Mikulinsky A, Gorfine L. Regenerative injection therapy: history of application in pain management. Part I. 1930s–1950s. *Pain Clin.* 2000;2(2):8–13.

Linetsky F, Saberski L, Miguel R, Snyder A. A history of the applications of regenerative injection therapy in pain management. Part II. 1960s–1980s. *Pain Clin.* 2001;3:32–36.

Liu Y, Tipton CM, Matthes RD, et al. An in situ study of the influence of a sclerosing solution in rabbit medial collateral ligaments and its junction strength. *Connect Tissue Res.* 1983;11:95–102.

Miller MR, Mathews RS, Reeves KD. Treatment of painful advanced internal lumbar disc derangement with intradiscal injection of hypertonic dextrose. *Pain Physician.* 2006 Apr;9(2):115–121.

Ongley MJ, Klein RG, Dorman TA, et al. A new approach to the treatment of chronic low back pain. *Lancet.* 1987;143–146.

Stanton-Hicks M. Cervicocranial syndrome: treatment of atlanto-occipital and atlanto-axial joint pain with phenol/glycerin injections. Paper presented at: 20th AAOM Annual Conference and Scientific Seminar: A commonsense approach to "hidden" pain generators; 2003; Orlando, Fl.

72 REHABILITATION EVALUATION AND TREATMENT IN PATIENTS WITH LOW BACK PAIN

Carmen M. Quinones, MD
Juan Carlos Robles, MD

LUMBAR ANATOMY

LUMBAR VERTEBRA

- Most patients have five lumbar vertebrae. The sacrum is composed of five vertebrae fused together and the coccyx of three or four rudimentary vertebrae.
- Vertebral Body—spongy bone covered by thin layer of hyaline cartilage, wedge-shaped with greater height anteriorly.

- Pedicles—They form the roots of the vertebral arch. Posteriorly, they connect to the laminae and they have a deep inferior and a less pronounced superior vertebral notch. On successive vertebrae, these two notches form the intervertebral foramen where the spinal nerve makes its exit.
- Lamina—The height of each lamina is less than that of the body so that a considerable space exists between adjacent laminae. Lumbar flexion widens the spaces between laminae.
- Transverse process—project laterally from the point of union of pedicle and lamina for attachment of muscles.
- Spinous process—midline posterior projections from the laminae for attachment of muscles.
- Joints—There are two types of joints in the lumbar spine: synovial, formed by the opposition of the articular processes, and cartilaginous, formed by the union of intervertebral discs with the bodies.
- Facet joint—diarthrodial articulations—They are paired in both sides of the spine and represent the junction of superior articulating process (SAP) (concave, posteromedially) and inferior articular process of the vertebra (smaller, anterolaterally). The SAP in the upper lumbar has sagittal orientation and in the lower lumbar it has a coronal orientation.
  - The facet joint forms the posterior aspect of the neural foramen.
  - The capsule is lined by a synovial membrane. It encloses a space with a maximal volume capacity of 1–2 mL of synovial fluid.
  - The ventromedial aspect is contiguous with the ligamentum flavum. The adipose tissue overlying the ligamentum flavum in the superior aspect of the facet joint is intimately related to the neural root sleeve → can produce pain down the leg.

LIGAMENTS

- Supraspinous—It stretches across the tips of the spinous processes.
- Interspinous—It is localized between the spinous process.
- Ligamentum flavum—It is a paired ligaments that connect the adjacent laminae. Laterally it blends with the capsule of the synovial joints.
- Anterior longitudinal ligament (ALL)—extends anteriorly from the sacrum to the occipital bone of the skull, partly covering the bodies and intervertebral discs; gives support and is of great clinical importance in fractures of the column.
- Posterior longitudinal ligament (PLL)—travels along the posterior aspect of the bodies. It becomes narrow on the lumbar spine and expands over the intervertebral discs.

INTERVERTEBRAL DISCS

- Five lumbar intervertebral discs—They are responsible for approximately 25% of the total length of the vertebral column above the sacrum. They bind vertebral body together anteriorly. On the lumbar spine, they have greater thickness anteriorly contributing to the lumbar lordosis. Two portions—annulus fibrosus, which is thinner posteriorly (reason why herniations are more likely to occur posteriorly—most common herniations are posterolateral around the thin lateral edge of the PLL). The second portion of the disc is the nucleus pulposus, which is a semigelatinous mass situated slightly closer to the posterior edge of the disc. They contain a very high percentage of water, 70%-80%. They are subject to dehydration as a result of pressure placed upon them.

MUSCLES

- Posterior muscles of the back are innervated by the dorsal rami of the spinal nerves. A thick thoracolumbar fascia covers the muscles in the lumbar spine. The main function of the back muscles when one is erect is to resist gravity.
- Erector spinae—originates from the posterior surface of the sacrum, iliac crest and spinous processes of the lumbar, and last two thoracic vertebrae. It divides into the iliocostalis system (laterally), longissimus, and spinalis (medial). Its action is extension of the vertebral column and lateral flexion.
- Multifidus—It originates from the sacrum and transverse processes and inserts on the spinous processes, obliquely placed in relation to the column. Its action is to extend, rotation to the opposite side, and lateral flexion of the column. It is innervated by the dorsal rami of the spinal nerves.
- Psoas major—limb muscle with direct action upon the vertebral column; originates from the bodies and transverse processes; helps flex a partially flexed vertebral column.
- Quadratus lumborum—a posterior abdominal muscle. It attaches to the transverse processes of the lumbar spine. It is a lateral flexor.

SPINAL NERVES

- There are five lumbar, five sacral, and one coccygeal nerves.
- Thoracic and lumbar spine—Each nerve leaves the vertebral canal below the vertebra of the same number.
- Each nerve is attached to the spinal cord by a sensory dorsal root and a motor ventral root.

- Dorsal root ganglion—accumulation of cell bodies of the sensory fibers. It lies on the dorsal root at the level of the intervertebral foramen.
- The motor and sensory roots join at the distal end of the ganglion to form the mixed spinal nerve.
- The spinal nerves exit through the foramen and divide into the dorsal and ventral ramus. The dorsal turns posteriorly to supply the back muscles. The ventral goes lateral and anteriorly to form the lumbosacral plexus.
- Dorsal ramus—divides into medial, lateral, and intermediate branches.
- The medial branch supplies the lower pole of the facet joint at its own level and the upper pole of the one below.
- A branch from the posterior opening of the S1 root in the sacrum runs cephalad to supply the L5–S1 joint. The L5–S1 joint is innervated by three nerves.
- Medial branch also supplies the multifidus, interspinalis, and the intertransversarii mediales muscles, the ligaments, and periosteum of the neural arch.

SACROILIAC JOINT

- Largest axial joint in the body; the average surface area of 17.5 cm².
- Diarthrodial synovial joint—hyaline cartilage on the sacral side and fibrocartilage on the iliac side.
- Its ligamentous structure is more extensive dorsally—limits motion in all planes; also supported by a network of muscles. Functionally these muscles are connected to the sacroiliac ligaments: gluteus maximus, piriformis, and biceps femoris → their actions affect joint mobility.
- Innervation—subject of much debate. General consensus—posterior joint is innervated by lateral branches of L4–S3 dorsal rami and anterior joint is innervated by L4–S2 ventral rami.

SACROILIAC JOINT PAIN

- Fifteen to twenty-five percent of patients with axial low back pain.
- The SIJ is designed primarily for stability → main motion in males tends to be translation and in females rotation. Maximum range of motion was 1.2 degrees in men and 2.8 degrees in women.

MECHANISM OF INJURY

- Combination of axial loading and abrupt rotation.
- Intra-articular causes → arthritis and infections. Age-related changes in the sacroiliac joint (SIJ) begin in puberty. In the sixties, motion of the joint may become markedly restricted as the capsule becomes increasingly collagenous and fibrous ankylosis occurs.
- Extra-articular causes → enthesopathy, fracture, ligamentus injury, and myofascial pain. The psoas and piriformis muscle pass anteriorly to the SIJ; imbalance of these muscles may affect its function.

RISK FACTORS

- Leg length discrepancy, gait abnormalities, prolonged vigorous exercise, scoliosis, spinal fusion to the sacrum and pregnancy, and all seronegative spondyloarthropathies.

CLINICAL PRESENTATION

- Pain and tenderness over the SIJ posteriorly. Pain referral patterns—buttock, lower lumbar region, lower extremity → back of thigh, groin area, and even calf. Pain is worse with long periods of sitting or standing, turning in bed or stepping on the affected leg and walking on uneven surfaces. Maximal pain—medial buttock, 10 cm caudally and 3 cm laterally from the PSIS.

PHYSICAL EXAM

- Sensory, motor, and reflex exam should be normal.
- Evaluation of true and apparent leg length discrepancies (LLD).
- Motion tests—standing flexion test, seated flexion test, Gillet's test (see SIJ dysfunction chapter).
- Pain tests—Gaenslen's test, Patrick's test, Distraction test, Compression test.

DIAGNOSTIC STUDIES

- Plain x rays—typically reveals no abnormalities.
- Bone Scan—may demonstrate increased uptake; poor screening test.
- CT scan—found to be 57.5% sensitive and 69% specific in diagnosing SIJ pain.
- Joint Block—assumed to be the most reliable method to diagnose SI join pain.

TREATMENT

- Medications—acetaminophen or NSAID.
- Manipulative treatment to restore functional symmetry during the gait cycle.
- Pelvic stabilization exercises—single and double leg bridges, claim rotary stability exercises, side bends,

plank series (side planks), lateral hip circuits, lateral hip, and gluteal strengthening exercises.

- Core and lower extremity strengthening and postural correction exercises.
- Self-mobilization exercises—seated and standing trunk rotational exercises combined with passive elongation of the affected leg.
- Sacroiliac belts—mainly used in young hypermobile patients. Older patients are usually hypomobile.
- Correction of LLD—heel lifts or orthotics.
- Fluoroscopically guided injections are considered to be "gold standard" in diagnoses and treatment.

LUMBAR FACET JOINT SYNDROME

- Lumbar facet arthropathy—acquired, traumatic, or degenerative process that distorts the normal anatomy and function of a facet joint.
- These changes result in hyaline cartilage damage and periarticular hypertrophy.
- Intervertebral disc degeneration produces loss of segmental integrity, narrowing of the intervertebral disc space, and increasing the load on the posterior elements producing joint degeneration.
- May be the source of pain in 10%-15% of patients with chronic LBP.

CLINICAL PRESENTATION

- Pain is produced during three-dimensional movements that lock the facets → extension, side bending, and ipsilateral rotation. Pain relief is with partial lumbar flexion. If there is underlying disc disease (common) there might also be pain on flexion.
- Referral pattern for the high lumbar facet joints are more frequently observed in the lumbar area—dull ache in the paraspinal region, whereas the lower joints referred pain into the gluteal region, groin area, and posterolateral thigh in a nonradicular pattern. Due to the relation to the neural root, sleeve can produce pain down the leg. Pain rarely radiates below the knee.
- Pain is reduced in the morning and worsens as the day progresses.
- Pain increases with prolonged standing, walking, twisting, and prone-lying.

PHYSICAL EXAM

- Observation of lumbar ROM, patient's gait, movement patterns, posture—patient might walk and prefer a flex posture.
- Spinal palpation may reveal paraspinal pain and spasms of the paravertebral muscles.

- In the absence of a coexisting pathology, strength, sensation, and deep tendon reflex should be normal.
- Straight leg raise may produce low back pain.
- Pain increases with downward pressure over the lumbar region with the patient in the prone position—increasing lumbar lordosis.

DIAGNOSTIC STUDIES

- Fluoroscopically guided anesthetic intra-articular or medial branch blocks are considered "gold standard."
- Bone scan, magnetic resonance imaging (MRI), or computed tomography (CT) scans have not been shown to correlate with facet joint pain.

TREATMENT

- Local pain control with ice, oral analgesics, and NSAIDs and local peri-articular corticosteroid injections.
- Avoidance of activities that increase lordosis.
- Temporary use of lumbosacral corsets can be considered.

REHABILITATION

- Modalities to control pain, traction.
- Back school exercises—neutral spine, hamstring stretch, leg slides, curl-ups, hip rolls, spine curls, roll downs, and gluteal exercises.
- Instruction in body mechanics and posture.
- Flexibility training and articular mobilization techniques.
- Williams flexion exercises.

SPONDYLOLISTHESIS

- Forward or backward translation subluxation of the body of the superior vertebra upon the adjacent inferior vertebra.
- Seventy percent L5 on sacrum, 25% L4 on L5, and 4% above L4.
- Spondylolysis—anatomic defect that causes discontinuity in the pars interarticularis; may be unilateral or bilateral, usually asymptomatic. Weakness in the neural arch predisposes to ultimate listhesis.
- Classification:
  - I. Dysplastic—congenital abnormality of the upper sacrum or L5 arch.
  - II. Isthmic—lesion of the pars interarticularis; most common at L5–S1.

- ▪ Lytic fatigue fracture
- ▪ Elongated but intact pars
- ▪ Acute fracture
- ○ III. Degenerative—caused by degeneration and alterations in the facet joints in conjunction with degenerative changes in the intervertebral discs. It can result in narrowing of the neuroforamina and central spinal canal stenosis. Lamina and pars are intact. Most common at L4–5. Increase incidence in black women over 40 years old.
- ○ IV. Traumatic—fracture or dislocation of the facet joint.
- ○ V. Pathological—pathological destruction of facets and pars interarticularis.
- Grades—based on amount of body slippage. Grade I—up to 25%, Grade II—26%-50%, Grade III—51%-75%, Grade IV—75%.

CLINICAL PRESENTATION

- Dull low back pain. It can often radiate into the SIJ region, buttocks, and thighs. The pain is worse with standing. No specific dermatomal pattern. Pain radiating to the lower extremities can be secondary to neuroforaminal narrowing.

PHYSICAL EXAM

- A palpable ledge may be felt at the upper aspect of the listhesis.
- Segmental lordosis, which when aggravated by the examiner increases the pain.
- Limited flexibility, mainly at the hamstrings.
- A waddling gait has been described, but is not a characteristic positive sign.

DIAGNOSTIC STUDIES

- Oblique x rays can detect a defect in the pars interarticularis—absent neck in the "Scotty dog." Lateral x rays demonstrate forward translation → document the degree of slippage.
- CT Scan—most accurate means for demonstrating spondylolysis.
- MRI—helpful in evaluating possible neuroforaminal compression or central canal stenosis.

TREATMENT

- Lordosis must be decreased.
- Symptomatic children with acute spondylolysis—spinal immobilization with an antilordotic brace for

approximately six months has shown improvement in symptoms and healing of fracture.
- Adults may also benefit from a corset or brace depending on symptom severity.
- Flexion type exercises—extension exercises are contraindicated.
- Stretching exercises of lower extremities.
- Strengthening of back and abdominal oblique muscles.
- Activity modification—activities that increase lordosis should be avoided.
- Shock-absorbing shoe inserts may be indicated.
- The value of surgical intervention is questionable and is usually indicated when there is progression of neurological symptoms.

LUMBAR DEGENERATIVE DISC DISEASE

- It is the result of normal aging.
- Nutrition of disc cells is dependent on the movement of nutrients and wastes through the matrix.
- Seventy-five percent of the lumbosacral spine motion occurs at L5–S1, restriction at this segment will cause excessive motion at L4–5 and levels above, with degenerative changes of these segments enhanced from increased shear.
- Most extensive age-related changes occur in the nucleus pulposus. Proteoglycan and water concentration decrease and collagenous and noncollagenous protein concentrations increase.
- Associated with vertebral body osteophytes, sclerosis of the vertebral bodies, and facet joint osteoarthritis.
- Degenerative discs have sensory fibers that penetrate deeper into the annulus fibrosus than healthy discs making them more sensitive to pain.
- May contribute to back pain through two mechanisms: (1) loss of disc structure and mechanical properties resulting in abnormal loading of facet joints, spinal ligaments, and muscles and (2) release of mediators that may sensitize nerve endings.

CLINICAL PRESENTATION

- Might be completely asymptomatic.
- Low back pain that radiates to one or both buttocks, aggravated by bending, lifting, stooping, or twisting. Typically relieved with lying down.
- Stiffness.

PHYSICAL EXAMINATION

- Complete low back examination—flexibility, lower extremity muscle strength, and functional strength testing, sensory exam, DTRs, and evaluation of upper motor neuron signs.

DIAGNOSTIC STUDIES

- X rays—AP, lateral, flexion/extension films.
- MRI/CT scan.
- Discography—remains the only test that correlates symptoms with pathology when compared to CT scans and MRIs. Simultaneously evaluates radiographic evidence of disc degeneration and reproduction of concordant pain with injection at specific levels. May provoke pain in normal discs. May also fail to provoke pain in markedly degenerated discs—15%-25% of degenerated discs fail to elicit concordant pain.

TREATMENT

- Intermittent use of NSAIDs or other non-narcotic pain medications.
- Exercise therapy has been shown to have modest benefits in patients with subacute and chronic LBP.
- Flexibility exercises aim at improving disc nutrition.
- Traction.
- Core-strengthening, aerobic exercises.
- "McKenzie Method"—directional preference end-range flexion/extension stretches.
- Back school exercises.
- Proper body mechanics, postural control.
- In cases where there is associated spondylolisthesis, a lumbar brace might be beneficial.
- Footwear modifications to decrease impact.

LUMBAR SPINAL STENOSIS

ANATOMY

- Spinal stenosis is defined as an anatomical condition that is characterized by narrowing of the spinal canal.
- The narrowing of the spinal canal can occur at the intraspinal (central) canal, lateral recess, and/or neural foramen. The spinal stenosis could be acquired or congenital.
- Congenital spinal stenosis is present only in approximately 9% of the population. Patients may become symptomatic at ages 20–40. It is characterized by narrowing of the spinal canal in the presence of short pedicles.
- Acquired spinal stenosis is the most common type of stenosis and is usually related to degenerative changes of facet joints and disc. The degenerative process leads to a loss of disc height with associated bulging of the disc

and infolding of the ligamentum flavum. Facet osteoarthritis and hypertrophy (from the increased stresses associated with disc degeneration) often lead to osteophyte formation and thickening of the joint capsule.
- Other causes of spinal stenosis could be related to spondylolisthesis, surgery (fibrosis), Paget's disease, vertebral fracture, bone retropulsion, tumor, infection, and Tarlov cyst.

CLINICAL PRESENTATION

- The hallmark of lumbar spinal stenosis (LSS) is neurogenic claudication. This is defined as a discomfort or pain in the lower back that radiates to the buttock, groin, and/or legs. The pain is exacerbated by walking or standing and is relieved by sitting or flexion at the waist.
- Often the patient presents with limited ambulation with no difficulty riding a bicycle. The patient may also have discomfort when lying in the prone position.
- A history of back pain while the patient was standing but no pain at all when the patient was sitting had a specificity for LSS of 93% and a sensitivity of 46%.
- Unlike peripheral arterial disease, which occurs with any kind of physical exertion, neurogenic claudication may not occur during stair-climbing since it involves slight lumbar flexion.

PHYSICAL EXAMINATION

- Observe for scoliosis or any sign of spinal dysraphism. Also, observe for posture, often patient walks or stands up with flexion at the hips and knees.
- Evaluate for any hip joint pathology, greater trochanter bursitis, SIJ dysfunction, peripheral arterial disease, or peripheral neuropathy that could mimic LSS.
- Often neurological examination is normal. A sensory or motor deficit occurs in about half of patients with symptomatic lumbar stenosis; the specificity of this finding is approximately 80%. The deficit may occur bilaterally and in a polyradicular pattern. Motor findings are typically mild, and functionally limiting weakness is uncommon. A wide-based gait and/or positive Romberg in the setting of low back pain had a specificity of more than 90% for LSS.
- The patient may have a positive "stoop test." To perform this test the patient walks with an exaggerated lumbar lordosis until claudication symptoms appear or are worsened. At the point of increased symptomatology, the patient is allowed to lean forward. Reduction of symptoms is a positive response and is suggestive of neurogenic claudication.

DIAGNOSTIC STUDIES

- MRI, CT, or CT myelogram can detect the presence of spinal stenosis.
- MRI is preferred over CT myelogram since it is less invasive.

TREATMENT

- Goal of treatment is to relieve pain and improve function.
- In addition to modalities and manual therapy, a flexion-based stabilization exercise and flexibility program should be considered. Also, posture exercises to decrease lumbar lordosis may be beneficial.
- Clinical experience indicates that exercises performed during lumbar flexion, such as bicycling, are typically better tolerated than walking. Exercises that strengthen the abdominal musculature may help patients avoid excessive lumbar extension. Although there are no trial data to guide decisions about the use of lumbar corsets in patients with symptomatic spinal stenosis, corsets may help patients maintain a posture of slight lumbar flexion and are worth trying. To avoid atrophy of paraspinal muscles, the corset should be worn only for a limited number of hours per day.
- Conservative treatment with pharmacotherapy such as aspirin, NSAID, and opiates in severe cases. Gabapentin may also be helpful for paresthesias associated with lumbar stenosis.
- In acute exacerbations, lumbar epidural steroid injection may be helpful.
- Minimal invasive lumbar decompression (MILD) procedure and traditional surgical decompression could be considered when conservative treatment fails to provide pain relief.

LUMBAR RADICULOPATHY

- Radiculitis refers to inflammation of the nerve root.
- Lumbar radiculopathy refers to the compression and/ or irritation of nerve roots. It can present with a combination of pain, and sensory and motor loss.
- The most common cause of radiculopathy is disc herniation.
- More common levels of disc herniation and radiculopathies are at L4–5 and L5–S1.
- Other causes of radiculopathy could also be related to infection, malignancy, bone encroachment, or inflammation.
- The location of the disc herniation will determine the level of nerve root affected:
  - Central—may compress multiple nerve roots if affecting the cauda equina, eg, L4–5 HNP may cause S1 radiculopathy.
  - Posterolateral—may affect the nerve root below the level of the disc herniation, eg, L4–5 affects the L5 nerve root.
  - Foraminal or far lateral—may affect the nerve root at that level. Seen more often from L2 to L4 levels.

CLINICAL PRESENTATION

- Patient usually presents with pain, numbness, and weakness in the distribution of the affected nerve root.
- Clinical presentation varies according to the nerve root involved:
  - L1—rare; this radiculopathy causes pain in the inguinal region.
  - L2—pain and sensory deficit in the anterior thigh. May cause Iliopsoas weakness.
  - L3—pain in anterior and lateral thigh; quadricep weakness.
  - L4—pain and paresthesias in the medial leg, knee, and medial malleolus. L2/L3/L4 radiculopathies are more common in patient with spinal stenosis.
  - L5—most common radiculopathy of the lumbar spine. Could present with EHL weakness and pain in the buttock, lateral leg, and dorsum of the foot.
  - S1—Usually causes pain in posterior thigh and calf, plantar flexors weakness. Absence of ankle reflex can also be normal in patient above 60 years old.

PHYSICAL EXAMINATION

- Careful neurological and musculoskeletal examination. Evaluate the gait and look for any sign of weakness such as foot drop indicating a L5 radiculopathy.
- Specific maneuvers to address dural tension:
  - Straight leg raise (SLR) or Lasègue's sign—patient in supine or sitting position. The examiner raises the leg with knee straight and foot in dorsiflexion. The test is positive if patient complains of pain at 30–60 degrees. Usually positive in lower lumbosacral radiculopathies.
  - Reverse SLR—contralateral leg is raised. The test is positive if it reproduces pain in the affected side.
  - Bowstring test—Examiner performs a straight leg raise, and then the knee is flexed to release pressure. The examiner applies pressure in popliteal fossa to provoke symptoms.
  - Femoral stretch test or reverse SLR—Patient is in the prone position with knee in flexion and hip extended. Positive for higher lumbar radiculopathies, L2–4.

DIAGNOSTIC STUDIES

- MRI, CT, or CT myelogram could be helpful to identify the level affected. MRI is preferred since it can identify other spinal pathology such as tumors and vascular abnormalities. Also, MRI is safer since it does not use ionizing radiation.
- Nerve conduction studies (NCS) and electromyography (EMG) could be of high diagnostic value when imaging studies do not correlate with clinical presentation or with a patient with persistent unexplainable symptoms.

TREATMENT

- Treatment goal is to reduce inflammation and pain and to improve function.
- Patient education about radiculopathies including the causes, prognosis, proper body mechanics, and treatment. It is also very important to educate the patient about the red flags for cauda equina, malignancy, and infection.
- Medications—nonopioids analgesics: NSAID, Cox-II inhibitor, or acetaminophen.
- Systemic glucocorticoids could be considered in acute radiculopathies.
- Gabapentin is commonly used in the treatment of acute/chronic radiculopathy; however, there are limited studies to support this.
- Modification of activities that exacerbates the symptoms.
- Relative bed rest limited to 24–48 hours in the acute phase.
- Physical therapy in the first two to three weeks is not recommended since the patient may not be able to tolerate it. Also, most radiculopathies improved within the first few weeks without any specific treatment.
- Extension exercises for disc herniation—Mckenzie approach.
- Back school for pain lasting 4–12 weeks.
- Modalities such as ultrasound, electrical stimulation, heat, and cryotherapy can temporarily relieve the pain associated to soft tissue.
- Some patients may respond to lumbar traction. Typically half of the body weight is necessary in order to attempt lumbar distraction.
- Lumbar epidurals steroid injections.
- Surgical intervention should be limited to patients with progressive neurological deficit, cauda equina, or those that failed conservative treatment.
- The following factors negatively affect the outcome in the conservative management of patients with acute lumbosacral radiculopathy:
  - Constitutional symptoms
  - History of back pain
  - Progressive neurological symptoms
  - Severity of SLR limitation
  - History of illness-related work absences
  - Physically demanding work
  - Low job satisfaction
  - Presence of secondary gain issues (ie, workers' compensation)
  - Psychiatric history

THERAPEUTIC EXERCISES FOR LOW BACK PAIN

- There is no strong evidence in the benefit of exercises on acute (less than four weeks) low back as compared to conservative treatment.
- In the absence of red flags, the treatment of acute low back pain should be limited to stretching exercises and modalities such as ice or heat.
- In contrast to the limited evidence of benefit from exercise for acute LBP, exercise therapy has been shown to have modest benefits in patients with subacute (4–12 weeks) and chronic (>12 weeks) LBP.
- Williams exercises—Set of exercises that focus on lumbar flexion. The goal is to reduce pain and provide lower trunk stability by strengthening the abdominal, gluteus maximus, and hamstring muscles as well as passive stretching of hip flexors and lower back muscles. These exercises include pelvic tilt, single knee-to-chest in supine position, double knee-to-chest, partial sit-up, hamstring stretch, hip flexor stretch, squat, and seated flexion. These exercises are commonly used in lumbar stenosis.
- McKenzie method—The McKenzie method is an assessment and treatment tool that helps identify the patient response to different dynamic loading strategies in the spine. The treatment is based on directional preferences, a series of sustained posture, or repeated movements. This technique emphasizes education and self-care. Some of the exercises are prone-lying, prone-lying on elbows, prone press-ups, progressive extension with pillows, standing extension, knee-to-chest in supine (flexion), and flexion-in-standing (bending forward).
- Core strengthening—The core muscles refer to the muscles that provides lumbar stability and proper body mechanics. These muscles work as a corset to support spine. The core muscles are anteriorly: transversus abdominis, rectus abdominis, and internal and external obliques. Posteriorly: multifidus, quadratus lumborum (primary stabilizer), erector spinae, and deep transverospinalis. Superiorly: diaphragm. Inferiorly: hip girdle musculature and pelvic floor muscles.

- Alexander technique—The Alexander technique involves individualized, hands-on instruction to improve balance, posture, and coordination, as well as recognition of harmful habits of muscle use in order to avoid painful movements.
- Pilates method—classified as a movement therapy. It focuses on proper posture alignment, core muscle strengthening, and breathing techniques.
- Tai chi—involves breathing, meditation, and slow controlled flowing movement with constant weight shifting from one leg to another. Very helpful in improving balance, coordination, body awareness, as well as stress reduction.
- Back schools—Back schools typically exist outside of the traditional healthcare system and are managed by large companies or occupational health centers. Generally, lessons are provided to groups of patients and supervised by a physical therapist or other therapist trained in back rehabilitation.
- Functional restoration programs—Functional restoration, also known as work hardening, involves simulated or actual onsite work testing in a supervised environment to improve strength, endurance, flexibility, and fitness for injured workers. This often involves a multidisciplinary component, including physical and occupational therapy. Functional restoration differs from back school in the emphasis on individualized exercise therapy compared to group educational training for back school programs.

PHYSICAL MODALITIES

- Modalities are physical agents that promote healing and analgesia. Modalities should only be used for short periods of time as an adjuvant treatment.
- Some of the modalities that are used in the treatment of low back are thermal agents and electrotherapy.
- The thermal agents are divided into cryotherapy and superficial or deep-heating agents. They may help decrease pain and improve range of motion.
  - Superficial heat—A conductive agent such as hydrocollator packs or hot moist packs are used. The heat promotes vasodilatation and promotes tissue healing.
  - Deep heating—Ultrasound, can increase the temperature up to 46°C (114.8° F) in deep tissue. The dose range from 0.5 to 2.0 W/cm^2 for 5–10 minutes.
  - Cryotherapy—cold packs, ice massage, and vapocoolant sprays.
- Electrotherapy—Transcutaneous electrical nerve stimulation (TENS). The TENS unit stimulates the nerve and provides pain relief based on the gate-control theory of Melzack and Wall.

- Manipulation is another commonly used treatment for low back pain. It can be used in the presence of somatic dysfunction such as in SIJ dysfunction, piriformis syndrome, lumbago, facet syndrome, sciatica, among others. Manipulation could be divided into thrusting vs. nonthrusting. Thrust spinal manipulation uses high-velocity and low-amplitude maneuvers. Nonthrust spinal manipulation involves controlled slow movement. It includes mobilization, muscle energy (isometrics), counterstrain, functional, myofascial release, and soft tissue and craniosacral therapy.
- Lumbar traction—not as effective as cervical traction.
- Massage is helpful to decrease muscle spasm. It is more beneficial when used with other therapeutic exercises.

BIBLIOGRAPHY

Bailey W. Observations on the etiology and frequency of spondylolisthesis and its precursors. *Radiol.* 1947; 48:107.

Bernard TN, Cassidy JD. The sacroiliac syndrome. Pathophysiology, diagnosis, and management. In: Frymoyer JW, ed. *The Adult Spine: Principles and Practice.* New York: Raven; 1991:2107–2130.

Bernard TN, Kirkaldy-Willis WH. Recognizing specific characteristics of nonspecific low back pain. *Clinic Orthopedic.* 1987;217:266–280.

Bogduk N. International Spine Injection Society Guidelines for the performance of spinal injection procedures. Part I. Zygapophysial joint blocks. *Clinical J Pain.* 1997;13:285–302.

Borenstein D, Wiesel S. *Low Back Pain: Medical Diagnosis and Comprehensive Management.* Philadelphia, Pa.: WB Saunders; 1989.

Brenner C, Kissling R, Jacob HA. The effects of morphology and histopathologic findings on the mobility of the sacroiliac joint. *Spine.* 1991;16:1111–1117.

Chiodo A, Haigh AJ. Lumbosacral radiculopathies: conservative approaches to management. *Phys Med Rehabil Clin N Am.* 2002, August;13(3):615–616.

Cohen SP, Larkin TM, Banna SA, et al. Lumbar discography: a comprehensive review of outcome studies, diagnostic accuracy, and principles. *Reg Anesth Pain Medicine.* 2005;30:163–183.

Coppes MH, Marani E, Thomeer RT, et al. Innervation of "painful" lumbar discs. *Spine.* 1997;22(20):2342–2349.

Cyron BM, Hutton WC. The tensile strength of the capsular ligaments of the apophyseal joints. *J Anat.* 1981;132:145–150.

Dyck P. The stoop-test in lumbar entrapment radiculopathy. *Spine.* 1979;4:89–92.

Elgfy H., Semaan H.B., Ebraheim N.A., et al. Computed tomography findings in patients with sacroiliac pain. *Clin Orthop.* 2001;382:112–118.

Hayden JA, van Tulder MW, Malmivaara A, et al. Exercise therapy for treatment of nonspecific low back pain. *Cochrane Database Syst Rev.* 2005, July;20(3):CD000335.

Katz JN, Harris MB. Clinical practice. Lumbar spinal stenosis. *N Engl J Med.* 2008;358(8):818.

Katz JN, Dalgas M, Stucki G, et al. Degenerative lumbar spinal stenosis. Diagnostic value of the history and physical examination. *Arthritis Rheum.* 1995;38:1236–1241.

Krawciw D, Atlas S. Occupational low back pain: treatment. *Uptodate.* March 07, 2013.

Maigne JY, Aivaliklis A, Pfefer F. Results of sacroiliac joint double block and value of sacroiliac pain provocation tests in 54 patients with low back pain. *Spine.* 1996;21(16):1889–1892.

Paris SV. Anatomy as related to function and pain. *Orthop Clin North Am.* 1983;14:475–489.

Schwarzer AC, Derby R, Aprill CN, et al. Pain from the lumbar zygapophysial joints: a test of two models. *J spinal Disord.* 1994;7: 331–336.

Sowa G, Deltto A. Exercise-based therapy for low back pain. *Uptodate.* January 03, 2013.

Steiner ME, Micheli LJ. Treatment of symptomatic spondylolisthesis and spondylolysis with a modified Boston brace. *Spine.* 1985;10:937–943.

Wiltse LL, Newman PH, Mac Nab I. Classification of spondylosis and spondylolisthesis. *Clin Orthop.* 1976;117:23.

73 INTRASPINAL DRUG DELIVERY FOR CHRONIC PAIN

Mark S. Wallace, MD
Peter S. Staats, MD, MBA

HISTORICAL PERSPECTIVES

- 1935 — Subarachnoid cannulation with five French ureteral catheter
- 1942 — Continous caudal anesthesia with a malleable Lemmon spinal needle
- 1942–1943 — Introduction of smaller catheters for continuous
- 1945 — Introduction of the Tuohy needle for intrathecal cannulation
- 1949 — Use of the Tuohy needle for epidural cannulation
- 1982 — First clinical implant, programmable pump, for intrathecal morphine
- 1984 — First clinical implant, programmable pump, for intrathecal baclofen
- 1988 — Market release of implantable, programmable pump for intrathecal morphine
- 2003, 2007, 2012 — Guidelines on the appropriate role of intrathecal therapy
- 2004 — Ziconotide is Food and Drug Administration (FDA) approved for intrathecal use to treat chronic pain
- 2015 — Expected 25,000 pumps implanted for pain and spasticity worldwide

INTRATHECAL DRUG DELIVERY (IDD) AND THE PAIN TREATMENT CONTINUUM

- IDD is considered an invasive and labor intensive therapy. Therefore, appropriate patient selection and failure of more conservative therapies are essential.
- The exact order of the pain treatment continuum is controversial; however, the following provides the basic foundation understanding that not all patients fit the continuum order, and the treatment needs to be individualized.
    - OTC Drugs
    - NSAIDS
    - PT, Manipulative Medicine, Acupuncture, TENS
    - Muscle Relaxants
    - Oral Analgesics
    - Nerve Blocks, Therapeutic
    - Nerve Blocks, Diagnostic
    - Behavioral Programs
    - Surgery
    - Spinal Cord Stimulation
    - Lower dose Chronic Opioid Therapy
    - Implantable Infusion Therapy
    - Destructive Neurosurgical Procedures

IDD VS. SPINAL CORD STIMULATION: WHICH THERAPY FOR WHICH PATIENT?

- Spinal cord stimulation is considered a much more conservative therapy than intrathecal therapy for the treatment of chronic pain and should be used before IDD when appropriate.
- Indications for spinal cord stimulation
    - Neuropathic pain
    - Low back or extremity pain
    - Cervical radiculopathy
    - Static pain
    - Examples
        - Adhesive arachnoiditis
        - Failed back surgery syndrome
        - Peripheral causalgia/neuropathy
        - Ischemic pain of vascular origin
        - Stump pain
        - Complex regional pain syndrome
    - If patient fails spinal cord stimulation, consider IDD
- Indications for IDD
    - Somatic/nociceptive pain
    - Neuropathic pain that has failed spinal cord stimulation
    - Multiple pain sites, truncal/axial pain
    - Static or changing

○ Examples
  ▪ Cancer pain
  ▪ Axial somatic pain
  ▪ Osteoporosis

SELECTION CRITERIA FOR IDD

- Malignant Pain
  ○ Life expectancy greater than three months
  ○ Inadequate pain relief and/or intolerable side effects from systemic agents
  ○ Favorable response to screening trial
- Nonmalignant Pain
  ○ Objective evidence of pathology
  ○ Psychological clearance
  ○ Inadequate pain relief and/or intolerable side effects from systemic agents at reasonable doses
  ○ Lack of drug-seeking behavior
  ○ Favorable response to screening trial

PSYCHOLOGICAL SCREENING

- Patients with a psychological profile deemed appropriate for implantable therapy have better outcomes than those deemed inappropriate (Kupers et al, 1994).
- Several studies state that depression, hysteria, and hypochondriasis are so common in pain patients and do not constitute a contraindication to implants (Burton, 1977; Shealy, 1975; Brandwin and Kewman, 1982; Simpson, 1999).
- Specialists with the most experience with implantables for pain relief agree that psychological screening is crucial to long-term success.
- Psychological Exclusion Criteria
  ○ Active psychosis
  ○ Active suicidality
  ○ Active homicidality
  ○ Major uncontrolled depression or other mood disorders
  ○ Somatization or other somatoform disorders
  ○ Alcohol or drug dependency
  ○ Unresolved compensation or litigation
  ○ Lack of appropriate social support
  ○ Neurobehavioral or cognitive deficits

SCREENING TRIAL FOR IDD

- The choice of screening technique for IDD is controversial. An early polyanalgesic consensus pain published the first recommendations for trialing IDD.
- In a retrospective review of 429 physicians:

TABLE 73-1   Recommended Doses for IDD Bolus Trialing

DRUG	RECOMMENDED IT BOLUS DOSE
Morphine	0.2–1.0 mg
Hydromorphone	0.04–0.2 mg
Ziconotide	1–5 mcg
Fentanyl	25–75 mcg
Bupivacaine	0.5–2.5 mg
Clonidine	5–20 mcg
Sufentanil	5–20 mcg

  ○ 33.7% used a single intrathecal injection technique
  ○ 18.3% used a multiple injection with blinded placebo technique
  ○ 35.3% used a continuous epidural infusion technique
- Currently, the most common technique appears to be a continuous intrathecal infusion technique, although all techniques are still used.
- Technique? (Table 73-1)
  ○ Single injection
    ▪ Recommended for patients who will not tolerate a prolonged infusion
    ▪ Advantages
      □ Lower cost
      □ Minimal time commitment
    ▪ Disadvantages
      □ Possible higher placebo response
      □ Does not adequately mimic the pharmacodynamics long-term continuous infusion therapy
  ○ Multiple injection
    ▪ There have been published reports of multiple injections with different doses of drug
    ▪ Not widely used and not currently recommended
  ○ Continuous infusion (Tables 73-2 and 73-3)
    ▪ If the patient can tolerate a prolonged infusion, generally recommended over single injection
    ▪ Advantages
      □ Closely approximates the drug delivery of an implanted pump

TABLE 73-2   Recommended Starting Dosage Range and Titration for IDD

DRUG	RECOMMENDED STARTING DOSE	INCREMENTAL INCREASE
Morphine	0.1–0.5 mg/d	0.5 mg
Hydromorphone	0.02–0.5 mg/d	0.1 mg
Ziconotide	0.5–2.4 mcg/d	0.5–1.2 mcg
Fentanyl	25–75 mcg/d	10 mcg
Bupivacaine	1–4 mg/d	1 mg
Clonidine	40–100 mcg/d	10 mcg
Sufentanil	10–20 mcg/d	10 mcg

Modified from Deer et al., Polyanalgesic Consensus Conference 2012: recommendations for the management of pain by intrathecal (intraspinal) drug delivery: report of an interdisciplinary expert panel. *Neuromodulation.* 2012;5:436–466. Modification based on the author's experience and does not fully represent the consensus.

TABLE 73-3 **Recommended Maximum Daily Dose and Concentration for IDD Therapy**

DRUG	MAXIMUM DOSE/24 h	MAXIMUM CONCENTRATION
Morphine	10 mg	20 mg/mL
Hydromorphone	10 mg	20 mg/mL
Fentanyl	1000 mcg	5 mg/mL
Sufentanil	500 mcg	2.5 mg/mL
Ziconotide	2.5 mcg	100 mcg/mL
Bupivacaine	10 mg	20 mg/mL
Clonidine	500 mcg	2000 mcg/mL

Modified from Deer et al., Polyanalgesic Consensus Conference 2012: recommendations for the management of pain by intrathecal (intraspinal) drug delivery: report of an interdisciplinary expert panel. *Neuromodulation.* 2012;5:436–466. Modification is based on the author's experience and does not fully represent the consensus.

- Disadvantages
  - Higher costs
  - Labor intensive
  - Risk of infection with externalized catheters and prolonged infusion
- Low volume vs. high volume?
  - There is controversy over the effects of delivered volume on drug kinetics and outcomes.
  - The lowest limit of drug infusion with currently available external pumps is 2.4 mL/d.
  - Chronic delivery with implanted IDD pumps ranges from 0.1 to 0.5 mL/d.
  - For trialing, it is recommended to keep total volume as low as possible.
- Epidural or intrathecal?
  - Systemic restribution of drugs is greater with epidural delivery than intrathecal delivery, which may confound results.
  - Intrathecal delivery is recommended over epidural when possible.
  - Only morphine and hydromorphone can be delivered epidurally for trialing. All the other drugs must be delivered intrathecally.
  - Epidural Delivery

- Advantages
  - No postdural puncture headache
- Disadvantages
  - Does not represent long-term intrathecal delivery
  - Different drug kinetics leading to possible false-positive and false-negative results
  - Intrathecal Delivery
    - Advantages
      - More representative of long-term intrathecal infusion
    - Disadvantages
      - Postdural puncture headache (if it occurs) can make interpretation of trial difficult
- Choice of drug? (Tables 73-4 and 73-5)
  - According to an Internet survey consisting of 413 physicians who represented management of 13,342 patients, responding physicians chose morphine most often, but many other drugs were selected without clear indications. There was evidence of wide variations in clinical practice.
  - The choice of drug depends on the pain etiology.
  - Nociceptive pain
    - Opioid
  - Neuropathic pain
    - Opioid
    - Ziconotide
- Withdrawal of systemic opioids?
  - It is controversial whether to withdraw systemic opioids prior to trialing of IDD.
  - Advantages
    - Reverses tolerance
    - Identifies patients with strong physical dependence
    - May identify patients with psychological dependence and addiction
    - May reduce total IDD dose over time
  - Disadvantages
    - Increase pain and suffering while off opioids
    - Delays initiation of IDD

TABLE 73-4 **2011 Polyanalgesic Consensus for IDD Drugs for Neuropathic Pain**

Line 1	Morphine	Ziconotide	Morphine + Bupivacaine
Line 2	Hydromorphone	Hydromorphone + Bupivaciane or Hydromorphone + Clonidine	Morphine + Clonidine
Line 3	Clonidine	Ziconotide + Opioid Fentanyl	Fentanyl + Bupivacaine or Fentanyl + Clonidine
Line 4	Opioid + Clonidine + Bupivacaine	Bupivacaine + Clonidine	
Line 5	Baclofen		

TABLE 73-5 **2011 Polyanalgesic Consensus for IDD Drugs for Nociceptive Pain**

Line 1	Morphine	Hydromorphone	Ziconotide	Fentanyl
Line 2	Morphine + Bupivacaine	Ziconotide + Opioid	Hydromorphone + Bupivacaine	Fentanyl + Bupivacaine
Line 3	Opioid (morphine, hydromorphone or fentanyl + clonidine)	Sufentanil	
Line 4	Opioid + Clonidine + Bupivacaine	Sufentanil + Bupivacaine or Clonidine	
Line 5	Sufentanil + Bupivacaine + Clonidine		

DRUGS USED FOR IDD

- Opioids
  - Pre- and postsynaptic mu receptor agonist in the dorsal horn
    - Reduce presynaptic neurotransmitter release
    - Hyperpolarize postsynaptic membrane
  - Currently used drugs
    - Morphine
      - Gold standard
      - FDA approved
    - Hydromorphone
    - Fentanyl
    - Sufentanil
  - Side effects
    - Respiratory depression with overdose
    - Nausea
    - Urinary retention
    - Pruritis
    - Peripheral edema
- Ziconotide
  - First nonopioid approved for IDD to treat chronic pain
  - Indicated for the management of severe chronic pain in patients for whom IDD is warranted, and who are intolerant of or refractory to other treatments, such as systemic analgesics, adjunctive therapies, or IDD morphine
  - Blocks presynaptic N-type calcium channels in the dorsal horn to reduce presynaptic neurotransmitter release.
  - Two fast titration trials
    - Malignant pain study showed a 53.1% vs. 18.1% reduction in pain (ziconotide vs. placebo)
    - Nonmalignant pain study showed a 31.2% vs. a 6% reduction in pain (ziconotide vs. placebo)
    - However, there was a high dropout rate due to side effects.
  - Slow titration trial
    - Three-week trial in chronic pain patients with preexisting implanted IDD pumps
    - Visual analogue spontaneous pain index improved from baseline to the end of week 3 (primary endpoint) by a mean of 14.7% in the ziconotide-treated group and 7.2% in the placebo group ($P = 0.036$)
    - Side effects much less than fast titration trial. Dropout between the ziconotide and placebo group not different.
  - Wide margin of safety in overdose
    - Highest overdose was 38 mcg/h × 24 h (912 mcg total)
      - Patient sedated but arousable, normal RR
    - Most symptoms resolved within 24 hours
- Side effects
  - Most side effects are cognition related
    - Cognitive impairment may appear after several weeks of treatment
    - May be dose dependent.
    - Reduce or discontinue PRIALT dose if signs or symptoms of cognitive impairment develop.
    - Other possible contributing causes should be considered.
    - The cognitive effects of PRIALT are generally reversible within two weeks after drug discontinuation.
  - Contains a black box warning precluding use in patients with preexisting psychosis
  - Elevation of serum creatine kinae (CK-MM)
    - In clinical studies (mostly open-label), 40% of the patients had serum creatine kinase (CK) levels above the upper limit of normal, and 11% had CK levels that were greater than or equal three-times ULN.
    - Recommend monitoring serum CK periodically in patients being treated with PRIALT
      - Every other week for first month and monthly as appropriate thereafter
    - If new neuromuscular symptoms develop (eg, myalgias, myasthenia, muscle cramps, asthenia) or reduction in physical activity is seen, clinical evaluation and CK measurement should be performed
    - Consider dose reduction or discontinuation if symptoms continue and CK levels remain elevated or continue to rise
- Local anesthetics
  - Block pre- and postsynaptic sodium channels
  - Commonly used in combination with opioids
  - Bupivacaine most commonly used
  - Side effects minimal
  - Sensory and motor disturbances with higher doses (above 20 mg/d)
  - Tachyphylaxis with higher doses
- Clonidine
  - Pre and postsynaptic Alpha2 receptor agonist
    - Reduces presynaptic neurotransmitter release
    - Hyperpolarizes postsynaptic membrane
  - FDA approved for epidural use in cancer patients only
  - Side effects
    - Hypotension, bradycardia, sedation
  - Proven efficacy in neuropathic pain with epidural use
  - Often used intrathecally in combination with opioids

- Baclofen
  - GABA-B agonist
    - Antispasmodic effects are through decreased release of excitatory neurotransmitters from IA, IB, and A alpha afferents in the spinal cord.
    - Analgesic effects may be the effects on voltage-sensitive calcium channels resulting in a reduction in neurotransmitter release.
  - FDA approval as antispasmotic
  - Case report series demonstrate efficacy in neuropathic pain at doses of 100–460 mg/d.

DRUG MIXING/COMPOUNDING

- Although none of the IDD drugs are FDA approved for combination therapy, it is common practice to mix and compound drugs.
- Decision to compound and mix drugs is based upon:
  - Availability of compounding
  - Refill intervals
    - As the drug dose increases, refill intervals will decrease.
    - Increasing drug concentrations will increase the time between refill intervals.
    - When using and mixing drugs, first try and use commercially available drugs to keep refill intervals at over 30 days (will depend on the size of the reservoir).
      - Commercially available concentrations
        - Morphine 20 mg/mL
        - Hydromorphone 10 mg/mL
        - Fentanyl/sufentanil 50 mcg/mL
        - Ziconotide 100 mcg/mL, 25 mcg/mL
        - Bupivacaine 7.5 mg/mL
        - Clonidine 500 mcg/mL
        - Baclofen 3000 mcg/mL
    - When refill intervals reach less than 30 days, consider compounding.
  - Side effects
    - If a side effect occurs in the presence of pain relief, reducing the dose and adding a second or third drug may be beneficial.
  - Risk of inflammatory mass formulation
    - Higher drug concentrations increase the risk of inflammatory mass. Mixing drugs will reduce the required drug dose and concentration.
- Advantages
  - Targets multiple mechanisms
  - May attenuate tolerance
  - Drug synergism
- Disadvantages
  - Drug compatability
    - May reduce drug potency

- May increase precipitation
  - More likely to occur at higher concentrations
- Granuloma formation with compounding higher concentrations
  - Changes in drug viscosity may affect delivered dose.

IDD SYSTEMS

- Programmable
  - Medtronic Synchromed II
    - 20- and 40-mL reservoirs
    - Programmable peristaltic roller system for variable rate delivery
    - Patient-controlled bolus dosing available by a remote-controlled device
    - 4 to 7 years battery life
    - FDA approved for morphine, baclofen, and ziconotide
  - Flowonix Prometra
    - Pressurized gas chamber as the driving force with a programmable flow-metering valve for variable rate delivery
      - Results in much lower energy requirements, thus longer battery life span
      - 10-year battery life
    - Patient-controlled bolus dosing available by a remote-controlled device
    - 20-mL reservoir
    - FDA approved for morphine
- Nonprogrammable Fixed Rate
  - Currently no fixed rate pumps on the market with FDA approval to treat chronic pain

MORBIDITY OF IDD

- Catheter-associated morbidity
  - Neurologic complications
  - Infection
  - Catheter fibrosis/inflammation
  - Catheter malfunction
  - Granuloma formation
    - Recent concern with chronic intraspinal drug delivery
    - Suggested that risk of granuloma formation is drug and concentration dependent
    - Exact drug concentration that will predispose to granuloma formation is unknown
    - Recommended that the lowest concentration possible be used
    - Detection
      - Prodromal or warning symptoms
        - LE motor, sensory, reflex functions
          - Important to establish baseline neurologic exam

> - Loss of drug effect (increase pain despite increasing dose)
> - CSF morphology
>   - WBC may be elevated
> - Symptoms that require immediate evaluation
> - New onset radicular pain/parasthesia
> - Spinal cord injury signs
> - Cauda equina syndrome
- Recommended actions
  - CT myelogram or MRI with contrast
  - If granuloma detected
    - Decrease drug infusion/concentration, or
    - Change drug, or
    - Stop infusion, or
    - Revise catheter
    - Surgical consult may be required
- Pump or port pocket-associated morbidity
  - Hematoma
  - Seroma
  - Infection
- Pump system-associated problems
  - Filling errors
  - Pump failure
  - Rotary stall
    - Can be assessed by examining rotary position before and after programming a bolus dose
  - Programming errors
  - Pump torsion with catheter occlusion

EFFICACY OF IDD FOR CHRONIC PAIN

- Challenges with Efficacy Studies on IDD
  - Lack of psychological assessment
  - Screening methods not described
  - No control groups, randomization, or blinding
  - Pain syndromes not defined
  - No standardization of methods used to determine outcome
  - No protocols for selecting, increasing, or changing drugs used
  - Studies are short to intermediate in follow-up
- Only one prospective randomized controlled trial on IDD
  - Randomized controlled trial
  - 202 cancer patients with uncontrolled pain randomized to either Intrathecal Drug Delivery System (IDDS) or Comprehensive Medical Management (CMM)
  - Clinical success defined as ≥20% reduction in VAS scores or equal scores with ≥20% reduction in toxicity
  - More IDDS patients achieved success (84.5% vs. 70.8%, $P = 0.05$)
  - More IDDS patients achieved ≥20% reduction in both pain VAS and toxicity
  - Nonsignificant change in mean VAS between groups (IDDS—52%, CMM—39%)
  - IDDS patients had significantly greater change in toxicity scores (52% vs. 17%, $P = 0.004$)
  - Approached statistical significance with improvement in survival in the group treated with an implanted pump

BIBLIOGRAPHY

Coffey RJ, Burchiel K. Inflammatory mass lesions associated with intrathecal drug infusion catheters: report and observations on 41 patients. *Neurosurgery.* 2002;50:78–87.

Hassenbusch SJ, Portenoy PK. Current practices in intraspinal therapy—a survey of clinical trends and decision making. *J Pain Sympt Manage.* 2000;20:S4–S11.

Oakley J, Staats P. The use of implanted drug delivery systems. In: Raj PP, ed. *The Practical Management of Pina.* St Louis, Mo.: Mosby; 2000:768–778.

Paice JA, Penn RD, Shott S. Intraspinal morphine for chronic pain: a retrospective, multicenter study. *J Pain Symptom Manage.* 1996;11(2):71–80.

Rauck RL, Wallace MS, Leong MS, et al. A randomized, double-blind, placebo-controlled study of intrathecal ziconotide in adults with severe chronic pain. *J Pain Symptom Manage.* 2006;31:393–406.

Smith TJ, Staats PS, Pool G, et al. Randomized clinical trial of an implantable drug delivery system compared to comprehensive medical management for refractory cancer pain: impact on pain, drug-related toxicity, and survival. *J Clin Oncol.* 2002;20:4040–4049.

Staats PS, Yearwood T, Charapata SG, et al. Intrathecal Ziconotide in the treatment of refractory pain in patients with cancer and AIDS: a randomized controlled trial. *J Am Med Assoc.* 2004;291:63–70.

Wallace MS, Charapata SG, Fisher R, et al. Intrathecal ziconotide in the treatment of chronic nonmalignant pain: a randomized, double-blind, placebo-controlled clinical trial. *Neuromodulation.* 2006;9:75–86.

Yaksh TL, Hassenbusch SJ, Burchiel K. Inflammatory masses associated with intrathecal drug infusion: a review of preclinical evidence and human data. *Pain Medicine.* 2002;3:300–312.

74 SYMPATHETIC BLOCKADE

Mazin Ellias, MD, FRCA

INTRODUCTION

- The sympathetic nervous system has been implicated in numerous pain syndromes.
- For over 100 years, sympathetic nerve blocks, which involve the interruption of the sympathetic outflow, have been used to diagnose and treat patients with sympathetically mediated (or maintained) pain (SMP).

- SMP may occur with many types of neuropathic pain. In addition, other pain states (ie, frostbite, upper abdominal malignancy, pelvic pain cluster headaches, and even angina) may respond to an appropriately performed sympathetic block.
- Diagnostic imaging studies are sometimes used to help diagnose various neuropathic pain states with SMP.
- There is no single gold-standard criterion to determine if a patient with neuropathic pain carries a diagnosis of SMP. Some have suggested a triple or quadruple test to determine.
  - Greater than 50% pain relief following an appropriately performed *sympathetic block.*
  - Response to the *phentolamine infusion test* (phentolamine is an alpha 1 antagonist which produces systemic sympathetic blockade).
  - Aggravation of the pain following local *injection of Norepinephrine* and finally the relief of the pain with local *injection of Clonidine* or *application of Clonidine patch.*
- The classical targets for sympathetic blockade are the *sphenopalatine* ganglia, *stellate* (cervicothoracic) sympathetic ganglia, *celiac/splanchnic* plexus (abdominal SMP and visceral pain), *lumbar* sympathetic ganglia (lower extremity SMP and related pain syndromes), *superior hypogastric* (pelvic pain), and *ganglia impar* (peri-anal and rectal pain and tenesmus).

Since complications are more common during the performance of sympathetic blockade of the cervicothoracic region, intravenous access should be considered.

SPHENOPALATINE GANGLIA BLOCK (SPG)

ANATOMY

- SPG is located in the pterygopalatine fossa (the sphenopalatine fossa), located posterior to the middle nasal conchae and anterior to the pterygoid canal. It lies in close proximity to the maxillary nerve.
- The sympathetic nerve passes through this ganglion to supply the sensory, vasomotor, and secretary fibers to the sphenopalatine, lacrimal, and nasal glands, and also to some of the sympathetic fibers along the cranial blood vessels.

TECHNIQUE OF SPG BLOCK

- The simplest technique is using two cotton-tip applicators, soft with cocaine or viscous lidocaine and then advanced through the nares along the middle turbinate posteriorly. A second applicator is then applied

superior and posterior to the first one, with both left in position for 30 minutes.
- Fluoroscopically guided block can be used for both temporary and for permanent block to the SPG, that is, neurolytic lesion or radiofrequency ablation (RFA).
  - The needle is inserted in between the mandibular rami, under fluoroscopy, and under the Zygoma, aiming at the sphenopalatine fossa.
  - Paresthesia to the maxillary nerve may occur and some local anesthetic agent may reduce the pain.
  - On AP view, the needle tip should lie just adjacent to the lateral nasal cavity wall.
  - Half to one milliliter of contrast dye or electrical stimulation using 2 Hz and 100 Hz through the RF needle can confirm the correct position of the needle tip.
  - Stimulation should produce a tingling sensation into the nasal area and nasal cavity. One milliliter of local anesthetic agent or neurolytic agent (in terminal patients only) can be applied. Alternatively, a RFA can be performed.
- **Indications:** This approach is commonly performed to diagnose headache disorders. Cluster headaches, among other headache disorders, which have been recalcitrant to many other forms of treatment, can respond favorably to this technique.

COMPLICATIONS

- Mechanical—traumatic injury to the maxillary nerve, intravascular injection, epistaxis, and pain at the site of the injection.
- Pharmacological—intravascular injection, damage to the maxillary nerve by the neurolytic agent, and seizure from the local anesthetic agent.

CERVICOTHORACIC/STELLATE GANGLION BLOCK

ANATOMY

- Sympathetic flow to the head, neck, and upper extremities is derived from the upper five to seven thoracic spinal segments.
- Preganglionic cell bodies of the sympathetic outflow tract are located in the gray matter of the dorsolateral spinal cord (intermediolateral cell column). These fibers pass through the anterior rami and exit as white rami communicante. The fiber ascends along the anterior lateral surface of the spinal column to synapse on postganglionic cell bodies in three cervical sympathetic ganglia (superior, middle, and inferior cervical sympathetic ganglia).

- In 80% of patients the inferior cervical and the first thoracic sympathetic ganglia fuse together to form the stellate ganglion (SG) also called the cervicothoracic ganglion.
- The SG lies in front of the neck of the first rib by the dome of the pleura.
- The SG supplies postganglionic sympathetic fibers to the head and neck, and most of the upper limb. One notable exception is the sympathetic nerve of Kuntz, which arises from the T2 spinal segment and may bypass the cervicothoracic/stellate ganglion and pass to the upper extremity. This may explain why an appropriately performed stellate ganglion block may not provide total sympathectomy to the upper extremity.

INDICATIONS

- Sympathetically maintained pain of the head and neck.
- CRPS type I and II and other sympathetically maintained pain syndromes to the upper extremities and to the anterior chest wall.
- Vascular insufficiency/vascular disorders, including Raynaud's disease, conditions to the upper extremities, head and neck, including some vascular type of headaches (migraine and cluster headaches).

TECHNIQUE OF CERVICOTHORACIC/STELLATE GANGLIA BLOCK (SGB)

- A SGB can be performed at either the C6 or C7 vertebrae using fluoroscopy or ultrasound guidance.
- Fluoroscopy can be used to identify the level, or the C6 transverse process (the Chassaignac's process) can be palpated and used as a landmark.
- The carotid artery is retracted laterally with the sternomastoid to avoid puncture. The periosteum is contacted using a short beveled needle at the junction of the C6 or C7 transverse process and the vertebral body. After contacting periosteum, the needle is withdrawn a few millimeters above the longus colli muscle. After negative aspiration for both blood and CSF, 1 mL of dye is injected to rule out intravascular or intrathecal spread. If negative and there is good spread along the sympathetic ganglion, 0.5 mL of local anesthetic is injected and after waiting for 2–3 minutes to exclude any signs of CNS toxicity (intravascular injection) or spinal analgesia (intrathecal injection), 2–5 mL of local anesthetic is injected.
- Sympathetic blockade to the head and neck is confirmed by the development of Horner's syndrome and to the upper extremity by measuring the skin temperature, which should increase by at least 2–3°C.

- Note: This is an evolving field and some physicians find safety in the use of ultrasound helpful in avoiding intravascular injection. Specifically, the vertebral artery can be visualized with ultrasound and visualization may improve the margin of safety.

COMPLICATIONS

- Mechanical—pain from the injection, hematoma, pneumothorax, pneumomediastinum, injury to the esophagus, brachial plexus, and vasovagal attacks.
- Pharmacological—spinal analgesia, brachial plexus, and phrenic nerve block leading to difficulty in breathing, recurrent laryngeal nerve block leading to hoarseness of voice (this is why bilateral stellate ganglion block/cervicothoracic ganglion block should not be attempted), and seizure because of intravascular injection.
- Contraindications include contralateral phenic nerve palsy, blood dyscrasia/coagulopathy, local sepsis, and patient refusal.

CELIAC/SPLANCHNIC NERVE PLEXUS BLOCK

ANATOMY

- Sympathetic supply to the abdominal viscera arises in the intermediolateral cell column.
- Preganglionic fibers from the T5–10 spinal segment give rise to the lesser splanchnic (T11–12), the greater splanchnic (T5–10), and the least splanchnic (T12). These nerves hug the thoracic vertebral body and then pass to form the celiac plexus.
- Celiac ganglia are a mesh-like structure which lies in front of the aorta. It measures about 1–4.5 cm in diameter at the approximate level of the first lumbar to T12 vertebra. From there, the postganglionic fibers travel to supply the abdominal viscera.
- Unlike sympathetic and sensory supply to nonvisceral structures, blockade of the sympathetic supply independent of the sensory supply to the viscera is not possible since the fibers all travel together. Therefore, sympathetic blockade to the viscera is usually to interrupt sensation rather than sympathetic supply.

CELIAC PLEXUS BLOCK

- Multiple approaches have been used to block the celiac plexus, including the anterior and posterior approaches and open techniques. The classical technique will be described here, which is the posterior approach.

- The posterior approach can be retrocrural or tran-scrural. Another approach is the transaortic, where the needle will lie in front of the aorta (celiac ganglion block), the transcrural deposits the agent directly on the celiac plexus block, while the retrocrural deposits the agent at the level of the splanchnic nerve block.
- Although all provide effective sympathetic blockade, the splanchnic block is reserved for those patients who have abdominal pathology such as widespread metastasis of tumor, which makes a transaortic approach difficult, or if there is a vascular anomaly, ie, aortic aneurysm, which prohibits the transcrural or transaortic approach.
- The posterior approach is performed with the patient in the prone position.
- It can be performed using fluoroscopy or CT scan.
- The needle is usually inserted at the edge of a triangle, which is formed from the T12 rib, L1 transverse process, and the tip of the T12 spinous process.
- The needle is then directed so that the final position will be either in front of the T12 (retrocrural) or the L1 vertebra (transcrural).
- For both approaches, bilateral needles should be inserted.
- The position is confirmed by both AP and lateral view and by the injection of dye.
- Following confirmation of the spread of dye, local anesthetic agent is injected (8–15 mL on each side).
- Alcohol or phenol is used in the terminally ill patient for more permanent blockades.
- Before lytic block is performed, a local anesthetic agent should be injected initially to provide anesthesia and block the pain of the lytic agent. It will also ensure no intravascular or intrathecal epidural spread, as confirmed by the development of spinal analgesia. This can be achieved by first injecting 5 cc of local anesthetic and after waiting 3–5 minutes, follow this with 100% alcohol.

INDICATIONS

- Acute/chronic pancreatitis and hepatobiliary disorder including biliary sphincteric disorder.
- Abdominal visceral pain syndrome including abdominal malignances.
- Abdominal angina.

COMPLICATIONS

- Mechanical—injury to the blood, kidney, ureter lung and pleura (pneumothorax, hemopneumothorax, pleurisy), and paraplegia because of intravascular/intrathecal injection or because of trauma to the blood supply to the spinal cord (artery of Adamkeiwicz).

- Pharmacological—Hypotention, and diarrhea because of sympathetic blockade, intravascular injection (seizure), and alcohol neurolytic block can cause alcohol withdrawal in people with disulfiram therapy for alcohol abuse therapy.
- Phenol should be avoided in patients who have vascular prosthesis as it can damage the prosthesis.
- IV access should be maintained and pre-load of fluid is also advisable to reduce the severity of hypotention.

LUMBAR SYMPATHETIC BLOCK

ANATOMY

- Preganglionic innervation to the lower extremities arises from the intermediolateral cell column (lower thoracic and upper two lumbar segments).
- They synapse into the lumbar sympathetic ganglion which is located in the anterior lateral surface of the L2 to the L4 vertebra, anterior to the psoas muscle. However, there is some individual variation in the position (Rocco).
- Most postganglionic sympathetic fibers accompany nerve roots to the lower extremity.

TECHNIQUE OF LUMBAR SYMPATHETIC BLOCK

- Performed using the lateral oblique approach, in the prone position at the level of L2.
- A 5-in. spinal needle is inserted, under fluoroscopy, and directed to avoid the transverse process of L2.
- Final tip of the needle will lie in front of and just lateral to the L2 vertebra (in the mid facetal line) or at the superior third of the L3 vertebra where in most individuals, the sympathetic ganglion is located (Rocco).
- Injection of dye should confirm the spread in front of and lateral to the vertebral body, both on AP and lateral view followed by 3–5 mL of local anesthetic.
- Sympathetic blockade confirmed with at least 3°C rise in the ipsilateral lower extremity temperature.

INDICATIONS

- CRPS type I and II (SMP).
- Vascular insufficiency/disorder to the lower extremity.
- Neuropathic pain, ie, postherpetic neuralgia.

COMPLICATIONS

- Mechanical—infection; trauma to the lumbar nerve and disc; intravascular, intrathecal, and epidural injection. Kidney trauma (hematuria).

- Pharmacological—intravascular or intrathecal injection of local anesthetic agent or neurolytic agent, hypotension, paraplegia, and in case of neurolytic block, genitofemoral neuralgia.

SUPERIOR AND INFERIOR HYPOGASTRIC PLEXUS BLOCK

ANATOMY

- The plexus is located retroperitoneally in the lower third of the fifth lumbar vertebral body and the upper third of sacrum in close proximity to the bifurcation of the common iliac vessel.
- It receives supply from the lumbar aortic and celiac sympathetic plexus.
- There are also some parasympathetic fibers from the ventral root of S2 to S4.
- The superior hypogastric plexus supplies the pelvic viscera, sigmoid colon, and rectum.
- It also communicates with the inferior hypogastric plexus which is located parallel to the pelvic floor in the presacaral tissues from S2–S4 spinal segment. Its afferent fibers originate from the sacral nerve roots from S2 or S4 (60%) and rarely S5. It is not easy to selectively block the inferior hypogastric plexus independently from the somatic fibers.

INDICATIONS

- Treatment of pelvic pain including malignancy, endometriosis, or pelvic inflammatory diseases/adhesions.

TECHNIQUE OF HYPOGASTRIC PLEXUS BLOCK

- With the patient in the prone position, with a pillow to flatten the lumbar lordosis, the x-ray beam is turned to 45 degrees lateral oblique view at the level of the L5 vertebra.
- A cephalocaudal view is then used to avoid hitting the iliac crest in such way that the view of the anterior lateral part of the L5 vertebra can be identified.
- A needle is inserted in such way that the tip will lie in front of the vertebral body of L5.
- If the transverse process of L4 or L5 is encountered, sometimes bending the needle tip by 50 degrees can be used to bypass that.
- Needle position is confirmed by AP and lateral view and also by injection of dye. This is followed by injecting 3–5 mL of local anesthetic or neurolytic solution (in terminal patients) on each side.
- A trans-discal approach has been used but does carry a small risk for discitis.

- A trans-sacral approach to block the inferior hypogastric plexus through the S1, S2, S3, or S4, has been described by Schultz. The S2 is preferred to avoid neural trauma.

GANGLION IMPAR (GANGLION OF WALTHER) BLOCK

ANATOMY

- This is a solitary retroperitoneal structure located at the level of the sacrococcygeal junction.
- Marks the termination of the paravertebral sympathetic chain.

INDICATION

- Peri-anal pain and rectal tenesmus (or spasm) which is presumed to be sympathetically maintained or visceral pain.

TECHNIQUE

- Two techniques have been described.
  - Trans-sacrococcygeal ligament
    - Easiest to perform
    - Needle is inserted through the ligament until it lies just a few millimeters in front of the curvature of the sacrum.
    - Confirmed by the injection of dye, followed by the injection of 2–4 cc of local anesthetic agent or neurolytic agent (in terminal patients).
  - Trans-anococcygeal ligament
    - Needle inserted between the coccygeal and the anal region, and then directed the curvature toward the coccyx until the needle is laid anterior to the surface of the bone.
    - Injection of dye confirmation should resemble an apostrophe.
- CT and ultrasound-guided methods were documented.

COMPLICATIONS

- Caudal/epidural spread, injury to the rectum or to the periosteum, and infection.

POSTSYMPATHECTOMY SYNDROME

- Following sympathetic blockade, especially following neurolytic agent (though can appear after RFA or surgical symapthectomy), the original pain may reappear.

- New neurological deficit and new pain syndromes may also appear.
- Causation: (1) reorganization and resprouting of the sympathic nerves with plasticity of the central and the peripheral nervous system; (2) injury to nearby somatic nerves by neurolytic agents and thus producing a new neuropathic syndrome.
- More common following sympathectomy for neuropathic pain, rather than following hyperhydrosis.
- Best prevention is to avoid neurolysis, use a smaller volume of neurolytic agent, or more localized RFA.

Bibliography

Elias M. The anterior approach for thoracic sympathetic ganglion block using a curved needle. *Pain Clinic.* 2000;12(1);17–24.

Hahn M, McQuollan P, Sheplock GJ. *Regional Anesthesia: An Atlas of Anatomy and Techniques.* 1st ed. Chicago, Il.: Mosby; 1996.

Livingstone JA, Atkins R. Intravenous regional sympathetic blockade in treatment of CRPS type I of the hand. *J. Bone Joint Surg. Brt.* 2002;84(3):380–386.

Raj SN, Campbell JN. Risk-benefit ratio for surgical sympathectomy: dilemmas in clinical decision-making. *J Pain.* 2000;1(4):261–264.

Rocco A. Radiofrequency: lumber sympatholysis. *Regional Anesth.* 1995;20(1):3–12.

Shultz D. Inferior hypogastric plexus blockade: a trans-sacral approach. *Pain Physician.* 2007;10(6):757–763.

Waldman W. *Interventional Pain Management.* 1st ed. Philadelphia, Pa.: W.B. Sanders; 2000.

75 TRANSCUTANEOUS ELECTRICAL NERVE STIMULATION

Gordon Irving, MD

WHAT IS IT?

- Transcutaneous electrical nerve stimulation (TENS) is current that is applied through electrodes placed on the skin that activates large-diameter sensory fibers.
- There are two main stimulation patterns: a low-frequency (also called acupuncture-like) 1-4 Hz, high-intensity, long pulse-width signal that causes visible muscle contractions, and a high-frequency 50-120 Hz, low-intensity signal that causes a tingling or buzzing sensation.
- A small, portable device with two or four leads is used to produce the low-voltage electrical current.
- An estimated 250,000 units are prescribed annually in the United States.

HOW DOES IT WORK?

- TENS is believed to work by changing an individual's perception of pain.
- The gate-control theory originally proposed by Melzak and Wall proposes that when large Aβ fibers are stimulated, Aδ and C fiber nociceptive input is inhibited at the interneuron level of the substantia gelatinosa of the dorsal horn.
- The high-frequency, low-intensity mode is thought to work by "closing the gate."
- The low-frequency, high-intensity mode works by recruiting both large- and small-diameter fibers and depends on supraspinal descending inhibitor mechanisms for its actions.

DOES IT WORK?

- Despite more than 600 published articles, the methodology of most studies is poor and recent meta-analyses have recommended more well-controlled trials.
- Specific evidence-based benefit include:
  - Labor pain
  - Chronic low back pain (Although there was a trend to greater pain reduction, better functional status, and better patient satisfaction with active TENS versus placebo, it was not statistically significant.)
- TENS was shown to be of benefit in:
  - Primary dysmenorrhea, where high-frequency but not low-frequency TENS worked
  - Osteoarthritis pain of the knee, where both high-frequency TENS and low-frequency TENS were found to be significantly better than placebo
- Indeterminate studies in which the efficacy of TENS could neither be refuted nor confirmed included chronic pain of more than three months duration, excluding angina, headache, migraine, and dysmenorrhea.
- There are many studies suggesting long-term efficacy of TENS, although these are not placebo controlled.
- A positive effect on almost 8000 patients over periods from 6 months to 4 years has been reported.
- Measures included improved sleep and socialization, decreased pain, as well as decreased medication and utilization of physical and/or occupational therapy.

HOW IS IT USED?

TRIALING

- Place the electrodes with the pads placed around the painful area.
- With the TENS connected and turned on, a sensation should be felt covering the painful area.
- Use the electrical stimulus pattern that by trial and error is found to be the most successful in decreasing pain. This is usually the high-frequency, low-intensity mode.
- With this mode the intensity is increased until a buzzing or tingling sensation is felt.
- The intensity is then reduced until it is barely felt.
- Continue this for 20–30 minutes.
- If the pain is decreased, 30 minutes or more of stimulation can be given.
- If there is no decrease in pain, move the pads to cover nearby trigger points or acupuncture points and retry the stimulation for an additional 20–30 minutes.
- If pain is felt along a nerve distribution, try placing the electrodes on the skin directly over the nerve.

LONG-TERM USE

- There are minimal side effects from the skin pads or use of the current.
- Tolerance may occur in the first few months with loss of efficacy.

HOW MUCH DOES IT COST?

- The medical insurance company usually covers the leasing and subsequent costs.
- Purchase costs are $350 to $400, with ongoing costs for renewing the pads and electrode wires.

BIBLIOGRAPHY

Brosseau L, Milne S, Robinson V, et al. Efficacy of the transcutaneaous electrical nerve stimulator for the treatment of chronic low back pain: a meta-analysis. *Spine.* 2002;27:596–603.

Carroll D, Moore RA, McQuay HJ, et al. Transcutaneous electrical nerve stimulation for chronic pain. *Cochrane Database Syst Rev.* 2001;CD003222.

Carroll D, Tramer M, McQuay HJ, et al. Transcutaneous electrical nerve stimulation in labour pain: a systematic review. *Br J Obst Gynaecol.* 1997;104:169–175.

Chabal C, Fishbain DA, Weaver M, et al. Long-term transcutaneaous electrical nerve stimulation use: impact on medication utilization and physical therapy costs. *Clin J Pain.* 1998;14:66–73.

Fishbain DA, Chabal C, Abbott A. Transcutaneaous electrical nerve stimulation treatment outcome in long-term users. *Clin J Pain.* 1996;12:201–214.

Osiri M, Welch V, Brosseau L. Transcutaneous electrical nerve stimulation for knee osteoarthritis. *Cochrane Database Syst Rev.* 2000;CD002823.

Proctor ML, Smith CA, Farquhar CM, et al. Transcutaneous electrical nerve stimulation and acupuncture for primary dysmenorrhoea. *Cochrane Database Syst Rev.* 2002;CD002123.

76 DISCOGRAPHY/INTRADISCAL THERMAL THERAPIES

Irina Melnik, MD
Richard Derby, MD
Sang-Heon Lee, MD, PhD

DISCOGRAPHY

CONCEPTS

- Discography is a provocative diagnostic test that attempts to evoke and reproduce the patient's typical pain, by injection of contrast medium into the nucleus of the intervertebral disc.
- Current concept of the discography relies on the assumption that evoked pain is a result of two pathways affecting intradiscal nerve endings: a chemical stimulation of sensitized disc tissue and a mechanical stimulus resulting from fluid-distending stress.
- Increased intradiscal pressure within a diseased disc is thought to stimulate over-sensitized nociceptors in the annulus fibrosis or/and the nerve endings within the pathologically innervated annular fissures.
- The test endeavors to confirm or refute the hypothesis that a particular disc is a source of patient's familiar (concordant) pain.
- Discography is an interventional procedure recommended only when other less invasive diagnostic tests are inconclusive.
- When combined with CT-discography, this test can also provide unique morphologic characteristics of the disc structure and degrees of annular and endplate disruption.
- Additional value of discography is in identification of asymptomatic discs. When a single disc is found to be symptomatic in the presence of adjacent asymptomatic discs, focused surgical therapy can be entertained.

- Although the diagnostic power of discography still remains controversial, when performed correctly, it is a relatively safe and sensitive test for identifying painful discs, which may predict therapeutic outcomes of surgical or other interventional treatments and may help patients avoid unnecessary surgical interventions.
- As a provocative test, discography is liable to false-positive results, which can be potentially lowered (to an acceptably low 6% rate), by adherence to strict operational standards, interpretation criteria, and proper patients selection.
- Discography is the diagnostic gold standard for diagnosing or excluding discogenic back pain.

DISCOGENIC PAIN

- Although the external outline of the disc may remain intact, there are many pathologic processes, including annular tears, degeneration, endplate injury, and inflammation, that can cause sensitization and stimulate pain nociceptors within the disc itself, independent of nerve-root stimulation symptoms.
- In a diseased disc, pain may be generated from deep within its own tissue, beyond normal innervation of the outer third of the annulus, with pain-carrying nerve fibers extending deep inward into the middle annulus and even deeper inward. This has been observed in degenerative discs, and has been linked to the discogenic back pain syndrome.
- Discogenic low back pain is considered to be one of the most common causes of chronic low back pain, accounting for approximately 26%–39% of its incidence.
- Pain response involves complex mechanisms, including amplification of the pain in the sensitized, diseased disc, through the secretion of pro-inflammatory mediators, including substance P, inflammatory cytokines, calcitonin gene-related peptide (CGRP), vasoactive intestinal peptide (VIP), tumor necrosis factor-alpha (TNF-a), nitric oxide, matrix metalloproteinases (MMPs), and increased number of mechanoreceptors and pain-producing neurons.
- Distinct from normally aging discs, "pathologically painful" discs show a process of neo-innervation extending along anular fissures as well as to the inner anulus and even nucleus pulposus, which likely explains the pain of provocation discography.
- Discogenic back pain is typically a "diagnosis by exclusion" when other potential sources of back pain have been eliminated.
- History, physical examination, and imaging studies have limited specificity for discogenic back pain, but can help navigate a diagnostic algorithmic process, and, most importantly, can help rule out and screen for potentially serious and rare spinal disorders.

INDICATION CRITERIA

- To test a diagnostic hypothesis of discogenic origin of pain when other sources of back pain have been eliminated in patients who failed conservative treatment lasting longer than four months.
- To confirm diagnosis of discogenic pain and to specify the exact levels of symptomatic discs when considering invasive intradiscal treatment options, including spinal fusion.
- To assess back or neck pain in patients with minimal or no findings on imaging studies, such as MRI or CT scan, and to analyze disc morphology.
- To determine symptomatic disc levels in patients with multilevel disc abnormalities on imaging studies.
- To identify normal and nonsymptomatic discs to minimize a chance of unnecessary surgical intervention.

CONTRAINDICATIONS

Absolute

- The patient is unable or unwilling to consent to the procedure, or to cooperate.
- Inability to assess patient response during the procedure.
- Untreated systemic or localized infections.
- Pregnancy.

Relative

- Allergy to contrast medium, local anesthetic, or anitibiotics.
- Anticoagulants or bleeding diathesis.
- Any psychological or anatomical problems that could compromise safety and success of the procedure (including spinal cord compromise and/or myelopathy at the level of proposed discography).

EVALUATION

- The patient response to disc stimulation needs to be accurately monitored, and include: the presence or absence of pain, the VAS score of the pain, the pressure at which the pain was produced, and concordance of pain.
- If the patient's pain intensity, location, and a character of pain during the disc provocation are similar to or

the same as the patient's typical, accustomed pain, the criteria for concordant pain are satisfied.

- A true positive response is concordant pain, ≥7/10, sustained for greater than 30–60 seconds, at a pressure of <50 psi above opening, volume ≤3.5 mL, and a presence of at least one negative control disc.

- Without an asymptomatic "control disc," there is no evidence that the patient can discriminate between a symptomatic and an asymptomatic discs, especially in case of multiple concordant pain levels.

- Most abnormal discs will be painful between 15 and 50 psi a.o. and are termed "mechanically-sensitive" based on a four-type classification introduced in the 1990s by Derby et al in respect to annular sensitivity. Discs which are painful at pressures <15 psi a.o. are termed low-pressure positive or "chemically-sensitive" discs; if discs are painful between 15 and 50 psi a.o., they are termed "mechanically sensitive" discs. Indeterminate discs are painful between 51 and 90 psi a.o., and normal discs are not painful on provocation.

- The degree of radial and annular disc disruption is commonly described using modified Dallas discogram scale. Grade 0 describes contrast contained within the nucleus pulposus; grades 1–3 describe degree of fissuring extending to the inner, middle, and outer annulus, respectively; grade 4 describes a grade 3 annular fissure with a greater than 30 degree circumferential arc of contrast; a grade 5 involves spread of contrast beyond the outer annulus on post-discography CT images.

LUMBAR DISCOGRAPHY

- Lumbar discography is usually approached posterolaterally, although lateral (extrapedicular), posterior, and midline approaches may be employed (Figure 76-1).

- Light sedation is advisable only during needles placement, and patient has to be responsive during the testing part of the procedure.

- Double needle approach is recommended to minimize the risk of disc infection and to assist in the needle placement technique (particularly at the L5–S1 interspace).

- The discography needle has to be ideally positioned within 4–5 mm of the center of the nucleus on both AP and lateral fluoroscopy views. An annular injection may give a false-positive, false-negative, or misleading pain response.

- Once the tip of needle has been properly placed in the center of the disc, contrast medium mixed with antibiotic is injected into each disc at slow velocity, using preferably a controlled injection syringe with digital pressure readout. Slow injection spead (~0.1 cc/s) is crucial to reduce false-positive findings.

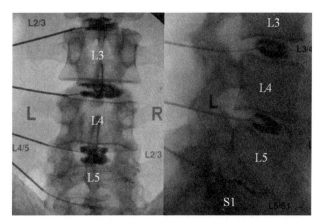

FIG. 76-1. Provocative Discography procedure at the L3–4, L4–5, and L5–S1 discs (AP and lateral fluoroscopy images). The L3–4 and 4–5 level discs exhibit a normal nucleus with bilobed "hamburger" patterns of contrast spread. The L5–S1 disc shows signs of disc degeneration with a contrast spread involving the nucleus pulposus with a relatively intact anulus fibrosus.

- Injection continues until one of the following endpoints is reached: pain response ≥7/10, intradiscal pressure >50 psi a.o. above opening in a disc with a grade 3 annular tear or 80-100 psi a.o. with a normal-appearing nucleogram, epidural or vascular pattern is evident, or a total of 3.5 mL of contrast has been injected (some severely degenerated discs may accept greater volume; however, the incidence of false-positive pain responses may increase).

- Typical opening pressures are 5–25 psi a.o., depending on the degree of nuclear degeneration; if it exceeds 30 psi a.o., this usually indicates that the needle tip is lodged within the inner anulus, and needs to be repositioned.

- A variety of patterns occur in abnormal discs, whereas the normal nucleus assumes a globular or bilobed ("hamburger") pattern. However, none of these patterns are indicative of discogenic pain. (See Figure 76-1).

- Positive diagnosis can be ascertained only by the patient's subjective response to disc injection.

CERVICAL DISCOGRAPHY

- Cervical discs are embryologically and morphologically different from lumbar discs and the pathology of painful cervical discs remains elusive.

- Besides the usual risks of discography, a cervical discography has the added risk of clinically significant hemorrhage, myelopathy, and esophageal puncture. A risk-benefit analysis prior to performing this procedure is highly advisable.

- During discography, the patient lies supine on the fluoroscopy table with gentle neck extension. As the esophagus lies to the left in the lower neck, the right-sided approach is preferable. Firm but gentle pressure applied at the point of needle insertion to displace the great vessels laterally and the laryngeal structures and trachea medially.

- The needle is advanced slowly into the substance of the disc under direct fluoroscopic visualization. Once the needle is passed several millimeters into the disc, the lateral view is recommended to guide further advancement, taking precaution to not pass the needle through the disc and into the epidural space or spinal cord.

- Once the tip of the needle has been correctly placed in the center of the disc, manual syringe pressure is increased slowly. Concordancy and pain intensity are recorded at the time of distention and at 0.1–0.2 mL increments. The volume of dye that the disc accepts should be noted. A normal cervical disc offers firm resistance and accepts 0.25–1.0 mL of solution.

COMPLICATIONS

- Vasovagal reactions, especially for cervical discography.
- Needle misplacement can result in penetration of the viscera and pneumothorax, arterial puncture, and damage of nerve roots, thecal sac puncture, and headaches.
- Infection is usually inocculated from skin surface organisms or midadventure through bowel perforation, and may involve epidural abscess, retropharyngeal abscess, and discitis and osteomyelitis.

PREVENTION OF DISCITIS

- To avoid infection, stringent attention to aseptic technique is critical. All the procedures should be performed under sterile conditions with double gloves.
- The causative organisms of discitis are typically *Staphylococcus aureus*, *Staphylococcus epidermidis*, and *Escherichia coli*.
- Prophylactic intravenous antibiotics (cefazolin 1 g, gentamicin 80 mg, clindamycin 900 mg, or ciprofloxacin 400 mg) are given right before the procedure.
- Along with IV antibiotics, many discographers mix antibiotics with contrast dye (between 1 and 6 mg/mL of cefazolin or an equivalent dose of another antibiotic) for intradiscal administration.

VALIDITY

- As a provocative test, discography has been criticized to have a potentially high false-positive rate. The reasons for that could be due to technical errors, due to neurophysiological phenomena, or due to psychosocial factors.
- Recent advances in discography technique, including use of pressure-controlled manometry and adherence to strict diagnostic criteria, help improve validity of this test significantly. If strict criteria are applied, lumbar discography is very specific in subjects with normal psychometric profiles without chronic pain.
- A recent meta-analysis of studies of asymptomatic subjects undergoing discography showed a high specificity of 0.94 (95% CI 0.89–0.98) and a relatively low false-positive rate of 6%.

UTILITY

- In patients with chronic intractable neck or back pain but negative or indeterminate imaging findings who are being considered for surgical intervention, discography can help localize the symptomatic level and potentially benefit patients by surgical intervention or help avoid an unnecessary intervention in case of negative discography results.
- Discography is an invasive test that can be associated with short- and long-term risks. When indicated and correctly performed, it is a safe and sometimes powerful complement to the overall clinical context and not intended to be a stand-alone test.

INTRADISCAL THERMAL THERAPIES

CONCEPTS

- Intradiscal thermal therapies refer to a group of percutaneous interventions that deliver heat energy to the intervertebral disc with the goal of reducing chronic back pain of discogenic origin.
- Inflammation, anatomic derangement of the disc tissue and abnormal disc mechanics are considered to be possible etiologic factors in developing discogenic back pain.
- Thermal destruction of nociceptive fibers, shrinking subannular disc protrusions, sealing annular tears, improving delaminated annular tissue by collagen modification, and stimulation of healing response have been proposed mechanisms of intradiscal thermal therapies in an attempt to alleviate discogenic pain. Scientific evidence to support such mechanisms of action in the literature is lacking
- The heat delivered with these therapies can be generated through a variety of means, including electrocautery, thermal cautery, laser, and radiofrequency energy. Variety of radiofrequency (RF) probes and catheters as well as resistive heating coils (such as

IDET, or intradiscal electrothermal therapy) have been developed and used.

- Most intradiscal thermal treatments are performed using radiofrequency energy, which may be applied with unipolar or bipolar probes, passed through an introducer needle into the outer postero-lateral annulus or passed across the posterior annulus.
- Bipolar probes are thought to allow for greater control and focus of the energy. One of the newer methods of increasing size or volume of the lesion is by cooling the RF electrodes internally, called intradiscal biacuplasty (IDB) procedure.
- Strict selection of patients with specific discogenic pain, possibly confirmed by provocative discography test, may improve results of intradiscal thermal therapies, and provide patients with minimally invasive approach, potentially avoiding spinal fusion surgery.

THEORY

- The precise mechanism of action of intradiscal heating in helping patients with back pain is unclear.
- Tissue modulation, including shrinkage, denaturation, and structural changes to collagen fibers in the annulus to increase annular stability and disc biomechanics, are some of the proposed hypothesis.
- Another possible mechanism of action is denervation of ingrown nociceptors by neuroablation of the posterior annulus and elimination of transmission of pain symptoms from the denervated disc.
- Targeted thermal therapy can induce collagen fibril shrinkage at temperatures greater than 60°C and destruction of neural tissue at temperatures above 42°C to 45°C.
- The typical IDET procedure can generate only sufficient heat to produce nerve ablation. Collagen modification may not be a primary effect.
- Current protocols might not cause either fissure closure or improved disc stability.
- The histologic findings are denaturation, shrinkage, and coalescence of annular collagen and stromal disorganization after IDET.

PROCEDURES

- Most intradiscal thermal therapy procedures target the outer and posterior annulus of the disc, using number of devices that deliver heat energy. The procedures are completed under fluoroscopy and minimal sedation.
- IDET uses a fluoroscopically guided intradiscal catheter inserted into the nucleus and circumferentially navigated to the outer annulus and heated

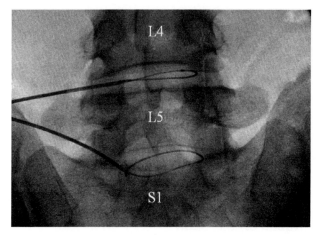

FIG. 76-2. IDET procedure (AP fluoroscopy image). The eletrothermal wires are positioned within the L4–5 and L5–S1 discs.

using either electrothermal energy or radiofrequency energy (RFE). The heating coil in the distal 5 cm of the catheter is heated to 90°C for 16–17 minutes. Proper catheter position is one of the key elements to obtaining good results. (Figure 76-2)

- Intradiscal radiofrequency treatment (IDRT) targets the outer annulus using an electrode passed through an introducer needle inserted into the outer posterior lateral annulus and passed across the posterior annulus.
- Cooled bipolar RFE or intradiscal biacuplasty (IDB) procedure uses a bipolar system that includes two radiofrequency probes placed on the posterolateral sides of the annulus 2.5–3 cm apart, and cooled using circulating water pumped through a cannula. The probes are heated to 45°C for 15 minutes while water is continuously circulated around the probes. The heating is typically less painful than heating using the IDET catheters (Figure 76-3).

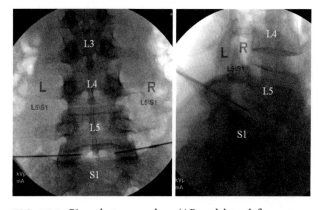

FIG. 76-3. Biacuplasty procedure (AP and lateral fluoroscopy images). Two water-cooled radiofrequency electrodes (Baylis Medical, Inc.) are placed on the posterolateral side of the annulus within the L5–S1 disc.

- Cooled RFE electrodes are thought to increase the lesion size and facilitate ablation when compared with standard RFE electrodes, whereas linear placement of the two electrodes makes the procedure easier to perform.
- The patient must be alert enough to be observed for the development of radicular pain during the procedure.
- To prevent discitis, the most serious potential complication of the procedures, pre-procedural intravenous antibiotics, and intradiscal antibiotic injection after heating (2–20 mg cefazolin) is recommended.

INCLUSION CRITERIA

- Unremitting, chronic axial low back pain of at least six months of duration.
- No improvement with aggressive nonoperative care.
- Absence of neural compressive lesions on MRI as well as instability or stenosis.
- Positive discography test with reproduction of concordant pain at low pressurization at one or two intervertebral disc levels.
- Preservation of greater than 50% of the disc height.

EXCLUSION CRITERIA

- Greater than 50% disc height loss.
- Major psychological impairment.
- Pregnancy.
- Extruded or sequestered herniation.
- Moderate to severe spinal stenosis and spondylolysthesis.
- Nerve root compression with motor deficit.
- Medical or metabolic disorder that would preclude appropriate follow-up and participation, as well as systemic infection and inflammatory arthritis.
- Prior surgery at the symptomatic level(s) (as a relative contraindication).

OUTCOMES

- The current peer-reviewed literature report conflicting evidence regarding the effectiveness of intradiscal heat treatments for chronic discogenic back pain.
- Two published randomized controlled trials (RCTs) evaluated annular heating using the IDET method. One found no effect of either the sham or IDET procedure; the other found statistical improvement in IDET group compared to sham control in VAS scores and the 36-item Short-Form Health Survey (SF-36), particularly in physical function, bodily pain, and sitting tolerance scores.

- There is a weak support in favor of using IDET over continued conservative care.
- Recent randomized placebo-controlled study of biacuplasty for treatment of discogenic pain showed statistically significant improvements in physical function, pain, and disability at six months follow-up as compared to sham group. Observational study showed a 50% decrease in VAS scores in 50% of patients at six months follow-up.
- Even though there is a lack of evidence that intradiscal heating is effective, it is significantly less invasive than conventional surgical options and may, therefore, be beneficial for a small subset of patients who fail to improve after conservative therapy or who are not appropriate surgical candidates.

COMPLICATIONS

- Serious complications following percutaneous intradiscal thermal procedures are infrequent.
- Possible complications include:
  - Catheter breakage (0.05%)
  - Nerve root injury
  - Discitis (0%-1.3%)
  - Osteonecrosis of the vertebral body
  - Epidural abscess
  - Acute lumbar disc herniation (0.3%)
  - Cauda equina syndrome

BIBLIOGRAPHY

Aprill C, Bogduk N. High-intensity zone: a diagnostic sign of painful lumbar disc on magnetic resonance imaging. *Br J Radiol.* 1992;65(773):361–369.

Bogduk N. Practice guidelines: spinal diagnostic and treatment procedures. In: Bogduk N, ed. *Lumbar Disc Stimulation (Provocation Discography).* San Francisco, Ca.: International Spine Intervention Society; 2004:20–46.

Carragee EJ, Don AS, Hurwitz EL, et al. Does discography cause accelerated progression of degeneration changes in the lumbar disc: a ten-year matched cohort study. *Spine (Phila Pa 1976).* 2009;13(21):2338–2345.

Coppes MH, Marani E, Thomeer RT, Groen Gj. Innervation of "painful" lumbar discs. *Spine.* 1997;22(20):2342–2349.

Derby R, Baker RM, Melnik I, et al. Chap 27. Intradiscal thermal therapies. In: Dagenais S, Haldeman S, eds. *Evidence-Based Management of Low Back Pain.* St. Louis, Mo.: Elsevier Mosby; 2012:364–388.

Derby R, Eek B, Chen Y, O'Neill C, Ryan D. Intradiscal electrothermal annuloplasty (IDET): a novel approach for treating chronic discogenic back pain. *Neuromodulation: Technology at the Neural Interface.* 2000;3(2):82–88.

Derby R, Howard MW, Grant JM, Lettice JJ, Van Peteghem PK, Ryan Dp. The ability of pressure-controlled discography to predict surgical and nonsurgical outcomes. *Spine*. 1999;24(4):364–371.

Derby R, Kim B-J, Chen Y, Seo K-S, Lee S-H. The relation between annular disruption on computed tomography scan and pressure-controlled diskography. *Arch Phys Med Rehab*. 2005;86(8):1534–1538.

Djurasovic M, Glassman SD, Dimar JR 2nd, Johnson Jr. Vertebral osteonecrosis associated with the use of intradiscal electrothermal therapy: a case report. *Spine*. 2002;27(13):E325–E328.

Freemont AJ, Peacock TE, Goupille P, Hoyland JA, O'Brien J, Jayson Mi. Nerve ingrowth into diseased intervertebral disc in chronic back pain. *Lancet*. 1997;350(9072):178–181.

Gill K, Blumenthal SL. Functional results after anterior lumbar fusion at L5-S1 in patients with normal and abnormal MRI scans. *Spine (Phila Pa 1976)*. 1992;17(8):940–942.

Guyer RD, Ohnmeiss DD. Lumbar discography. Position statement from the North American Spine Society Diagnostic and Therapeutic Committee. *Spine*. 1995;20(18):2048–2059.

Helm S, Hayek SM, Benyamin RM, Manchikanti L. Systematic review of the effectiveness of thermal annular procedures in treating discogenic low back pain. *Pain Physician*. 2009;12(1):207–232.

Kapural L, Ng A, Dalton J, et al. Intervertebral disc biacuplasty for the treatment of lumbar discogenic pain: results of a six-month follow-up. *Pain Med*. 2008;9(1):60–67.

Kapural L, Vrooman B, Sarwar S, et al. A randomized, placebo-controlled trial of transdiscal radiofrequency, biacuplasty for treatment of discogenic lower back pain. *Pain Medicine*. 2013;14(3):362–373.

Kleinstueck FS, Diederich CJ, Nau WH, et al. Acute biomechanical and histological effects of intradiscal electrothermal therapy on human lumbar discs. *Spine*. 2001;26(20):2198–2207.

Klessig HT, Showsh SA, Sekorski A. The use of intradiscal antibiotics for discography: an in vitro study of gentamicin, cefazolin, and clindamycin. *Spine*. 2003;28(15):1735–1738.

Manchikanti L, Singh V, Pampati V, et al. Evaluation of the relative contributions of various structures in chronic low back pain. *Pain Physician*. 2001;4(4):308–316.

Melnik I, Derby R, Baker R. Provocative discography (Chapter 45). In: Deer TR, Leong MS, Buvanendran A, et al., eds. *Comprehensive Treatment of Chronic Pain by Medical, Interventional, and Integrative Approaches the AAPM (American Academy of Pain Medicine): Textbook on Patient Management*. New York: Springer; 2013:461–478.

Osti OL, Fraser RD, Vernon-Roberts B. Discitis after discography. The role of prophylactic antibiotics. *J Bone Joint Surg. (British Volume)*. 1990;72(2):271–274.

Peng B, Wu W, Hou S, Li P, Zhang C, Yang Y. The pathogenesis of discogenic low back pain. *J Bone Joint Surg*. 2005;87(1):62–67.

Podichetty VK. The aging spine: the role of inflammatory mediators in intervertebral disc degeneration. *Cell Mol Biol (Noisy-le-grand)*. 2007;53(5):4–18.

Roberts S, Eisenstein SM, Menage J, Evans EH, Ashton Ik. Mechanoreceptors in intervertebral discs. Morphology, distribution, and neuropeptides. *Spine*. 1995;20(24):2645–2651.

Saal JA, Saal JS. Intradiscal electrothermal treatment for chronic discogenic low back pain: prospective outcome study with a minimum two-year follow-up. *Spine (Phila Pa 1976)*. 2002;27(9):966–973; discussion 73–74.

Sachs BL, Vanharanta H, Spivey MA, et al. Dallas discogram description. A new classification of CT/discography in low-back disorders. *Spine*. 1987;12(3):287–294.

Schwarzer AC, Aprill CN, Derby R, Fortin J, Kine G, Bogduk N. The prevalence and clinical features of internal disc disruption in patients with chronic low back pain. *Spine*. 1995;20(17):1878–1883.

Shah RV, Lutz GE, Lee J, Doty SB, Rodeo S. Intradiskal electrothermal therapy: a preliminary histologic study. *Arch Phys Med Rehab*. 2001;82(9):1230–1237.

Troussier B, Lebas JF, Chirossel JP, et al. Percutaneous intradiscal radio-frequency thermocoagulation. A cadaveric study. *Spine*. 1995;20(15):1713–1718.

Walsh TR, Weinstein JN, Spratt KF, Lehmann TR, Aprill C, Sayre H. Lumbar discography in normal subjects. A controlled, prospective study. *J Bone Joint Surg*. 1990;72(7):1081–1088.

Wolfer LR, Derby R, Lee J-E, Lee S-H. Systematic review of lumbar provocation discography in asymptomatic subjects with a meta-analysis of false-positive rates. *Pain Physician*. 2008;11(4):513–538.

77 MINIMALLY INVASIVE LUMBAR DISC DECOMPRESSION

Ramsin Benyamin, M.D.

INTRODUCTION

Percutaneous lumbar disc decompression (PLDD) refers to several techniques that are utilized for disc material extraction of patients with disc herniations. Mixter and Barr first described the surgical treatment for intervertebral disc ruptures in 1934 and since then, open surgical procedures for discectomies have become a popular procedure, despite the limited evidence to support its efficacy. Hemilaminectomies and discectomies were initially performed to address the pain and symptoms of intervertebral disc herniations. Open microdiscectomies that involve the dilation of paraspinus muscles, rather than stripping the muscles followed as an alternative technique to reduce morbidity rates. Minimally invasive percutaneous procedures for disc decompression were then developed as a less invasive way of performing microdiscectomies. This approach yields less tissue damage and has faster recovery times.

Pain as a result of disc herniations is likely due to ventral compression and vascular ischemia of nerve roots. The PLDD procedures are best suited for contained disc herniations with radiculopathy. Complications arise and the treatment can be less effective if used on uncontained disc herniations, patients who have narrowed intervertebral disc space or obstructive vertebral abnormalities, cauda equina syndrome, and severe paresis. Additionally, these techniques work best for those patients who have single-level herniations.

INDICATIONS

- Back and/or leg pain for at least three months with leg pain greater than back pain.
- Contained disc herniation that fails to respond to 6 weeks of conservative therapy.
- Unilateral leg pain with positive straight leg raise and/or bowstring sign.
- Disc height preservation of 60% original height.
- Corresponding positive imaging findings for subligamentous contained disc herniation.

CONTRAINDICATIONS

- Severe lateral recess stenosis, calcification of disc herniation, ligamentum flavum hypertrophy causing spinal stenosis, or severe degenerative facet disease with corresponding radiologic evidence.
- Cauda equina syndrome, free or extruded disc fragments in the spinal canal, or disc degeneration causing height loss of more than 50%.
- Disc herniation extending cephalad or caudad, grade V annular tear, or significant sclerotic end plate changes.
- Large, noncontained disc herniation, sequestration, or extension.
- Fractures, tumors, pregnancy, coagulopathy, or active systemic infection.

CHRONIC LOW BACK PAIN ALGORITHM (FIGURE 77-1)

- PLDD is reserved for patients that have failed more conservative therapies.
- Non-interventional therapies should be tried first.
- If non-invasive therapies fail, spine interventional therapies may be indicated with the therapy dependent upon the source of the pain (Figure 77-1).

TECHNICAL MODALITIES

Technical variations of percutaneous lumbar disc decompression include the DeKompressor, Automated Percutaneous Lumbar Discectomy (APLD), Hydrocision, and Nucleoplasty. Other means of PLDD include injections of Chymopapain, Nucleotome, and laser decompression including LASE and the Holmium YAG laser.

- Chymopapain was a very popular enzymatic injection, but in a small percentage of patients was associated with anaphylactic shock, transverse myelitis, subarachnoid hemorrhage, paraplegia, and postoperative back spasms. This led to its discontinuation in the United States.
- Nucleotome is a very safe technique that minimizes the risk of cutting the anterior annulus and endplate damage by using an enclosed guillotine cutting action that re-sects and aspirates the nucleus in one step.
- Percutaneous laser discectomy (LASE) vaporizes nuclear material using most commonly the Holmium YAG laser where a laser fiber is inserted through the cannula into the center of the nucleus pulposus and laser energy is then delivered into the nucleus. The Holmium YAG laser has a steerable catheter tip for more precise, directional therapy.

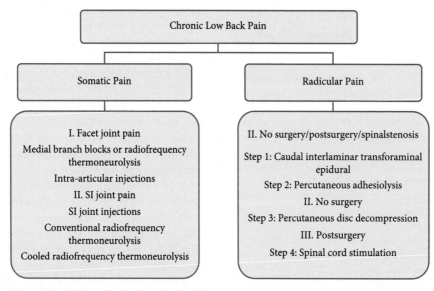

FIG. 77-1. Chronic low back pain algorithm.

DeKompressor

- It is a mechanical high revolutions per minute device that uses the Archimedes screw to selectively extract disc material from disc herniations without annular or nuclear disruption. When activated, the probe rotates creating suction and removal of the nucleus pulposus.
- Outcomes are relatively similar to nucleoplasty, in the long term, at reducing the use of oral opioid analgesics, disability, pain scores, and occupational incapacitation.
- A standard discography approached is used when performing the DeKompressor procedure. Fluoroscopy is used to guide a cannula and stylet into the targeted disc and confirm the needle position. The stylet is then removed and the DeKompressor probe is advanced through the cannula into the disc. The DeKompressor is then activated and the targeted amount intervertebral disc nucleus is removed, reducing the size of the disc herniation.
- This process relieves the nerve compression caused by the herniation, resulting in a reduction of pain.
- Literature reviews have shown reductions in pain in the short- and long-term are results of the DeKompressor procedure. In a multicenter study, Alo et al. determined that the DeKompressor technique results in a 65% pain reduction, 79% analgesic reduction, 90% functional improvement, and 88% patient satisfaction over one year.
- DeKompressor procedure, like most intradiscal procedures, has a slight risk of infection and mild back pain at the site is a common and short-lived complication of the procedure.
- Other risks that are uncommon include spinal cord compression, increased intra-cranial pressure from compression of spinal fluid, and bleeding.
- The rare but still notable complication of the DeKompressor procedure is that in a very small number of instances the probe broke while in the patient's body, having to be removed surgically. These patients were reported recovered with no further issues or complications related to the device or procedure.

Automated Percutaneous Lumbar Discectomy

- APLD is designed for patients with contained disc herniations; otherwise, the procedure is less likely to be effective.
- This is an outpatient procedure done under local anesthesia and fluoroscopic guidance. Using a guide needle under fluoroscopy, the physician guides the needle into the nucleus pulposus, where a 2.8-mm cannula is inserted. The needle is then withdrawn and a pneumatically driven, suction-cutting probe is placed through the cannula into the center of the disc. The cannula is then activated and extracts nuclear material, which is then cut loose. This relieves intradiscal pressure, which results in the alleviation of symptoms.
- One of the main reasons for reported APLD failure is using the technique for herniations that are not appropriate for the procedure.
- APLD only effectively relieves pain when performed on contained disc herniations. Additionally, patients treated with APLD have leg pain as the primary source of pain, rather than back pain.
- It has also been noted that outcomes with APLD are not as favorable as open microdiscectomies or chemonucleolysis.
- According to published evidence, APLD results in moderate relief for the short term and limited relief for the long term.

Hydrocision

- Percutaneous hydrodiscectomy using hydrocision removes disc material using a sterile thermal saline solution, applied at a high velocity, to perform disc decompression.
- Challenges include special detail to the safety of the device, assurances that the fluid is sterile, and the size and maneuverability of the tools to be able to successfully perform the procedure.
- The procedure is performed using a local anesthetic and mild sedation. Minimal tissue trauma, blood loss, and complications are expected.
- Hydrocision allows for the removal of soft tissue, specifically disc nucleus, with no potential damage to other tissues or vertebral endplates, making the procedure safe and allowing for a reduction of pain with minimal risk.
- In a multicenter retrospective review of patients who failed conservative management of their HNP and hydrocision was performed, 94% experienced significant improvement in back and radicular leg pain. Hydrocision, when compared to conventional tools used in the excision of disc material, results in greater disc area preparation and removal with no endplate damage over a shorter period of time.
- Hydrocision is a more effective technique for disc removal in preparation for bone grafting or fusion surgery. Hydrocision is not only effective for disc decompression, but the preservation of endplate material and the ability to remove the maximum amount of disc material makes it a superior technique to complement transforaminal lumbar interbody fusion (TLIF).

Nucleoplasty

- The nucleoplasty technique decreases disc protrusion and pressure, often allowing for alleviation of radicular symptoms associated with nerve impingement from the disc displacement.

- After a probe is placed into the disc, a small amount of the nucleus is removed using the Controlled Ablation (Coblation) technology. Coblation results in dissolving tissue by plasma created through a non-heat driven process. Nucleoplasty reduces disc pressure with minimum thermal damage to surrounding tissues, even though the equipment is capable of radiofrequency coagulation during the retraction of the wand. Radiofrequency is not required for disc decompression.
- Initial systematic reviews of the literature revealed that nucleoplasty is effective in relieving leg pain, but not back pain, and that these initial trials were not well controlled based on USPSTF guidelines. Later reviews focused more on the type of herniation. A systematic review focused on nucleoplasty for contained disc herniations revealed limited to fair evidence that nucleoplasty reduces or manages the radicular symptoms and pain associated with contained disc herniations.
- Research shows that the evidence for nucleoplasty as an effective treatment for low back pain and radicular symptoms is minimal. However, the treatment proves to be effective in removing the maximum amount of disc material with minimal damage to peripheral tissues and structures surrounding the disc.

SIDE EFFECTS AND COMPLICATIONS

- The side effects and complications are controlled with proper technique.
- Primary risks include bleeding, infection, and nerve injury.
- Nerve injury is caused by improper decompression or needle insertion and minimized by using image guidance and minimal sedation.
- Infections are minimized by proper sterilization and prophylactic use of antibiotics.
- Complications that result in the need for open discectomies include adjacent endplate damage, development of spinal instability, and/or progressive degeneration.

BIBLIOGRAPHY

Armin S, Holly L, Khoo L. Minimally invasive decompression for lumbar stenosis and disc herniation. *Neurosurg Focus.* 2008;25(2):E11.

Hardenbrook MA, Gannon DP Jr, Younan E, Amoroso ML, Rodriguez JE, Prvulovic TT. Clinical outcomes of patients treated with percutaneous hydrodiscectomy for radiculopathy secondary to lumbar herniated nucleus pulposus. *Internet J Spine Surg.* 2013;7(1).

Hirsch JA, Singh V, Falco FJ, Benyamin RM, Manchikanti L. Automated percutaneous lumbar discectomy for the contained herniated lumbar disc: a systematic assessment of evidence. *Pain Physician.* 2009, May–June;12(3):601–620.

Huh H-Y, Ji C, Ryu K-S, Park C-K. Comparison of SpineJet™ XL and conventional instrumentation for disk space preparation in unilateral transforaminal lumbar interbody fusion. *J Korean Neurosurg Soc.* 2010, May;47(5):370–376.

Javernick MA, Kuklo TR, Polly DW Jr. Transforaminal lumbar interbody fusion: unilateral versus bilateral disk removal—an in vivo study. *Am J Orthop (Belle Mead NJ).* 2003, July;32(7):344–348.

Lemcke J, Al-Zain F, Mutze S, Meier U. Minimally invasive spinal surgery using nucleoplasty and the Dekompressor tool: a comparison of two methods in a one year follow-up. *Minim Invasive Neurosurg.* 2010, October;53(5–6):236–242.

Manchikanti L, Derby R, Benyamin RM, Helm S., Hirsch JA. A systematic review of mechanical lumbar disc decompression with nucleoplasty. *Pain Physician.* 2009;12(3):561–572.

Manchikanti L, Falco FJ, Benyamin RM, et al. An update of the systematic assessment of mechanical lumbar disc decompression with nucleoplasty. *Pain Physician.* 2013;16(2 Suppl):SE25–SE54.

Schenka B, Brouwera PA, Peulb WC, van Buchema MA. Percutaneous laser disk decompression: A review of the literature. *Am J Neuroradiol.* 2006, January;27:232–235.

Singh V, Benyamin RM, Datta S, Falco FJ, Helm S 2nd, Manchikanti L. Systematic review of percutaneous lumbar mechanical disc decompression utilizing Dekompressor. *Pain Physician.* 2009, May–June;12(3):589–599.

Singh V, Manchikanti L, Benyamin R, Helm S, Hirsch J. Percutaneous lumbar laser disc decompression: a systematic review of current evidence. *Pain Physician.* 2009;12:573–588.

Singh V, Manchikanti L, Calodney A, et al. Percutaneous lumbar laser disc decompression: an update of current evidence. *Pain Physician.* 2013;16:SE229–SE260.

78 LYSIS OF ADHESIONS

Miles R. Day, MD
Gabor Racz, MD

INTRODUCTION

- Low back pain, with or without radicular symptoms, is a common medical condition that triggers mild to severe suffering, high health costs, and disability.
- The vast majority of low back pain sufferers recovers in a relatively short period and is left without sequelae.
- The less fortunate patients, in whom resolution of the condition does not occur despite aggressive therapy, find themselves without a definite or completely effective treatment.

- Developing an understanding of the pathophysiology underlying the pain and designing target-specific treatment modalities may enhance the occurrence of successful outcomes.
- The past 15–20 years have seen tremendous progress in the understanding of neural pathways and the extent of tissue involvement in back pain. This understanding has triggered the development of new treatment approaches.

HISTORY

- Cathelin performed one of the first documented epidural injections for chronic pain in 1901.
- Sicard and Forstier performed the first epidurography in 1921.
- In 1950, when Payne and Rupp combined hyaluronidase with a local anesthetic in an attempt to alter the rapidity of onset, extent, intensity, and duration of caudal anesthesia, they demonstrated maximal efficacy in a group receiving local anesthetic, hyaluronidase, and epinephrine. The hyaluronidase used in this study was relatively dilute at 6 U/mL, with an average volume of injection of 25 mL.
- In 1951, Moore added 150 U of hyaluronidase to enhance the spread of the local anesthetic that he used in 1,309 nerve blocks, including 20 caudal blocks. His work confirmed that hyaluronidase is relatively nontoxic.
- Liévre and coworkers reported the first injection of a corticosteroid into the epidural space for the treatment of sciatica in 1957. They injected a combination of hydrocortisone acetate (dose unknown) and radiopaque dye in 46 patients, with 31 positive results.
- In 1960, Goebert and colleagues reported good results after injecting 30 mL of 1% procaine with 125 mg hydrocortisone acetate hydrocortisone into the caudal epidural space.
- That same year, Brown injected 40–100 mL of normal saline followed by 80 mg methylprednisolone in an attempt to mechanically disrupt and prevent reformation of presumably fibrotic lesions in patients with sciatica. He reported complete resolution of pain for two months in his four patients. This investigation laid the theoretical foundation for therapies in which specific catheter placement is crucial to the effective treatment of epidural adhesions.
- Administration of cold hypertonic saline intrathecally was first described by Hitchcock in 1967 for the treatment of chronic pain. In 1969, he reported that the hypertonicity rather than the temperature of the solution was the determining factor in its therapeutic effect.
- Intrathecal hypertonic saline was subsequently employed by Ventafridda and Spreafico in 1974 for intractable cancer pain. All 21 patients in this study had pain relief at 24 hours, although only three reported relief at 30 days.
- Racz and Holubec in 1989 reported the first use of epidural hypertonic saline to facilitate the lysis of adhesions.
- Stolker et al. introduced hyaluronidase as an alternative agent in 1994.

WHY ADHESIONS?

- Connective tissues, or any kind of tissue, naturally form fibrous layers (scar tissue) after disruption of the intact milieu.
- The tissues surrounding neural structures behave in the same fashion, trapping nerve roots and exposing them to continuous pressures as well as to stretching, which sensitizes the nerves.
- In 1991, Kushlich et al. published their observation that sciatica-like pain was generated by pressure on the anulus fibrosus and posterior longitudinal ligament, as well as by swollen, stretched, or compressed nerve roots. All 193 of their patients who had undergone laminectomies under local anesthesia developed perineural fibrous tissue. While this scar tissue was never sensitive, the nerve root was frequently very tender. This led to the conclusion that pain to the nerve roots that are trapped by scar tissue might be associated with fixation of these affected nerve roots and susceptibility to tension and compression.

HOW TO DIAGNOSE EPIDURAL FIBROSIS?

- Radiologic studies, such as MRI and CT scan (including CT myelography), are of limited diagnostic value.
- Epidurography is more effective in diagnosing scar tissue because injected dye forms a filling defect. If this defect correlates with the neurologic abnormality, it helps formulate a diagnosis.

WHAT TO DO?

- These tissue changes can trigger back pain and radicular symptoms, for which treatment might seem difficult. Thus, a great many patients are labeled with a diagnosis of "intractable chronic low back pain syndrome."
- Attempts to treat this pain range from increasing medical treatment by escalating drug dosages and submitting the patient to unsuccessful and frustrating physical therapy trials to conducting interventions, such as epidural steroid injections and selective nerve

root blocks, both of which offer only very transient relief.
- If no attempt is made to release the neural structures from fibrous scar tissue, all of these treatment options are likely to be unsuccessful.
- This is why, in 1989, Dr. Gabor B. Racz developed the procedure known as "lysis of adhesions (epidural decompressive neuroplasty)" at Texas Tech University. Other synonyms include adhesiolysis and the Racz procedure.
- Lysis of adhesions can be performed in the cervical, thoracic, and lumbar epidural regions.
- The addition of a transforaminal catheter is sometimes necessary in patients with multilevel pathology.

CAUDAL EPIDURAL DECOMPRESSIVE NEUROPLASTY (LYSIS OF ADHESIONS)

INDICATIONS

- Failed back surgery
- Radiculopathy unresponsive to interlaminar or transforaminal epidural steroid injections
- Internal disc disruption
- Traumatic vertebral body compression fracture
- Metastatic carcinoma of the spine leading to compression fracture
- Multilevel degenerative arthritis
- Facet pain refractory to medial branch nerve blocks
- Epidural scarring following the resolution of infection or meningitis
- Pain unresponsive to spinal cord stimulation
- Pain unresponsive to spinal opioids
- Pathologic vertebral compression fracture
- Osteoporotic vertebral compression fracture

CONTRAINDICATIONS

- Sepsis
- Coagulopathy
- Local infection at the site of the procedure
- Arachnoiditis secondary to concerns with loculation
- Syrinx formation secondary to pressure concerns leading to cord ischemia.

TECHNIQUE

- After informed consent is obtained, this elective operative procedure is performed under monitored anesthesia care. General anesthesia should be avoided to decrease the possibility of complications, as communication with the patient is crucial.

- Prophylactic antibiotics are administered intravenously with ceftriaxone sodium (Rocephin) 1 g or cephazolin (Ancef) 1 g within 30 minutes of the start of the procedure. If the patient is allergic to penicillin, we prescribe oral quinolones (ciprofloxacin or levofloxacin) 1 hour prior to the start of the procedure and both cephalexin (Keflex) 500 mg orally every 12 hours or quinolones orally every day for five days.
- The patient is placed in the prone position with a pillow under the abdominal area and ankles.
- C-arm fluoroscopy is available.
- The lumbosacral region is prepped and draped.
- The sacral hiatus is palpated, and a skin wheal is raised 1 cm lateral and 2 cm caudal to the sacral hiatus on the side opposite the suspected epidural scarring.
- The skin is pierced with an 18-gauge needle, and a 16-gauge RX coudé needle is inserted through the sacral hiatus into the epidural canal.
- Correct needle positioning is confirmed with fluoroscopic views in the anteroposterior as well as the lateral planes. The tip of the needle should not be advanced beyond the S3 foramen as this will decrease the chance of puncturing a low-lying dura.
- If, at this point, cerebral spinal fluid is aspirated or withdrawn from the needle, the needle should be removed and the procedure aborted and rescheduled.
- After any negative aspiration of fluid (cerebral spinal fluid, blood, etc.), we inject 5–10 mL of iohexol (Omnipaque 240 mg/mL or Isovue M 200 mg/mL).
- If venous runoff occurs, the needle should be repositioned, and additional iohexol should be injected for confirmation. In a patient without pathology, the outline of the caudal epidural canal resembles a Christmas tree, with the branches being the nerve roots. In contrast, a patient with fibrosis of any origin will exhibit the filling defects (areas without contrast spread) that indicate adhesions potentially created by scar tissue.
- A Tun-L-Kath/24 or a stiffer Tun-L-XL/24 (which will facilitate directional control) epidural catheter is inserted through the needle and guided ventrally utilizing continuous fluoroscopy to the area of the filling defect. Before insertion, we bend the catheter about 30 degrees approximately 2.5 cm from the tip to aid with directional control. The target is the ventral lateral epidural space.
- A lateral view should be obtained to assist in placing the catheter in the ventral epidural space.
- When the position is confirmed, inject 1–2 additional mL of Omnipaque to further assess the epidural space at the target level.
- Next, 10 mL of preservative-free normal saline with 1500 U of hyaluronidase or 300 U of human

recombinant hyaluronidase (Hyelenex) is slowly injected.

- The final position of the tip of the catheter is confirmed by injecting 2–5 mL of iohexol, with fluoroscopic observation of the contrast spread into the previously nonvisualized area of the epidural space opened by removal of the scar tissue.
- This is followed by injection of 3 mL of a solution of 9 mL 0.2% ropivacaine and 1 mL of 4–10 mg/mL dexamethasone. After 5 minutes, if there is no evidence of motor–sensory block, the remaining 7 mL of mixture is injected.
- The epidural needle is then removed under fluoroscopic guidance to ensure that the catheter remains at the site of adhesions, and the catheter is anchored to the skin with a nylon suture. Triple antibiotic ointment is applied at the catheter site, which is covered with a sterile dressing. A microfilter is connected to the end of the catheter hub, and the three pieces are taped together.
- In the postanesthesia care unit, after 20 minutes have passed, 10 mL 10% hypertonic saline is infused for a minimum of 30 minutes after administration of local anesthesia, and the catheter is flushed with 2–3 mL of normal saline and recapped sterile.
- If the patient complains of severe discomfort, the infusion is stopped, and 2–3 mL of 0.2% ropivacaine is administered. After 5 minutes, the infusion is restarted.
- In our institution, the patient is admitted for a 23-hour observation period. The second and third infusions of 10 mL, 0.2% ropivacaine and 10 mL, 10% hypertonic saline are performed the following day, following the same guidelines as with the first infusion. The additional infusions should be separated by a minimum of 4 hours.
- Follow-up at our clinic is within 4 to 6 weeks post procedure for general assessment and reinforcement to continue the physical therapy exercises. The procedure may be repeated in three months if necessary.

TRANSFORAMINAL APPROACH

- A transforaminal approach is indicated when the suspected scar tissue cannot be reached through the caudal epidural approach or when severe scar tissue does not allow the caudal epidural catheter to open up the most cephalic areas (lumbar 3, lumbar 4 in most cases) that require this technique.
- When both caudal and transforaminal catheters are placed, the volume of injectate is 7 mL for each of the earlier mentioned solutions, through each catheter.

CERVICAL AND THORACIC LYSIS OF ADHESIONS

This technique can also be applied to the cervical and thoracic regions. The major differences are the amount of hyaluronidase, and the volumes of local anesthetic and hypertonic saline used. In the cervical region, volumes of 5–6 mL are used for each of the aforementioned substances, with 900 U of hyaluronidase dissolved in 5–6 mL of preservative-free normal saline. In the thoracic region, volumes of 8 mL are used and the dose of hyaluronidase is 1200 U. Transforaminal catheters are not used in these areas.

EPIDUROSCOPY

- Epiduroscopy has utility as an adjuvant technique to assist in the specific placement of catheters at the caudal epidural level because it allows for direct visualization of the type of scar tissue and creates a bigger path of lysis of scar tissue.
- At present, epiduroscopy is considered an experimental technique by medical insurers and, thus, is not covered under any policy.

COMPLICATIONS

- Any reaction to the medications.
- Unintended subdural or subarachnoid injection of local anesthetics or of any of the medications used for this procedure (this is avoidable when the practitioner has enough experience to recognize the fluoroscopic patterns that these injections cause).
- Spinal canal loculation of injected medications can occur if adequate runoff is not observed during the injection of the contrast media. Ischemia may occur secondary to direct compression of the nerve roots and/or spinal cord at the target level. This is especially worrisome in the cervical region where the epidural space is smaller. Fluid can spread from the injection site to the opposite side of the spinal canal along the epidural veins, and is prevented from spreading cephalad or caudad and through the neuroforamina, thus compressing the spinal cord from both sides. This is termed perivenous counter spread. If not recognized, intraoperative, disastrous consequences may occur.
- Bowel or bladder dysfunction from damage to neural structures.
- Bleeding.
- Infection.
- Shearing of the catheter.

RELEVANT LITERATURE

- Several recent articles have evaluated the lysis of adhesions procedure.
- Park et al. retrospectively evaluated epidural neuroplasty for cervical disc herniation in 128 patients who failed conservative therapy. Compared with preprocedural values, the pain numerical rating scale score demonstrated significant improvement at 1 day, and 1, 3, 6, and 12 months after the procedure ($P < 0.001$). The neck disability index was significantly reduced at 3, 6, and 12 months after the procedure ($P < 0.001$).
- Gerdesmeyer's group performed a randomized, double-blinded, placebo-controlled trial evaluating percutaneous adhesiolysis in chronic lumbar radicular pain. Ninety patients were randomized to two groups. In this study, one group received the lysis procedure and the other group a placebo consisting of a subcutaneously placed catheter. Both the primary outcome measure (percent change of Oswestry Disability Index scores at three months) and secondary measures (percent change of ODI and Visual Analogue Score at 6 and 12 months) improved significantly in the active treatment arm (>50% improvement over baseline) ($P < 0.01$).
- Manchikanti et al. published a randomized, controlled trial with two-year follow-up comparing percutaneous adhesiolysis versus caudal epidural injections in managing postlumbar surgery syndrome in 120 patients. Primary outcome was defined as 50% improvement in pain and Oswestry Disability Index. Eighty-two percent of patients in the adhesiolysis group at two years showed significant improvement compared to 5% in the control group receiving caudal epidural injections.
- Another study by Manchikanti's group assessed the effectiveness of percutaneous adhesiolysis in managing chronic low back pain secondary to central spinal stenosis. Seventy-one percent of patients ($n = 70$) at the end of two years achieved greater than 50% improvement in pain scores and ODI.
- Based on a systematic review published in *Pain Physician*, there is fair evidence that percutaneous adhesiolysis is effective in relieving low back and/or leg pain caused by postlumbar surgery syndrome and that there is fair evidence that percutaneous adhesiolysis is effective in relieving low back and/or leg pain caused by spinal stenosis.
- Park and Lee evaluated the effectiveness of percutaneous transforaminal adhesiolysis in 35 patients with lumbar neuroforaminal spinal stenosis. Improvement defined as little pain, moderate pain, or no pain was observed in 25 patients at 2 weeks and in 22 patients at 3 months after the procedure.

BIBLIOGRAPHY

Anderson G. Epidemiology of low back pain. *Acta Orthop Scand.* 1998;69:28.

Brown J. Pressure caudal anesthesia and back manipulation. *Northw Med.* 1960;59:905.

Burn J. Treatment of chronic lumbosciatic pain. *Proc R Soc Med.* 1973;66:544.

Gerdesmeyer L, Wagenpfeil S, Birkenmaier C, et al. Percutaneous epidural lysis of adhesions in chronic lumbar radicular pain: a randomized, double-blind, placebo-controlled study. *Pain Physician.* 2013;16:185–196.

Goebert H, Jallo S, Gardner W, et al. Sciatica: Treatment with epidural injections on procaine and hydrocortisone. *Cleve Clin Q.* 1960;27:191.

Helm S, Benyamin R, Chopra P, et al. Percutaneous adhesiolysis in the management of chronic low back pain in post lumbar surgery syndrome and spinal stenosis: a systematic review. *Pain Physician.* 2012;15:E435–E462.

Hitchcock E. Hypothermic subarachnoid irrigation for intractable pain. *Lancet.* 1967;1:1133.

Hitchcock E. Osmolytic neurolysis for intractable facial pain. *Lancet.* 1969;1:434.

Kushlich S, Ulstrom C, Michael C. The tissue origin of low back pain and sciatica. *Orthop Clin North Am.* 1991;22:181.

Lewandowski E. The efficacy of solutions used in caudal neuroplasty. *Pain Digest.* 1997;7:323.

Liévre J, Block-Michel H, Attali P. L'injection transsacrée, etude clinique et radiologique. *Bull Soc Med Paris.* 1957;73:110.

Lou L, Racz G, Heavner J. Percutaneous epidural neuroplasty. In: Waldman SD, Lambert R, eds. *Interventional Pain Management.* 2nd ed. Philadelphia, Pa.: WB Saunders; 2002.

Manchikanti L, Cash K, McManus C, Pampati V. Assessment of effectiveness of percutaneous adhesiolysis in managing chronic low back pain secondary to central spinal stenosis. *Int J Med Sci.* 2013;10:50–59.

Manchikanti L, Singh V, Cash K, Pampati V. Assessment of effectiveness of percutaneous adhesiolysis and caudal epidural injections in managing post lumbar surgery syndrome: 2-year follow-up of a randomized, controlled trial. *J Pain Res.* 2012;5:597–608.

Moore D. The use of hyaluronidase in local and nerve block analgesia other than spinal block: 1520 cases. *Anesthesiology.* 1951;12:611.

Park E, Park S, Lee S, et al. Clinical outcomes of epidural neuroplasty for cervical disc herniation. *J Korean Med Sci.* 2013;28:461–465.

Park C, Lee S. Effectiveness of percutaneous transforaminal adhesiolysis in patients with lumbar neuroforaminal spinal stenosis. *Pain Physician.* 2013;16:E37–E43.

Payne J, Rupp N. The use of hyaluronidase in caudal block anesthesia. *Anesthesiology.* 1951;2:164.

Racz G, Heavner J. Cervical spinal canal loculation and secondary ischemic cord injury—PVCS—perivenous counter spread—danger sign! *Pain Practice.* 2008;8:399–403.

Racz G, Heavner J, Diede J. Lysis of epidural adhesions utilizing the epidural approach. In: Waldman SD, Winnie AP, eds. *Interventional Pain Management*. Philadelphia, Pa.: WB Saunders; 1996.

Racz G, Heavner J, Raj P. Nonsurgical management of spinal radiculopathy by the use of lysis of adhesions (neuroplasty). In: Aronoff GM, ed. *Evaluation and Treatment of Chronic Pain*. 3rd ed. 1999:533.

Racz G, Holubec J. Lysis of adhesions in the epidural space. In: Raj P, ed. *Techniques of Neurolysis*. Boston, Ma.: Kluwer Academic; 1989:57.

Racz G, Noe C, Heavner J. Selective spinal injections for lower back pain. *Curr Rev Pain*. 1999;3:333–341.

Sicard J, Forestier J. Méthode radiographique d'exploratione de la cavité épidurale par le lipiodol. *Rev Neurol*. 1921;28:1264.

Stolker R, Vervest A, Gerbrand J. The management of chronic spinal pain by blockades: a review. *Pain*. 1994;58:1.

Ventafridda V, Spreafico R. Subarachnoid saline perfusion. *Adv Neurol*. 1974;4:477.

79   DISABILITY/IMPAIRMENT

Gerald M. Aronoff, MD

PAIN IMPAIRMENT AND DISABILITY ISSUES

- Chronic pain is a major public health problem that inflicts tremendous personal suffering and, in the United States, has an annual cost exceeding $125 billion. Estimates suggest that up to 50% of the adult population reports continuous pain for at least three of the last six months.
- Between 1971 and 1981, the number of people with disabling back problems increased by 168%, whereas the population increased only by 12.5%.
- In the United States and other countries where entitlement programs are viewed as appealing alternatives to gainful employment, advances in technology and increased emphasis on interventional techniques to pain management have not appreciably improved the problem of pain-related disability.
- Often, no direct correlation exists between objective impairment and an individual's request for disability status. When economic conditions diminish job satisfaction and financial security, a "disability epidemic" can become a major public health problem.
- To reverse the "disability epidemic," our compensation and disability systems must offer incentives toward rehabilitation that encourage early intervention, prevention of chronicity, a functional restoration approach to treatment and timely return to work.

PHYSICIAN-RELATED DISABILITY ISSUES

- Compounding this epidemic is the failure of some medical practitioners to distinguish between impairment and disability, as well as confusion about what constitutes maximal medical improvement (MMI).
- Clinically, physicians cannot prove the existence of a patient's pain because there is no objective way to quantify pain. The "pain behavior" exhibited on examination may represent symptom embellishment or submaximal effort and may also represent conditioned, and goal-directed dysfunctional behavior.
- Excessive pain behavior may lead to unnecessary diagnostic testing or invasive procedures and result in iatrogenic complications and prolonged disability.
- Recipients of workers' compensation who have significant financial, psychosocial, and/or environmental reinforcement for their disability and little incentive to return to work may exhibit excessive pain behavior and be at increased risk of developing chronic pain syndromes unresponsive to conventional treatment.
- By overestimating impairment and imposing senseless activity limitations or restrictions, physicians and other healthcare providers can reinforce a disability syndrome. In vulnerable individuals, this is a major factor leading to iatrogenic disability.
- Maladaptive pain behavior may be modified or replaced by adaptive wellness behavior through behavioral intervention and psychotherapy. Therefore, patients with a chronic pain syndrome may need psychosocial treatment to achieve MMI.

IMPAIRMENT AND DISABILITY ASSESSMENT

- Despite the need to adopt a biopsychosocial–economic perspective for evaluation and treatment of chronic pain, disability evaluation systems often continue to apply a biomedical perspective.

KEY DEFINITIONS

- A "disability conviction" is the sufferer's belief that chronic pain impedes the ability to meet occupational demands, fulfill domestic and social responsibilities, or engage in avocational and recreational activities. A disability conviction is often based on cognitive distortions and abnormal behavior conditioned by being enmeshed in the healthcare system. However, the disability conviction may also be iatrogenic related to the healthcare providers imposing excessive limitations and restrictions, and not using a functional restoration approach to treatment.

- "Chronic pain syndrome" describes persistent pain accompanied by dysfunctional pain behavior, self-limitation in activities, delayed recovery from what would normally be anticipated, and a degree of life disruption disproportional to the pathophysiology. A chronic pain syndrome occurs when pain becomes the focal point of a patient's life.
- Impairment is "A loss, loss of use, or derangement of any body part, organ system, or organ function."
- Disability is "Alteration of an individual's capacity to meet personal, social, or occupational demands or statutory or regulatory requirements because of impairment. Disability is a relational outcome, contingent on the environmental conditions in which activities are performed."
- Maximal medical improvement (MMI) is "A condition or state that is well stabilized and unlikely to change substantially in the next year, with or without medical treatment. Over time, there may be some change; however, further recovery or deterioration is not anticipated."
- The "chronic disability syndrome," in which individuals who are capable of working choose to remain disabled, and demonstrate little motivation to even attempt to return to work needs to be considered in situations of delayed recovery with little or no medical basis.

CLINICAL IMPAIRMENT ASSESSMENT

- *The AMA Guides to Impairment and Disability Assessment* offers "a blend of evidence-based medicine and specialty consensus recommendations" for evaluating permanent impairment and is used throughout most of the United States and, increasingly, in other countries.
- The AMA Guides indicate that in evaluating the reliability and credibility of pain behaviors among patients undergoing pain-related assessment, examiners should consider

1. Congruence with establish conditions
2. Consistency over time and situation
3. Consistency with anatomy and physiology
4. Agreement between observers
5. Inappropriate illness behavior.

- Physicians who evaluate patients in a clinical setting become the patients' advocates.
- Physicians evaluating individuals for impairment or disability are *not* patient advocates and ideally should not rate impairment/disability in their own patients because it may represent an ethical conflict.
- Disability evaluators should avoid being overly influenced by subjective complaints, rate impairment on objective findings, and never refer to or consider the evaluee as a "patient."
- Evaluators should emphasize this situation to claimants prior to the assessment and should document this discussion in writing.
- Motivation should be evaluated as a very important link between impairment and disability. Attitude, motivation, and support systems are often more important prognosticators of disability and delayed recovery than are physical findings.
- There is no linear relationship between the degree of medical or psychiatric impairment and a disability rating.
- It is essential to take a detailed medical, developmental, behavioral, and psychosocial history to assess an individual's current and premorbid level of functioning.
- Information about stressors, such as traumatic events, patterns of disability in the patient or other family members, patterns of self-defeating behavior, unmet dependency needs, childhood deprivation, and substance abuse, is important in understanding how the patient became the person being evaluated and prognosis, as well as in making statements about vocational matters and disability.
- It should be determined if there appears to be significant suffering and demonstrable pain behavior.
- How the individual was functioning prior to the incident should be established.

MEASURING AND RATING PAIN

- Despite inherent limitations in self-report measures of pain, they are considered the most reliable tool.
- Three useful questions are:

1. What is the extent of the patient's disease or injury?
2. To what extent is the patient suffering, disabled, and unable to enjoy usual activities?
3. Is the illness behavior appropriate to the disease or injury or is there evidence of amplification of symptoms for psychologic or social reasons?

USING THE *AMA GUIDES* AND GENERAL ISSUES RELATED TO IMPAIRMENT FROM CHRONIC PAIN

- The *AMA Guides* and other rating systems (Social Security, Workers' compensation, private insurance companies, Veterans Administration) consider underlying medical (both organic and psychiatric) conditions rather than pain to be the cause of impairment.
- Despite the fact that this traditional biomedical model does not account for the subjective experience of the

patient in pain, the *Guides* acknowledges that the reality of subjective experience challenges their system of impairment rating.

- The *Guides* chapter on pain presents an alternative conceptual model for painful conditions not based in mechanical failure and when the conventional rating system is inadequate for assessing the patient's actual activities of daily living (ADLs) and assumes that:

  1. Pain is influenced significantly by psychosocial factors.
  2. There is often no direct correlation between pain and mechanical dysfunction.
  3. Pain may significantly impact patients' ability to perform ADLs.

- The pain chapter guidelines are meant to evaluate pain-related impairment characterized by:

  1. Excess pain in the context of verifiable conditions that cause pain.
  2. Well-established pain syndromes without significant, identifiable organ dysfunction to explain the pain.
  3. Associated pain syndromes (neuropathic pain states).

- The pain chapter guidelines should not be applied to rate pain-related impairment in situations when:

  1. Conditions are adequately rated in other chapters of the *Guides*.
  2. Evaluees have low credibility.
  3. The pain syndromes are ambiguous or controversial.

- The guidelines may be used to rate ambiguous or controversial pain syndromes only if:

  1. The symptoms and/or physical findings match a known medical condition.
  2. The individual's presentation is typical of a widely accepted diagnosed condition with a well-defined pathophysiologic basis.
  3. The pain chapter provides detailed protocols for assessing mild, moderate, moderately severe, and severe pain-related impairments.
  4. Although the pain chapter emphasizes that some pain may be real but not ratable, the chapter guidelines may frequently be used in a contrary attempt to rate such pain based on conditioned dysfunctional pain behavior, poor coping, and embellished self-reports.
  5. To make an impairment rating, the pain-related condition must have reached MMI and the pain must result in significant diminished capacity to carry out ADLs (does not merely make daily activity painful).

- Individuals with chronic pain should not be considered to have reached maximum medical improvement unless they have:

  1. Been evaluated by physicians knowledgeable about chronic pain
  2. Had a multidisciplinary evaluation
  3. Had an adequate trial of adjuvant analgesics in addition to primary analgesics
  4. The *AMA Guides* recognizes that emotional factors alter mental health, and rather than being the same as chronic pain, "psychogenic" pain is a psychiatric disorder that should be treated by specialists.

RETURN-TO-WORK ISSUES

- When a directive return-to-work approach is incorporated into the treatment of chronic pain patients receiving workers' compensation, most return to work and continue to work.
- A less successful prognosis for successful return to work is a physician's recommendation for restricted or light duty.
- Patients' physical, emotional, social, and spiritual well-being is more likely to be realized with the self-esteem that results from feeling useful because of gainful employment than with a disability award.
- The probability of return to work is 50% after more than six months of disability, 25% after more than one year, and extremely unlikely after more than two years.
- When chronic pain patients are treated in an interdisciplinary setting that combines treatment principles from physical, behavioral, and rehabilitation medicine using a biopsychosocial approach, return-to-work probability increases to the range of 68% despite prolonged absenteeism.

TREATMENT ISSUES

- The initial noxious stimulus leading to nociception seems to be less important in the management of chronic pain syndromes than the patient's suffering, which reflects emotional distress, and pain behavior. Thus, central factors may be more responsible than peripheral factors for delaying recovery and contributing to disability. Nociception, if present, may not be directly treatable by conventional techniques.
- If pain is intractable, both the healthcare professional and the patient become increasingly uncertain about the appropriate course of treatment and develop a sense of impotence and frustration that strains their interaction.

- It is essential that treating physicians use established principles of behavioral and rehabilitation medicine to get to know their patients.
- Many patients with delayed recovery from chronic headaches, myalgias, or nonspecific pain syndromes are actually saying "my life hurts," and, instead of medicalizing their suffering, we should channel them into appropriate treatment.
- Disability is more difficult to treat when it has continued for six months or longer. Thus, early recognition of features predicting poor prognosis and prompt intervention is important.
- Malingering should be considered in medical legal situations involving delayed recovery in contested injury or illness where a clinical diagnosis is uncertain and the subjective complaints are grossly disproportionate to objective findings.

BIBLIOGRAPHY

American Medical Association. *American Medical Association Guides to the Evaluation of Permanent Impairment.* 4th ed. Chicago, Il: AMA Press; 1993.

Aronoff GM. The role of the pain center in the treatment of intractable suffering and disability from chronic pain. *Semin Neurol.* 1983;3:377.

Aronoff GM. The disability epidemic (editorial). *Clin J Pain.* 1986;1:187.

Aronoff GM. Chronic pain and the disability epidemic. *Clin J Pain.* 1991;7:330.

Aronoff GM, Feldman JB. Preventing iatrogenic disability from chronic pain. *Curr Rev Pain.* 1999;3:67.

Aronoff GM, Feldman JB, Campion T. Chronic pain: Controlling disability. In: Randolph DC, ed. *Occupational Medicine.* 2000.

Aronoff GM, Livengood J. Pain: Psychiatric aspects of impairment and disability. *Curr Pain Headache Rep.* 2003;7:105.

Aronoff GM, Mandel S, Genovese E, et al. Evaluating malingering in contested injury or illness. *Pain Pract.* 2007;7(2):178–204.

Aronoff GM, Tota-Foucette M, Phillips L, et al. Are pain disorder and somatization disorder valid diagnostic entities? *Curr Rev Pain.* 2000;4:309.

Catchlove R, Cohen K. Effects of a directive return to work approach in the treatment of workers' compensation patients with chronic pain. *Pain.* 1982;14:181.

Flor H, Fydrich T, Turk DC. Efficacy of multidisciplinary pain treatment centers: A meta-analytic review. *Pain.* 1992;49:221.

Gatchel RJ, Polatin PB, Mayer TG, et al. Psychopathology and the rehabilitation of patients with chronic low back pain disability. *Arch Phys Med Rehabil.* 1994;75:666.

Hall H, McIntosh G, Melles T, et al. Effect of discharge recommendations on outcome. *Spine.* 1994;19:2033–2037.

Hebben N. Toward the assessment of clinical pain in adults. In: Aronoff GM, ed. *Evaluation and Treatment of Chronic Pain.* Baltimore, Md: William & Wilkins; 1992:384.

Hinnant DW. Psychological evaluation and testing. In: Tollison CD, ed. *Handbook of Pain Management.* 2nd ed. Baltimore, Md: Williams & Wilkins; 1994:18.

Loeser J. In: Stanton-Hicks M, Boas R, eds. *Chronic Low Back Pain.* New York: Raven Press; 1982:145.

Okifuji A, Turk DC, Kalauokalani D. Clinical outcome and economic evaluation of multidisciplinary pain centers. In: Block A, Kremer E, Fernandez E, eds. *Handbook of Pain Syndromes.* Mahwah, Nj: Lawrence Erlbaum; 1999:77.

Rondinelli RD, Genovese E, Katz RT, et al. *American Medical Association Guides to the Evaluation of Permanent Impairment.* 6th ed. Chicago, Il: AMA Press; 2008.

Strang JP. The chronic disability syndrome. In: Aronoff GM, ed. *The Evaluation and Treatment of Chronic Pain.* Baltimore, Md: Urban & Schwarzenberg; 1985.

Turk DC. Evaluation of pain and disability. *J Disability.* 1991;2:24.

Turk DC, Melzack R, eds. *Handbook of Pain Assessment.* New York: Guilford Press; 1992:111.

Turk DC, Rudy TE. Persistent pain and the injured worker: Integrating biomechanical, psychosocial, and behavioral factors in assessment. *J Occup Rehabil.* 1991;1(2),159–179.

Waddell G. Biopsychosocial analysis of low back pain. *Baillieres Clin Rheumatol.* 1992;6:523.

80 MEDICAL/LEGAL EVALUATION

Richard L. Stieg, MD, MHS

INTRODUCTION

- It is difficult to practice medicine in the 21st-century America and not be exposed to medical/legal activity.
- To believe that we can practice in the isolated environment of an office or medical facility without regard to the legal ramifications of what we do is to invite potential harm to ourselves and our patients.

INFORMAL MEDICAL/LEGAL ACTIVITIES, AVOIDING LEGAL CONFLICT

MEDICAL RECORDS/REPORTS

- The importance of careful, comprehensive, and timely recordkeeping of patient interactions cannot be overemphasized.
- The medical record/report has far-reaching legal implications.
- It may become a legal document that will be scrutinized by fellow healthcare professionals, patients, payers, attorneys, or other third parties.

- A careful and thoughtful report reflects positively on the physician and serves that professional well in ongoing treatment planning.
- On the contrary, a sloppy, poorly written report, particularly one that is generated days, weeks, or months after a patient encounter, may imply to all who read it (assuming that it is legible) that the doctor practices substandard medicine.
- The consequences of inadequate recordkeeping for doctor and patient may include:
  o delayed payment of benefits to patients
  o delayed reimbursement to physicians and hospitals
  o an increased chance of peer review
  o increased risk of medical malpractice action
  o loss of patients
- When writing or dictating a medical report, it may be useful to imagine presenting it to a jury or peer review panel.
- In this day of electronic recordkeeping, it may be tempting to generate reports that represent nothing more than a reiteration of previously obtained historical and physical examination data. That does not document, however, that the physician has paid attention to new information, reexamined the patient, or altered treatment plans in a timely fashion. Consider the frustration of any peer reviewer or legal agent in reading such reports that repeatedly say nothing new and how that may negatively impact the treating physician. Electronic records may save time but are not without significant liabilities.

REQUEST FOR MEDICAL RECORDS/REPORTS

- An increase in business and regulatory demands now take an enormous amount of time. This, coupled with legal requirements about how patient information may be shared, has changed the landscape and the nature of cooperation among medical personnel and third parties. For example, Federal HIPAA regulations that often supersede or interfere with state laws or with internal health plan demands and personal ethics are requiring of practitioners' more diligence in recordkeeping.
- In addition to requests for patient records, summarizing reports from the physician are also frequently required.
- Workers' compensation and long-term disability insurance carriers or personal injury protection insurance seem to request more than traditional medical health plans. Such requests may come from individuals hired by these companies to help manage claims or from their legal representatives. These demands often appear to be onerous to physicians. Responding to them in a thoughtful and timely manner, however, is generally good business and may be helpful in securing

appropriate benefits for your patients and timely payments for the physicians and hospital or ambulatory surgery centers. Before responding, it is wise to:
o understand your legal requirements;
o arrange for appropriate payment of your services. Fees may be dictated by a Fee Schedule as with workers' compensation insurance, or by the terms of a contract that you or your facility have with a requesting party. It is generally appropriate to ask in advance for your fee when such contractual arrangements do not exist. For example, most long-term disability insurance carriers do not pay for clinical reports or for legal reports not requested by their own attorneys. In such cases, your advance fee may have to be collected from your patient or their legal representative and it is wise to always do so via a written agreement.
o be sure that your patient has signed a release to permit you to communicate information to specific parties. It is advised to establish a good working rapport with all of your patients and have each one sign specific releases so that you can share your records with whomever you feel needs to help with patient care, medical claims management, or other benefits;
o explain to the patient that you are trying to fulfill what may be competing business/regulatory/legal demands on you and that failure or delays in doing so could result in delayed or denied benefits. It is appropriate to ask patients to assume responsibility in understanding what their benefits are with plans that you have no contractual obligations to (eg, a long-term disability plan) and communicating that to you and your support staff. Many larger practices may have resources to do that for you and on behalf of the patient but most smaller practices have neither the time nor expertise to do so. If your patient refuses, it would be wise to let other parties know why you are not sending records or reports.

PRESENCE OF THIRD PARTIES DURING OFFICE VISITS

- Third parties such as family members, friends, nurse case managers, insurance adjusters, "medical witnesses" or lawyers may pay unannounced or unrequested visits to your office during the course of a patient visit. You and your patient each have the right to refuse such interventions.
- Make it a point to:
  o be sure you have the patient's permission for such individuals to be present;
  o reserve the right to refuse admission into your office or exam room or excuse them from any portion of an interview or examination;

○ disallow any electronic recording of the visit by patients or third parties unless specifically required to do so by law (as may be the case in some workers' compensation encounters) or agreed to in writing by all parties.

- When the party present is viewed as an ally or may be important to patient care, you may wish to actually encourage such visits. Examples are family members who wish to be present or case managers who may be better able than you to secure medical benefits from the insurer for your patient.

- In the case of complex chronic-pain patients, you may also wish to facilitate case conferences at your office or via conference calling so that all parties playing a role in the patient's life can have a better understanding of the medical issues, including treatment plans. The medical/legal ramifications of this type of activity are self-evident. A carefully crafted document of such visits should include the names of the persons present and the purpose of their presence.

- Unfortunately, payment for this additional time and effort by pain medicine physicians varies considerably and must sometimes be viewed as a noncompensated add-on service.

- Once again, you have the right to request payment in advance for such activity and, I believe, the ethical obligation to offer to participate whenever possible.

MEDICAL CREDENTIALS AND QUALIFICATIONS

- Many physicians have little or no interest in participating in more formal medical/legal activities such as being deposed or serving as a medical witness at a trial. They may even have an aversion to such activity. They may find themselves forced into such roles, however, by subpoena or by feeling morally obligated to participate on behalf of their patient or a medical colleague (as in the case of peer review activity or medical malpractice actions). It is wise to document your credentials and qualifications for such activity to insulate yourself as much as possible from legal attack. Such documentation should appear in your reports and will no doubt be asked for during legal activities such as depositions or trial.

- You may sometimes be asked to produce new material such as a clinical summary on a patient or an updated curriculum vitae (CV), old records, or documents in the medical file. Copies may already be in the hands of legal parties and altered documents can be personally very damaging. Maintain an accurate CV that is absolutely factual, truthful, and contains no exaggerations or material omissions. You may be questioned about your CV by professionals who know much more about you than you might imagine (eg, calling yourself a "fellow" or a "diplomat" of organizations that offer no such qualifications can be cannon fodder to an attorney seeking to discredit you).

FORMAL MEDICAL/LEGAL EVALUATIONS

- As with any other professional activity, training and/or credentialing for medical/legal evaluations is highly desirable and can be obtained from a number of different resources. Many specialty professional organizations such as the American Board of Independent Medical Examiners, the American Academy of Disability Evaluating Physicians, the American Academy of Pain Medicine, and the American Medical Association offer both live and online training in this arena. So, too, do independent organizations such as SEAK that offer training for medical legal experts.

- Engaging in medical/legal work, particularly if it involves peer review activity, carries a unique set of ethical standards and problems and is not for the faint hearted. For Pain Medicine physicians, ethical standards have been articulated both by the American Academy of Pain Medicine and the American Medical Association. It would be wise to consult these before considering more formal medical/legal work.

PEER REVIEW ACTIVITY

- All peer review activity has medical/legal implications. This work may include participating in medical society ethics committees, credentialing or utilization review committees and similar services for a variety of health-related institutions/organizations, conducting independent medical examinations, or doing medical file reviews. These may require answers to questions about the reasonableness and appropriateness of colleagues' treatment.

- Such activity can be onerous but has long been recognized as acceptable and necessary to organized medicine.

- The American Medical Association advises that individuals engaging in such work "act ethically as long as principles of due process are observed" and that they "balance the physician's right to exercise medical judgment freely with the obligation to do so wisely and temperately."

- Peer review activity can at times lead to personal negative consequences. A colleague of mine recently issued an opinion (shared by two fellow physicians) during the course of a formal utilization review for the State Workers Compensation Board that a treating physician should be removed from a case because of unsound medical practice. Despite the fact that the panel members had been assured that they were immune from legal attack because their activity was part of the State Workers' Compensation administrative process dictated by regulations, the physician being reviewed sued the panel members. Although the case was dismissed, my colleague had to pay for her legal defense.

- There are few guarantees that peer review examiners whose opinions reflect unfavorably on their peers are immune from counterattack.
- Physicians engaging in peer review, then, should understand the risks they face and determine whether such activities are worth their time.
- Before engaging in a peer review, it would be wise to contact your medical malpractice carrier, as well as the organization requesting the review. You should ask for a copy of their insurance policy that protects you in the course of your work for them. All parties should be informed in writing about the scope of your expected activities and responsibilities. Any contract should be reviewed, preferably by a business or legal expert representing you. Do not assume that others have taken precautions for you. A little personal risk management in this regard could save you a lot of time, effort, and even money, should you find yourself under counterattack.

EXPERT TESTIMONY

- Expert testimony is an art and skill requiring expertise and, ideally, additional appropriate training. Such training is available through scientific and professional organizations as discussed above. The following brief remarks are in no way intended to substitute for such training and are only meant by the author as an introduction to the topic.
- At deposition or trial, answer questions simply, succinctly, and truthfully. The more unnecessary detail you add, the more likely you are to prolong your time and discomfort in the legal "hot seat."
- Always stay within your area of expertise and do not try to overwhelm an examining lawyer or judge.
- Avoid jargon, editorial commentary, or illogical conclusions.
- Your examiner is usually much better informed about medical/legal matters than you are.
- It is better to say "I don't know" or "that is beyond my area of expertise" than to have someone publicly demonstrate your weakness.

- Come prepared: review the documents that are likely to be the foundation for your testimony (including that CV) and think through what you are going to talk about.
- The lawyer who has summoned you can and should help you prepare and you should insist upon them doing so and billing them on an hourly basis for your time.
- The AMA believes that "As a citizen and as a professional with special training and experience the physician has an ethical obligation to assist in the administration of justice" and that "medical witnesses should testify honestly and truthfully to the best of their medical knowledge."
- The medical witness must be nonpartisan and should not "accept compensation that is contingent upon the outcome of litigation."
- That statement raises the issue about accepting cases on a lien basis. It is wise to have a written, signed Fee Agreement with attorneys requesting your medical expert services on a lien. Such an agreement may include delayed payments but should not waiver payment in the event of an unfavorable outcome to the requesting party.

THE INDEPENDENT MEDICAL EXAMINATION

- The Independent Medical Examination (IME) is a relatively recent phenomenon in the American healthcare system.
- Medical and legal professional organizations such as the American Academy of Disability Evaluating Physicians (AADEP), the American Board of Independent Medical Examination (ABIME), and SEAK offer such services as training, credentialing, and ongoing educational resources for IME physicians.
- Among the problems and challenges facing IME physicians and their clients, articulated by a taskforce of 50 physicians in 1998 under the joint sponsorship of SEAK and the American College of Occupational and Environmental Medicine, are:
  - objectively assessing and evaluating work capacity;
  - addressing malingering and symptom magnification;
  - obtaining needed medical reports in a timely manner;
  - preparing a cost-effective and time-efficient report;
  - obtaining appropriate and desirable comprehensive training in this highly specialized area (doing so adds respect from colleagues, clients, and business associates and may decrease to some degree legal scrutiny of the examiner's practice and credentials).

CONCLUSIONS

- We live in a highly litigious society where medical activities are highly regulated. This makes medical/legal activity unavoidable to the practicing physician.
- Many have found formal medical/legal activities such as peer review work, independent medical examinations, and professional witnessing to be challenging, interesting, and rewarding; others dread it.
- Training and certification programs are available to medical professionals who choose to add this to their repertoire.
- The recognition that legal activity may be part of everyday practice will serve our patients and us well.
- Patients also must cope with medical/legal issues while we are acting as their advocates or as independent reviewers of their care by others.
- We can better serve justice and the American healthcare system by being as familiar as possible with our medical/legal responsibilities.

BIBLIOGRAPHY

American Academy of Disability Evaluating Physicians. Available at: www.aadep.org. Accessed on 28th October, 2014.

American Academy of Pain Medicine. Available at: www.painmed.org. Accessed on 28th October, 2014.

American Board of Independent Medical Examiners. Available at: www.abime.org. Accessed on 28th October, 2014.

American Medical Association. *Code of Medical Ethics: Current Opinions with Annotations.* 1996/1997.

American Medical Association. Available at: www.ama-assn.org. Accessed on 28th October, 2014.

Babitsky S, Mangraviti JJ Jr, Todd CJ. *The Comprehensive Forensic Services Manual: The Essential Resources for all Experts.* Falmouth, Ma: SEAK Inc., Legal and Medical Information Systems; 2000.

SEAK, Inc. Legal and Medical Information Systems. Available at: www.seak.com. Accessed on 28th October, 2014.

INDEX

Page numbers in *italics* indicate figures or tables.